Get ready. Get set. Get moving!

Access to exercise videos and news clips included with any new book.

Registration will let you:

– Access over 80 exercise demonstration videos and safety tips

– Select from resistance band, free weight, machine, stability ball, and flexibility exercises

– Exercise at your own pace in the comfort of your own home

– View *ABC News* clips that bring fitness and wellness topics to life

www.pearsonhighered.com/powers

TO REGISTER

1. Go to www.pearsonhighered.com/powers
2. Click "See It."
3. Click "Register."
4. Follow the on-screen instructions to create your login name and password.

Your Access Code is:

Note: If there is no silver foil covering the access code, it may already have been redeemed, and therefore may no longer be valid. In that case, you can purchase access online using a major credit card or PayPal account. To do so, go to www.pearsonhighered.com/powers, click on "Buy Access," and follow the on-screen instructions.

TO

1. Go ... /powers
2. Cl...
3. Enter your login name and password.
4. Click "Log In."

D1530563

Hint:
Remember to bookmark the site after you log in.

Technical Support:
http://247pearsoned.custhelp.com

Behavior Change Contract

Choose a health behavior that you would like to change, starting this quarter or semester. Sign the contract at the bottom to affirm your commitment to making a healthy change and ask a friend to witness it.

My behavior change will be:

_____

My long-term goal for this behavior change is:

_____

Barriers that I must overcome to make this behavior change are   (things that I am currently doing or situations that contribute to this behavior or make it harder to change):

    1. _____

    2. _____

    3. _____

The strategies I will use to overcome these barriers are:

    1. _____

    2. _____

    3. _____

Resources I will use to help me change this behavior include:

    a friend/partner/relative: _____

    a school-based resource: _____

    a community-based resource: _____

    a book or reputable website: _____

In order to make my goal more attainable, I have devised these short-term goals

short-term goal	target date	reward
short-term goal	target date	reward
short-term goal	target date	reward

When I make the long-term behavior change described above, my reward will be:

_____ target date: _____

I intend to make the behavior change described above. I will use the strategies and rewards to achieve the goals that will contribute to a healthy behavior change.

Signed: _____   Witness: _____

Behavior Change Contract

Choose a health behavior that you would like to change, starting this quarter or semester. Sign the contract at the bottom to affirm your commitment to making a healthy change and ask a friend to witness it.

My behavior change will be:

_____

My long-term goal for this behavior change is:

_____

Barriers that I must overcome to make this behavior change are   (things that I am currently doing or situations that contribute to this behavior or make it harder to change):

     1. _____
     2. _____
     3. _____

The strategies I will use to overcome these barriers are:

     1. _____
     2. _____
     3. _____

Resources I will use to help me change this behavior include:

    a friend/partner/relative: _____
    a school-based resource: _____
    a community-based resource: _____
    a book or reputable website: _____

In order to make my goal more attainable, I have devised these short-term goals

_____	_____	_____
short-term goal	target date	reward
_____	_____	_____
short-term goal	target date	reward
_____	_____	_____
short-term goal	target date	reward

When I make the long-term behavior change described above, my reward will be:

_____ target date: _____

I intend to make the behavior change described above. I will use the strategies and rewards to achieve the goals that will contribute to a healthy behavior change.

Signed: _____   Witness: _____

5 e

TOTAL FITNESS & WELLNESS
Media Update

Scott K. Powers
University of Florida

Stephen L. Dodd
University of Florida

Erica M. Jackson
College of William and Mary

CONTRIBUTOR

Marilyn K. Miller *Bloomsburg University*

Benjamin Cummings

Boston   Columbus   Indianapolis   New York   San Francisco   Upper Saddle River
Amsterdam   Cape Town   Dubai   London   Madrid   Milan   Munich   Paris   Montréal   Toronto
Delhi   Mexico City   São Paulo   Sydney   Hong Kong   Seoul   Singapore   Taipei   Tokyo

Acquisitions Editor: Sandra Lindelof
Development Manager: Claire Alexander
Developmental Editor: Cheryl Cechvala
Project Editor: Kari Hopperstead
Project Editor, Ancillaries: Susan Scharf
Editorial Assistant: Jacob Evans
Marketing Manager: Neena Bali
Managing Editor: Wendy Earl
Production Supervisors: Sharon Montooth, Dorothy Cox
Text Design: tani hasegawa
Cover Design: Marilyn Perry
Composition: Progressive Information Technologies
Manufacturing Buyer: Jeffrey Sargent

Art Coordinator: Linda Jupiter
Illustrations: Precision Graphics
Photo Researcher: Kristin Piljay
Permissions Editor: Caroline Gloodt
Director, Image Resource Center: Melinda Patelli
Image Rights and Permissions Manager: Zina Arabia
Copyeditor: Sally Peyrefitte
Proofreader: Martha Ghent
Indexer: Katherine Pitcoff
Text Printer: Worldcolor, Dubuque
Cover Printer: Phoenix Color Corporation
Cover Photo: Getty Images/Plustwentyseven

Photography credits appear on page CR-1

Library of Congress Cataloging-in-Publication Data
Powers, Scott K. (Scott Kline), 1950–
  Total fitness and wellness / Scott K. Powers, Stephen L. Dodd, Erica M. Jackson;
contributor, Marilyn K. Miller.—5th ed., media update.
    p. cm.
  Includes bibliographical references and index.
  ISBN-13: 978-0-321-67654-2 (alk. paper)
  ISBN-10: 0-321-67654-8 (alk. paper)
  1. Physical fitness—Textbooks. 2. Health—Textbooks. I. Dodd, Stephen L. II. Jackson,
Erica M. III. Miller, Marilyn K. IV. Title. V. Title: Total fitness and wellness.
  RA781.P66 2011c
  613.7—dc22

2009046905

Benjamin Cummings
is an imprint of

ISBN 10: 0-321-67654-8; ISBN 13: 978-0-321-67654-2 (student edition)
ISBN 10: 0-321-67655-6; ISBN 13: 978-0-321-67655-9 (professional copy)
ISBN 10: 0-321-67633-5; ISBN 13: 978-0-321-67633-7 (a la carte edition)

www.pearsonhighered.com   1 2 3 4 5 6 7 8 9 10—QWD—14 13 12 11 10

To Jen, Haney, and Will. Your love and encouragement have always meant more than you will ever know.
  Stephen L. Dodd

To my mother, who encouraged me to pursue academic endeavors.
  Scott K. Powers

Brief Contents

Contents

2 General Principles of Exercise for Health and Fitness   31

4 Improving Muscular Strength and Endurance   95

9 Preventing Cardiovascular Disease   269

11 Exercise and the Environment   325

15 Addiction and Substance Abuse   413

Preface

Good health is our most precious possession. Although we tend to appreciate it only in times of illness or injury, more and more of us are realizing that good health is not simply the absence of disease. Indeed, there are degrees of health, or wellness, and lifestyle can have a major impact on many of its components.

Intended for an introductory college course, *Total Fitness and Wellness* focuses on helping students effect positive changes in their lifestyles, most notably in exercise and diet. The interaction of exercise and diet and the essential role of regular exercise and good nutrition in achieving total fitness and wellness are major themes of the text.

Total Fitness and Wellness, Fifth Edition, was built on a strong foundation of both exercise physiology and nutrition. The text provides clear, objective, research-based information to college students during their first course in physical fitness and wellness. By offering a research-based text, we hope to dispel many myths associated with exercise, nutrition, weight loss, and wellness. In particular, we show students how to evaluate their own wellness level with respect to the various wellness components, such as fitness level and nutritional status. Indeed, the title of the book reflects our goals.

Numerous physical fitness and wellness texts are available today. Our motivation in writing *Total Fitness and Wellness*, Fifth Edition, was to create a unique, well-balanced physical fitness text, one that not only covers primary concepts of physical fitness and wellness but also addresses important issues such as behavior change, exercise-related injuries, exercise and the environment, and prevention of cardiovascular disease.

Foundation in Exercise Physiology

We believe it is imperative that students develop an understanding of the basic physiological adaptations that occur in response to both acute exercise and regular exercise training. Without this understanding, it is impossible to plan, modify, and properly execute a lifetime exercise program.

Strong Emphasis on Behavior Change

We recognize that one of the most important aspects of teaching students about personal fitness is presenting them with ways to alter their own behaviors and make fitness and health a part of their own lives. In this fifth edition of *Total Fitness and Wellness*, we have expanded our coverage of behavior change and relocated it to the first chapter. Presenting the concepts of behavior change at the outset encourages students to think about strategies for incorporating fitness and wellness principles into their own lives as they progress through the chapters and the course.

Steps for Behavior Change boxes throughout the text present students with quick evaluations of their current health behaviors and offer simple and practical ways to modify those behaviors and work toward lasting change. Laboratories at the end of each chapter are exercises and activities that encourage the immediate development of healthy lifestyle choices and a core fitness plan. The Behavior Change Log Book with Wellness Journal, packaged with each new copy of the text, further motivates behavior change by providing students with hands-on material to track daily exercise and food intake and to create personal, long-term fitness and nutrition programs. New journaling activities and an updated table listing nutritional content of common foods have also been added.

Coverage of the Latest Scientific Research on Physical Fitness, Nutrition, and Wellness

We firmly believe that college physical fitness and wellness texts should contain the latest scientific information and include references for scientific studies to support key information about physical fitness, nutrition, and wellness. Accordingly, we offer the most current research in the arena of fitness and wellness in *Total Fitness and Wellness*, Fifth Edition. For example, it is now clear that exercise plays a role in reducing the risk of some cancers and can contribute to a longer life. Although it has long been speculated that exercise brings about significant health benefits, evidence has only recently become available. In the area of nutrition, scientific data now suggest that vitamins may play a new role in preventing certain diseases and combating the aging process. In addition, whereas it has been well accepted that fat in the diet increases our risk of heart disease, it has just lately been shown that dietary fat plays a greater role than other nutrients in weight gain. Source information documenting the validity of the content presented, along with suggestions for further reading, appear at the end of each chapter.

New to the Media Update

- **New coauthor,** Erica Jackson, provides a fresh voice and a wealth of experience teaching fitness and wellness courses that enhances and revitalizes the text.
- **An extensively updated Companion Website** features content reorganized into a new format:
  - **New RSS feeds of health articles** (Read It)
  - **More than 80 new exercise videos and related** *ABC News* **videos** (See It)
  - **New audio case studies** (Hear It)
  - **New online labs and self-assessments** available in Microsoft® Word, and accompanied by a comprehensive pre- and post-fitness assessment for students to take at the beginning and end of the course (Do It)
  - **New updated flashcards** that are exportable to cell phones, as well as study quizzes (Review It)
  - **Behavior Change resources** to help students come up with behavior change goals and plans, and to track their progress (Live It)
- **New MyFitnessLab website** includes all of the same organization and content as the Companion Website in addition to
  - **New Pearson eText with live links to various media** in the Read It section
  - *Live Right!* and *Eat Right!* content in the Live It section
  - **Course management features** for assigning and submitting coursework (Do It and Review It)
- **Statistics and data, references, and resources** updated and/or replaced throughout the text.
- **A new "video" icon** in the text indicates labs and exercises that have videos on the Companion Website and MyFitnessLab. Lists of related videos are also included at the end of each chapter.
- **A Pre-/Post-course fitness assessment** has been added at the front of the book.

Unique to the Fifth Edition

- **Contributing author,** Marilyn Miller, brings additional expertise in fitness and first-hand knowledge of the challenges finess and wellness instructors face in the classroom.
- **A new chapter, Body Composition** (Chapter 6), emphasizes the importance of body composition as one of the five major components of physical fitness.
- **Behavior change material** has been expanded and moved up from Chapter 10 to Chapter 1, to reflect the standard organization of the course.
- **Steps for Behavior Change** boxes focus students on evaluating their own behaviors (e.g., Are you a fast food junkie? Are you reluctant to strength train?) and present them with practical steps they can take to make meaningful behavior change.
- **True or False? chapter-opening quizzes** addressing common fitness myths and misperceptions combine with a fresh new design throughout to make the text more accessible, engaging, and visually appealing than ever before.
- **Consider This!** features grab students' attention with surprising statistics, prompting them to consider the consequences of specific health behaviors.
- **Integration of fitness assessment material** throughout the book aligns the assessments with the topics to which they are relevant.
- **Updated exercise photos** serve as a valuable reference for students, who often take their book with them to the fitness center and use it when completing a Laboratory.

Continuing Features

- **Unique topics.** Several chapters in the Fifth Edition address topics not contained in other introductory fitness and wellness texts. For example, this book includes chapters on exercise and the environment and on preventing and rehabilitating exercise-related injuries. Further, in several chapters we have incorporated an elementary discussion of the physiology of exercise to improve students' knowledge of how the body operates and responds to regular exercise.
- **Updated coverage.** Citing references to new research, we have expanded our coverage of current topics of student interest, such as eating disorders, stress management strategies, Pilates, diabetes and prediabetes, ergogenic dietary supplements,

at-home fitness equipment, antioxidants, and emotional health.

- **Informational boxes.** Each chapter features a variety of informational boxes. **A Closer Look** boxes give the reader insight into special topics, such as the effects of caffeine, the search for a cure for AIDS, road rage, muscle cramps, and anabolic steroids. **Appreciating Diversity** boxes present current health research, covering issues such as how the risk of cancer varies across the United States and how the incidence of drug abuse varies across populations. **Consumer Corner** boxes teach students to be smart and discerning health and fitness consumers, guiding them to make the best fitness and wellness decisions in a market full of fads, gimmicks, and gadgets.

- **Laboratories.** Each chapter contains easy-to-follow, application-based lab exercises that allow students to apply textual information to practical issues, encouraging the immediate development of healthy lifestyle choices and a core fitness plan. New and revised labs reflect current trends in fitness and incorporate activities that students can do at home or outdoors and with less costly equipment. New topics include assessing tobacco use, selecting a health insurance plan, and measuring core strength and stability.

- **Pedagogical aids.** Throughout the text, **Make Sure You Know** features summarize key points, prompting students to recall and process main concepts covered. To emphasize and support understanding of material, important terms are boldfaced in the text and defined in a **running glossary** at the bottom of text pages. For students' review, the **Chapter Summary** sections succinctly restate the most significant ideas presented in the chapter. **Study Questions** encourage analysis of chapter discussions and prepare students for tests. **Suggested Readings, Web links,** and **References** offer quality information sources for further study of fitness and wellness.

- **Food appendix.** To help students track and modify their food intake, we present caloric and nutrient content of common foods and fast foods in the Appendix.

Supplemental Materials

Instructor Supplements

Teaching Tool Box

Developed to support adjunct and part-time faculty teaching the fitness and wellness course, and also to be invaluable to veteran instructors, this kit offers all the

tools instructors need to guide students through the course. The box includes the Course-at-a-Glance Quick Reference Guide, Fitness Support Manual (with First-Time Teaching Tips), Instructor Resource Manual and Printed Test Bank, Media Manager with *ABC News* Lecture Launcher videos and TestGen, MyFitnessLab Instructor Access Kit, *Great Ideas: Active Ways to Teach Health and Wellness*, and transparency acetates. The Tool Box also includes the supplemental materials for students, such as the Behavior Change Logbook and Wellness Journal, Take Charge of Your Health! Worksheets, *Eat Right!*, and *Live Right!*

- **Course-at-a-Glance Quick Reference Guide.** This fold-out quick reference guide provides sample syllabi for both quarter- and semester-based fitness and wellness courses. A useful planning tool for both beginning and experienced instructors, this concise grid gives an at-a-glance overview of where multiple course resources are located for both student and instructor support.

- **Fitness Support Manual: First Time Teaching Tips and Visual Lecture Outlines.** Organized chapter by chapter, this key manual provides a step-by-step guide to all the resources available to instructors. It provides information on available PowerPoint lectures with the accompanying figures and art; integrated *ABC News* Lecture Launcher videos; suggested classroom discussion questions; in-class activities, tips, and strategies for large classrooms; and the best strategies to promote active learning.

- **Instructor Resource Manual and Test Bank.** The Instructor Resource Manual and Test Bank includes suggestions for class discussion, student activities, readings, lecture outlines, learning objectives, chapter summaries, Web references, and media resources. The Test Bank includes over 1,000 multiple-choice, true-or-false, short-answer, and matching questions to use for student review or testing.

- **Media Manager.** This cross-platform CD-ROM includes all the PowerPoint lecture outlines with embedded links to *ABC News* Lecture Launcher video clips and new exercise videos that can be customized for any lecture presentation. In addition, quiz show and classroom-response "clicker" questions are included, as well as all figures and tables from the book, Microsoft Word files of the Instructor Resource Manual and Test Bank, and the TestGen computerized test bank, which enables instructors to create lists, edit questions, and add their own material to existing exams.

- **Transparency Acetates.** Over 180 full-color transparency acetates include all figures and tables from the main text. The transparencies are excellent for presenting information in a clear manner consistent with the text.

- **Great Ideas! Active Ways to Teach Health and Wellness.** This booklet is loaded with teaching tips from instructors on how to make class come alive, including collaborative and active learning techniques and effective use of technology in the classroom.

MyFitnessLab

(**www.pearsonhighered.com/myfitnesslab**) MyFitnessLab, powered by CourseCompass™, provides a one-stop spot for accessing a wealth of preloaded content and tools, making it easier than ever to organize your fitness & wellness class, personalize your students' educational experience, and push their learning to the next level. MyFitnessLab includes a variety of content organized by learning area: Pearson eText with live links, as well as RSS feeds of articles in the news (Read It); more than 80 exercise videos plus *ABC News* videos (See It); MP3 case studies (Hear It); electronic versions of labs, self-assessments, and comprehensive pre- and post-course fitness assessments (Do It); practice quiz questions and Flashcards downloadable to mobile phones (Review It); as well as behavior change resources and electronic versions of *Live Right!* and *Eat Right!* (Live It).

Student Supplements

Behavior Change Log Book and Wellness Journal

This assessment tool helps students track their daily exercise and nutritional intake and create a long-term nutritional and fitness prescription plan. Packaged with each new copy of the text, it also includes a Behavior Change Contract and journal topics.

Live Right! Beating Stress in College and Beyond

Live Right! gives students useful tips for coping with stressful life challenges both during college and for the rest of their lives. Topics include sleep, managing finances, time management, coping with academic pressure, and relationships.

Eat Right! Healthy Eating in College and Beyond

Eat Right!, a handy, full-color 80-page booklet, provides students with practical guidelines, tips, shopper's guides and recipes that turn healthy eating principles into blueprints for action. Topics include healthy eating in the cafeteria, dorm room, and fast-food restaurants; planning meals on a budget; weight management; vegetarian alternatives; and the effects of alcohol on health.

MyFitnessLab

(**www.pearsonhighered.com/myfitnesslab**) MyFitnessLab features online access to a selection of the print and media supplements for students and makes studying convenient and fun. The preloaded content on this website includes interactive labs from the book, an interactive Pearson eText, self-assessment worksheets, Behavior Change Log Book and Wellness Journal, audio case studies, flashcards that can be downloaded to mobile phones, and the *ABC News* Lecture Launcher video clips. There are also new exercise videos demonstrating proper techniques for a variety of muscular strength and flexibility exercises.

Companion Website

(**www.pearsonhighered.com/powers**) The Companion Website has been extensively updated and reorganized in the same manner as MyFitnessLab to help make student learning fun. Students can check out RSS feeds of fitness- and health-related news stories (Read It); view *ABC News* video clips and more than 80 new demonstration exercise videos (See It); listen to MP3 case studies (Hear It); fill in electronic versions of labs, self-assessments, and pre- and post-course fitness assessments (Do It); take practice quizzes as well as download flashcards to their mobile phone (Review It), and access behavior change resources (Live It).

Take Charge of Your Health! Worksheets

A total of 50 self-assessment exercise worksheets give more opportunities for assessment.

MyDietAnalysis

Powered by ESHA Research, Inc., MyDietAnalysis features a database of nearly 20,000 foods and multiple reports. This easy-to-use program allows students to track their diet and activity for up to three profiles and to generate and submit reports electronically.

Acknowledgments

First and foremost, this edition of *Total Fitness and Wellness* reflects the valuable feedback provided by many people throughout the country. Most notably, our contributing author, Marilyn Miller, deserves great accolades. Her insights and skills have made major contributions to the content, as well as making the text very user-friendly.

As always, this edition could not have been completed without the work of an enormous number of people at Benjamin Cummings. From the campus sales representatives to the president of the company, they are truly first rate, and our interaction with them is always delightful.

There were several key people in the process. Our Acquisitions Editor, Sandra Lindelof, has been the primary force behind assembling the team and directing the process, and her input has been invaluable. Several new additions to the team have been important in both the revisions of the text and the production process. Claire Alexander has been a guiding presence over several editions, and her involvement is always appreciated. Specifically for this edition, Cheryl Cechvala has been a major force in the development of the text. She has directly supervised the revision, and has made contributions to the writing. Her input has been most valuable, and it has been a pleasure to work with her. Kari Hopperstead and Susan Scharf have also been major contributors to the editorial process and the development of ancillary materials. Their efforts have been most appreciated. Sharon Montooth has again served as Production Supervisor and has expertly guided the manuscript through each stage of production. Linda Jupiter again has coordinated the artwork for this edition, and, as before, her efforts have enhanced the look of the book and helped convey a message. Other specific duties were expertly handled by the following list of professionals. We offer them our utmost appreciation for their efforts: Erik P. Fortier, Media Producer; Jacob Evans, Editorial Assistant; Wendy Earl, Managing Editor; Renn Sminkey of Creative Digital Visions, Photographer; Kristin Piljay, Photo Researcher; Precision Graphics, Illustrator; tani hasegawa, Cover and Text Designer; Sally Peyrefitte, Copyeditor; Martha Ghent, Proofreader; Progressive Information Technologies, Compositor; Kathy Pitcoff, Indexer; Dorothy Cox, Manufacturing Supervisor; Caroline Gloodt, Permissions Editor.

For the Media Update, we are grateful for the contributions of Dorothy Cox as Production Supervisor, Kelly Reed as Media Producer, Brianna Paulson as Editorial Assistant, and Linda Kern at Progressive Publishing Alternatives.

Quinlyn Soltow at the University of Florida has made major contributions to the ancillaries. Her technical and editing work, informed by her expert knowledge of fitness and wellness, was exceptional.

Finally, there is a long list of professionals whose reviews of the text's content and style or participation in a fitness and wellness forum have helped to shape this book. We owe these individuals a tremendous debt of gratitude:

George Abboud,	*Salem State College*
Roxanne Allen,	*McNeese State University*
Arturo Arce,	*Louisiana State University*
Kym Atwood,	*University of West Florida*
J. Sunshine Cowan,	*University of Central Oklahoma*
Mandi Dupain,	*Millersville University*
Michael Dupper,	*University of Mississippi*
Ken Grace,	*Chabot College*
Peg Hamlett,	*University of Idaho*
Todd Hammonds,	*Lansing Community College*
Jerry Hawkins,	*Lander University*
Mary Kemp,	*Carroll Community College*
Gary Ladd,	*Southwestern Illinois College*
Rosemary Lindle,	*University of Maryland*
Amanda Nelson,	*University of Illinois*
Karen Poole,	*University of North Carolina-Greensboro*
Christopher Rasmussen,	*Baylor University*
Tammy Sabourin,	*Valencia Community College East*
Andrea Willis,	*Abraham Baldwin Agricultural College*

Many thanks to all!

Scott K. Powers
University of Florida

Stephen L. Dodd
University of Florida

Erica M. Jackson
College of William and Mary

Understanding Fitness and Wellness

1

true or false?

F **1.** Your physical activity as a college student has no effect on your health later in life.

F **2.** You definitely have a high level of wellness if you exercise and eat a healthy diet.

T **3.** As little as 30 minutes of brisk walking most days of the week can improve your health.

F **4.** Most people do not need help to make a health behavior change.

T **5.** Smoking is the leading cause of preventable death in the United States.

Answers appear on the next page.

aria is a college freshman who is away from home for the first time and starting to gain a little weight. In high school, Maria had been active with after-school sports, and her mother kept healthy food around the house and cooked meals for the family. After soccer or softball practice, Maria would go home, have dinner with her family, and study. Since coming to college, Maria has not been involved in sports and rarely finds time to go to the gym. Her eating habits are erratic, and she's spending more time partying with her friends, forgoing much study and sleep time in the process. Like many college students, Maria is excited to be away from home and "on her own," but she is a little overwhelmed by all of the choices she now has to make about what to eat and how to spend her time.

Do you relate to Maria? Are you less physically active now than when you were in high school? Has your diet changed for the worse since you've assumed control of what you eat? Do you think your level of wellness is better or worse than when you left home?

In this book, you will learn about behaviors that can put you on the path to optimal wellness. In this first chapter, we present the concept of wellness, discuss the health benefits of exercise, and outline the major components of physical fitness. Understanding the role that exercise plays in your own health and wellness can help motivate you to sustain a lifetime of physical fitness.

What Is Wellness?

Not so long ago, *good health* was defined as the absence of disease. But then, in the 1970s and 1980s, many exercise scientists and health educators became dissatisfied with this limited definition. These visionary health professionals believed that health includes physical fitness and emotional and spiritual health as well. Their revised concept of good health is called **wellness** (1). You can achieve a state of wellness by practicing a healthy lifestyle that includes regular physical activity, proper nutrition, eliminating unhealthy behaviors (that is, avoiding high-risk activities such as reckless driving, smoking, and drug use), and maintaining good emotional and spiritual health (1). Let's discuss the components of wellness, and what it means to enjoy a healthy lifestyle, in more depth now.

Six Components of Wellness

To enjoy an optimal state of wellness, you need to achieve physical, emotional, intellectual, spiritual, social, and environmental health. Do you get regular physical and dental exams? Do you stay close to and communicate with friends and family? Do you recycle? These choices and habits can all contribute to a healthy lifestyle, and they all fall under the components of wellness.

Wellness is also a dynamic concept in that the choices you make each day move you along a continuum. At one end is optimal well-being associated with a high level of functioning. At the other end is a low level of wellness that likely includes poor physical and mental health (Figure 1.1). You can move toward optimal well-being by eliminating unhealthy behaviors and adopting healthy ones.

Physical Health Physical health refers to all the behaviors that keep your body healthy. One of the key aspects for maintaining a healthy body is physical fitness. Physical fitness can have a positive effect on your

Answers

1. FALSE What you do as a college student will affect your health as you get older. Students who are active in college have lower risk for heart disease later in life.

2. FALSE Although exercising and eating a healthy diet are very positive wellness habits, they don't cover everything. There are six components that determine overall wellness, which you will learn about as you read this chapter.

3. TRUE Regular moderate exercise can produce a lot of health benefits. However, for certain goals, such as improving fitness, you will have to do more than 30 minutes of moderate activity.

4. FALSE To adopt and maintain a healthy behavior, you will need information, as well as support from friends, family, and possibly support groups.

5. TRUE Approximately 430,000 deaths per year are attributed to smoking. Most people are aware of the relationship between smoking and lung cancer. Moreover, smoking is also a major risk factor for heart disease.

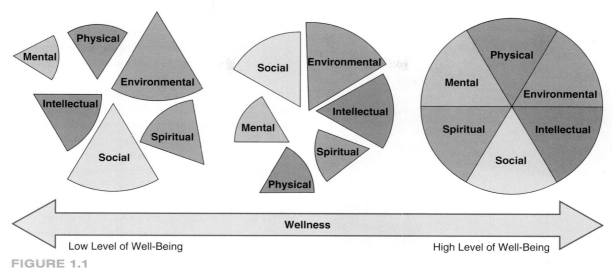

FIGURE 1.1
When the wellness components are well integrated and working together, you can enjoy the benefit of optimal well-being.

health by reducing your risk of disease and improving your quality of life. Proper nutrition, performing self-exams, and practicing personal safety are other important physical health behaviors.

Emotional Health   Emotions play an important role in how you feel about yourself and others. Emotional health (also called mental health) includes your social skills and interpersonal relationships. Your levels of self-esteem and your ability to cope with the routine stress of daily living also are aspects of emotional health.

The cornerstone of emotional health is emotional stability, which describes how well you deal with the day-to-day stresses of personal interactions and the physical environment. Most people are well equipped to handle life's ups and downs, but the inability to handle everyday situations can lead to poor emotional health or mental health disorders, such as depression and anxiety disorders, in many people. In fact, mental disorders are the leading cause of disability for people aged 15–44 years (2). Emotional wellness means being able to respond to life situations in an appropriate manner and not remaining in extreme high or low emotional states.

CONSIDER THIS!

Approximately one in four adults between the ages of 18 and 44 has a diagnosable mental disorder in a given year.

Intellectual Health   You can maintain intellectual health by keeping your mind active through lifelong learning. College is the ideal place to develop this wellness component, partly because it exposes you to new ideas and ways of thinking about life. Attending lectures, engaging in thoughtful discussions with friends or teachers, and reading are excellent ways to promote intellectual health. Maintaining good intellectual health can also increase your ability to define and solve problems, and continuous learning and thinking can provide you with a sense of fulfillment. Take advantage of opportunities to broaden your mind. Listen to audio books in the car, keep up with current events by reading the newspaper, and do not shy away from friendly debate.

Spiritual Health   The term *spiritual* means different things to different people. Most definitions of *spiritual health* include having a sense of meaning and purpose. Many people define spiritual health according to their religious beliefs, but it is not limited to religion. People

> **wellness** The state of healthy living achieved by the practice of a healthy lifestyle, which includes regular physical activity, proper nutrition, eliminating unhealthy behaviors, and maintaining good emotional and spiritual health.

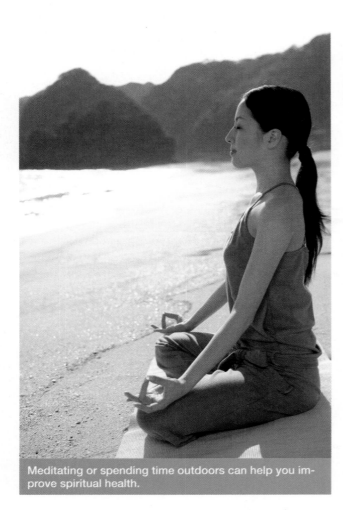
Meditating or spending time outdoors can help you improve spiritual health.

people in your support network that matters, but the quality of those relationships that is important. Developing strong communication skills is one behavior that is crucial for maintaining a strong social network.

Environmental Health Environmental health includes the influence of the environment on your health, as well as your behaviors that affect the condition of the environment. Our environment can have a positive or negative impact on our total wellness. For example, air pollution and water contamination are two important environmental factors that can harm physical health. Breathing polluted air can lead to a variety of respiratory disorders (e.g., asthma). Drinking water that has been contaminated with harmful bacteria can lead to infection, and drinking water that contains carcinogens (cancer-producing agents) increases the risk of certain types of cancers.

Your environment can also have a positive influence on wellness. For example, a safe environment invokes feelings of comfort and security, which impact your emotional health. Moreover, if your environment is safe, you are more likely to spend time outside being active and improving your physical health.

Our relationship with our environment is a two-way street. We discussed the positive and negative impacts the environment can have on our health. Now, let's discuss some examples of how people's behaviors might influence the environment. Think about your own behaviors: Do you recycle regularly, or does much of your trash end up in a landfill? Do you carpool or take public transportation when you can, or are you leaving a large carbon footprint? Achieving total wellness requires learning about the environment and protecting yourself against environmental hazards that threaten your health and well-being, as well as being aware of your impact on the environment.

Interaction of Wellness Components

None of the components of wellness works in isolation; in fact, all six work closely together. For example, people with an anxiety or depressive disorder who also have a chronic physical illness report more physical symptoms than those who do not have a mental health disorder (4). Also, strong spirituality is associated with lower rates of mental disorders, better immune function, and greater participation in health-promoting behaviors (3, 5). Although the wellness components are interrelated, practicing healthy behaviors related to one aspect of wellness is not a guarantee of a high level of total wellness. Rather, total wellness is achieved through a balance of physical, intellectual, social, emotional, spiritual, and environmental health.

may also find meaning in helping others and being altruistic, through prayer, or enjoying the beauty of nature. Whether you define spiritual health as religious beliefs or the establishment of personal values, it is an important aspect of wellness, is closely linked to emotional health, and also influences physical health (3).

Optimal spiritual health includes the ability to understand your basic purpose in life; to experience love, joy, pain, peace, and sorrow; and to care for and respect all living things. Anyone who has experienced a beautiful sunset or smelled the first scents of spring can appreciate the pleasure of maintaining optimal spiritual health.

Social Health Social health is the development and maintenance of meaningful interpersonal relationships. The result is the creation of a support network of friends and family. Good social health helps you feel confident in social interactions and provides you with emotional security. It is not necessarily the number of

Make sure you know...

> *Wellness* is defined as a state of optimal health achieved by living a healthy lifestyle.

> There are six interacting components of wellness: physical health, emotional health, intellectual health, spiritual health, social health, and environmental health.

Wellness Goals for the Nation

All countries, including the United States, have a vested interest in having a healthy population. A nation of unhealthy people drains national resources by reducing worker productivity and increasing the amount of money the governments have to spend on health care. To improve the overall well-being of Americans, the U.S. government has established a set of wellness goals known as Healthy People.

The Healthy People initiative seeks to prevent unnecessary disease and improve the quality of life for all Americans. The wellness goals were first presented in *Healthy People* reports published in 1980 and have since been revised every 10 years based on the progress toward meeting the objectives. Each report includes a broad range of health and wellness objectives based on 10-year agendas. *Healthy People 2020* is currently under development. The overreaching goals will be to eliminate preventable disease, disability, injury, and premature death; to achieve health equity, eliminate disparities, and improve the health of all groups (see the Appreciating Diversity box below); to create social and physical environments that promote good health for all; and to promote healthy development and healthy behaviors across every stage of life. For more details on the current goals and objectives, *Healthy People 2010*, see the Closer Look box on the next page, or visit www.healthypeople.gov.

Make sure you know...

> *Healthy People* is a set of wellness goals set by the U.S. government for the American people.

> The main goals of *Healthy People 2020* will be to eliminate preventable disease, disability, injury, and premature death; achieve health equity, eliminate disparities, and improve the health of all groups; create environments that promote good health; and promote healthy development and healthy behaviors across every stage of life.

What Is Exercise, and Why Should I Do It?

When you hear the word *exercise*, do you picture someone in a gym running on a treadmill? Or, do you imagine hiking up a scenic mountain with a group of friends? Actually, both activities can be exercise, and both are good for your health. In fact, there are numerous fun and interesting ways to exercise. So if going to the gym is not your thing, there are many other ways you can be active and improve your health. One part of designing your personal fitness program is to find out what works best for *you*.

APPRECIATING DIVERSITY WELLNESS ISSUES ACROSS THE POPULATION

Your behaviors have a significant impact on your level of health and wellness. However, there are factors beyond your control that contribute to your wellness and your risk for certain chronic diseases and conditions. Ethnicity, sex, age, family history, and socioeconomic status affect the risk of developing diabetes, cancer, cardiovascular disease, obesity, and other conditions.

For example, black Americans have a higher risk of developing hypertension (high blood pressure) compared to the U.S. population as a whole. Similarly, diabetes is more common in Native Americans and Latinos than people from other ethnic backgrounds. Further, men and women differ in their risk for heart disease, osteoporosis, and certain types of cancer.

Aging also can affect the ability to achieve wellness. For instance, the risk of chronic diseases (e.g., heart disease and cancer) increases with age. Finally, people with low socioeconomic status often have less access to quality health care and experience higher rates of obesity, heart disease, and drug abuse. The goal for everyone is to achieve optimal wellness, but individual and demographic differences can present special challenges in achieving wellness. This important issue will be discussed throughout this book.

Selected *Healthy People 2010* objectives include the following:

- Increase the proportion of people who engage in daily physical activity.
- Reduce activity limitations due to chronic back conditions.
- Reduce the prevalence of cigarette smoking.
- Increase the consumption of fruits and vegetables.
- Reduce the lung cancer death rate.

- Reduce the prostate cancer death rate.
- Reduce the melanoma death rate.
- Reduce the number of college students engaging in heavy drinking of alcoholic beverages.
- Reduce the proportion of people who experience adverse health effects from stress each year.
- Reduce the prevalence of overweight people (aged 20 and older).

Government agencies and public health professionals are in the process of assessing the nation's progress in meeting the *Healthy People 2010* goals. Based on the progress, they will work toward developing the *Healthy People 2020* objectives needed to meet the new overreaching goals for the nation.

Source: U.S. Department of Health and Human Services, Office of Disease Prevention and Health Promotion, www.healthypeople.gov.

Exercise Is One Type of Physical Activity

Although the terms *physical activity* and *exercise* are often used interchangeably, they do not mean the same thing. **Physical activity** includes all physical movement, regardless of the level of energy expenditure or the reason you do it (6). Physical activity can be occupational, lifestyle, or leisure time. Occupational activity is the activity that you carry out in the course of your job as, for example, a restaurant server or construction worker. Lifestyle activity includes housework, walking to class, or climbing the stairs to get to your apartment or dorm room. Leisure-time physical activity is any activity you choose to do in your free time.

Exercise is a type of leisure-time physical activity (6). Virtually all conditioning activities and sports are considered exercise because they are planned and help maintain or improve physical fitness. The main thing that distinguishes exercise from other types of physical activity is that exercise is done specifically for health and fitness.

When we use the term *physical activity*, it encompasses exercise, but exercise does not include all types of physical activity. For example, riding your bike to work for transportation is lifestyle physical activity, and lifting heavy boxes at work is occupational physical activity. Both of these activities will improve health and are examples of how an active lifestyle or job can affect health even when a person does not participate in a regular structured exercise program. Typically, exercise produces the greatest health benefits (you'll learn more about this in Chapter 2), but you still can receive a lot of health benefits with regular physical activity.

There Are Numerous Health Benefits of Physical Activity

If you ask people whether they exercise regularly, the answer often is no. People have many reasons for not exercising. However, most of us are aware there are many health benefits of regular physical activity and exercise. In addition to making us look better by improving muscle tone and levels of body fat, regular exercise helps improve our energy levels and our ability to perform everyday tasks. Perhaps even more important, it can help you achieve total wellness (2, 7–15).

The importance of regular physical activity in promoting good health and wellness is emphasized in the 1996 Surgeon General's report on physical activity and health (16). This report concludes that lack of physical activity is a major public health problem in the United States and that all Americans can improve their health by engaging in as little as 30 minutes of light-to-moderate-intensity physical activity most days of the week. The Surgeon General's report recognizes numerous health benefits of physical activity and exercise (Figure 1.2), which we will discuss next. Keep in mind that different levels of physical activity or exercise are needed for different health benefits. You will learn more about the recommended amounts of activity needed for health and fitness throughout the book.

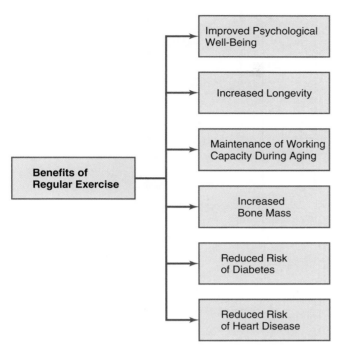

FIGURE 1.2
Regular exercise can yield several long-term benefits for your health.

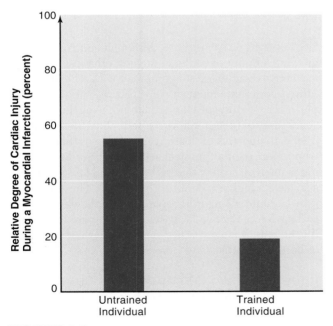

FIGURE 1.3
Regular endurance exercise protects the heart against injury during heart attack. This figure illustrates that during a myocardial infarction (a heart attack), exercise-trained individuals suffer less cardiac injury compared to untrained individuals.

Source: Data from Yamashita, N. et al. Exercise provides direct biphasic cardioprotection via manganese superoxide dismutase activation. *Journal of Experimental Medicine* 189:1699–1706, 1999.

Reduced Risk of Heart Disease   **Cardiovascular disease (CVD)** (i.e., any ailment of the heart and blood vessels) is a major cause of death in the United States. In fact, one of every two Americans dies of CVD (17). Regular physical activity and exercise can significantly reduce your risk of developing CVD (1, 7, 8, 10, 11, 17–21). Further, strong evidence suggests that regular physical activity reduces the risk of dying during a heart attack (Figure 1.3) (22–25). Note from Figure 1.3 that exercise training can reduce the magnitude of cardiac injury during a heart attack by more than 60% (23, 24). Many preventive medicine specialists argue that these facts alone are reason enough for engaging in regular physical activity and exercise (7, 18, 26). Chapter 9 provides a detailed discussion of exercise and CVD.

Reduced Risk of Diabetes   **Diabetes** is a disease characterized by high blood sugar (glucose) levels. Untreated diabetes can result in numerous health problems, including blindness and kidney dysfunction. Regular physical activity and exercise can reduce the risk of a specific type of diabetes, called type 2, by improving the regulation of blood glucose (9, 27, 28). We will discuss diabetes in more detail in Chapter 6.

Increased Bone Mass   The bones of the skeleton provide a mechanical lever system to permit movement and protect internal organs. Clearly, then, it is important to maintain strong and healthy bones. Loss of bone mass and strength is called **osteoporosis,** and it increases the risk of bone fractures. Although osteoporosis can occur in men and women of all ages, it is more common in older adults, particularly women.

Exercise can improve bone health by strengthening your bones. Mechanical force applied by muscular

physical activity Any movement of the body produced by a skeletal muscle that results in energy expenditure, especially through movement of large muscle groups.

exercise Planned, structured, and repetitive bodily movement done to improve or maintain one or more components of fitness.

cardiovascular disease (CVD) Any disease of the heart and blood vessels.

diabetes A metabolic disorder characterized by high blood glucose levels. Chronic elevation of blood glucose is associated with increased incidence of heart disease, kidney disease, nerve dysfunction, and eye damage.

osteoporosis A condition that results from the loss of bone mass and strength.

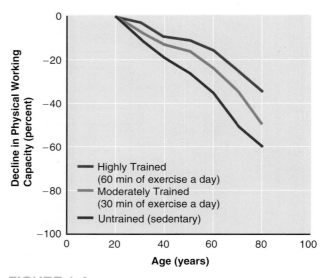

FIGURE 1.4
Regular exercise can reduce the natural decline in working capacity that occurs as we age.

Regular weight-bearing exercise can prevent loss of bone mass.

activity is a key factor in regulating bone mass and strength. Numerous studies have demonstrated that regular exercise increases bone mass, density, and strength in young adults (29–31). In particular, weight-bearing activities, such as running, walking, and resistance training, are important for bone health. Further, research on osteoporosis suggests that regular exercise can prevent bone loss in older adults and is also useful in treating osteoporosis (29).

Easier Aging   As people age, they gradually lose their physical capacity to do work. As we grow older, our ability to perform strenuous activities (e.g., running, cycling, or swimming) progressively declines. Although this decline may begin as early as the 20s, the most dramatic changes occur after about age 60 (32–34). Regular exercise training can reduce the rate of decline in physical working capacity as we age (32, 35, 36). Notice the differences in physical working capacity among highly trained, moderately trained, and inactive individuals in Figure 1.4. The key point is that

although physical working capacity declines with age, regular exercise can reduce the rate of this decline, increasing your ability to enjoy a lifetime of physical recreation and an improved quality of life that comes with it.

Increased Longevity   Although controversial, a growing amount of evidence suggests that regular physical activity and exercise (combined with a healthy lifestyle) increase longevity (7, 8, 25, 37–39). For example, a classic study of Harvard alumni over the past 30 years reported that men with a sedentary lifestyle have a 31% greater risk of death from all causes than men who report regular physical activity (8). Studies including women also show that sedentary and low-fit women also have a higher risk of death (40, 41). These findings translate into a longer life span for people who exercise and have more active lifestyles. The primary factor for this increased longevity is thought to be their lower risk of both heart attack and cancer (7, 8).

Improved Psychological Well-Being   Strong evidence indicates that regular exercise improves psychological well-being in people of all ages. The mental health benefits of regular exercise include reduced risk for anxiety disorders and depression (42). Also, people report feeling less anxious and stressed after an exercise session, even up to 8 hours afterward. These mental benefits lead to an improved sense of well-being in the physically active individual. We will further discuss the role of exercise as a method for reducing psychological stress in Chapter 10.

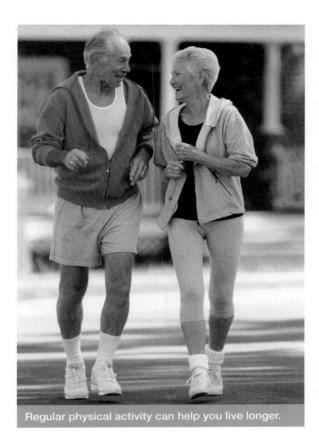

Regular physical activity can help you live longer.

Make sure you know...

> Regular physical activity and exercise reduce the risk of both heart disease and diabetes.

> Exercise increases bone mass in young people and strengthens bone in older adults.

> Regular exercise maintains physical working capacity as the person ages.

> Regular physical activity and exercise have been shown to increase longevity and improve quality of life.

> Exercise promotes psychological well-being and reduces risk of depressive and anxiety disorders.

Exercise and Activity for Health-Related Fitness

Exercise conditioning programs can be divided into two broad categories according to their goals: (1) health-related physical fitness and (2) sport or skill-related physical fitness. This textbook focuses on health-related fitness. The overall goal of a total health-related physical fitness program is to optimize the quality of life (1, 42). The specific goals of this type of

fitness program are to reduce the risk of disease and to improve total physical fitness so that daily tasks can be completed with less effort and fatigue. In contrast, the single goal of sport and skill-related fitness is to improve physical performance in a specific sport. Note though, that the "weekend warrior" engaged in a total health-related physical fitness program will likely also improve physical performance in many sports.

Most fitness experts agree that there are five major components of total health-related physical fitness:

1. Cardiorespiratory endurance
2. Muscular strength
3. Muscular endurance
4. Flexibility
5. Body composition

In addition to these, some fitness experts include motor skill performance as a sixth component. Motor skills are movement qualities, such as agility and coordination, that help athletes improve their performance. Although motor skills are important for sport performance, they are not directly linked to improving health in young adults and are therefore not considered a major component of health-related physical fitness. However, these motor skills might increase in importance as people age, because good balance, coordination, and agility may help reduce the risk for falls in older adults.

Let's examine each of the five components of fitness in more depth.

Cardiorespiratory Endurance

Cardiorespiratory endurance (sometimes called *aerobic fitness* or *cardiorespiratory fitness*) is often considered the key component of health-related physical fitness. Cardiorespiratory endurance is a measure of the heart's ability to pump oxygen-rich blood to the working muscles during exercise and of the muscles' ability to take up and use the oxygen. The oxygen delivered to the muscles is used to produce the energy needed for prolonged exercise.

In practical terms, cardiorespiratory endurance is the ability to perform endurance-type exercises such as distance running, cycling, and swimming. Someone who has achieved a high measure of cardiorespiratory endurance is generally capable of performing 30 to 60

cardiorespiratory endurance A measure of the heart's ability to pump oxygen-rich blood to the working muscles during exercise and of the muscles' ability to take up and use the oxygen.

Cyclists who bike for long distances exhibit strong cardiorespiratory endurance.

minutes of vigorous exercise without undue fatigue. Chapter 3 discusses the details of exercise training designed to improve cardiorespiratory fitness.

Muscular Strength

Muscular strength is evaluated by how much force a muscle (or muscle group) can generate during a single maximal contraction. Practically, this means how much weight an individual can lift during one maximal effort.

Muscular strength is important in almost all sports. Sports such as football, basketball, and events in track and field require a high level of muscular strength. Even nonathletes require some degree of muscular strength to function in everyday life. For example, routine tasks around the home, such as lifting bags of groceries and moving furniture, require muscular strength. Even modest amounts of resistance training (commonly performed as weight training) can improve muscular strength and increase ease of everyday tasks. The principles of developing muscular strength are presented in Chapter 4.

Muscular Endurance

Muscular endurance is the ability of a muscle to generate a submaximal force over and over again. Although muscular strength and muscular endurance are related, they are not the same. These two terms can be best distinguished by examples. A person lifting a 150-pound barbell during one maximal muscular effort demonstrates high muscular strength. If she lifts a 75-pound barbell a dozen times, she demonstrates muscular endurance. As one develops muscular strength, endurance typically improves. However, strength does not generally improve with muscular endurance training.

Most sports require muscular endurance. For instance, tennis players, who must repeatedly swing their racquets during a match, require a high level of muscular endurance. Many everyday activities (e.g., carrying your backpack across campus all day) also require some level of muscular endurance. Techniques of developing muscular endurance are discussed in Chapter 4.

Flexibility

Flexibility is the ability to move joints freely through their full range of motion. Flexible individuals can bend and twist at their joints with ease. Without routine stretching, muscles and tendons shorten and become tight, retarding the range of motion around joints and impairing flexibility.

Individual needs for flexibility vary. Certain athletes (such as gymnasts and divers) require great flexibility to accomplish complex movements. The average individual requires less flexibility than an athlete. However, everyone needs some flexibility for activities of daily living such as reaching for something on the back of the top shelf. Research suggests that flexibility is useful in preventing some types of muscle–tendon injuries and may be useful in reducing low back pain (43, 44). Techniques for improving flexibility are discussed in Chapter 5.

Body Composition

The term **body composition** refers to the relative amounts of fat and lean tissue in your body. The rationale for including body composition as a component of health-related physical fitness is that having a high percentage of body fat (a condition known as obesity) is associated with an increased risk of developing CVD, type 2 diabetes, and some cancers. It also contributes to joint stress during movement. In general, being "over-fat" elevates the risk of medical problems.

Lack of physical activity has been shown to play a major role in gaining body fat. Conversely, regular ex-

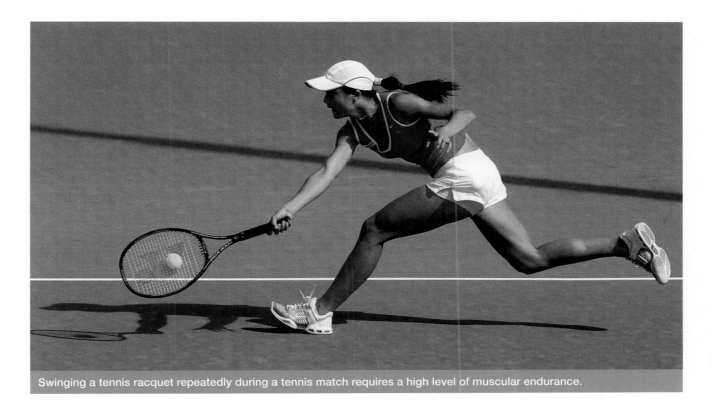

Swinging a tennis racquet repeatedly during a tennis match requires a high level of muscular endurance.

ercise is an important factor in promoting the loss of body fat. You will learn more about body composition in Chapter 6.

Make sure you know...

> Health-related physical fitness consists of five components: cardiorespiratory endurance, muscular strength, muscular endurance, flexibility, and body composition.

How Can You Make Healthier Behavior Choices?

Remember Maria? She needs to change several behaviors to improve her wellness. Her exercise, eating, sleeping, and time management habits could all be improved. Changing her current behaviors will require some effort on her part, and it will not happen overnight. Unhealthy habits and patterns develop over time, so she cannot expect to change them without time and effort. Fortunately, Maria is committed to improving her health, and she is going to use strategies she learned in her wellness course to make lifestyle behavior changes.

The Stages of Change Model

The **Stages of Change Model** suggests that there are a series of five stages to behavior change:

1. Individuals in the *precontemplation* stage of behavior change do not plan to change their unhealthy behavior. They might not realize the need to change, or they just might not want to change.

2. In the *contemplation* stage, a person is aware of the need to change and intends to do so within the next 6 months. People in these first two stages need information about healthy behaviors and the small steps they can make to get closer to changing.

3. During the *preparation* stage, the person is getting ready to make the change within the next 30 days.

muscular strength The maximal ability of a muscle to generate force.

muscular endurance The ability of a muscle to generate a submaximal force over and over again.

flexibility The ability to move joints freely through their full range of motion.

body composition The relative amounts of fat and fat-free tissue (muscle, organs, bone) found in the body.

Stages of Change Model A framework for understanding how individuals move toward adopting and maintaining health behavior changes.

In some cases, the person might already be making some changes (e.g., increasing lifestyle activity before starting an exercise program). People also begin to take practical steps, such as buying a daily planner to list and prioritize daily tasks.

4. In the *action* stage, the behavior change has occurred, but for fewer than 6 months.

5. After sustaining the behavior change for 6 months, the person enters the *maintenance* stage. During this stage, the behavior change is more of a habit and requires less conscious effort. As this stage progresses, the temptation to resume old habits steadily decreases. In the last three stages, it is important to use the behavior modification strategies discussed in the next sections to advance through the stages and to maintain the change long term.

The length of time that one spends in each stage is highly individual, and progression through the stages is not usually linear. Often, people move back and forth between the stages multiple times before they are able to make the behavior change permanent. Note that a setback does not mean failure. If you experience a lapse to an earlier stage, evaluate why you had the setback, and develop a new plan. Learn from this experience, and do not let it discourage you.

The key element in any behavior change plan is the desire to change. Without a genuine desire to make lifestyle changes, the best behavior change plan is doomed to fail. The rest of this section discusses specific strategies and steps to help you adopt and maintain healthy behaviors.

Behavior Modification

Behavior modification is using the cues that precede a behavior or the consequences of the behavior to change it. For example, packing a bag of workout clothes before you go to bed at night and leaving it by your front door is a reminder to take your bag with you the next day so you can stop by the gym after work. If you enjoy the relaxed feeling that results from a good workout, you are likely to keep exercising. Seven commonly used behavior modification strategies are outlined below.

1. *Behavior change contracts* (like the one in the front of this book) include your goals and plans for changing your behavior and are signed by you and a person close to you. Filling out the contract will help you think through your plan, and having another person sign the contract will provide a partner for support and accountability.

2. *Setting realistic short-term and long-term goals* is essential for effective behavior change. The details of goal setting are outlined at length in Chapter 2.

3. *Self-monitoring* involves analyzing your behavior to determine what influences your unhealthy behaviors and patterns. Self-monitoring helps you see the things that trigger and reinforce your unhealthy choices so you can make changes.

4. *Counter conditioning* is replacing an unhealthy behavior choice with a healthier one. Something as simple as keeping fresh fruits and vegetables for snacks instead of potato chips can help you make dietary changes.

5. *Self-reinforcement* is developing a system to reward yourself when you meet your goals.

6. *Decisional balance* involves weighing the positives and negatives of the behavior you want to change. This strategy is usually more helpful for people in the last three stages of change, when they are expecting or experiencing positive outcomes of the new behaviors. In the first two stages, you are more likely to see the negatives of the behavior, so decisional balance might be counterproductive for changing your behavior.

7. *Relapse prevention* is used to keep you from lapsing back to your unhealthy behavior. This strategy involves identifying the "high-risk" situations that are likely to trigger your unhealthy choice and then developing a specific plan of action to avoid or eliminate those situations. If you are trying to drink less alcohol on the weekend and you know that you are likely to drink too much at a campus keg party, you might skip the party and go to a restaurant with your friends instead. Then you might take only enough money for one or two drinks, and rotate the responsibility of being the designated driver.

Assessing Your Habits

Before you can change a wellness-related behavior, you must recognize that the behavior is unhealthy and that you can make changes. You also need to identify alternative behaviors for your unhealthy behavior. A good place to begin is a personal assessment of your health risk status. You can use the lifestyle assessment inventory in Laboratory 1.1 to increase your awareness of factors that affect your health. As you complete the lab, develop a list of your less-than-optimal behaviors. Can you identify where you are in the stages of change? Do you need to gather more information before you initiate your behavior change plan? Remember, to be successful in changing the behavior, you must be ready, physically and mentally. Keep in mind that you can control each of these health behaviors but that being aware of them is not enough to bring about change.

After you determine which behaviors you want to change, you can use self-monitoring to study your

STEPS FOR BEHAVIOR CHANGE

Do you have trouble making healthy behavior changes?

Answer the following questions about your typical efforts to change a health behavior.

Y N

☐ ☐ Do you have a specific game plan?

☐ ☐ Do you get help from your friends and family?

☐ ☐ Do you set goals?

☐ ☐ Do you reward yourself for your successes?

If you answered no to most or all of the questions, then you should consider using the behavioral contract in the front of the text.

BENEFITS OF USING A BEHAVIORAL CONTRACT

☑ Helps you think through and assess your behavior.

☑ Helps you develop specific plans in writing.

☑ Provides you with accountability and support from another person.

☑ Shows strong commitment and motivation to change.

---

habits to make the best plan of action. When you assess your patterns, consider why you make the choices you make and why you want to change. Do you have poor dietary habits because you do not know healthy nutrition recommendations, or do you overeat to deal with stress or emotional problems? Also, you need to assess the things and people in your life that facilitate healthy decisions and that present barriers for healthy decisions.

Lastly when assessing your habits, consider why it is important for you to change. Do you want to change to improve your health and feel better about yourself, or do you want to change to please someone else? Understanding the motivations for your choices will help you develop the best plan to make your changes permanent.

Identifying Behavior Change Barriers

After you have assessed your current behavior patterns, you can focus on the barriers that may prevent you from changing your behavior. For example, you want to

start an exercise program, but you have a full load of classes and work part-time in the evening—you may feel that lack of time is a barrier. You want to stop smoking, but all your friends smoke when you hang out together—your barrier would be the social pressure you feel from your friends. Your goal is to reduce or eliminate your barriers, and this is the perfect opportunity to use relapse prevention.

Some barriers are easy to work with. Others are complicated, especially when they are influenced by people who are important to you. To go back to our examples, getting up a half-hour earlier might help you overcome the barrier of a perceived lack of time, but to address the social barrier to your quitting smoking you will need some help from your friends. People who care about you will typically be supportive if they know about your goals, but they cannot help if you do not communicate your desire to change. Telling your friends you want to stop smoking and that you do not want to be with them when they smoke will help them support your decision. Relapse prevention can be very effective in changing behaviors.

CONSUMER CORNER

FINDING CREDIBLE HEALTH INFORMATION

With all of the health information out there, how do you know what to believe? "Experts" endorse products and plans on infomercials and in magazines, but some of the claims seem too good to be true. To avoid becoming overwhelmed—or worse, being scammed—you have to develop a "healthy skepticism." The next time you visit a website, read a supplement label, or watch an infomercial, ask yourself the following questions:

- Do the claims made about this product seem too good to be true?
- Has all of the supporting research been conducted or funded by the company that makes the product or offers the service?
- Are the claims made about the product supported by quality scientific research?
- Is there information available about short- and long-term effects?
- Does the information fit with the information I am learning in class?
- Are potential risks and side effects of products and services mentioned?
- Are the experts endorsing the product or service really experts in that field? (For example, a doctor who is a podiatrist might not be the best source for a weight loss pill.)
- Is there any opposing information available?

Answering yes to the first two questions should always raise a red flag. If you can answer yes to the remaining questions, the product or service might be worth considering. Get the opinion of a trusted professional, such as your instructor or a health care worker at your student health center for further evaluation.

Changing Unhealthy Behaviors

Now you can begin to develop a game plan for changing your behaviors. After you complete Laboratory 1.1, you might see multiple behaviors you could change to improve your wellness. Do not let your results overwhelm you. Recognize that you do not need to change all of your unhealthy behaviors at the same time. Trying to make too many changes at once is usually very difficult and reduces your chances for success. Setbacks can reduce your motivation to change, but keep in mind that a setback does not mean failure.

Before you can develop your plan of action, you need to have accurate information about the behaviors. You will get a lot of information from this book and your instructor. However, you might also need to seek out additional resources, such as counselor at the student health center, a fitness specialist, or a support group. Make sure any outside resources are reputable groups or individuals who are qualified to give you the information and guidance you need (see Consumer Corner for how to identify credible sources of health information).

When deciding which changes you want to make first, consider the number of behaviors you want to change and the effort it will take to change them. Some behaviors, such as flossing your teeth regularly or performing monthly self-exams, are simple and do not require as much effort. However, starting a new exercise program, quitting smoking, or changing your diet require more effort. Most people can successfully make more than one simple change at a time. However, for the more complex behaviors, making them one at a time is recommended. Also, breaking them into smaller steps, or **shaping,** is also recommended to make the change seem less intimidating. Your success with the simple behaviors and the small steps on the way to the complex behavior will increase your confidence and motivate you to work toward total wellness.

Finally, you need to set goals and develop your specific plan for changing the behavior. Something as simple as putting a monthly reminder on your personal digital assistant (PDA) to do a self-exam and hanging a plastic tag on your shower head might do the trick. Or, using counter conditioning by trading a sedentary choice for an active one will increase lifestyle physical activity. However, for many behaviors you will need a more detailed plan of action. For example, changing your eating habits might include meeting with a dietitian, making grocery lists, planning meals ahead of time, and having an accountability partner. Also, these changes will likely be made in stages. Using shaping will make the change seem more manageable.

Make sure you know...

> Knowing your stage of change will help you develop the best plan of action for changing your behavior.

> Behavior modification strategies are very helpful in successfully changing your behavior.

> Assessing your current habits and addressing your barriers are essential before developing your plan for behavior change.

Specific Application of Behavior Modification

Let's apply behavior modification to two common behaviors that can be a challenge to address: quitting smoking and losing weight.

Smoking Cessation

As previously mentioned, cigarette smoking increases the risk of cancer and heart disease. Research shows that smoking is the largest cause of preventable death in the United States (45). Although millions of people have quit smoking, the number of smokers has increased since the late 1960s because of an increase in young smokers, particularly young women. Smoking is a difficult behavior to change because it involves an addiction to nicotine, so outside assistance might be necessary to help overcome the addiction.

The first step in quitting smoking is having the desire to stop. You may want to quit because you recognize the negative health effects of smoking, or you may have important people in your life who want you to quit. When you analyze your smoking behavior, pay attention to the times you smoke. Think about the reasons you decide to smoke. Is it automatic after a meal, or when you are with certain friends? Note the times you do not have the desire to smoke or when you choose other behaviors over smoking, and note your barriers for quitting smoking.

After you have a good idea of when and why you smoke, it is time to set goals and make a plan. Relapse prevention and counter conditioning can be very helpful. Mobilize your support network by telling your friends and family what you plan to do—and, specifically, how they can help.

When you set your goals, be very specific so you can assess your progress. Also, be sure to set both short-term and long-term goals. Obviously, the long-term goal is to stop permanently, but you should set goals for the things you will do to prepare for and maintain cessation. For example, you might sign a behavioral contract with your roommate and agree to check in after meals to maintain accountability. If you smoke after meals, plan to brush your teeth or chew gum instead of smoking; this is an example of counter conditioning. Relapse prevention might involve eating lunch in a no-smoking restaurant. Planning ahead and

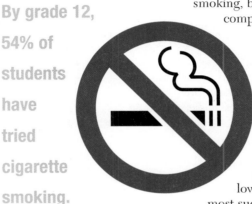

CONSIDER THIS!

By grade 12, 54% of students have tried cigarette smoking.

having an alternate behavior will decrease the likelihood of smoking at your high-risk times.

Quitting smoking "cold turkey" is the most commonly reported method for smoking cessation (45, 46). Continue using behavior modification strategies to move from the action to the maintenance stage. If you smoke even one cigarette during the action stage, you move back into the preparation or possibly the contemplation stage, but remember that lapse does not mean failure. Reevaluate your behavior and why you had the lapse, and revise your plan. As you maintain your new healthy behavior of not smoking, be sure to reward yourself for accomplishing your goal.

Weight Loss

Losing weight and keeping it off are difficult for many people. Applying behavior modification principles and using behavior change models are essential. Although no single weight-loss program works for all people, the following are common components of most successful efforts:

1. Make sure that you want to lose weight for yourself. If you want to lose weight to please someone else, your chances for success are not as high.

2. Assess your eating habits, including the kind and amount of food you eat as well as the environmental and social circumstances involved. Also assess your physical activity and exercise patterns.

3. Establish short- and long-term goals. Do not limit your goals to a specific number of pounds to lose; set goals for changing your exercise and eating habits as well.

4. Establish your support network and accountability partners. A behavioral contract can be helpful.

5. Develop your specific plan, including dietary and activity changes. Remember to make it very detailed and to include specific steps. For example, a goal to "prepare healthier meals" is not specific enough. Instead, spell out what you will do to prepare healthier meals. Find recipes for dishes that are low in calories and dense in nutrients. Plan meals for an entire week, and make a grocery list for only the foods needed for your menus. Prepare meals according to

shaping Breaking a behavior or task into small steps to accomplish the larger goal.

the plan, and consider portion size. Each step might seem minor, but each takes effort. With this level of detail, you are using shaping, and you can experience success at each level to increase your confidence. (See Chapter 8 for more on weight management.)

6. Relapse prevention and counter conditioning will help plan for situations that might make you slip from your dietary changes and exercise plans. For example, knowing healthy menu options before you get to the restaurant and planning to exercise as soon you get home instead of watching television can help keep you on track.

7. Use your support network and any other outside assistance.

8. Reward yourself for successes along the way (self-reinforcement). Make sure your rewards do not undermine your success. Rewarding yourself with chocolate cake for a week is not the best choice, but a dessert once in a while is not unreasonable.

There is a lot of good and bad information out there about ways to lose weight. You need to check information for accuracy when you consider a weight-loss plan. Unsound plans often produce rapid weight loss, but they might leave you missing key nutrients and can cause you to gain more weight later. These plans may also lighten your wallet, but not your body. Stay away from products or services that do not have information about long-term effects. Refer to Chapter 8 and your instructor to help you evaluate a plan.

Remember that the key elements in a weight-loss program are the desire to lose weight for oneself, establishing goals, developing a plan, and getting support from your friends and family. As you develop your plan, assess your readiness for change as well as the benefits, barriers, and other factors that will contribute to your success.

Make sure you know...

> Behavior modification can be applied to many health behaviors.

> A detailed plan of action is essential for using behavior modification to change your unhealthy behaviors.

Summary

1. The term *wellness* means "healthy living." Wellness is achieved by practicing a healthy lifestyle, which includes regular physical activity, proper nutrition, eliminating unhealthy behaviors (avoiding high-risk activities such as smoking and drug use), and maintaining emotional and spiritual health.

2. Total wellness can be achieved only by a balance of physical, emotional, intellectual, spiritual, social, and environmental health. The components of wellness do not work in isolation; they interact strongly. For example, poor physical health can lead to poor emotional health.

3. Exercise offers many health benefits. Regular exercise has been shown to reduce risk of CVD and diabetes, increase bone mass, and maintain physical working capacity as one ages.

4. The five major components of "total" health-related physical fitness are cardiorespiratory endurance, muscular strength, muscular endurance, flexibility, and body composition.

5. Used correctly, behavior modification strategies can be very helpful for changing health behaviors.

Study Questions

1. _____ is any body movement produced by skeletal muscles that results in energy expenditure.
   a. Exercise
   b. Physical fitness
   c. Physical activity
   d. Health-related fitness

2. _____ is *not* a dimension of wellness.
   a. Exercise
   b. Spiritual health
   c. Social health
   d. Mental health

3. Which of the following is *not* a component of health-related fitness?

   a. muscular strength

   b. body composition

   c. agility

   d. flexibility

4. Which of the following is a health benefit of regular physical activity?

   a. reduced risk for osteoporosis

   b. reduced risk for heart disease

   c. improved mental health

   d. all of the above

5. The main goals for *Healthy People 2010* include

   a. increasing quality and quantity of healthy years and eliminating health disparities.

   b. eliminating physical inactivity and reducing obesity.

   c. increasing wellness of all and eliminating smoking.

   d. increasing fitness for all and improving healthy eating.

6. A person in the _____ stage of change has been fully participating in the new health behavior for less than 6 months.

   a. maintenance

   b. action

   c. contemplation

   d. new activity

7. Which of the following is an important step in initiating a health behavior change?

   a. making a specific plan

   b. mobilizing your support network

   c. getting outside help if needed

   d. all of the above

8. Which of the following should be considered when you are planning to make a behavior change?

   a. number of behaviors you want to change and effort involved

   b. motive for behavior change

   c. current behavior patterns

   d. all of the above

9. What is wellness?

10. Name at least one behavior associated with each of the six components of wellness.

11. List and discuss the five components of health-related fitness.

12. Outline the strategies for setting exercise goals.

13. Discuss the importance of the *Healthy People* goals and objectives.

Suggested Reading

Blair, S., and M. Moore. Surgeon General's report on physical fitness. The inside story. *ACSM's Health and Physical Journal* 1:14–18, 1997.

Brooks, G. A., N. Butte, W. Rand, J. Flatt, and B. Caballero. Chronicle of the Institute of Medicine physical activity recommendation: How a physical activity recommendation came to be among dietary recommendations. *American Journal of Clinical Nutrition* 79:921S–930S, 2004.

Brown, D., D. Brown, G. Heath, L. Balluz, W. Giles, E. Ward, and A. Mokdad. Associations between physical activity dose and health-related quality of life. *Medicine and Science in Sports and Exercise* 36:890–896, 2004.

Franklin, B. Improved fitness = Increased longevity. *ACSM's Health and Fitness Journal* 5:32–33, 2001.

Haskell, W. L., et al. Physical activity and public health: Updated recommendation for adults from the American College of Sports Medicine and the American Heart Association. *Medicine and Science in Sports and Exercise* 39:1423–1434, 2007.

Howley, E., and D. Franks. *Fitness Professional's Handbook*, 5th ed. Champaign, IL: Human Kinetics Publishers, 2007.

Powers, S., and E. Howley. *Exercise Physiology: Theory and Application to Fitness and Performance*, 7th ed. New York: McGraw-Hill, 2009.

Powers, S., S. Lennon, J. Quindry, and J. Mehta. Exercise and cardioprotection. *Current Opinion in Cardiology* 17:495–502, 2002.

For links to the organizations and websites listed below, visit The Total Fitness and Wellness Website at www.pearsonhighered.com/powers.

American Heart Association

Contains latest information about ways to reduce your risk of heart and vascular diseases. Site includes information about exercise, diet, and heart disease.

American College of Sports Medicine

Contains information about exercise, health, and fitness.

WebMD

Contains the latest information on a variety of health-related topics, including diet, exercise, and stress. Links to nutrition, fitness, and wellness topics.

Healthy People

Contains information about the U.S. government's initiative to improve health and wellness for the American people.

References

1. Margen, S., et al., eds. *The Wellness Encyclopedia.* Boston: Houghton Mifflin, 1995.

2. National Institute of Mental Health. The Numbers Count: Mental Disorders in America. Fact Sheet. www.nimh.nih.gov/publicat/numbers.cfm#MajorDepressive

3. Koeing, H. G. Religion, spirituality and medicine: Research findings and implications for clinical practice. *Southern Medical Journal* 97:1194–1200, 2004.

4. Katon, W., E. H. B. Lin, and K. Kroenke. The association of depression and anxiety with medical symptom burden in patients with chronic medical illness. *General Hospital Psychiatry* 29:147–155, 2007.

5. Weaver, A. J., and K. J. Flannelly. The role of religion/spirituality for cancer patients and their caregivers. *Southern Medical Journal* 97:1210–1214, 2004.

6. Caspersen, C. J., K. E. Powell, and G. M. Christenson. Physical activity and exercise: Definitions and distinctions for health related-fitness research. *Public Health Reports* 100:126–130, 1985.

7. Paffenbarger, R., J. Kampert, I-Min Lee, R. Hyde, R. Leung, and A. Wing. Changes in physical activity and other lifeway patterns influencing longevity. *Medicine and Science in Sports and Exercise* 26:857–865, 1994.

8. Paffenbarger, R., R. Hyde, A. Wing, and C. Hsieh. Physical activity, all-cause mortality, longevity of college alumni. *New England Journal of Medicine* 314:605–613, 1986.

9. Helmrich, S., D. Ragland, and R. Paffenbarger. Prevention of non-insulin-dependent diabetes mellitus with physical activity. *Medicine and Science in Sports and Exercise* 26:824–830, 1994.

10. Wood, P. Physical activity, diet, and health: Independent and interactive effects. *Medicine and Science in Sports and Exercise* 26:838–843, 1994.

11. Morris, J. Exercise in the prevention of coronary heart disease: Today's best buy in public health. *Medicine and Science in Sports and Exercise* 26:807–814, 1994.

12. Blair, S. N., M. LaMonte, and M. Nichaman. The evolution of physical activity recommendations: How much is enough? *American Journal of Clinical Nutrition* 79:913S–920S, 2004.

13. Thompson, P., et al. Exercise and physical activity in the prevention and treatment of atherosclerotic cardiovascular disease. *Circulation* 107:3109–3116, 2003.

14. Brooks, G. A., N. Butte, W. Rand, J. Flatt, and B. Caballero. Chronicle of the Institute of Medicine. Physical activity recommendation: How a physical activity recommendation came to be among dietary recommendations. *American Journal of Clinical Nutrition* 79:921S–930S, 2004.

15. Brown, D., D. Brown, G. Heath, L. Balluz, W. Giles, E. Ward, and A. Mokdad. Associations between physical activity dose and health-related quality of life. *Medicine and Science in Sports and Exercise* 36:890–896, 2004.

16. U.S. Department of Health and Human Services. *Physical activity and health: A report of the Surgeon General.* Atlanta, GA: U.S. Department of Health and Human Services, Centers for Disease Control and Prevention, National Center for Chronic Disease Prevention and Health Promotion, 1996.

17. American Heart Association. *Heart Disease and Stroke Statistics—2009 Update (At-a-Glance Version).* Dallas, TX: American Heart Association, 2009.

18. Barrow, M. *Heart Talk: Understanding Cardiovascular Diseases.* Gainesville, FL: Cor-Ed Publishing, 1992.

19. Williams, P. T. Relationship between distance run per week to coronary heart disease risk factors in 8283 male runners: The National Runners Health Study. *Archives of Internal Medicine* 157:191–198, 1997.

20. Fagard, R. Physical activity in the prevention and treatment of hypertension in the obese. *Medicine and Science in Sports and Exercise* 31:S624–S630, 1999.

21. Williams, P. Physical fitness and activity as separate heart disease risk factors: A meta-analysis. *Medicine and Science in Sports and Exercise* 33:754–761, 2001.

22. Lennon, S., J. Quindry, K. Hamilton, J. French, J. Staib, J. Mehta, and S. K. Powers. Loss of cardioprotection after cessation of exercise. *Journal of Applied Physiology* 96: 299–1305, 2004.

23. Powers, S., M. Locke, and H. Demirel. Exercise, heat shock proteins, and myocardial protection from I-R injury. *Medicine and Science in Sports and Exercise* 33:386–392, 2001.

24. Hamilton, K., J. Staib, T. Phillips, A. Hess, S. Lennon, and S. Powers. Exercise, antioxidants, and HSP72: Protection against myocardial ischemia-reperfusion. *Free Radicals in Biology and Medicine* 34:800–809, 2003.

25. Lee, I. M., and R. Paffenbarger. Associations of light, moderate, and vigorous intensity physical activity with longevity: The Harvard Alumni Health Study. *American Journal of Epidemiology* 151:293–299, 2000.

26. Powell, K., and S. Blair. The public health burdens of sedentary living habits: Theoretical but realistic estimates. *Medicine and Science in Sports and Exercise* 26:851–856, 1994.

27. Rodnick, K., J. Holloszy, C. Mondon, and D. James. Effects of exercise training on insulin-regulatable glucose-transporter protein levels in rat skeletal muscle. *Diabetes* 39:1425–1429, 1990.

28. Pan, X. R., et al. Effects of diet and exercise in preventing NIDDM in people with impaired glucose tolerance. *Diabetes Care* 20:537–544, 1997.

29. Rankin, J. Diet, exercise, and osteoporosis. *Certified News* (American College of Sports Medicine) 3:1–4, 1993.

30. Wheeler, D., J. Graves, G. Miller, R. Vander Griend, T. Wronski, S. K. Powers, and H. Park. Effects of running on the torsional strength, morphometry, and bone mass on the rat skeleton. *Medicine and Science in Sports and Exercise* 27:520–529, 1995.

31. Taaffe, D., T. Robinson, C. Snow, and R. Marcus. High impact exercise promotes bone gain in well-trained female athletes. *Journal of Bone and Mineral Research* 12:255–260, 1997.

32. Hagberg, J. Effect of training in the decline of VO_{2max} with aging. *Federation Proceedings* 46:1830–1833, 1987.

33. Fleg, J., and E. Lakatta. Role of muscle loss in the age-associated reduction in VO_2max. *Journal of Applied Physiology* 65:1147–1151, 1988.

34. Nakamura, E., T. Moritani, and A. Kanetaka. Effects of habitual physical exercise on physiological age in men and women aged 20–85 years as estimated using principal component analysis. *European Journal of Applied Physiology* 73:410–418, 1996.

35. Hammeren, J., S. Powers, J. Lawler, D. Criswell, D. Martin, D. Lowenthal, and M. Pollock. Exercise training–induced alterations in skeletal muscle oxidative and antioxidant enzyme activity in senescent rats. *International Journal of Sports Medicine* 13:412–416, 1992.

36. Powers, S., J. Lawler, D. Criswell, Fu-Kong Lieu, and D. Martin. Aging and respiratory muscle metabolic plasticity: Effects of endurance training. *Journal of Applied Physiology* 72:1068–1073, 1992.

37. Holloszy, J. Exercise increases average longevity of female rats despite increased food intake and no growth retardation. *Journal of Gerontology* 48:B97–B100, 1993.

38. Lee, I., R. Paffenbarger, and C. Hennekens. Physical activity, physical fitness, and longevity. *Aging—Milano* 9:2–11, 1997.

39. Franklin, B. Improved fitness = increased longevity. *ACSM's Health and Fitness Journal* 5:32–33, 2001.

40. Blair, S. N., and M. Wei. Sedentary habits, health, and function in older men and women. *American Journal of Health Promotion* 15:1–8, 2000.

41. Blair, S. N., H. W. Kohl, R. Paffenbarger, D. Clark, K. Cooper, and L. Gibbons. Physical fitness and all-cause mortality: A prospective study of healthy men and women. *Journal of the American Medical Association* 262:2395–2401, 1989.

42. Penedo, F. J., and J. R. Dahn. Exercise and well-being: A review of mental and physical health benefits associated with physical activity. *Current Opinion in Psychiatry* 18:198–193, 2005.

43. Jones, M. A., G. Stratton, T. Reilly, and V. B. Unnithan. Biological risk indicators for recurrent non-specific low back pain in adolescents. *British Journal of Sports Medicine* 39:137–140, 2005.

44. Mikkelson, L. O., H. Nupponen, J. Kaprio, H. Kautiainen, and U. M. Kujala. Adolescent flexibility, endurance strength, and physical activity as predictors of adult tension neck, low back pain and knee injury: A 25 year follow up. *British Journal of Sports Medicine* 40:107–113, 2006.

45. Edwards, R. ABC of smoking cessation: The problem of smoking. *British Medical Journal* 328:217–219, 2004.

46. Doran, C. M., L. Valenti, M. Robinson, H. Britt, and R. P. Mattick. Smoking status of Australian general practice patients and their attempts to quit. *Addictive Behaviors* 31:758–766, 2005.

47. Ridner, L. S., and E. J. Hahn. The pros and cons of cessation in college-age smokers. *Clinical Excellence for Nurse Practitioners* 9:81–87, 2005.

Videos

Log on to www.pearsonhighered.com/powers to view these chapter-related videos.

Personal Fitness and Exercise
Promoting Healthy Behavior Change

NAME _____ DATE _____

Lifestyle Assessment Inventory

The purpose of this lifestyle assessment inventory is to help you identify areas in your life that increase your risk of disease, injury, and possibly premature death. Awareness is the first step in making change.

Put a check by each statement that applies to you. You may select more than one choice per category.

Physical Health

A. Physical Fitness

_____ I exercise for a minimum of 20 to 30 minutes at least 3 days per week.

_____ I walk for 15 to 30 minutes (3 to 7 days per week).

_____ I get lifestyle or occupational physical activity most days of the week.

B. Body Fat

_____ There is no place on my body where I can pinch more than 1 inch of fat.

_____ I am satisfied with the way my body looks.

C. Car Safety

_____ I always use a seat belt when I drive.

_____ I rarely drive above the speed limit.

_____ I do not drink and drive, and I do not ride in a car with someone who has been drinking.

D. Sleep

_____ I always get 7 to 9 hours of sleep.

_____ I do not have trouble going to sleep.

_____ I generally do not wake up during the night.

E. Diet

_____ I generally eat balanced meals and a variety of food.

_____ I eat fruits and vegetables daily.

_____ I rarely overeat.

_____ I rarely eat large quantities of fatty foods and sweets.

F. Alcohol Use

_____ I consume fewer than two drinks per day.

_____ I never get intoxicated.

_____ I do not binge drink.

G. Tobacco and Drug Use

_____ I never smoke (cigarettes, pipe, cigars, etc.).

_____ I do not use smokeless tobacco.

_____ I use prescription medications only for their intended purpose.

_____ I do not use illegal drugs.

H. Sexual Practices

_____ I always practice safe sex (e.g., always using condoms or being involved in a monogamous relationship).

_____ I am not sexually active.

Social Health

_____ I have a happy and satisfying relationship with my spouse or boyfriend/girlfriend.

_____ I have good relationships with my close friends.

_____ I get a great deal of love and support from my family.

_____ I work to have good communication skills.

_____ I am able to express my feelings and emotions to people close to me.

Emotional Health

A. Stress Level

_____ I find it easy to relax.

_____ I rarely feel tense or anxious.

_____ I am able to cope with daily stresses without undue emotional stress.

_____ I have not experienced a major stressful life event in the past year.

B. Mental Health

_____ I do not suffer from depressive or anxiety disorders.

_____ I do not have an eating disorder.

Intellectual Health

_____ I attend class regularly.

_____ I keep informed about current events.

_____ I seek opportunities to learn new things.

_____ I have an open mind about ideas that might be different from mine.

Environmental Health

_____ I am not exposed to second-hand smoke on a regular basis.

_____ I use sunscreen regularly or limit my sun exposure.

_____ I carpool or use physical activity for transportation when possible.

_____ I recycle regularly.

_____ I limit my exposure to harmful environmental contaminants.

Spiritual Health

_____ I have a sense of meaning and purpose in my life.

_____ I am satisfied with my level of spirituality.

_____ I work to develop my spiritual health.

Evaluating Your Responses

1. What area of wellness is your strongest area? What do you do to maintain healthy behaviors for that wellness component?

   _____

   _____

2. What area of wellness is your weakest area? What behaviors can you change to improve that area?

   _____

   _____

3. Write a long-term and a short-term goal for improving one wellness behavior you seriously want to change this semester.

   _____

   _____

NAME _____ DATE _____

Changing Your Behavior

Select a health behavior you want to change, and use the steps below to indicate how you will accomplish the change. Use additional paper if needed.

1. Select a behavior to change. _____

2. Assess your behavioral patterns.
State at least one barrier you will face.

   _____

   _____

   State at least one thing that will support your change.

   _____

   _____

3. Name the people you will be able to count on for support and accountability. Will one of them be willing to sign the behavior change contract with you?

   _____

   _____

4. What behavior modification strategies will you use? For each strategy you list, write out a specific plan for how you will use it.

   _____

   _____

5. Write out your long-term goal and at least two short-term goals that will help you get there.

   Long-term goal: _____

   _____

   Short-term goals: _____

   _____

6. How will you reward yourself when you achieve your short- and long-term goals?

   _____

   _____

   _____

NAME _____ DATE _____

Medical History Check

Most people can safely begin an exercise program and significantly increase their physical activity. However, certain medical conditions require clearance from a physician or alternative prescriptions for exercise and physical activity. Therefore, it is important to assess your health before making significant physical activity changes. Respond honestly to the following questions to assess your medical history.

Do you currently have or have you ever had any of the following? Check any of the following that apply.

_____ Heart murmur

_____ Elevated cholesterol

_____ High blood pressure

_____ Irregular heart beat

_____ Coronary heart disease

_____ Chest pain

_____ Blood clots

_____ Abnormal rest or exercise electrocardiogram (ECG)

_____ Stroke

_____ Diabetes

_____ Heart attack

_____ Shortness of breath

_____ Family history of heart disease (blood relative)

_____ Arthritis

_____ Chronic back pain

_____ Obesity

_____ Asthma

_____ Any other heart, metabolic, or respiratory conditions

_____ Any other joint problems

Check any of the following that apply to you:

_____ 45 years or older

_____ Smoker or quit smoking within last 6 months

_____ Currently taking prescription medication

Please list: _____

Please explain any items you checked.

_____

_____

Please explain any reasons you feel it would be unsafe for you to exercise.

_____

_____

NAME _____ DATE _____

Par-Q and You

The following questionnaire can also be used to determine your readiness to engage in a fitness program.

Physical Activity Readiness
Questionnaire - PAR-Q
(revised 2002)

PAR-Q & YOU

(A Questionnaire for People Aged 15 to 69)

Regular physical activity is fun and healthy, and increasingly more people are starting to become more active every day. Being more active is very safe for most people. However, some people should check with their doctor before they start becoming much more physically active.

If you are planning to become much more physically active than you are now, start by answering the seven questions in the box below. If you are between the ages of 15 and 69, the PAR-Q will tell you if you should check with your doctor before you start. If you are over 69 years of age, and you are not used to being very active, check with your doctor.

Common sense is your best guide when you answer these questions. Please read the questions carefully and answer each one honestly: check YES or NO.

YES	NO		
☐	☐	1.	**Has your doctor ever said that you have a heart condition <u>and</u> that you should only do physical activity recommended by a doctor?**
☐	☐	2.	**Do you feel pain in your chest when you do physical activity?**
☐	☐	3.	**In the past month, have you had chest pain when you were not doing physical activity?**
☐	☐	4.	**Do you lose your balance because of dizziness or do you ever lose consciousness?**
☐	☐	5.	**Do you have a bone or joint problem (for example, back, knee or hip) that could be made worse by a change in your physical activity?**
☐	☐	6.	**Is your doctor currently prescribing drugs (for example, water pills) for your blood pressure or heart condition?**
☐	☐	7.	**Do you know of <u>any other reason</u> why you should not do physical activity?**

If

you

answered

YES to one or more questions

Talk with your doctor by phone or in person BEFORE you start becoming much more physically active or BEFORE you have a fitness appraisal. Tell your doctor about the PAR-Q and which questions you answered YES.

- You may be able to do any activity you want — as long as you start slowly and build up gradually. Or, you may need to restrict your activities to those which are safe for you. Talk with your doctor about the kinds of activities you wish to participate in and follow his/her advice.
- Find out which community programs are safe and helpful for you.

NO to all questions

If you answered NO honestly to <u>all</u> PAR-Q questions, you can be reasonably sure that you can:
- start becoming much more physically active — begin slowly and build up gradually. This is the safest and easiest way to go.
- take part in a fitness appraisal — this is an excellent way to determine your basic fitness so that you can plan the best way for you to live actively. It is also highly recommended that you have your blood pressure evaluated. If your reading is over 144/94, talk with your doctor before you start becoming much more physically active.

DELAY BECOMING MUCH MORE ACTIVE:
- if you are not feeling well because of a temporary illness such as a cold or a fever — wait until you feel better; or
- if you are or may be pregnant — talk to your doctor before you start becoming more active.

PLEASE NOTE: If your health changes so that you then answer YES to any of the above questions, tell your fitness or health professional. Ask whether you should change your physical activity plan.

<u>Informed Use of the PAR-Q</u>: The Canadian Society for Exercise Physiology, Health Canada, and their agents assume no liability for persons who undertake physical activity, and if in doubt after completing this questionnaire, consult your doctor prior to physical activity.

No changes permitted. You are encouraged to photocopy the PAR-Q but only if you use the entire form.

NOTE: If the PAR-Q is being given to a person before he or she participates in a physical activity program or a fitness appraisal, this section may be used for legal or administrative purposes.

"I have read, understood and completed this questionnaire. Any questions I had were answered to my full satisfaction."

NAME _____

SIGNATURE _____   DATE_____

SIGNATURE OF PARENT _____   WITNESS _____
or GUARDIAN (for participants under the age of majority)

Note: This physical activity clearance is valid for a maximum of 12 months from the date it is completed and becomes invalid if your condition changes so that you would answer YES to any of the seven questions.

Source: The Canadian Society for Exercise Physiology, developed by the British Columbia Ministry of Health.

General Principles of Exercise for Health and Fitness

2

true or false?

1. Establishing fitness goals is a key part of the exercise prescription.

2. Exercise must be hard and boring to improve physical fitness.

3. Too much exercise can increase your risk of illness.

4. As little as 30 minutes of physical activity per day will have health benefits.

5. Use it or lose it! If you stop exercising, you'll lose fitness.

Answers appear on the next page.

Everyone can improve his or her level of physical fitness. Whether your idea of exercise is getting out of a chair to go grab a soda or going for a daily run, you can improve your fitness level by analyzing your routine and making gradual improvements.

The purpose of this chapter is to discuss the general principles behind improving your physical fitness. The basic concepts presented here apply to both men and women of all ages and fitness levels. You will find out more about the individual components of health-related physical fitness—that is, cardiorespiratory fitness, muscular strength and endurance, flexibility, and body composition—in the next few chapters.

Principles of Exercise Training to Improve Physical Fitness

Although everyone's exercise training program will vary according to personal needs, the general principles of physical fitness are universal. The more you exercise, and the greater the variety of activities you do, the more fit you'll be. In the following sections we describe the training concepts of over-

CONSIDER THIS!

More than 67% of Americans do not get enough physical activity, and 45% engage in almost no physical activity during the day.

load, progression, specificity, recuperation, and reversibility, all of which affect the progress you'll make as you design and carry out your exercise training program.

Overload Principle

To improve physical fitness, systems of the body (e.g., the muscular and cardiorespiratory systems) must be stressed. For example, for a skeletal muscle to increase in strength, the muscle must work against a heavier load than normal. This concept is part of the **overload principle,** and it's a key component of all conditioning programs (1, 2) (Figure 2.1). We achieve an overload by increasing the intensity of exercise, such as by using heavier weights.

You can also achieve overload by increasing the duration (or time) of exercise. For instance, to increase muscular endurance, a muscle must be worked over a longer duration than normal, such as by performing a higher number of exercise repetitions. To improve flexibility and increase the range of motion at a joint, we must either stretch the muscle to a longer length than normal or hold the stretch for a longer time.

Although overload is important to attaining physical fitness, your workouts should not be exhausting. The often-heard bodybuilding adage "No pain, no gain," is not accurate. In fact, you can improve your physical fitness without punishing training sessions.

Principle of Progression

The **principle of progression** is an extension of the overload principle. It states that overload

FLEXIBILITY — Stretch farther or longer

STRENGTH — Increase weight loads

ENDURANCE — Perform more repetitions

CARDIO-RESPIRATORY — Run farther

FIGURE 2.1
You can use the overload principle to increase your fitness level in each of the key training areas.

FIGURE 2.2
If you're starting a new exercise training program, you'll begin slowly and progress toward doing more exercise at a greater intensity until you reach your desired fitness level. Then, you'll develop a maintenance program to sustain your new level of fitness.

Source: From Pollack, Wilmore, and Fox, *Health and Fitness through Physical Activity.* Copyright © 1978. Reprinted by permission of Pearson Education, Inc.

should be increased gradually during the course of a physical fitness program. For example, Becky, a sedentary college-aged student who is slightly overweight, might begin her new fitness program with a daily 10-minute walk/jog, then move up to an 11-minute walk/jog in week 2, and by week 5, do a 16-minute jog.

The overload of a training program should generally be increased slowly during the first 4 to 6 weeks of the exercise program. After this initial period, the overload can be increased at a steady but progressive rate during the next 18–20 weeks of training. For best results, the overload should not be increased too slowly or too rapidly. Progressing too slowly may not result in the desired improvement in physical fitness, and progressing too quickly may cause chronic fatigue or injuries.

What is a safe rate of progression during an exercise training program? Although people vary in their tolerance for exercise overload, a commonsense guideline to improve physical fitness and avoid overuse injuries is the **ten percent rule** (2). In short, this rule says that the training intensity or duration of exercise should be increased by no more than 10% per week. For example, a runner running 20 minutes per day

could increase his or her daily exercise duration to 22 minutes per day (10% of 20 = 2) the following week.

Once you reach your desired level of physical fitness, you no longer need to increase the training intensity or duration of your physical conditioning. You should instead focus on designing a **maintenance program** to maintain your new fitness level with regular exercise (Figure 2.2).

Specificity of Exercise

Another key concept of training is the **principle of specificity,** which states that the exercise training effect is specific to those muscles involved in the activity (3). If you perform leg curls, for example, you wouldn't expect your upper arms to benefit, and likewise, your

overload principle A basic principle of physical conditioning that states that in order to improve physical fitness, the body or specific muscles must be stressed.

principle of progression A principle of training that states that overload should be increased gradually.

ten percent rule The training intensity or duration of exercise should not be increased by more than 10% per week.

maintenance program Exercising to sustain a desired level of physical fitness.

principle of specificity The effect of exercise training is specific to those muscles involved in the activity.

BUYING THE BEST RUNNING SHOE FOR YOU

Choosing the correct running or exercise shoe is an important decision. All runners need flexible, durable shoes that protect the foot. Moreover, good running shoes should absorb shock and control foot motion. In selecting running shoes, remember that there is no best running shoe for all people. Every individual is different, and each model of running shoe is different. Because of the complexity of individual foot shapes and biomechanics (i.e., running style), it usually is a good idea to buy running shoes at a specialty shoe store with a well-trained, expert staff that can help you find the best shoe to meet your exercise needs.

Here are some tips for choosing your optimal running shoe:

- Shop for shoes late in the day. The swelling your feet experience by the end of the day is similar to the swelling they experience during running (swelling is due to increased blood flow and fluid collection). Trying on shoes at the end of the day will help you find the best-fitting shoe.

- Wear the socks that you will wear when running. This will also help you find the best-fitting shoes.

- Bring an old pair of running shoes with you to the store so that the running shoe expert can see where your shoes wear the most. The salesperson will use this information to recommend the types of running shoes that you should consider.

Here are some tips on how to make sure the shoe fits:

- Make sure that there is a full thumb length between the end of your longest toe and the end of the shoe. This ensures that the shoe is long enough for your foot.

- Make sure the front section of the shoe (the "toe box") allows the toes to move around.

- The shoe should not feel too tight, but the foot should not slide around in the shoe.

- Many running shoe specialty stores will have a treadmill so you can try walking or running in the shoes you're thinking of buying. If your shoe store has a treadmill, use it. This will help you see the shoes in action.

- Do not rely on a break-in period for your shoes to stretch—running shoes should feel good on the day you buy them.

- If in doubt about the correct size, buy the larger size.

Because running involves the use of the leg muscles, doing it regularly will improve the endurance of those muscles. This is an example of specificity of training.

biceps curls aren't going to improve your calf muscles. This is part of the reason why a varied set of exercises is so important to overall physical fitness improvement.

Specificity of training also applies to the types of adaptations that occur in the muscle. For example, strength training, such as with free weights, results in an increase in muscle strength but does not greatly improve the endurance of the muscle. Therefore, strength training is specific to improving muscular strength (4). Similarly, endurance exercise training, such as distance running, results in improved muscular endurance without altering muscular strength much (5). Suppose you want to improve your ability to run a distance of 3 miles. In this case, specific training should include running 3 or more miles several times a week. This type of training would improve muscular endurance in your legs but would not result in large improvements in leg strength (3).

Principle of Recuperation

Overloading your muscles means stressing them, and they need a period of rest before your next workout. During the recovery period, the body adapts to the exercise stress by increasing endurance or becoming

FIGURE 2.3
To avoid injury and maximize benefits, allow adequate rest periods between sessions in your exercise training program.

FIGURE 2.4
Stopping exercise training will reverse gains made in both muscular strength and muscular endurance.

stronger. In fact, a rest period, usually 24 hours or more, is essential for achieving maximal benefit from exercise. This needed rest period between exercise training sessions is called the **principle of recuperation** (2) (Figure 2.3).

Failure to get enough rest between sessions may result in a fatigue syndrome referred to as **overtraining.** Overtraining may lead to chronic fatigue and/or injuries. Common symptoms of overtraining include sore and stiff muscles or a feeling of general fatigue the morning after an exercise training session, sometimes called a "workout hangover." The cure is either to increase the duration of rest between workouts, to reduce the intensity of workouts, or both. Although too much exercise is the primary cause of the overtraining syndrome, an inadequate diet, particularly if it's short on carbohydrates, can also contribute (we will cover more about the effects of good nutrition on exercise in Chapter 7).

CONSIDER THIS!
Among people who start an exercise program, 50% will drop out within 6 months.

How quickly is fitness lost after training has stopped? The answer depends on which component of physical fitness you are referring to. For example, if you stop strength training, you will lose muscular strength relatively slowly (4, 7). In contrast, after you stop performing endurance exercise, you will lose muscular endurance relatively rapidly (6) (Figure 2.4). Note that 8 weeks after strength training is stopped, only 10% of muscular strength is lost (7). In contrast, 8 weeks after cessation of endurance training, 30–40% of muscular endurance is lost (6).

Reversibility of Training Effects

Although rest periods are important to maximizing your benefits from exercise, going too long between exercise sessions (such as days or weeks), or being too inconsistent in your routine, can result in losing the progress you've made (6). To maintain physical fitness, you need to exercise regularly. In other words, physical fitness cannot be stored. The loss of fitness due to inactivity is an example of the **principle of reversibility.**

---

principle of recuperation The body requires recovery periods between exercise training sessions to adapt to the exercise stress. Therefore, a period of rest is essential for achieving maximal benefit from exercise.

overtraining The result of failure to get enough rest between exercise training sessions.

principle of reversibility The loss of fitness due to inactivity.

A CLOSER LOOK TOO MUCH EXERCISE INCREASES YOUR RISK OF ILLNESS

Research indicates that intense exercise training (or overtraining) reduces the body's immunity to disease (14). In contrast, light to moderate exercise training boosts the immune system and reduces the risk of infections (15). The relationship between exercise training and the risk of developing an upper respiratory tract infection (e.g., a cold) is shown in the figure in this box. The J-shaped curve indicates that moderate exercise training reduces the risk of infection, whereas high-intensity and long-duration exercise training increase the risk of infection.

The explanation for this relationship is complex, but it appears that too much exercise increases levels of stress hormones in the body that weaken the immune system. Depressed immune function increases your risk for developing an infection when you are exposed to bacteria or viruses.

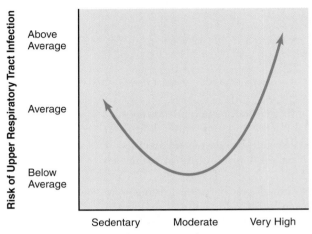

This J-shaped curve illustrates the relationship between physical activity and colds. Note that moderate physical activity reduces your risk of infection, whereas long-duration or high-intensity exercise increases your risk of disease.

Source: Redrawn from Nieman, D. Moderate exercise boosts the immune system: Too much exercise can have the opposite effect. *ACSM's Health and Fitness Journal* 1(5):14–18, 1997. Reprinted by permission of Lippincott Williams & Wilkins, http://lww.com.

Make sure you know . . .

> Five key principles of exercise training are overload principle, principle of progression, specificity of exercise, principle of recuperation, and reversibility of training effects.

> The overload principle states that to improve physical fitness, the body or the specific muscle group used during exercise must be stressed.

> The principle of progression is an extension of the overload principle and states that overload should be increased gradually over the course of a physical fitness training program.

> The principle of specificity refers to the fact that exercise training is specific to those muscles involved in the activity.

> The requirement for a rest period between training sessions is called the principle of recuperation.

> The principle of reversibility refers to loss of physical fitness due to inactivity.

Designing Your Exercise Program

If you go to a doctor with a bacterial infection and she prescribes you an antibiotic as treatment, chances are good that the dose she asks you to take is going to be different from the dose she might prescribe for your 10-year-old brother. Similarly, for each individual there is a correct "dose" of exercise to effectively promote physical fitness, called an **exercise prescription** (6). Exercise prescriptions should be tailored to meet the needs of the individual (3, 6, 9). They should include fitness goals, mode of exercise (or type of activity), a warm-up, a primary conditioning period, and a cool-down. The following sections provide a general introduction to each of these components.

Setting Goals

If you don't know what you're working toward, you are not likely to achieve it. Thus, setting goals (both short-term and long-term goals) is an essential part of an exercise prescription. Visualizing your leaner, stronger body or your improved competitive performance (if these were your goals, for example) would help motivate you to begin your exercise program. Further, attaining your fitness goals improves self-esteem and provides the incentive needed to make a lifetime commitment to regular exercise.

One common type of fitness goal is a performance goal. You can establish performance goals in each component of health-related physical fitness. Figure 2.5 illustrates a hypothetical example of how Susie Jones might establish short-term and long-term performance goals using fitness testing to determine when she has reached her objective. The column labeled "current status" contains Susie's fitness ratings based on tests performed prior to starting her exercise program. After consulting with her instructor, Susie has established short-term goals that she hopes to achieve within the first 8 weeks of training. Note that the short-term goals are not "fixed in stone" and can be modified if the need arises. Susie's long-term goals are fitness levels that she hopes to reach within the first 18 months of training. Similar to short-term goals, long-term goals can be modified to meet changing needs or circumstances.

In addition to performance goals, consider establishing exercise adherence goals. That is, set a goal to exercise a specific number of days per week. Exercise adherence goals are important because fitness will improve only if you exercise regularly!

The following guidelines can help you set achievable fitness goals:

- *Be realistic.* This is perhaps the most important rule in goal setting—set goals that you can reach. Consider your current fitness level, consult with your instructor, and write down goals you know you can achieve. Setting goals that are unachievable is likely to frustrate you and may result in your giving up on your program.
- *Establish short-term goals first.* Reaching short-term fitness goals will motivate you to continue exercising. Therefore, establishing realistic short-term goals is critical. After you reach a short-term goal, pat yourself on the back, and then establish a new one.
- *Set realistic long-term goals.* When setting your long-term goals, take into account your physical limitations and any hereditary factors that may affect your fitness limits. Set goals that are realistic for you and not based on performance scores of other people.

FIGURE 2.5
As you begin thinking about your short-term and long-term goals for each of the five fitness components, fill out a worksheet like this so you can track your progress.

Name: Susie Jones			
FITNESS GOALS			
FITNESS CATEGORY	CURRENT STATUS	SHORT-TERM GOAL (8 weeks)	LONG-TERM GOAL (18 months)
Cardiorespiratory fitness	Poor	Average	Excellent
Muscular strength	Poor	Average	Excellent
Muscular endurance	Very poor	Average	Good
Flexibility	Poor	Average	Good
Body composition	High fat	Moderately high	Optimal

- *Establish lifetime maintenance goals.* In addition to short-term and long-term goals, consider establishing a fitness maintenance goal. The purpose of this goal will be to maintain your new fitness level by remaining physically active.
- *Put goals in writing.* A key to meeting goals (and to not forgetting them) is to write them down and post them where you will see them every day. You should revisit and revise your goals periodically as your routine or schedule changes so that they continue to be realistic and up-to-date. Remember, just because goals are in writing does not mean that they cannot be changed.

exercise prescription The individualized amount of exercise that will effectively promote physical fitness for a given person.

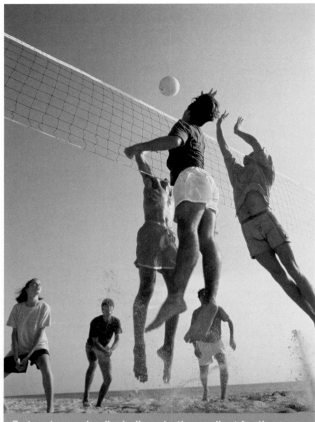

Swimming and volleyball are both excellent for the cardiovascular system. Swimming puts less stress on the joints and is considered a low-impact activity, whereas volleyball puts more stress on joints and is considered a high-impact activity.

- *Make your goals specific and measurable.* You need a way to determine whether you met your goal. Be sure to avoid unfocused goals, such as, "I want to lose weight by spring break. To lose weight I will eat healthy and exercise regularly." Establish focused goals instead: "I want to lose 15 pounds by spring break. I will exercise 3 times a week for at least 20 minutes and follow the healthy eating plan outlined by my dietitian. With these changes I should lose 1.5 pounds a week for 10 weeks."
- *Establish a time frame.* Setting a date for reaching the goal will help you stay focused.
- *Use a reward system.* Reaching a goal is an accomplishment that you should acknowledge with a reward that is meaningful to you.
- *Recognize obstacles to achieving goals.* Once you begin your fitness program, be prepared for setbacks (such as skipping workouts and losing motivation) and to backslide a bit (and have your fitness level decline temporarily). This is normal. How-

ever, once you realize that you have stopped making progress toward your goals, you must get back on track and start making progress again as soon as you can.

The importance of fitness goals cannot be overemphasized. Goals provide structure and motivation for a personal fitness program. Keys to maintaining a lifelong fitness program are discussed again in Chapter 16.

Selecting Activities

Every exercise prescription includes at least one **mode of exercise**—that is, a specific type of exercise to be performed. For example, to improve cardiorespiratory fitness, you could select from a wide variety of activities, such as running, swimming, or cycling. To ensure that you'll engage in the exercise regularly, you should choose activities that you will enjoy doing, that are available to you, and that carry little risk of injury.

Physical activities can be classified as being either high impact or low impact, based on the amount of stress placed on joints during the activity. Low-impact activities put less stress on the joints than high-impact activities. Because of the strong correlation between high-impact activities and injuries, many fitness experts recommend low-impact activities for fitness beginners or for people susceptible to injury (such as people who are older or overweight). Examples of low-impact activities include walking, cycling, swimming, and low-impact aerobic dance. High-impact activities include running, basketball, and high-impact aerobic dance.

The Importance of a Warm-Up

A **warm-up** is a brief (5- to 15-minute) period of exercise that precedes a workout. It generally involves light calisthenics or a low-intensity form of the exercise and

An Example of the FIT Principle	
Frequency	3–5 times per week
Intensity	Moderate
Time (Duration)	30 minutes

often includes stretching exercises. The purpose of a warm-up is to elevate muscle temperature and increase blood flow to those muscles that will be engaged in the workout (1). A warm-up can also reduce the strain on the heart imposed by rapidly engaging in heavy exercise and may reduce the risk of muscle and tendon injuries. You can find specific some warm up exercises in Laboratory 2.1.

THE WORKOUT

Regardless of the activity, the major components of the exercise prescription that make up the workout (also called the primary conditioning period) are frequency, intensity, and duration (time) of exercise (see box above), often called the *FIT principle*. The **frequency of exercise** is the number of times per week that you intend to exercise. The recommended frequency of exercise to improve most components of health-related physical fitness is 3 to 5 times per week (10–12).

The **intensity of exercise** is the amount of physiological stress or overload placed on the body during the exercise. The method for determining the intensity of exercise varies with the type of exercise performed. For example, as you use more energy during exercise, your heart rate will increase, so measuring heart rate has become a standard means to determine exercise intensity during cardiorespiratory fitness training.

Whereas heart rate can also be used to gauge exercise intensity during strength training, the number of repetitions performed before muscular fatigue occurs is more useful for monitoring intensity during weight lifting. For instance, a load that can be lifted only 5 to 8 times before complete muscular fatigue is an example of high-intensity weight lifting. In contrast, a load that can be lifted 50 to 60 times without resulting in muscular fatigue is an illustration of low-intensity weight training.

Finally, flexibility is improved by stretching muscles beyond their normal lengths. Intensity of stretching is monitored by the degree of tension felt during the stretch. Low-intensity stretching results in only minor tension on the muscles and tendons. In contrast, high-intensity stretching places great tension or moderate discomfort on the muscle groups being stretched.

A key aspect of the primary conditioning period is the **duration of exercise**—that is, the amount of time invested in performing the primary workout. Note that the duration of exercise does not include the warm-up or cool-down. Research has shown that 30 minutes per exercise session (performed 3 or more times per week) is the minimum amount of time required to significantly improve physical fitness. Figure 2.6 shows a physical activity pyramid that can help you identify types of physical activities that increase your fitness level, and how frequently you should perform them.

The Importance of the Cool-Down

The **cool-down** is a 5- to 15-minute period of low-intensity exercise that immediately follows the primary conditioning period. For instance, a period of slow walking might be used as a cool-down following a running workout. A cool-down period accomplishes several goals. In addition to lowering body temperature after exercise, the cool-down allows blood to return from the muscles toward the heart (3–6). During exercise, large amounts of blood are pumped to the working muscles. Once exercise stops, blood tends to pool in large blood vessels located around the exercised muscles. Failure to redistribute pooled blood after exercise could result in your feeling lightheaded or even fainting. You can prevent blood pooling by doing low-intensity exercise that uses the same muscles you used during the workout.

Personalizing Your Workout

Although the same general principles of exercise training apply to everyone, no two people are the same, and everyone's exercise prescription will be slightly different. Your exercise prescription should be based on your

mode of exercise The specific type of exercise to be performed.

warm-up A brief (5- to 15-minute) period of exercise that precedes a workout.

frequency of exercise The number of times per week that one exercises.

intensity of exercise The amount of physiological stress or overload placed on the body during exercise.

duration of exercise The amount of time invested in performing the primary workout.

cool-down A 5- to 15-minute period of low-intensity exercise that immediately follows the primary conditioning period; sometimes called a *warm-down*.

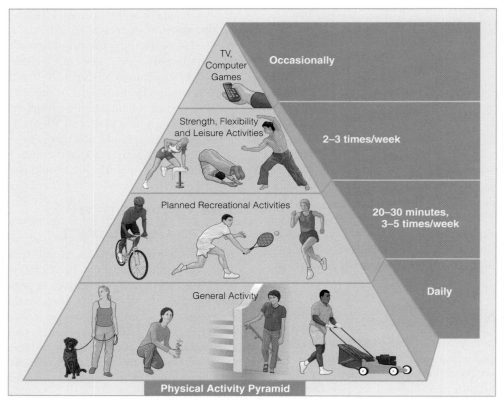

FIGURE 2.6
A physical activity pyramid like this one shows examples of activities you can incorporate into your fitness program and can help guide the frequency and time you plan for each activity.

Source: Corbin, C. B., and R. D. Pangrazi. Physical activity pyramid rebuffs peak experience. *ACSM's Health and Fitness Journal* 2(1), 1998. Copyright © 1998. Used with permission.

general health, age, fitness status, musculoskeletal condition, and body composition. You will learn more about individualizing workouts in the next several chapters.

Make sure you know . . .

> The "dose" of exercise required to effectively promote physical fitness is called the exercise prescription.

> The components of the exercise prescription include fitness goals, mode of exercise, the warm-up, the workout, and the cool-down. You can use the FIT principle (frequency, intensity, and duration or time of exercise) to help you design your fitness program.

> Exercise training programs should be individualized by considering such factors as age, health, and fitness status of the individual.

Health Benefits of Exercise: How Much Is Enough?

As discussed in Chapter 1, exercise training to improve sport performance differs from exercise performed to achieve health benefits. Exercise training for sport performance typically includes long workouts (60–180 minutes/day) involving high-intensity exercise. In contrast, exercising to obtain health benefits does not need to be as high in intensity, or performed as long, as exercise to improve performance.

Although even low levels of physical activity can provide some health benefits, evidence indicates that moderate-to-high levels of physical activity are required to provide major health benefits (10, 12–14, 16, 19, 20). The theoretical relationship between physical activity and health benefits is illustrated in Figure 2.7. Note that the minimum level of exercise required to achieve some of the health benefits is the **threshold for health benefits.** Most experts believe that 30–60

STEPS FOR
BEHAVIOR
CHANGE

Are you a couch potato?

Answer the following questions to find out whether you could use more daily physical activity.

Y   N

☐ ☐   Do you usually drive to your destinations, even for short trips to the corner store?

☐ ☐   Do you tend to take the elevator instead of the stairs?

☐ ☐   Does your evening routine involve hours of inactivity (e.g., sitting in front of the computer or television)?

☐ ☐   When you drive to a store for shopping, do you tend to park as close to the store entrance as possible?

☐ ☐   Do you always use a remote control to adjust the volume on your stereo or change the channel on your television?

If you answered "yes" to more than one question, you may be a bit too sedentary.

TIPS TO INCORPORATE MORE PHYSICAL ACTIVITY INTO YOUR DAILY ROUTINE

☑   Walk or ride your bike for short trips and errands; walk to class if you live close to or on campus.

☑   Get off the bus a stop early, and walk the rest of the way.

☑   Forgo an hour of Internet time every day to walk the dog, or play a round of basketball or tennis with a friend.

☑   Take the stairs instead of the elevator.

☑   Instead of settling in with the television after dinner, go for a bike ride with a friend or family member.

FIGURE 2.7

The relationship between physical activity and improved health benefits. Note that as the level of regular physical activity increases, the theoretical risk of disease (or death) decreases.

Source: Data are from References 17–19.

minutes of moderate-to-high-intensity exercise performed 3–5 days per week will surpass the threshold for health benefits and will reduce risk of all causes of death (19–22, 24–26). (See Laboratory 2.3 for one way to determine whether you're engaging in enough physical activity to achieve health benefits—counting your steps with a pedometer.)

The U.S. government has recently issued new physical activity guidelines for Americans. These guidelines recommend that adults aged 18–64 perform at least 150 minutes of moderate-intensity exercise or 75 minutes of vigorous-intensity aerobic physical activity per week (28). Fortunately, the activity doesn't need to be done all at once and can be divided into two to three segments of exercise throughout the day (22–29). If you walk briskly for 15 minutes to

threshold for health benefits The minimum level of physical activity required to achieve some of the health benefits of exercise.

get to your class in the morning and then take a 15-minute bike ride to get to your job in the afternoon, you've attained the goal of incorporating 30 minutes of moderate exercise into your day.

However, this dose of exercise may be insufficient to prevent weight gain in some individuals who need additional exercise and calorie restriction to prevent weight gain (see Chapter 8 for more details). Further, people who get 30 minutes of moderate-intensity exercise per day are likely to achieve additional health benefits if they exercise for longer periods of time (24, 28).

Are some forms of exercise better than others for obtaining health benefits? There is no short answer to this question. Nonetheless, numerous activities, including running, swimming, cycling, and walking, can help achieve exercise-related health benefits. Details on how to achieve health-related aspects of physical fitness will be discussed in Chapters 4 through 6.

Make sure you know . . .

> Although low levels of physical activity can provide some health benefits, moderate-to-high levels of physical activity are required to provide major health benefits.

> The threshold for health benefits is the minimum level of exercise required to achieve some health benefits of exercise.

Summary

1. The overload principle, which is the most important principle of exercise training, states that to improve physical fitness, the body or muscle group used during exercise must be stressed.

2. The principle of progression states that overload should be increased gradually during the course of a physical fitness program.

3. The need for a rest period between exercise training sessions is called the principle of recuperation.

4. Physical fitness can be lost due to inactivity; this is often called the principle of reversibility.

5. The components of the exercise prescription include fitness goals, type of activity, the warm-up, the workout, and the cool-down.

6. All exercise training programs should be tailored to meet the objectives of the individual. Therefore, the exercise prescription should consider the individual's age, health, fitness status, musculoskeletal condition, and body composition.

7. The minimum level of physical activity required to achieve some of the health benefits of exercise is called the threshold for health benefits.

Study Questions

1. Which one of the following is NOT a key principle of exercise training?
   a. overload principle
   b. principle of progression
   c. principle of recuperation
   d. principle of supercompensation

2. The current public health recommendation is for adults to achieve a minimum of _____ minutes of moderate-intensity physical activity each day.
   a. 15
   b. 20
   c. 30
   d. 60

3. A primary purpose of a warm-up is to
   a. elevate muscle temperature and increase blood flow to the active muscles.
   b. remove lactic acid from the blood.
   c. reduce the level of stress hormones in the blood.
   d. none of the above.

4. What is the difference between overtraining and the principle of recuperation?

5. What are the general purposes of a cool-down and a warm-up?

6. What are the components of the exercise prescription?

7. How does the principle of progression apply to the exercise prescription?

8. What is the overload principle, and what is one practical example?

9. Why is the threshold for health benefits an important concept?

10. What happens to physical fitness if you stop training?

11. Why should the exercise prescription be individualized?

12. Why is goal setting important when beginning an exercise program?

Suggested Reading

Blair, S. N. Physical inactivity: The biggest public health problem of the 21st century. *British Journal of Sports Medicine* 43:1–2, 2009.

Humphrey, R. Activity and fitness in health risk. *ACSM's Health and Fitness Journal* 11:36–37, 2007.

Murphy, M. H., S. N. Blair, and E. M. Murtagh. Accumulated versus continuous exercise for health benefit: A review of empirical studies. *Sports Medicine* 39:29–43, 2009.

Powers, S., and E. Howley. *Exercise Physiology: Theory and Application to Fitness and Performance,* 7th ed. New York: McGraw-Hill, 2009.

Swain, D. Moderate or vigorous-intensity exercise: What should we prescribe? *ACSM's Health and Fitness Journal* 10:42–43, 2006.

U.S. Department of Human Services. *2008 Physical Activity Guidelines for Americans.* 2008. www.health.gov/paguidelines.

Warburton, D., C. Nicol, and S. Bredin. Prescribing exercise as preventative therapy. *Canadian Medical Association Journal* 28:961–974, 2006.

For links to the organizations and websites listed below, visit The Total Fitness and Wellness Website at www.pearsonhighered.com/powers.

American Heart Association

Contains the latest information about ways to reduce your risk of heart and vascular diseases. Includes information about exercise, diet, and heart disease.

American College of Sports Medicine

Contains information about exercise, health, and fitness.

WebMD

Contains the latest information on a variety of health-related topics, including diet, exercise, and stress. Includes links to nutrition, fitness, and wellness topics.

Medline Plus

Contains up-to-date information on a variety of health-related issues including exercise and physical fitness.

References

1. Howley, E., and B. D. Franks. *Health Fitness: Instructors Handbook.* Champaign, IL: Human Kinetics, 2003.

2. Powers, S., and E. Howley. *Exercise Physiology: Theory and Application to Fitness and Performance,* 6th ed. St. Louis, MO: McGraw-Hill, 2007.

3. Stone, M., S. Plisk, and D. Collins. Training principles: Evaluation of modes and methods of resistance training—A coaching perspective. *Sports Biomechanics* 1:79–103, 2002.

4. Abernethy, P., J. Jurimae, P. Logan, A. Taylor, and R. Thayer. Acute and chronic response of skeletal muscle to resistance exercise. *Sports Medicine* 17:22–28, 1994.

5. Powers, S., D. Criswell, J. Lawler, L. Ji, D. Martin, R. Herb, and G. Dudley. Influence of exercise and fiber type on antioxidant enzyme activity in rat skeletal muscle. *American Journal of Physiology* 266:R375–R380, 1994.

6. Coyle, E., W. Martin, D. Sinacore, M. Joyner, J. Hagberg, and J. Holloszy. Time course of loss of adaptations after stopping prolonged intense endurance training. *Journal of Applied Physiology* 57:1857–1864, 1984.

7. Costill, D., and A. Richardson. *Handbook of Sports Medicine: Swimming.* London: Blackwell Publishing, 1993.

8. Lamb, D., and M. Williams. *Ergogenics: Enhancement of Performance in Exercise and Sport.* Vol. 4. Madison, WI: Brown and Benchmark, 1991.

9. McGlynn, G. *Dynamics of Fitness: A Practical Approach.* Dubuque, IA: Wm. C. Brown, 1996.

10. Bouchard, C., R. Shephard, T. Stephens, J. Sutton, and B. McPherson, eds. *Exercise, Fitness, and Health: A Consensus of Current Knowledge.* Champaign, IL: Human Kinetics, 1990.

11. Barrow, M. *Heart Talk: Understanding Cardiovascular Diseases.* Gainesville, FL: Cor-Ed Publishing, 1992.

12. Morris, J. Exercise in the prevention of coronary heart disease: Today's best buy in public health. *Medicine and Science in Sports and Exercise* 26:807–814, 1994.

13. Warburton, D., C. Nicol, and S. Bredin. Prescribing exercise as preventative therapy. *Canadian Medical Association Journal* 28:961–974, 2006.

14. Nieman, D. Immune response to heavy exertion. *Journal of Applied Physiology* 82:1385–1394, 1997.

15. Nieman, D. Moderate exercise boosts the immune system: Too much exercise can have the opposite effect. *ACSM's Health and Fitness Journal* 1(5):14–18, 1997.

16. Paffenbarger, R., J. Kampert, I-Min Lee, R. Hyde, R. Leung, and A. Wing. Changes in physical activity and other lifeway patterns influencing longevity. *Medicine and Science in Sports and Exercise* 26:857–865, 1994.

17. Blair, S., H. W. Kohl, N. Gordon, and R. Paffenbarger. How much physical activity is good for health? *Annual Review of Public Health* 13:99–126, 1992.

18. Lee, I., and R. Paffenbarger. Associations of light, moderate, and vigorous intensity physical activity with longevity. *American Journal of Epidemiology* 151:293–299, 2000.

19. Williams, P. Physical fitness and activity as separate heart disease risk factors: A meta-analysis. *Medicine and Science in Sports and Exercise* 33:754–761, 2001.

20. Pollock, M., G. Gaesser, J. Butcher, J. P. Despres, R. Dishman, B. Franklin, and C. Garber. The recommended quantity and quality of exercise for developing and maintaining cardiorespiratory fitness, muscular fitness, and flexibility in healthy adults. *Medicine and Science in Sports and Exercise* 30:975–991, 1998.

21. Howley, E. T. You asked for it: Is rigorous exercise better than moderate activity in achieving health-related goals? *ACSM's Health and Fitness Journal* 4(2):6, 2000.

22. Thompson, P. et al. Exercise and physical activity in the prevention and treatment of atherosclerotic cardiovascular disease. *Circulation* 107:3109–3116, 2003.

23. Swain, D. Moderate or vigorous intensity exercise: What should we prescribe? *ACSM's Health and Fitness Journal* 10:21–27, 2006.

24. Blair, S., M. LaMonte, and M. Nichman. The evolution of physical activity recommendations: How much exercise is enough? *American Journal of Clinical Nutrition* 79: 913S–920S, 2004.

25. Brooks, G., N. Butte, W. Rand, J.P. Flatt, and B. Caballero. Chronicle of the institute of medicine physical activity recommendation: How a physical activity recommendation came to be among dietary recommendations. *American Journal of Clinical Nutrition* 79:921S–930S, 2004.

26. Brown, D., D. Brown, G. Heath, L. Balluz, W. Giles, E. Ford, and A. Mokdad. Associations between physical activity dose and health-related quality of life. *Medicine and Science in Sports and Exercise* 36:890–896, 2004.

27. Ishikawa-Takata, K., T. Ohta, and H. Tanaka. How much exercise is required to reduce blood pressure in essential hypertensive: A dose-response study. *American Journal of Hypertension* 16:629–633, 2003.

28. U.S. Department of Human Services. *2008 Physical activity guidelines for Americans.* 2008. www.health.gov/paguidelines.

29. Blair, S.N. Physical inactivity: The biggest public health problem of the 21st century. *British Journal of Sports Medicine* 43:1–2, 2009.

Videos

Log on to www.pearsonhighered.com/powers to view these chapter-related videos.

Personal Fitness and Exercise

Calf Stretch

Hamstrings Stretch (Seated)

Low Back Knee-to-Chest Stretch

Side Stretch

NAME _____ DATE _____

Warming Up

Use the following activities to warm up your body for aerobic activities such as jogging, walking, or cycling. Perform the exercises slowly, holding each stretch for 20 to 30 seconds. Do not bounce or jerk the muscle. Do each stretch at least once and up to three times.

(▷) Log on to **www.pearsonhighered.com/powers** to view demonstration videos of these stretches.

Cardiovascular Warm-Up

Walk briskly or jog slowly for 5 minutes.

Stretches

Calf Stretch for Gastrocnemius and Soleus

Stand with your right foot about 1 to 2 feet in front of your left foot, with both feet pointing forward. Keeping your left leg straight, lunge forward by bending your right knee and pushing your left heel backward. Hold this position. Then pull your left foot in slightly and bend your left knee. Shift your weight to your left leg and hold. Repeat this entire sequence with the left leg forward.

Sitting Toe Touch for Hamstrings

Sit on the ground with your right leg straight and your left leg tucked close to your body. Reach toward your outstretched right foot as far as possible with both hands. Repeat with the left leg.

Step Stretch for Quadriceps and Hip

Step forward and bend your front knee about 90 degrees, keeping your knee directly above your ankle. Stretch the opposite leg back so that it is parallel to the floor. Rotate your hips forward and slightly down to stretch. Your arms can be at your sides or resting on top of your forward thigh. Repeat on the other side.

Leg Hug for the Hip and Back Extensors

Lie flat on your back with both legs straight. Bending your knees, bring your legs up to your torso, and grasp both legs behind the thighs. Pull both legs in to your chest and hold.

Side Stretch for the Torso

Stand with feet shoulder-width apart, knees slightly bent, and pelvis tucked under. Raise one arm over your head, and bend sideways from the waist. Support your torso by placing the hand of your resting arm on your hip or thigh for support. Repeat on the other side.

You can also repeat these same exercises after a workout to cool down.

1. Did you notice an increase in heart rate during the cardiovascular warm-up? _____

2. In which stretch did you feel the most tightness? _____

3. Do you think the sample warm-up is adequate for the activities you plan to do as part of your exercise program? If not, what exercises would you add?

   _____

   _____

NAME _____ DATE _____

Which Physical Activities Work Best for You?

As you design your personal fitness program, think about the activities you currently enjoy most and least and about new activities you would like to try. Which can you incorporate into your program?

Answer the following questions in the spaces provided.

1. List the fitness/wellness activities in which you have participated or are currently participating. Examples include recreational tennis, high school basketball, or yoga classes.

   _____

2. Which of these activities did you enjoy the most? Why?

   _____

3. What are some new activities you might enjoy? (See the list at the end of the lab for additional options.)

   _____

   _____

4. What components of physical fitness do you think these activities affect? For instance, jogging improves cardiovascular fitness, whereas weight lifting increases muscular strength.

   _____

   _____

5. What areas of physical and mental health would you like to improve? Can you think of any physical activities that would aid in this goal?

   _____

   _____

Examples of Exercise and Physical Activity

- Walking or jogging on a treadmill
- Walking to work instead of driving
- Cycling on an upright or recumbent exercise bike
- Cycling to work instead of driving
- Outdoor walking or jogging
- Outdoor cycling
- Aerobics class
- Kickboxing class
- Weight or resistance training
- Yoga
- Martial arts
- Pilates
- Hiking
- Rock climbing
- Elliptical trainer
- Sport activities (e.g., soccer, basketball, tennis, racquetball)

NAME _____ DATE _____

Using a Pedometer to Count Your Steps

One way to determine your level of daily physical activity is to use a pedometer to measure the number of steps you take in a day. A pedometer is a small portable device that contains a sensor and, often, software applications to estimate the distance walked and the number of calories expended. The accuracy of pedometers can vary from device to device, but many pedometers are reasonably accurate if they are worn in the optimal position (such as on a belt clip). However, carrying a pedometer in a pocket or handbag tends to reduce its accuracy. Moreover, some pedometers record movement other than walking (e.g., bending to tie your shoes), and therefore some "false steps" may show up on your daily step count.

Experts currently recommend 10,000 steps per day to reach a level of physical activity that is considered to be an active lifestyle with positive health benefits. Do you think you meet this goal?

A pedometer worn at the waist.

Directions:

Wear a pedometer for a day and note your number of steps. Write in the total number below. Then, set a goal for the number of steps you want to take per day, and list some strategies for incorporating more steps into your day. Track the number of steps you take every day for the next 2 weeks, and note your progress toward your goal.

Number of steps for day 1: _____

Number of steps for day 2: _____

Number of steps for day 3: _____

Number of steps for day 4: _____

Number of steps for day 5: _____

Number of steps for day 6: _____

Number of steps for day 7: _____

Number of steps for day 8: _____

Number of steps for day 9: _____

Number of steps for day 10: _____

Number of steps for day 11: _____

Number of steps for day 12: _____

Number of steps for day 13: _____

Number of steps for day 14: _____

Goal number of steps/day: _____

Analysis

1. Did you meet your goal for number of daily steps on most days?   Yes/No

2. Are you walking at least the recommended 10,000 steps per day? Yes/No

3. If not, think about how you can incorporate more steps into your daily routine. List below four ways to increase the amount of walking you do daily:

_____

_____

_____

_____

Cardio-respiratory Endurance: Assessment and Prescription

3

true or false?

1. Performing aerobic exercise is the best way to improve your cardiorespiratory endurance.

2. People with disabilities cannot do exercises to improve their cardiorespiratory endurance.

3. Including a warm-up and cool-down with your aerobic workout is very important.

4. Cross training can help reduce your risk for injury.

5. All people beginning a cardiorespiratory fitness program should start with the same program.

Answers appear on the next page.

Are there any hills on your campus? Have you ever trudged up one of them, only to be winded and out of breath by the time you got to the top? Do you notice that some of your fellow students, and probably many of your professors, can perform the activity without exertion? If you answered yes to these questions, you are already familiar with the concept of cardiorespiratory endurance. The low cardiorespiratory endurance that often accompanies a lack of regular exercise can make even common everyday tasks difficult. In this chapter, we will explore the basics of cardiorespiratory endurance and the types of exercise that will improve it.

In Chapters 1 and 2, we discussed the health benefits of exercise and the general principles of exercise training. In this and the next three chapters, we describe how to assess your level of each health-related fitness component and how to design a comprehensive, scientifically based exercise program to meet your health and fitness goals. Before we discuss the assessment and prescription for cardiovascular fitness, we need to define cardiorespiratory endurance and to cover some basic cardiovascular physiology.

The Need for Cardiorespiratory Endurance in Daily Living

Developing cardiorespiratory endurance is beneficial for a number of everyday activities. Walking around your campus to get to class or the library requires cardiorespiratory fitness. Other everyday activities, such as cleaning your dorm room or apartment, or yard work if you live in a house, are easier when you have a higher level of cardiorespiratory fitness. Your leisure time and social activities, such as a weekend hiking or camping trip with friends or a night out dancing, are more enjoyable with higher cardiorespiratory fitness.

What Are Cardiorespiratory Endurance and the Cardiovascular System?

Cardiorespiratory endurance is the ability to perform **aerobic exercises,** such as swimming, jogging and cycling, for a prolonged period of time, and is effective in promoting weight loss and reducing the risk of cardiovascular disease. Because of this, many exercise scientists consider cardiorespiratory endurance to be the most important component of health-related physical fitness (2, 3).

The most valid measurement of cardiorespiratory fitness is $\dot{V}O_2max,$ or maximal aerobic capacity, which is the maximum amount of oxygen the body can take in and use during exercise. In simple terms, $\dot{V}O_2max$ is a measure of the endurance of both the cardiorespiratory system and exercising skeletal muscles.

The cardiorespiratory system is made up of the cardiovascular system (the heart and blood vessels) and the respiratory system (the lungs and muscles involved in respiration). Together these systems deliver oxygen and nutrients throughout the body and remove waste products (e.g., carbon dioxide) from tissues. Exercise challenges the cardiorespiratory system because it in-

Cycling, whether outside or at the gym, is one popular type of exercise that will improve cardiorespiratory endurance.

creases the demand for oxygen and nutrients in the working muscles.

The Cardiovascular System

The heart is a pump, about the size of your fist, that contracts and generates pressure to move blood through the blood vessels throughout the body. Actually, the heart is considered two pumps in one. The right side pumps oxygen-depleted (deoxygenated) blood to the lungs in a pathway called the **pulmonary circuit,** and the left side pumps oxygen-rich (oxygenated) blood to tissues throughout the body through a pathway called the **systemic circuit.** Figure 3.1 illustrates the path of blood through the heart and lungs.

There are different types of blood vessels in the circulatory system. With the exception of the pulmonary artery (which carries oxygen-depleted blood from the heart to the lungs), **arteries** carry oxygen-rich blood away from the heart and to the rest of the body. Except for the pulmonary vein (which carries oxygen-rich blood from the lungs to the heart), **veins** carry oxygen-depleted blood from the body's tissues back to the heart.

Blood is pumped from the left side of the heart into the aorta, the largest artery in the body. From the aorta, arteries branch into smaller vessels called *arterioles*, which further branch into **capillaries.** The capillaries have walls that are one cell thick through which oxygen and nutrients can easily pass. Through capillaries, oxygen and nutrients are delivered to the tissues, and carbon dioxide and waste are picked up from the tissues and taken back to the heart. The capillaries branch into bigger vessels called *venules*, and then into veins. From the veins the blood enters the right side of the heart and is pumped to the lungs.

Every time your heart pumps (or beats), you can feel a pulse. People often measure the number of times their heart beats per minute (commonly called the

heart rate), to gauge their exercise intensity (more on this later in the chapter). When people say they are "taking their pulse," they are referring to their heart rate. The easiest places to take your heart rate are your radial and carotid arteries. The radial artery is located on the inside of your wrist just below your thumb, and the carotid artery can be found along the neck (Figure 3.2). The amount of blood that is pumped with each heartbeat is called **stroke volume.** The product of heart rate and stroke volume is **cardiac output,** which is the amount of blood that is pumped per minute.

The Respiratory System

The respiratory system controls our breathing. In the lungs, carbon dioxide and waste from the oxygen-depleted blood pass into tiny air sacs called **alveoli.** When we exhale, the carbon dioxide and waste are released into the air. Then, as we inhale, we bring oxygen into the lungs, where oxygen enters the alveoli and passes into the capillaries. From the lungs the oxygen-rich blood travels to the left side of the heart to start the process again.

Make sure you know...

> Cardiorespiratory endurance, which refers to how well you can perform aerobic exercises, is considered one of the most important health-related fitness components.

---

cardiorespiratory endurance The ability to perform aerobic exercises for a prolonged period of time.

aerobic exercise A common term to describe all forms of exercises that primarily use the aerobic energy system and that are designed to improve cardiorespiratory fitness.

VO2max The maximum amount of oxygen the body can take in and use during exercise.

pulmonary circuit The vascular system that circulates blood from the right side of the heart, through the lungs, and back to the left side of the heart.

systemic circuit The vascular system that circulates blood from the left side of the heart, throughout the body, and back to the right side of the heart.

arteries The blood vessels that carry blood away from the heart.

veins The blood vessels that transport blood toward the heart.

capillaries Thin-walled vessels that permit the exchange of gases (oxygen and carbon dioxide) and nutrients between the blood and tissues.

stroke volume The amount of blood pumped per heartbeat (generally expressed in milliliters).

cardiac output The amount of blood the heart pumps per minute.

alveoli Tiny air sacs in the lungs that receive carbon dioxide and other wastes from oxygen-depleted blood.

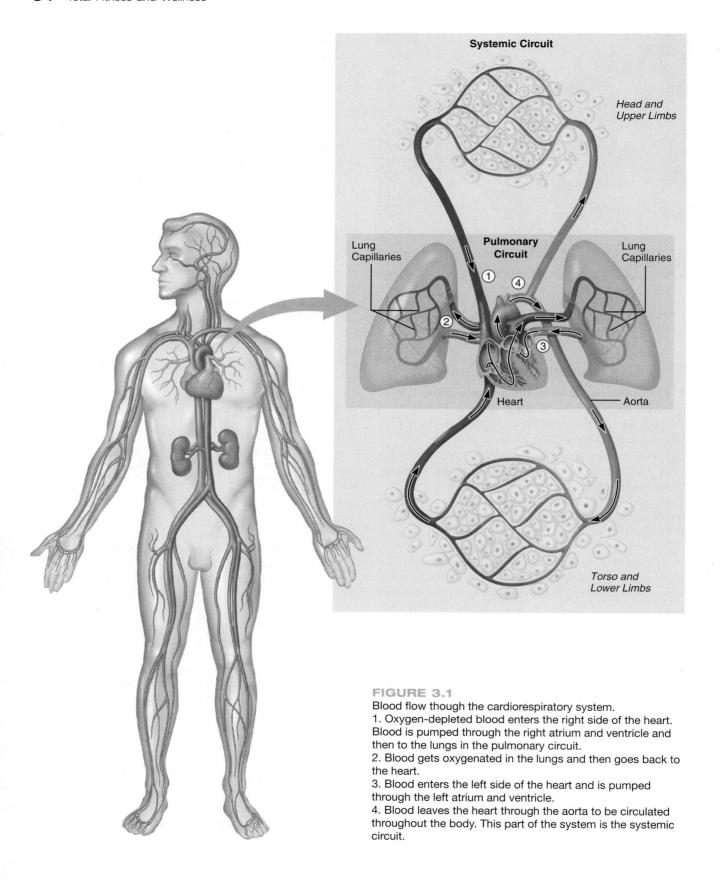

FIGURE 3.1

Blood flow though the cardiorespiratory system.
1. Oxygen-depleted blood enters the right side of the heart. Blood is pumped through the right atrium and ventricle and then to the lungs in the pulmonary circuit.
2. Blood gets oxygenated in the lungs and then goes back to the heart.
3. Blood enters the left side of the heart and is pumped through the left atrium and ventricle.
4. Blood leaves the heart through the aorta to be circulated throughout the body. This part of the system is the systemic circuit.

(a)   (b)

FIGURE 3.2

You can measure heart rate at either the radial artery in the wrist **(a)** or at the carotid artery in the neck **(b)**.

▷ Log on to **www.pearsonhighered.com/powers** to view demonstration videos of locating the radial and carotid pulses.

> $\dot{V}O_2max$ is a measure of cardiorespiratory endurance.

> The cardiorespiratory system consists of the cardiovascular and respiratory systems.

> The heart and blood vessels make up the cardiovascular system, and the lungs and muscles used for breathing make up the respiratory system.

> The pulmonary circuit pumps blood to the lungs, and the systemic circuit pumps blood throughout the body.

How Do We Get Energy for Exercise?

We have discussed the importance of getting oxygen to the muscles and having energy for prolonged exercise. But why is it important to get more oxygen to the muscles, and what do we mean by *energy*? Energy is the fuel needed to make the muscles move for activity, and we get that energy from the breakdown of food. However, food energy cannot be used directly by the muscles. Instead, the energy released from the breakdown of food is used to make a biochemical compound, called **adenosine triphosphate (ATP).** ATP is made and stored in small amounts in muscle and other cells. The breakdown of ATP releases energy that your muscles can use to contract and make you move. ATP is the only compound in the body that can provide this immediate source of energy. Therefore, for muscles to contract during exercise, a supply of ATP must be available.

The body uses two "systems" in muscle cells to produce ATP. One system does not require oxygen and is called the **anaerobic** ("without oxygen") system. The second system requires oxygen and is called the **aerobic** ("with oxygen") system. The aerobic system is the primary system for developing cardiorespiratory endurance, which is why we need to get oxygen to the muscles.

Anaerobic Energy Production

Most of the anaerobic ATP production in muscle occurs during **glycolysis,** the process that breaks down carbohydrates in cells. In addition to ATP production, glycolysis often results in the formation of **lactic acid.** Because of this lactic acid by-product, this pathway for ATP production is often called the *lactic acid system.* This system can use only carbohydrates as an energy source. Carbohydrates are supplied to muscles from blood sugar (glucose) and from muscle stores of glucose called *glycogen*.

The anaerobic energy pathway provides ATP at the beginning of exercise and for short-term (30–60 seconds) high-intensity exercise. Exercise that is intense and less than 2 minutes in duration, such as a 60- to 80-second 400-meter sprint, primarily relies on this system. During this type of intense exercise, muscles produce large amounts of lactic acid because the lactic acid system is operating at high speed.

Aerobic Energy Production

After about a minute of high-intensity exercise, anaerobic production of ATP begins to decrease, and aerobic production of ATP starts to increase. The aerobic system needs oxygen for the chemical reactions to make ATP. Activities of daily living and many types of exercise depend on ATP production from the aerobic system.

Whereas the anaerobic system uses only carbohydrates as a food source, aerobic metabolism can use fats, carbohydrates, and protein to produce ATP. However, for a healthy person who eats a balanced diet,

adenosine triphosphate (ATP) A high-energy compound that is synthesized and stored in small quantities in muscle and other cells. The breakdown of ATP results in a release of energy that can be used to fuel muscular contraction.

anaerobic "Without oxygen"; in cells, pertains to biochemical pathways that do not require oxygen to produce energy.

aerobic "With oxygen"; in cells, pertains to biochemical pathways that use oxygen to produce energy.

glycolysis A process during which carbohydrates are broken down in cells. Much of the anaerobic ATP production in muscle cells occurs during glycolysis.

lactic acid A by-product of glucose metabolism, produced primarily during intense exercise (i.e., greater than 50–60% of maximal aerobic capacity).

FIGURE 3.3
After about 60 minutes of exercise, the body begins to use more fat and fewer carbohydrates for ATP production.

proteins have a limited role during exercise—carbohydrates and fats are the primary sources. In general, at the beginning of exercise, carbohydrates are the main fuel broken down during aerobic ATP production. During prolonged exercise (i.e., longer than 20 minutes), there is a gradual shift from carbohydrates to fat as an energy source (Figure 3.3).

The Energy Continuum

Although we often speak of aerobic versus anaerobic exercise, in reality many types of exercise use both systems. Figure 3.4(a) illustrates the anaerobic–aerobic energy continuum as it relates to exercise duration. Anaerobic energy production is dominant during short-term exercise, and aerobic energy production is greatest during long-term exercise. For example, a 100-meter dash sprint uses anaerobic energy sources almost exclusively. At the other end of the energy spectrum, running a marathon uses mostly aerobic production of ATP, because the exercise involves 2 or more hours of continuous activity. Running a maximal-effort 800-meter race (exercise of 2–3 minutes' duration) is an example of an exercise duration that uses almost an equal amount of aerobic and anaerobic energy sources.

Figure 3.4(b) applies the anaerobic–aerobic energy continuum to various sports activities. Weight lifting, gymnastics, and wrestling are examples of sports that use anaerobic energy production almost exclusively. Boxing and skating (1500 meters) require an equal contribution of anaerobic and aerobic energy production. Finally, during cross-country skiing and jogging, aerobic energy production dominates.

> ATP is used for energy during exercise.
> Anaerobic energy production does not require oxygen, uses carbohydrates for fuel, and supplies energy for short-term and high-intensity exercises.
> Aerobic energy production requires oxygen to make ATP; can use carbohydrates, fats, or proteins for fuel; and is used for longer-duration exercises.
> Many activities use both energy systems at some level.

What Happens to the Cardiorespiratory System with Exercise and Training?

You have probably noticed that when you go for a run or spend more than a few minutes on an exercise bike, your heart rate increases and you start to sweat. These reactions are due to specific needs of your body during exercise. We'll discuss these next.

During an exercise session and after a regular exercise program, your cardiorespiratory system undergoes several **responses** and **adaptations.** Responses are the changes that occur during and immediately after exercise. For example, your increased heart rate and heavy breathing after you walk up a hill is a response. Adaptations are the changes you will see if you stick with a regular exercise program. Your ability to walk up that hill without getting winded after a few weeks of regular aerobic exercise is the result of adaptations to the cardiorespiratory system. As the cardiorespiratory system gets stronger, it does not have to work as hard for the same level of exercise.

Responses to Exercise

When you exercise, the exercising muscles need more oxygen and nutrients to maintain their activity, so your cardiac output has to increase. The faster heart rate you experience during exercise contributes to the increased cardiac output. Stroke volume also increases to increase cardiac output, enabling your working muscles to get enough oxygen to produce energy. The arteries going to the working muscles dilate (or expand) to deliver the increased blood and oxygen to the exercising muscles.

The respiratory system also has to respond to the demand of exercise by maintaining constant levels of oxygen and carbon dioxide in the blood. Exercise increases the amount of oxygen the body uses and the amount of carbon dioxide produced. Therefore,

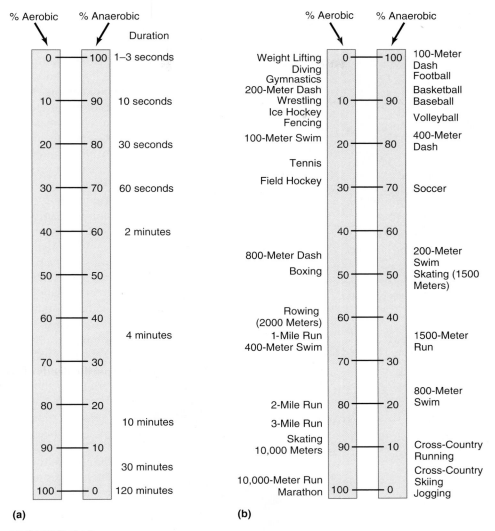

FIGURE 3.4
Contributions of aerobically and anaerobically produced ATP to energy metabolism during exercise. **(a)** Contributions as a function of exercise duration. **(b)** Contributions for various sport activities.

breathing rate increases to bring more oxygen into the body and to remove the carbon dioxide. As you exercise at higher intensities, breathing increases rapidly to enhance removal of carbon dioxide.

Adaptations to Exercise

Regular endurance exercise training results in adaptations in the cardiovascular and respiratory systems, skeletal muscles, and the energy-producing systems.

Endurance training results in several adaptations in the cardiovascular system (4). One thing you will notice as your cardiorespiratory fitness level increases is that your resting heart rate decreases. This occurs because your heart is able to pump more blood per heartbeat, so it does not have to beat as many times per

minute to get the same amount of blood throughout the body. The maximum number of times your heart beats per minute does not increase with aerobic exercise training, but your maximal stroke volume does. As maximal stroke volume increases, maximal cardiac output increases. Remember that cardiac output is the amount of blood that is pumped through the body per

responses The changes that occur during exercise to help you meet the demand of the exercise session. These changes return to normal levels shortly after the exercise session.

adaptations Semipermanent changes that occur over time with regular exercise. Adaptations can be reversed when a regular exercise program is stopped for an extended period of time.

FIGURE 3.5

The relationship between training intensity and improvements in $\dot{V}O_2$max following a 12-week training period.

minute. Because the maximal amount of blood your heart can pump per minute increases, the maximal amount of oxygen you can use during exercise, or your $\dot{V}O_2$max increases.

Aerobic exercise training does not alter the structure or function of the respiratory system, but it does increase the endurance of the muscles involved in the breathing process (5). The diaphragm, located below the lungs, and other key muscles of respiration can work harder and longer without fatigue. This improvement in respiratory muscle endurance may reduce the feeling of being out of breath during exercise and eliminate the pain in the side (often called a stitch) that people sometimes experience when beginning an aerobic exercise program.

Endurance training also increases the muscles' capacity to produce aerobic energy. The practical results of this adaptation are that the body is better able to use fat to produce energy and that muscular endurance increases (4). Note that these changes occur only in those muscles used for exercise or activity. For example, endurance training using a stationary exercise cycle results in improved muscular endurance in leg muscles, but it has little effect on arm muscles. Also, although

CONSIDER THIS!

$\dot{V}O_2$max begins to decrease around the age of 25 and decreases at a rate of approximately 1% per year.

endurance training improves muscle tone, you will not see significant increases in muscle size or strength.

Recall that many exercise physiologists consider $\dot{V}O_2$max to be the best single measure of cardiorespiratory fitness. Therefore, improved $\dot{V}O_2$max is an important adaptation of regular aerobic exercise training. In general, 12 to 15 weeks of endurance exercise produce a 10–30% improvement in $\dot{V}O_2$max (4). A combination of the adaptations of the cardiorespiratory system, improved aerobic capacity of the aerobic muscles, and increased maximal cardiac output produce the increase in $\dot{V}O_2$max. The benefits of the increase are that your body can deliver and use more oxygen during exercise, muscular endurance improves, and you experience less fatigue during routine daily activities.

In general, a person with an initial low $\dot{V}O_2$max will have greater increases than a person who starts an aerobic exercise program with a high $\dot{V}O_2$max. The increase in $\dot{V}O_2$max is directly related to the intensity of the training program, with high-intensity training programs producing greater increases than low-intensity and short-duration programs (6) (Figure 3.5). Note though, that poor nutritional habits will impede improvements in $\dot{V}O_2$max. You will learn more about developing a healthy diet in Chapter 7.

Body Composition

Endurance training generally produces a loss of body fat and healthier body composition (4). However, a loss of body fat is not guaranteed. If you begin an aerobic exercise program with the goal of losing weight, you also need to consider the amount of exercise you do and your dietary habits. You will learn more about body composition and weight management in Chapters 6 and 8.

Make sure you know...

> Responses are the short-term changes that occur during exercise, and adaptations are the changes that occur over time as a result of regular exercise.

> Responses to exercise include increases in heart rate, stroke volume, cardiac output, and breathing rate.

> Adaptations to regular aerobic exercise include decreased resting heart rate, increased stroke volume and $\dot{V}O_2$max, improved ability to use fat for fuel, and improved body composition.

What Are the Health Benefits of Cardiorespiratory Endurance?

As you learned in Chapter 1, health and fitness are not the same. You also learned the differences between physical activity and exercise. Regular physical activity can lead to health improvements (e.g., reduced risk for heart disease) even if you do not have a structured exercise program. However, without a structured exercise program, you probably will not see significant changes in your cardiorespiratory endurance level.

Among the most significant health benefits of cardiorespiratory fitness are a lower risk of cardiovascular disease (CVD) and increased longevity. Also, people who exercise to improve their cardiorespiratory fitness have a reduced risk of type 2 diabetes, lower blood pressure, and increased bone density in weight-bearing bones (7).

In addition to physical health benefits, there are also psychological health benefits associated with regular aerobic exercise training, including higher self-esteem and a more positive body image (8). This relationship is due to multiple factors. First, there is a sense of accomplishment that comes from starting and maintaining a regular exercise program and meeting personal goals. Regular exercise also improves muscle tone and helps with weight management, both of which can have positive impact on appearance. Improved sleep quality is another psychological benefit of regular exercise (9). Fit individuals tend to sleep longer without interruptions (i.e., they enjoy more restful sleep) than do less-fit people. A better night's rest will likely translate to a more complete feeling of being mentally restored.

Benefits of cardiorespiratory endurance also extend to activities of daily living. More energy for work and play is a commonly reported benefit; fit individuals can perform more work with less fatigue. People with high levels of cardiorespiratory fitness often say they exercise because it makes them feel better. The box on this page summarizes the benefits you can expect to experience from the improved cardiovascular fitness that results from a regular exercise program.

Make sure you know...

> Regular exercise is needed to improve your cardiorespiratory endurance.

> There are numerous physical and psychological health benefits of regular aerobic exercise, including reduced risk of CVD, increased longevity, and improved self-esteem and body image.

Benefits of Improved Cardiorespiratory Fitness

- Lower risk of heart disease
- Reduced risk of type 2 diabetes
- Lower blood pressure
- Increased bone density
- Increased energy for work and play
- Increased feeling of well-being
- Improved self-esteem
- Increased muscle tone and endurance
- Easier weight control
- Improved sleep

Evaluation of Cardiorespiratory Endurance

The most accurate means of measuring cardiorespiratory fitness is the laboratory assessment of $\dot{V}O_2$max (4,10). However, direct measurement of $\dot{V}O_2$max requires expensive equipment and is very time-consuming, so it is not practical for general use. Fortunately, there are numerous field tests for estimating $\dot{V}O_2$max (11–13). Each of these tests has a margin of error, but they are valid measures, and the practical advantages outweigh the disadvantages. This section will explain some of the common ways you can easily estimate your $\dot{V}O_2$max. You can use Laboratory 3.1A–D at the end of the chapter to estimate your $\dot{V}O_2$max.

One of the simplest and most accurate assessments of cardiorespiratory fitness is the **1.5-mile run test.** This test is based on the idea that people with a higher level of cardiorespiratory fitness can run 1.5 miles faster than those with a lower level of cardiorespiratory fitness (11, 12).

The objective of the test is to complete a 1.5-mile run in the shortest possible time. Regular exercisers and people with active lifestyles can probably complete the 1.5-mile distance running or jogging. Because this test requires you to run the 1.5 miles as fast as you can, it is not the best option for sedentary people over age 30, for people who have a very low fitness level due to medical reasons, for individuals with joint problems, or for obese individuals. For less active individuals, a

1.5-mile run test One of the simplest and most accurate assessments of cardiorespiratory fitness.

FIGURE 3.6
A cycle ergometer can be used to assess cardiorespiratory endurance.

1.5 mile run/walk test is better suited. Laboratory 3.1A at the end of the chapter provides instructions for performing the test and recording the score.

The 1-mile walk test is another common field test to estimate cardiorespiratory fitness. The walk test is based on the same idea as the 1.5-mile run test: that people who have higher cardiorespiratory fitness will be able to complete the test faster than those with low cardiorespiratory fitness. This test is particularly good for sedentary individuals (14–16). However, people with joint problems should consider a non-weight-bearing test, such as the cycle test described next. See Laboratory 3.1B for instructions on how to perform the 1-mile walk test and how to determine your score.

Two other tests that can be used to assess your cardiorespiratory endurance are the cycle ergometer test and the step test. A **cycle ergometer** test (Figure 3.6) is ideal for people with joint problems because, unlike walking or jogging, it does not involve weight bearing. The cycle ergometer test is a submaximal cycle test based on the principle that individuals with high cardiorespiratory fitness levels have a lower exercise heart rate at a standard workload than less-fit individuals (13, 17). You can use Laboratory 3.1C to estimate your $\dot{V}O_2$max according to your heart rate and the workload used during the cycle ergometer test.

Finally, the step test can be performed by people at all fitness levels. Additionally, this test does not require expensive equipment, and it can be performed in a short amount of time. However, the step test is not recommended for overweight individuals or for people with joint problems. The step test is based on the principle that your heart rate "recovers," or returns to resting levels, faster after exercise when you have a high level of cardiorespiratory fitness. Therefore, individuals with a higher cardiorespiratory fitness will have a lower heart rate during a 3-minute period immediately following the test compared to less-fit individuals (4). Also, be aware that this test requires stepping at a consistent rate and accurately taking your heart rate multiple times, so there is more chance for error. You can use Laboratory 3.1D to perform the step test and to find the norms for step test results in a college-aged population (18–25 years).

Make sure you know...

> Common tests to assess cardiorespiratory fitness include the 1.5-mile run, the 1-mile walk, the cycle ergometer test, and the step test.

> Obese individuals and people with joint problems should avoid weight-bearing cardiorespiratory assessment tests. Sedentary individuals should avoid the 1.5-mile run test.

Designing Your Aerobic Exercise Program

After you know your level of cardiorespiratory fitness, you can design an appropriate exercise plan to meet your goals. As we discussed in Chapter 2, setting long- and short-term goals is key to making a healthy behavior change. Starting and maintaining your aerobic exercise program will be much easier if you set goals first and then plan your program specifically to meet your goals. Many fitness experts agree that lack of goals is a major contributor to the high dropout rates seen in many organized fitness programs (18).

As you learned from Chapter 2, each exercise session will include the warm-up, workout, and cool-down phases. Within the workout phase you need to consider the frequency, intensity, time, and type (mode) of exercise. Also, it is important to consider the stage of the program. These stages include the initial conditioning, progression, and maintenance phases.

The Warm-Up

Every workout should begin with a warm-up of 5 to 10 minutes of low-intensity exercise and some light stretching. If you take a class such as step aerobics or spinning, your instructor will lead you though an appropriate warm-up. If you do other aerobic exercises, such as jogging or swimming, then you will need to plan your own warm-up. Typically, the warm-up will include a lower-intensity activity that is similar to or the same as your activity of choice for your workout. For example, you might walk or jog as warm-up for a run or swim a couple of laps more slowly than you would for the rest of your swim workout. You might also include some light stretching (see Chapter 5). Then, as you start the workout phase, you will gradually increase your intensity to the desired level.

The Workout

The components of an exercise prescription to improve cardiovascular fitness include the components of the FITT principle: frequency, intensity, time (or duration), and type of exercise.

Frequency   The general recommendation for exercise frequency is 3 to 5 sessions per week to achieve near-optimal gains in cardiorespiratory fitness with minimal risk of injury. However, cardiorespiratory fitness gains can be achieved with as few as 2 exercise sessions per week (10). You typically will not see significantly greater improvements in your cardiorespiratory fitness if you exercise more than 5 days per week. Additionally, greater exercise frequency entails a greater risk for injury, which generally does not outweigh any added benefit of a greater frequency.

You might have to start with 2 or 3 days per week and increase the frequency as you progress through your program. You should also consider the rest between exercise sessions. A general rule is to exercise no more than 3 days in a row and to rest no more than 3 days in a row, especially if you are doing the same exercise each session.

Intensity   Cardiorespiratory fitness improves when the training intensity is at least 50% of $\dot{V}O_2$max (this level is often called the **training threshold**). Training at exercise intensities close to $\dot{V}O_2$max does not produce significantly greater benefits and increases risk for injury. Therefore, the recommended range of exer-

CONSIDER THIS!

Up to 50% of college students do not get the recommended amount of exercise.

cise intensity for improving health-related physical fitness is between 50% and 85% $\dot{V}O_2$max.

You cannot readily assess your percent $\dot{V}O_2$max during exercise, but you can use heart rate to monitor exercise intensity. $\dot{V}O_2$max and heart rate both increase linearly as exercise intensity increases. We also know that maximal heart rate is reached at $\dot{V}O_2$max. This relationship, coupled with the fact that heart rate is easily monitored, make heart rate a practical way to monitor exercise intensity.

How do you know what your heart rate should be during exercise? We can calculate a **target heart rate (THR)** range. Figure 3.7 illustrates the pattern of heart rate during an exercise session in the THR. Because the tests we described to assess cardiorespiratory endurance are submaximal tests, we have to estimate maximal heart rate. *Maximal heart rate (HR_{max})* decreases with age and can be estimated by this formula:

$$HR_{max} = 220 - \text{age (in years)}$$

For example, we can estimate a 20-year-old college student's maximal heart rate by the formula

$$HR_{max} = 220 - 20 = 200 \text{ beats/min}$$

To determine your THR, we next have to determine your **heart rate reserve (HRR)**. Heart rate reserve is the difference between your maximal heart rate and resting heart rate:

$$HRR = HR_{max} - \text{resting HR}$$

Let's assume that our 20-year-old college student's resting heart rate is 60 beats per minute (bpm). Then,

$$HRR = 200 - 60 = 140 \text{ beats/min}$$

After determining the HRR, we can calculate 50% and 85% of his HRR. This range will place him at the desired percentage of his $\dot{V}O_2$max.

$$0.50 \times 140 = 70 \text{ bpm}$$
$$0.85 \times 140 = 119 \text{ bpm}$$

cycle ergometer A stationary exercise cycle that provides pedaling resistance so the amount of work can be measured.

training threshold The training intensity above which there is an improvement in cardiorespiratory fitness. This intensity is approximately 50% of $\dot{V}O_2$max.

target heart rate (THR) The range of heart rates that corresponds to an exercise intensity of approximately 50–85% $\dot{V}O_2$max. This is the range of training heart rates that results in improvements in aerobic capacity.

heart rate reserve (HRR) The difference between your maximal heart rate and resting heart rate.

FIGURE 3.7
Sample workout in the target heart rate range.

FIGURE 3.9
Borg's Rating of Perceived Exertion (RPE) scale. The perception of exertion depends mainly on the strain and fatigue in your muscles and on your feelings of breathlessness or aches in the chest. Try to appraise your feeling of exertion as honestly as possible, without thinking about what the actual physical load is. Don't underestimate it, but don't overestimate it either.

Source: Borg-RPE-scale® from G. Borg, (1998), *Borg's Perceived Exertion and Pain Scales.* Champaign, IL: Human Kinetics. © Gunnar Borg, 1970, 1985, 1994, 1998. Used with permission of Dr. G. Borg. For correct usage of the scale the exact design and instructions given in Borg's folders must be followed: The BORG-RPE SCALE®, a method for measuring perceived exertion. © G. Borg, 1994, 2003. Order folders and scales from: Borg Products, Inc., "BPU," Joseph V. Myers III, 1579F, Monroe Drive, #416, Atlanta, GA 30324.

The final step in determining the THR is to add your resting heart rate back to the values you just calculated. This step is done because your resting heart rate is the starting point. Our student's THR is calculated as follows:

$$70 + 60 = 130 \text{ bpm}$$
$$119 + 60 = 179 \text{ bpm}$$
$$\text{THR} = 130 - 179 \text{ bpm}$$

You can calculate your THR using Laboratory 3.3 at the end of the chapter. Because your maximal heart rate decreases with age, your THR will change as you get older (Figure 3.8). Also, remember that a lower resting heart rate is an adaptation of aerobic exercise

training. As you get older and see changes in your resting heart rate, you should recalculate your THR.

Another way to estimate exercise intensity is the **Borg Rating of Perceived Exertion (RPE)** scale in Figure 3.9.(19). Perceived exertion is how hard you think you are working during exercise. To determine your RPE, take into consideration your efforts of breathing, how much you are sweating, and feelings in your muscles. Because your heart rate increases as your exercise intensity increases, your perception of effort assessed by the RPE scale typically correlates with heart rate during exercise. An RPE value between 12 and 16 will correspond with the target heart rate range for most people.

Time (Duration) Recall that the duration of exercise does not include the warm-up or cool-down. In general, exercise durations most effective in improving cardiorespiratory fitness are between 20 and 60 minutes (10). The time you need to obtain your desired benefits will be specific to your initial level of fitness and your training intensity. For example, a poorly conditioned individual may see improvement in his cardiorespiratory endurance with 20 to 30 minutes of exercise 3 to 5 days per week at his THR. In contrast, a highly trained person may need regular exercise sessions of 40 to 60 minutes' duration to improve cardiorespiratory fitness.

When determining your exercise duration, you also have to consider your exercise intensity. If you choose

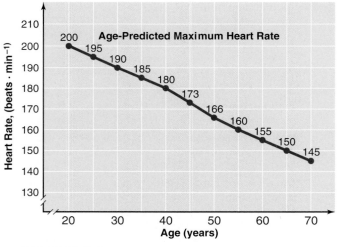

FIGURE 3.8
As you age, your maximal heart rate will decrease.

A CLOSER LOOK

AEROBIC WORKOUTS—FAQS

Which is better, exercising for a brief period several times, or exercising for one longer period?
Both approaches can work. You do need to warm up for 5 to 10 minutes and cool down for 5 to 10 minutes, regardless of the session length. Short sessions last typically at least 10 minutes for the workout phase. After you add the time for the warm-up and cool-down, you are looking at a 20-minute session. Keep in mind that if you choose multiple sessions, your total workout time should be the same as with one longer session. Also, shorter sessions should not be less intense. You still have to maintain your prescribed exercise intensity to maximize the benefits.

What is the best time of day to exercise?
It doesn't matter whether you exercise in the morning or afternoon, but it does matter that you stick with your routine. So, the best time of day to exercise is whenever you're most likely to do it consistently.

Should I train if I'm sick?
Generally, if the sickness is above the neck (e.g., sinus problem, headache, sore throat), light exercise might not be a problem. Just take it easy, and be sure to respect others who are not sick by wiping off any equipment that you use and by washing your hands frequently. If you are not sure whether you should exercise, listen to your body. If you feel you need to rest, then you should take the day off.

Can I do aerobic exercise if I have asthma?
People with asthma can, in general, safely participate in all types of exercise. However, it is important to have a prescribed medication program to control your asthma (21). When asthma is under control, your exercise prescription need not be different from those for individuals without asthma. Exercise with other people present, and keep your inhaler readily available while exercising in case of an asthma attack. Additionally, you should avoid exercise in cold weather and in polluted environments. If you live in an area with a high level of pollution, exercising in a place with properly filtered indoor air may be preferable to exercising outdoors.

lower-intensity exercise rather than higher-intensity exercise, you will need to factor in a longer duration. For example, training at the lower end of your target heart rate range, around 50% of HRR, might require an exercise duration of 40 to 50 minutes to improve cardiorespiratory fitness. However, if you exercise at a moderate or higher intensity, such as 70% of HRR, you might see similar improvements with only 20 to 30 minutes.

Type   Any type of aerobic activities that you enjoy enough to do consistently will help improve and maintain your cardiorespiratory fitness. Also, any activity that uses a large muscle mass (e.g., the legs) in a slow, rhythmic pattern can improve cardiorespiratory endurance. These activities can be performed at a duration and intensity that will use the aerobic energy system. The box at right lists several activities that have been shown to improve cardiorespiratory fitness.

Because there are many exercises and activities that will improve your cardiorespiratory endurance, it is important to select activities you will enjoy. Another consideration is the risk of injury associated with high-impact activities, such as running. Listen to your body when it comes to choosing a high-impact exercise. If

Exercises and Activities That Can Improve Cardiorespiratory Fitness

- Aerobics classes
- Bicycling
- Cross-country skiing
- Hiking
- Skipping rope
- Rowing
- Running
- Skating (ice or roller)
- Spinning classes
- Stair climbing
- Swimming
- Brisk walking

Borg Rating of Perceived Exertion A subjective way of estimating exercise intensity based on a numerical scale of 6 to 20.

Frequency	3–5 times per week
Intensity	50–85% of HRmax
Time	20–60 minutes per session
Type	Jogging

FIGURE 3.10
An example of the FITT principle for improving cardiorespiratory fitness.

you experience joint pain or discomfort with high-impact activities, you should see a physician. You might need to find lower-impact exercises, such as swimming or cycling. Cross training, discussed later in the chapter, is another option to reduce your risk for injury if you enjoy a high-impact exercise. For an example of how to use the FITT principle in designing an exercise program, see Figure 3.10.

Consumer CORNER
HOW GOOD ARE EXERCISE GADGETS?

Trends and fads come and go in the fitness industry, and right up with diet trends and workout fads are the gadgets that tend to get sold on late-night infomercials and in fitness magazines. Some gadgets work, and others do not. Before buying a new gadget, do your homework. If you have not used the equipment before, try to find someone who has to get an honest opinion. If you are concerned with which modality burns the most calories, the best piece is the one that you use consistently and for the longest amount of time.

For home exercise, treadmills and exercise bikes are excellent choices, but they can be very expensive. The most expensive is not always the best, but you often get what you pay for. Lower-priced treadmills or exercise bikes might not be sturdy enough for long-term use. For outside exercise, bicycles or rollerblades/inline skates are great options. You can usually get good assistance from the sporting goods staff to determine the most appropriate bike or skates for your fitness goals.

Don't forget what you learned in this chapter about aerobic exercise. Abdominal machines or equipment that promise great results in "just 5 minutes" per day are not going to give you an aerobic workout. Keep in mind no gadget will work if you do not use it, so make sure whatever you are considering is something you will put to good use.

The Cool-Down

Every training session should conclude with a cool-down of light exercises and stretching. Allowing your cardiovascular system to slow down gradually is important: Stopping your workout abruptly can cause blood to pool in the arms and legs, which could result in dizziness and/or fainting. A cool-down may also decrease the muscle soreness and cardiac irregularities that sometimes appear after a vigorous workout. Although cardiac irregularities are rare in healthy individuals, a cool-down period is still wise to minimize the risk.

A general cool-down of at least 5 minutes (e.g., light exercise such as walking, or a lighter intensity of the activity you did for your exercise session) should be followed by 5 to 30 minutes of flexibility exercises. If you take an exercise class, your instructor will lead you through the cool-down. In general, stretching exercises should focus on the muscles used during training. The type and duration of the stretching session depends on your flexibility goals (Chapter 5).

Make sure you know...

> Establishing both short-term and long-term fitness goals is essential before beginning a fitness program.
> Each workout should include warm-up, workout, and cool-down phases.
> You need to consider the exercise frequency, intensity, time (duration), and type (mode) for the workout phase.
> Intensity can be monitored using the target heart rate range or Rating of Perceived Exertion.
> Aerobic exercise performed 3 to 5 days per week at 50–85% of your heart rate reserve for 20–60 minutes is recommended to improve your cardiorespiratory endurance.

Developing an Individualized Exercise Prescription

As we discussed in Chapter 2, anyone beginning a new aerobic exercise program, regardless of initial fitness level or exercise mode, will usually go through three stages: initial conditioning, improvement, and maintenance. In this section we will show you how you can individualize these stages to meet your specific needs and goals.

Initial Conditioning Phase

The initial conditioning stage is to your program what the warm-up is to your workout. Starting slowly will allow the body to adapt gradually to exercise and to avoid soreness, injury, and discouragement. Generally this stage lasts 4 weeks, but it can be as short as 2 weeks or as long as 6 weeks, depending on your initial fitness level (10). For example, if your cardiorespiratory fitness is poor, this stage will likely last closer to 6 weeks, but if you start at a relatively high cardiorespiratory fitness level, a 2-week initial conditioning stage might be sufficient.

You should include 10- to 15-minute warm-up and cool-down phases with each workout. In the initial conditioning period of your workout, exercise intensity will be low, typically 40–60% HRR or RPE of 11–13 (10). For people who have never been involved in a regular exercise program or who have very low fitness, the initial intensity might even be less than the 50% HHR we calculated earlier. It is acceptable to start at an intensity of 40–50% HRR if that is comfortable for you (10). The duration of the session will likely be short. Initial sessions for a person with very low fitness might be as short as 10 to 15 minutes. At these intensity and duration recommendations, an exercise frequency of 3 or 4 days is ideal (10).

Here are some key points to remember for your initial conditioning stage:

- Start at an exercise intensity that is comfortable for you.
- Increase your training duration or intensity when you are comfortable, but do not increase intensity and duration at the same time. Gradually increase your duration, and then work on increasing the intensity. Your goal should be 20 to 30 minutes of continuous low to moderate (40–60% HHR) activity at the end of the initial conditioning phase (10).
- Be aware of new aches or pains. Pain is a symptom of injury and indicates that the body needs rest to repair itself. (See Chapter 12 for a discussion of injury prevention and treatment.)

Improvement Phase

The improvement phase can range from 12 to 40 weeks, and your program will progress more rapidly during this period than in the initial conditioning phase (10). The duration and frequency are increased first, and then the intensity is increased toward the upper end of the THR (60–85% HRR or RPE of 13–16). The changes should be gradual, with increases in the duration of no more than 20% per week until you can do 20 to 30 minutes at a moderate to vigorous intensity (10). Frequency of 3 to 4 days might still be appropriate, but if you want greater changes in your cardiorespiratory endurance, increasing to 5 days might be necessary. A general recommendation is to increase the intensity by no more than 5% of your HRR every sixth exercise ses-

sion (10). If you are exercising 3 days per week, that means an increase every 2 weeks. As you can see, the changes are gradual, and you should not feel pressure to make increases faster than you feel comfortable doing so.

Maintenance Phase

The average college-aged student will generally reach the maintenance phase of the exercise prescription after 16 to 28 weeks of training, but it might take longer for those who started at a low fitness level. In the maintenance stage, you have achieved your fitness goal, and your new goal is to maintain this level of fitness. You still need to exercise regularly, but you do not need to keep increasing all of the components of your exercise prescription.

Several studies have shown that the key factor in maintaining cardiorespiratory fitness is exercise intensity (6). If you keep your intensity at the same level you reached in the final weeks of the improvement stage, you can reduce your frequency. Exercising as little as 2 days per week can still maintain your fitness level. If you keep to the same frequency and intensity as you achieved during the final weeks of the improvement stage, you can reduce duration to 20 to 25 minutes per session. However, if you hold frequency and duration constant, decreasing intensity by even one-third can significantly decrease your cardiorespiratory endurance. So, if you keep up your exercise intensity, you can cut back the duration or frequency to keep your hard-earned benefits.

Sample Exercise Prescriptions

Your exercise program should be tailored to your individual needs to meet the goals you set. An important consideration in designing a personal training program is your current fitness level. People with good or excellent cardiorespiratory fitness can start at a higher level and progress more rapidly than people with low cardiorespiratory endurance. The boxes on pages 66–68 illustrate three sample cardiorespiratory training programs designed for college-aged people with varying initial cardiorespiratory fitness levels. Note that these programs are sample programs to give you an idea of how to start and develop your program. You can use Laboratory 3.4 at the end of this chapter to develop your personal exercise prescription.

Make sure you know...

> Regardless of your initial fitness level, an exercise prescription to improve cardiorespiratory fitness has three phases: initial conditioning, improvement, and maintenance.

Sample Exercise Program for Someone with an Initial Low Level of Cardiorespiratory Fitness

General guidelines:

1. Begin each session with a warm-up.
2. Don't progress to the next level until you feel comfortable with your current level of exercise.
3. Monitor your heart rate during each training session.
4. End each session with a cool-down.
5. Be aware of aches and pains. If you are injury prone, choose a low-impact activity mode, and limit your exercise duration to 20 to 30 minutes per day.

Week No.	Phase	Duration (min/day)	Intensity (% of HR_{max})	Frequency (days/wk)
1	Initial conditioning	10	60	3
2	Initial conditioning	10	60	3
3	Initial conditioning	12	60	3
4	Initial conditioning	12	70	3
5	Initial conditioning	15	70	3
6	Initial conditioning	15	70	3
7	Improvement	20	70	3
8	Improvement	20	70	3
9	Improvement	25	70	3
10	Improvement	25	70	3
11	Improvement	30	70	3
12	Improvement	30	70	3
13	Improvement	35	70	3
14	Improvement	35	70	3
15	Improvement	40	70	3
16	Improvement	40	70	3
17	Improvement	40	75	3
18	Improvement	40	75	3
19	Improvement	40	75	3
20	Improvement	40	75	3–4
21	Improvement	40	75	3–4
22	Improvement	40	75	3–4
23	Maintenance	30	75	3–4
24	Maintenance	30	75	3–4
25	Maintenance	30	75	3–4
26	Maintenance	30	75	3–4

> Your exercise program should be tailored to your individual needs and should take into account your current fitness level.

Training Techniques

Endurance training is a generic term that refers to any type of exercise aimed at improving cardiorespiratory endurance. However, there are numerous endurance training methods that you can use to improve your cardiorespiratory endurance. Most common is the use of a continuous activity, such as walking or jogging at a constant exercise intensity. Cross training and interval training are two techniques for people who need some variety or want to make faster gains.

Cross Training

Cross training is the use of multiple training modes. To cross-train, you might take an aerobic class one day, run one day, and swim another day. Some people use cross training to reduce the boredom of performing the same kind of exercise day after day. Cross training also

Sample Exercise Program for Someone with an Initial Average Level of Cardiorespiratory Fitness

General guidelines:

1. Begin each session with a warm-up.

2. Don't progress to the next level until you feel comfortable with your current level of exercise.

3. Monitor your heart rate during each training session.

4. End each session with a cool-down.

5. Be aware of aches and pains. If you are injury prone, choose a low-impact activity mode, and limit your exercise duration to 20 to 30 minutes per day.

Week No.	Phase	Duration (min/day)	Intensity (% of HR_{max})	Frequency (days/wk)
1	Initial conditioning	10	70	3
2	Initial conditioning	15	70	3
3	Initial conditioning	15	70	3
4	Initial conditioning	20	70	3
5	Improvement	25	70	3
6	Improvement	25	75	3
7	Improvement	25	75	3
8	Improvement	30	75	3
9	Improvement	30	75	3
10	Improvement	35	75	3
11	Improvement	35	75	3
12	Improvement	40	75	3
13	Improvement	40	75	3
14	Improvement	40	75	3
15	Improvement	40	80	3
16	Improvement	40	80	3–4
17	Improvement	40	80	3–4
18	Improvement	40	80	3–4
19	Maintenance	30	80	3–4
20	Maintenance	30	80	3–4
21	Maintenance	30	80	3–4
22	Maintenance	30	80	3–4

might reduce the risk and occurrence of overuse injuries. However, cross training does not provide training specificity. Your cardiorespiratory endurance will improve, but jogging will not improve your swimming, because jogging does not train the arm muscles. Cross training might not be ideal if you are looking to improve your ability in a specific activity, but if you like variety and simply want to increase your cardiorespiratory fitness, cross training is a great option.

Interval Training

Interval training is typically used by athletes and others who are at a higher fitness level. This type of training includes repeated sessions, or intervals, of relatively intense exercise alternated with lower-intensity periods to rest or recover. Runners, swimmers, and cy-

clists use interval training to improve their times in competition. People exercising to improve fitness might use interval training to make more rapid increases in their exercise intensity during the improvement stage. Interval workouts are intense training sessions and should not be used on a daily basis: rather, they should be alternated with continuous moderate-intensity exercise sessions.

cross training The use of a variety of activities for training the cardiorespiratory system.

interval training Type of training that includes repeated sessions or intervals of relatively intense exercise alternated with lower-intensity periods to rest or recover.

Sample Exercise Program for Someone with an Initial High Level of Cardiorespiratory Fitness

General guidelines:

1. Begin each session with a warm-up.
2. Don't progress to the next level until you feel comfortable with your current level of exercise.
3. Monitor your heart rate during each training session.
4. End each session with a cool-down.
5. Be aware of aches and pains. If you are injury prone, choose a low-impact activity mode, and limit your exercise duration to 20 to 30 minutes per day.

Week No.	Phase	Duration (min/day)	Intensity (% of HR_{max})	Frequency (days/wk)
1	Initial conditioning	15	75	3
2	Initial conditioning	20	75	3
3	Improvement	25	75	3
4	Improvement	30	75	3
5	Improvement	35	75	3
6	Improvement	40	75	3
7	Improvement	40	75	3–4
8	Improvement	40	75	3–4
9	Improvement	40	80	3–4
10	Improvement	40	80	3–4
11	Improvement	40	80	3–4
12	Improvement	40	80–85	3–4
13	Improvement	40	80–85	3–4
14	Improvement	40	80–85	3–4
15	Maintenance	30	80–85	3–4
16	Maintenance	30	80–85	3–4
17	Maintenance	30	80–85	3–4
18	Maintenance	30	80–85	3–4

The duration of the intervals can vary, but a 1- to 5-minute duration is common. Each interval is followed by a rest period, which should be equal to or slightly longer than the interval duration. For example, if you are running 400-meter intervals on a track and it takes you approximately 90 seconds to complete each run, your rest period between efforts should be at least 90 seconds. An "active rest" period is recommended. If you are running, your rest would be an easy jog or brisk walk to prevent muscle tightness. You do not have to use a track for interval training. You can use a stop watch and do an interval workout anywhere you usually train.

Make sure you know...

> Cross training can prevent you from becoming bored with an exercise program and reduce your risk for injury.

> Interval training is used by athletes and more advanced exercisers to produce faster gains in cardiorespiratory endurance.

How Can You Get Motivated to Be Active?

Every year, millions of people make the decision to start an exercise program. Unfortunately, over half of those who begin an aerobic exercise program quit within the first 6 months (18). There are many reasons for this high dropout rate, but lack of time is the most commonly cited reason (18). Although finding time for exercise in a busy schedule is difficult, it is not impossible. The key is to schedule a regular time for exercise and to stick with it. A small investment in time to exercise can reap large improvements in fitness and health.

Think about how much time you have in a week and how much of that time is needed to improve your cardiorespiratory endurance. There are 168 hours in every week, and all you need is three 30-minute workouts to improve cardiorespiratory fitness. Of course you need to

APPRECIATING DIVERSITY

DON'T LET A DISABILITY STOP YOU!

A temporary or permanent disability can discourage you from exercising, but you can take comfort in knowing that even with most disabilities you can obtain all of the benefits of cardiovascular exercise. If you have an injury that temporarily keeps you from performing your exercise of choice, your physical therapist or physician can help you find suitable alternative exercises to maintain your fitness level. Consulting a physical therapist, physician, or exercise specialist for the best exercise options is also recommended if you have a permanent disability. Additionally, these health pro-

fessionals will be able to make you aware of any medical complications associated with your disability and how you can address them.

In general, swimming and other water activities are excellent ways to decrease the need to support your body weight and safely exercise capable muscle groups. Other benefits of water exercise include the following:

- They pose little to no risk of falling.

- Flexibility exercises are much easier to do in water.

- Water provides resistance to capable muscle groups. This resistance enables you to progressively overload the intensity and improve the cardiorespiratory system.

- A variety of water aids, including hand paddles, pull-buoys, flotation belts, and kickboards can be used to help maintain buoyancy and balance as well as help you work in the water.

Basic water safety rules still apply, so be sure to perform water activities with a workout partner or with a lifeguard present.

A CLOSER LOOK

SPINNING—REV IT UP?

Do you like to exercise with a group? Do you like biking but find it hard to do around campus or in your city? Find a spinning class! Spinning is an aerobic exercise performed on stationary bikes in an indoor group ride led by an instructor. The bike is specially designed so you can quickly change the speed and resistance of pedaling. Being able to make the quick changes enables you to mimic cycling in outdoor settings, such as a long country road or up a mountain. The spinning bikes also are designed to be much more

comfortable than typical stationary bikes and feature multiple ways to adjust the seats and handlebars.

Spinning is led by an instructor, so you have the benefit of someone guiding you through your session. The instructor's direction is especially important if you are a beginner, because the instructor can tell you how to make the changes in intensity to fit your experience and fitness level. The classes usually last 30 to 60 minutes, have music for motivation, and use visualization techniques so

you can feel as though you were cycling over hills and through valleys.

Spinning is an excellent exercise for improving cardiorespiratory endurance. You can burn up to 600 calories in an hour depending on the speed and resistance, and it is a low-impact activity that is easy on your joints. Additional benefits of spinning include a group setting for support and encouragement and an indoor setting so weather is not a barrier.

STEPS FOR BEHAVIOR CHANGE

How good is your level of cardiorespiratory fitness?

Answer the following questions to assess your level of cardiorespiratory fitness.

Y N

☐ ☐ Do you participate in recreational or competitive sports?

☐ ☐ Can you perform at least 20 minutes of continuous aerobic exercise?

☐ ☐ Can you do your regular household chores without getting out of breath (e.g., cleaning your apartment, walking your dog, mowing the lawn)?

☐ ☐ Can you walk across campus to your classes with little effort?

If you answered yes to either of the first two questions, your cardiorespiratory fitness level is probably above average. If you answered yes only to the last two questions or to none of the questions, you might need to make some improvements.

TIPS TO BECOME MORE ACTIVE

☑ Take the stairs when possible.

☑ Walk to class instead of driving or taking the bus.

☑ Find a friend to take a walk with you.

☑ Join a club or intramural sport team.

☑ Visit your campus recreation center for options for activity and exercise programs.

☑ Get a pedometer to see how many steps per day you walk. Fewer than 5000 per day indicates a sedentary lifestyle.

---

add warm-ups, cool-downs, and showers, which still totals only about 3 hours per week. That leaves you with 165 hours per week to accomplish all of the other things you need to do. The bottom line is that with proper time management, anyone can find time to exercise.

Consider the strategies you learned for behavior change in Chapter 1, and apply them to your aerobic exercise program. Setting long- and short-term goals is important. Changes happen slowly, and short-term goals will help you monitor your progress to stay on track. Keeping a record of your training program will help you see the small changes that occur on the way to your long-term goal. Keeping your program enjoyable also is important. Exercising with a partner can make your workout more fun and maintain your commitment to a regular exercise routine. Just make sure you choose a partner who is committed and a good exercise role model.

Finally, some discomfort and soreness after your first several exercise sessions is normal. Do not let these feelings discourage you. In a short time the soreness will fade, and the discomfort associated with exercise will disappear. As your fitness level improves, you will feel better and look better. Although reaching and maintaining a healthy level of cardiorespiratory fitness requires time and effort, the rewards are well worth the labor.

Make sure you know...

> You should apply the behavior strategies you learned in Chapter 1 to help maintain your new aerobic exercise program.

> Discomfort and soreness are normal with a new exercise routine but will last only for a brief period.

Summary

1. Benefits of cardiorespiratory fitness include a lower risk of disease, feeling better, increased capacity to perform everyday tasks, and improved self-esteem and body image.

2. Adenosine triphosphate (ATP) provides the energy muscles need to move. It is produced by two systems: anaerobic (without oxygen) and aerobic (with oxygen).

3. Anaerobic energy production is the primary source of energy for short-term exercise, and aerobic energy production dominates during prolonged exercise.

4. The term *cardiorespiratory system* refers to the cooperative work of the circulatory and respiratory systems. The primary function of the circulatory system is to transport blood carrying oxygen and nutrients to body tissues. The principal function of the respiratory system is to load oxygen into and remove carbon dioxide from the blood.

5. Responses to exercise are the short-term changes that occur during exercise to meet the immediate demand of exercise. Adaptations are developed over the long term through regular exercise training and will remain if you continue your exercise program.

6. Many exercise physiologists consider $\dot{V}O_2$max (which is the maximum capacity of the cardiorespiratory system to transport and use oxygen during exercise) to be the most valid measurement of cardiorespiratory endurance.

7. Cardiac output, stroke volume, and heart rate increase as a function of exercise intensity. Breathing rate also increases in proportion to exercise intensity.

8. There are many field tests that can be used to estimate $\dot{V}O_2$max. These tests are practical and can be performed with little equipment.

9. Establishing both short-term and long-term fitness goals is essential before beginning a fitness program.

10. These primary elements make up the exercise prescription: warm-up, workout (primary conditioning period), and cool-down.

11. The components of the workout are the frequency, intensity, time (duration), and type (mode) of exercise (FITT).

12. In general, the FITT principle for improving cardiorespiratory endurance calls for a type of exercise that uses large-muscle groups in a slow, rhythmic pattern for 20 to 60 minutes 3 to 5 times per week.

13. The target heart rate is the range of exercise heart rates that lie between 50% and 85% of heart rate reserve.

14. Regardless of your initial fitness level, an exercise prescription for improving cardiorespiratory fitness has three phases: initial conditioning, improvement, and maintenance.

15. Cross training and interval training provide alternatives to a continuous workout of the same mode. Cross training can be done by individuals of all fitness levels, but interval training is for those who are more experienced with exercise.

16. Maintaining a regular exercise routine requires proper time management and choosing physical activities that you enjoy.

Study Questions

1. Which of the following is not an example of an aerobic exercise?
   a. running
   b. swimming
   c. abdominal toning class
   d. spinning class

2. The anaerobic energy pathway is predominantly responsible for production of ATP during which of the following activities?
   a. wrestling
   b. 800-meter run
   c. 400-meter swim
   d. 30-minute brisk walk

3. _____ is an adaptation of a regular aerobic exercise program.

   a. Lower maximal heart rate

   b. Lower resting heart rate

   c. Faster breathing rate

   d. All of the above

4. Exercise intensity should be at least _____ % of heart rate reserve to improve cardiorespiratory endurance.

   a. 85

   b. 70

   c. 50

   d. 25

5. _____ is a response during exercise.

   a. Faster heart rate

   b. Increased cardiac output

   c. Faster breathing

   d. All of the above

6. _____ are the blood vessels that take blood away from the heart.

   a. Arteries

   b. Veins

   c. Capillaries

   d. Venules

7. What is meant by the term *cardiorespiratory system*?

8. List the major functions of the circulatory and respiratory systems.

9. Why is the heart considered "two pumps in one"?

10. Define the following terms:

    adenosine triphosphate (ATP)

    cross training

    target heart rate

Suggested Reading

Blair, S. N., M. J. LaMonte, and M. Z. Nichaman. The evolution of physical activity recommendations: How much is enough? *American Journal of Clinical Nutrition* 79(5):913S–920S, 2004.

Brisswalter J., M. Collardeau, and A. Rene. Effects of acute physical exercise characteristics on cognitive performance. *Sports Medicine* 32(9):555–566, 2002.

Chobanian, A. V., G. L. Bakris, H. R. Black, W. C. Cushman, L. A. Green, J. L. Izzo Jr, D. W. Jones, B. J. Materson, S. Oparil, J. T. Wright Jr, and E. J. Roccella. National Heart, Lung, and Blood Institute Joint National Committee on Prevention, Detection, Evaluation, and Treatment of High Blood Pressure; National High Blood Pressure Education Program Coordinating Committee. The seventh report of the Joint National Committee on Prevention, Detection, Evaluation, and Treatment of High Blood Pressure: The JNC 7 report. *Journal of the American Medical Association* 289(19):2560–2572, 2003.

Haskell, W. L., et al. Physical activity and public health: Updated recommendation for adults from the American College of Sports Medicine and the American Heart Association. *Medicine and Science in Sports and Exercise* 39:1423–1434, 2007.

Pollock, M. L., and J. H. Wilmore. *Exercise in Health and Disease*, 3rd ed. Philadelphia: W. B. Saunders, 1998.

Powers, S., and E. Howley. *Exercise Physiology: Theory and Application to Fitness and Performance*, 7th ed. New York: McGraw-Hill, 2009.

Robertson, Robert. *Perceived Exertion for Practitioners: Rating Effort With the OMNI Picture System*. Champaign, IL: Human Kinetic Publishers, 2004.

Spriet, L. L., and M. J. Gibala. Nutritional strategies to influence adaptations to training. *Journal of Sports Science* 22(1):127–141, 2004.

Warburton, D. E., N. Gledhill, and A. Quinney. Musculoskeletal fitness and health. *Canadian Journal of Applied Physiology* 26(2):217–237, 2001.

For links to the organizations and websites listed below, visit The Total Fitness and Wellness Website at www.pearsonhighered.com/powers.

WebMD
General information about exercise, fitness, and wellness. Great articles, instructional information, and updates.

ACSM
Comprehensive website providing information, articles, equipment recommendations, how-to articles, books, and position statements about all aspects of health and fitness.

FitnessOnline
Provides information, tools, and support to achieve health and fitness goals.

Sympatico: Health
Includes numerous articles, book reviews, and links to nutrition, fitness, and wellness topics.

The Running Page
Contains information about racing, running clubs, places to run, running-related products, magazines, and treating running injuries.

Meriter Fitness
Contains information on injury prevention and treatment, weight training, flexibility, exercise prescriptions, and more.

References

1. Cooper, K. H. *Aerobics*. New York: Bantam Books, 1968.

2. Ross, R., and I. Janssen. Physical activity, total and regional obesity: Dose-response considerations. *Medicine and Science in Sports and Exercise* 33(6):S345–S641, 2001.

3. Kohl, H. W. Physical activity and cardiovascular disease: Evidence for a dose response. *Medicine and Science in Sports and Exercise* 33(6):S472–S483, 2001.

4. Powers, S., and E. Howley. *Exercise Physiology: Theory and Application to Fitness and Performance*, 4th ed. St. Louis, MO: McGraw Hill, 2004.

5. Powers, S., and E. Howley. *Exercise Physiology: Theory and Application to Fitness and Performance*, 7th ed. New York: McGraw-Hill, 2009.

6. Laursen, P. B., and D. G. Jenkins. The scientific basis for high-intensity interval training: Optimising training programmes and maximising performance in highly trained endurance athletes. *Sports Medicine* 32(1):53–73, 2002.

7. Kesaniemi, Y. A., E. Danforth, M. D. Jensen, P. G. Kopelman, P. Lefebvre, and B. A. Reeder. Dose-response issues concerning physical activity and health: An evidence-based symposium. *Medicine and Science in Sports and Exercise* 33(6):S351–S358, 2001.

8. Dunn, A. L., M. H. Trivedi, and H. A. O'Neal. Physical activity dose-response effects on outcomes of depression and anxiety. *Medicine and Science in Sports and Exercise* 33(6):S587–S597, 2001.

9. Gambelunghe, C., R. Rossi, G. Mariucci, M. Tantucci, and M. V. Ambrosini. Effects of light physical exercise on sleep regulation in rats. *Medicine and Science in Sports and Exercise* 33(1):57–60, 2001.

10. American College of Sports Medicine. *ACSM's Guidelines for Exercise Testing and Prescription*, 7th ed. Philadelphia: Lippincott Williams, & Wilkins, 2006.

11. Cooper, K. *The Aerobics Program for Total Well-Being*. New York: M. Evans, 1982.

12. Cooper, K. *The Aerobics Way*. New York: Bantam Books, 1977.

13. Fox, E. A simple technique for predicting maximal aerobic power. *Journal of Applied Physiology* 35:914–916, 1973.

14. Rippe, J., A. Ward., J. Porcari, and P. Freedson. Walking for fitness and health. *Journal of the American Medical Association* 259:2720–2724, 1988.

15. Rippe, J. Walking for fitness: A roundtable. *Physician and Sports Medicine* 14:144–159, 1986.

16. Ward, A., and J. Rippe. *Walking for Health and Fitness*. Philadelphia: J. B. Lippincott, 1988.

17. Pollock, M., J. Wilmore, and S. Fox. *Health and Fitness Through Physical Activity.* New York: John Wiley and Sons, 1978.

18. Mullineaux, D. R., C. A. Barnes, and E. F. Barnes. Factors affecting the likelihood to engage in adequate physical activity to promote health. *Journal of Sports Sciences* 19(4):279–288, 2001.

19. Borg, G. *Borg's Perceived Exertion and Pain Scales*. Champaign, IL: Human Kinetics, 1998.

20. Keating, X. D., J. Guan, J. C. Pinero, D. M. Bridges. A meta-analysis of college students' physical activity behaviors. *Journal of American College Health* 54(2):116–125, 2005.

21. Storms, W. W. Review of exercise-induced asthma. *Medicine and Science in Sports and Exercise* 35 (9):1464–1470, 2003.

Videos

Log on to www.pearsonhighered.com/powers to view these chapter-related videos.

Heart Rate: Carotid Pulse

Heart Rate: Radial Pulse

Step Test

NAME _____ DATE _____

Measuring Cardiorespiratory Fitness: The 1.5-Mile Run Test

The objective of the test is to complete the 1.5-mile distance as quickly as possible. You can complete the run on an oval track or any properly measured course. If the run will take place outside, the test is best conducted in moderate weather conditions; avoid running it on very hot or very cold days. A good strategy is to try to keep a steady pace during the entire distance. Performing a practice test is a good way to get familiar with the distance and determine the ideal pace you can maintain. You should use a stopwatch to get an accurate time. You should attempt this test only if you have met the medical clearance criteria discussed in Chapter 1 of this text.

Before the test, perform a 5- to 10-minute warm-up. If you become extremely fatigued during the test, slow your pace or walk—do not overstress yourself! If you feel faint or nauseated or experience any unusual pains in your upper body, stop and notify your instructor.

After you complete the test, cool down and record your time and fitness category from Table 3.1 included in this lab. Find your age group along the top of the table, and then locate your time range according to your sex. The fitness classifications are along the left of the table.

Test date: _____

Finish time: _____

Fitness category: _____

1. Is your fitness classification what you expected based on your current level of activity? If not, why do you think it was higher or lower than expected?

   _____

   _____

2. Write fitness goals for maintaining or improving your cardiorespiratory endurance. You might have to refer to Chapter 2 for a reminder on how to set goals.

   _____

   _____

LABORATORY

TABLE 3.1
Fitness Categories for Cooper's 1.5-Mile Run Test

Fitness Category	Age (years)					
	13–19	20–29	30–39	40–49	50–59	60+
Men						
Very poor	>15:30	>16:00	>16:30	>17:30	>19:00	>20:00
Poor	12:11–15:30	14:01–16:00	14:46–16:30	15:36–17:30	17:01–19:00	19:01–20:00
Average	10:49–12:10	12:01–14:00	12:31–14:45	13:01–15:35	14:31–17:00	16:16–19:00
Good	9:41–10:48	10:46–12:00	11:01–12:30	11:31–13:00	12:31–14:30	14:00–16:15
Excellent	8:37–9:40	9:45–10:45	10:00–11:00	10:30–11:30	11:00–12:30	11:15–13:59
Superior	<8:37	<9:45	<10:00	<10:30	<11:00	<11:15
Women						
Very poor	>18:30	>19:00	>19:30	>20:00	>20:30	>21:00
Poor	16:55–18:30	18:31–19:00	19:01–19:30	19:31–20:00	20:01–20:30	20:31–21:31
Average	14:31–16:54	15:55–18:30	16:31–19:00	17:31–19:30	19:01–20:00	19:31–20:30
Good	12:30–14:30	13:31–15:54	14:31–16:30	15:56–17:30	16:31–19:00	17:31–19:30
Excellent	11:50–12:29	12:30–13:30	13:00–14:30	13:45–15:55	14:30–16:30	16:30–18:00
Superior	<11:50	<12:30	<13:00	<13:45	<14:30	<16:30

Times are given in minutes and seconds. (> = greater than; < = less than)

Source: From Cooper, K. *The Aerobics Program for Total Well-Being.* Bantam Books, New York, 1982. Copyright © 1982 by Kenneth H. Cooper. Used by permission of Bantam Books, a division of Random House, Inc.

NAME _____ DATE _____

Measuring Cardiorespiratory Fitness:
The 1-Mile Walk Test

The objective of the test is to walk the 1-mile distance as quickly as possible. You can complete the walk on an oval track or any properly measured course. You should attempt this test only if you have met the medical clearance criteria discussed in Chapter 1 of this text.

Before the test, perform a 5- to 10-minute warm-up. If you become extremely fatigued during the test, slow your pace—do not overstress yourself! If you feel faint or nauseated or experience any unusual pains in your upper body, stop and notify your instructor.

After you complete the test, cool down and record your time and fitness category from Table 3.2 included in this lab. Find your age group along the top of the table, and then locate your time range according to your sex. The fitness classifications are along the left of the table.

Test date: _____

Finish time: _____

Fitness category: _____

1. Is your fitness classification what you expected based on your current level of activity? If not, why do you think it was higher or lower than expected?

   _____

   _____

2. Write fitness goals for maintaining or improving your cardiorespiratory endurance. You might have to refer to Chapter 2 for a reminder on how to set goals.

   _____

   _____

TABLE 3.2
Fitness Classification for 1-Mile Walk Test

Fitness Category	Age (years)			
	13–19	20–29	30–39	40+
Men				
Very poor	>17:30	>18:00	>19:00	>21:30
Poor	16:01–17:30	16:31–18:00	17:31–19:00	18:31–21:30
Average	14:01–16:00	14:31–16:30	15:31–17:30	16:01–18:30
Good	12:30–14:00	13:00–14:30	13:30–15:30	14:00–16:00
Excellent	<12:30	<13:00	<13:30	<14:00
Women				
Very poor	>18:01	>18:31	>19:31	>20:01
Poor	16:31–18:00	17:01–18:30	18:01–19:30	19:31–20:00
Average	14:31–16:30	15:01–17:00	16:01–18:00	18:01–19:30
Good	13:31–14:30	13:31–15:00	14:01–16:00	14:31–18:00
Excellent	<13:30	<13:30	<14:00	<14:30

Because the 1-mile walk test is designed primarily for older or less conditioned individuals, the fitness categories listed here do not include a "superior" category.

Source: Modified from *Rockport Fitness Walking Test.* Copyright © 1993. The Rockport Company, Inc. All rights reserved. Reprinted by permission of The Rockport Company, Inc.

NAME _____ DATE _____

Measuring Cardiorespiratory Fitness: Submaximal Cycle Test

This lab test is performed with a partner. While you are exercising, your partner will help by setting the workload for the test, checking your pedal rate, and taking your heart rate. The work performed on a cycle ergometer is commonly expressed either in *kilopond meters per minute (KPM)* or in watts. Your instructor will explain how to use the KPM and watts settings to adjust the workload.

Warm up for 3 minutes without using any resistance (unloaded pedaling). Your instructor will tell you how to adjust the workload. Set the appropriate load for your age, sex, and level of conditioning (Table 3.3), and begin pedaling at the rate of 50 revolutions per minute (RPM). Your instructor will set a metronome so you know how fast to pedal. Exercise for a 5-minute period. Your partner will take your heart rate during a 15-second period between minutes 4.5 and 5 of the test.

Cool down for 3 to 5 minutes without resistance. Record your heart rate (15-second count) below, and calculate your relative $\dot{V}O_2$max using Table 3.4. After calculating your relative $\dot{V}O_2$max, locate your fitness category in Table 3.5.

Test date: _____

Heart rate (15-second count) during minute 5 of test: _____

Fitness category: _____

1. Is your fitness classification what you expected based on your current level of activity? If not, why do you think it was higher or lower than expected?

   _____

   _____

2. Write fitness goals for maintaining or improving your cardiorespiratory endurance. You might have to refer to Chapter 2 for a reminder on how to set goals.

   _____

   _____

TABLE 3.3
Work Rates for Submaximal Cycle Ergometer Fitness Test

Gender	Age (years)	Pedal Speed (RPM)	Load	(watts)
Men				
	Up to 29	50	150	(900 KPM)
	30 and up	50	50	(300 KPM)
Women				
	Up to 29 (or well conditioned)	50	100	(600 KPM)
	30 and up (or poorly conditioned)	50	50	(300 KPM)

TABLE 3.4

Cycle Ergometer Fitness Index for Men and Women

Locate your 15-second heart rate in the left-hand column; then find your estimated $\dot{V}O_2max$ in the appropriate column on the right. For example, the second column from the left contains the absolute $\dot{V}O_2max$ (expressed in mL/min) for male subjects using the 900-KPM work rate. The third column from the left contains the absolute $\dot{V}O_2max$ (expressed in mL/min) for women using the 600-KPM work rate, and so on. After determination of your absolute $\dot{V}O_2max$, calculate your relative $\dot{V}O_2max$ (mL/kg/min) by dividing your $\dot{V}O_2max$ expressed in mL/min by your body weight in kilograms (1 kilogram = 2.2 pounds). For example, if your body weight is 70 kilograms and your absolute $\dot{V}O_2max$ is 2631 mL/min, your relative $\dot{V}O_2max$ is approximately 38 mL/kg/min (i.e., 2631 divided by 70 = 37.6). After computing your relative $\dot{V}O_2max$, use Table 3.5 to identify your fitness category.

15-Second Heart Rate	Estimated Absolute $\dot{V}O_2max$ (mL/min)		
	Men: 900-KPM Work Rate (mL/min)	Women: 600-KPM Work Rate (mL/min)	Men or Women: 300-KPM Work Rate (mL/min)
28	3560	2541	1525
29	3442	2459	1475
30	3333	2376	1425
31	3216	2293	1375
32	3099	2210	1325
33	2982	2127	1275
34	2865	2044	1225
35	2748	1961	1175
36	2631	1878	1125
37	2514	1795	1075
38	2397	1712	1025
39	2280	1629	—
40	2163	1546	—
41	2046	1463	—
42	1929	1380	—
43	1812	1297	—
44	1695	1214	—
45	1578	1131	—

TABLE 3.5
Cardiorespiratory Fitness Norms for Men and Women Based on Estimated $\dot{V}O_2max$ Values Determined by the Cycle Ergometer Fitness Test

After determining your relative $\dot{V}O_2max$ (mL/kg/min) in Table 3.4, find your appropriate fitness category.

Age Group (years)	Fitness Categories Based on $\dot{V}O_2max$ (mL/kg/min)					
	Very Poor	Poor	Average	Good	Excellent	Superior
Men						
18–25	<30	30–39	40–45	46–60	61–64	>64
26–35	<29	29–38	39–43	44–55	56–59	>59
36–45	<27	27–35	36–40	41–49	50–55	>55
46–45	<25	25–31	32–35	36–45	46–49	>49
56–65	<22	22–28	29–33	34–40	41–43	>43
>65	<20	20–25	26–28	29–34	35–38	>38
Women						
18–25	<30	30–38	39–43	44–54	55–58	>58
26–35	<28	28–33	34–41	42–53	54–58	>58
36–45	<24	24–32	33–36	37–46	47–50	>50
46–55	<22	22–28	29–31	32–41	42–45	>45
56–65	<19	19–25	26–29	30–36	37–40	>40
>65	<17	17–21	22–25	26–30	31–34	>34

Source: Data reprinted from Golding, L., (ed.). *YMCA Fitness Testing and Assessment Manual,* 4th Edition. With permission of the YMCA of the USA, Chicago IL. Copyright © 2000.

LABORATORY

NAME _____ DATE _____

Measuring Cardiorespiratory Fitness: Step Test

To complete this test, you need a step or bench that is approximately 18 inches high, such as a locker room bench or a sturdy chair. The step test lasts for 3 minutes, and then heart rate is assessed in the 3.5 minutes following the test. You will need a metronome to help you maintain the step rate.

   To perform this test, you will step up and down at a rate of 30 complete steps per minute. If you set the metronome to 60 tones per minute, you will step with each tone making a complete step (up, up, down, down) every 2 seconds. Note that it is important that you straighten your knees during the "up" phase of the test. After you complete the test, sit quietly in a chair or on the step bench, and take your heart rate for 30 seconds at the following times:

1 to 1.5 minutes post exercise

2 to 2.5 minutes post exercise

3 to 3.5 minutes post exercise

▷ Log on to **www.pearsonhighered.com/powers** to view a demonstration video of the step test.

Subject steps up onto an 18-inch surface and then down once every 2 seconds. Set metronome to 60 tones per minute.

Maintaining the 30-step-per-minute cadence and accurately taking your heart rate are very important for getting a good estimate from the step test. To determine your fitness category, add the three 30-second heart rates obtained during the period after exercise.

Record your heart rates below, and use Table 3.6 on this page to determine your fitness category.

Test date: _____

Recovery heart rate post exercise (bpm)

1–1.5 min: _____

2–2.5 min: _____

3–3.5 min: _____

Total (recovery index): _____

Fitness category: _____

TABLE 3.6
Norms for Cardiorespiratory Fitness Using the Sum of Three Recovery Heart Rates Obtained Following the Step Test

Fitness Category	3-Minute Step Test Recovery Index	
	Women	Men
Superior	95–120	95–117
Excellent	121–135	118–132
Good	136–153	133–147
Average	154–174	148–165
Poor	175–204	166–192
Very Poor	205–233	193–217

Fitness categories are for college-aged men and women (aged 18–25 years) at the University of Florida who performed the test on an 18-inch bench.

1. Is your fitness classification what you expected based on your current level of activity? If not, why do you think it was higher or lower than expected?

   _____

   _____

2. Write fitness goals for maintaining or improving your cardiorespiratory endurance. You might have to refer to Chapter 2 for a reminder on how to set goals.

   _____

   _____

NAME _____ DATE _____

Assessing Cardiorespiratory Fitness for Individuals with Disabilities

This test uses arm exercise and is for people who cannot perform exercise that requires use of the legs (people in wheelchairs or with leg or foot injuries). To perform this assessment, you will need an arm crank ergometer. Your instructor will adjust the ergometer to the correct height and position for the test.

First, do a warm-up with no resistance. Then your instructor will increase the resistance, and you will perform a 2-minute stage. Rest 5 to 10 minutes. Then, after your instructor increases the workload, perform another 2-minute period of arm exercise. Repeat this cycle until you cannot complete 2 minutes of exercise at a given workload. Your instructor will tell you the workload for the last stage in which you completed the full 2 minutes of exercise. You can use that number, along with Table 3.7 included in this lab, to determine your $\dot{V}O_2$max. After you find your weight and workload on the table, find the corresponding number and multiple that value by 3.5 to get your $\dot{V}O_2$max. If your weight is not on the table, you can use the following equation to calculate your $\dot{V}O_2$max:

$$\dot{V}O_2\text{max} = 3 \times (\text{work rate*})/\text{body weight in kg} \dagger + 3.5$$

Table 3.5 in Laboratory 3.1C has the fitness classifications that correspond to your $\dot{V}O_2$max. Because this test uses arm exercise, which involves a smaller muscle mass than leg or whole body exercise, your $\dot{V}O_2$max estimate will be a slight underestimate.

Fitness category: _____

1. Is your fitness classification what you expected based on your current level of activity? If not, why do you think it was higher or lower than expected?

   _____

   _____

2. Write fitness goals for maintaining or improving your cardiorespiratory endurance. You might have to refer to Chapter 2 for a reminder on how to set goals.

   _____

   _____

* Your instructor will give you this value.
† Weight in kg = weight in lbs ÷ 2.2

TABLE 3.7

Approximate Energy Requirements in METs* during Arm Ergometry

Body Weight		Power Output (kg/g/min and W†)					
		150	300	450	600	750	900 (kg/m/min)
kg	lb	25	50	75	100	125	150 (W)
50	110	3.6	6.1	8.7	11.3	13.9	16.4
60	132	3.1	5.3	7.4	9.6	11.7	13.9
70	154	2.8	4.7	6.5	8.3	10.2	12.0
80	176	2.6	4.2	5.8	7.4	9.0	10.6
90	198	2.4	3.9	5.3	6.7	8.1	9.6
100	220	2.3	3.6	4.9	6.1	7.4	8.7

* 1 MET=3.5 ml/kg/mín. This value is your $\dot{V}O_2$ at rest.

† W = watts.

Source: From American College of Sports Medicine. *ACSM's Guideline for Exercise Testing and Prescription,* 7th ed. Philadelphia: Lippincott, Williams, & Wilkins, 2006.

NAME _____ DATE _____

Determining Target Heart Rate

Practice taking your heart rate at both the carotid and radial locations. You can feel the carotid pulse next to the larynx, beneath the lower jaw. The radial pulse is located on the inside of the wrist, directly in line with the base of the thumb. Use a stopwatch to count for 15, 30, and 60 seconds. To determine your heart rate in beats per minute (bpm), multiply your 15-second count by 4, and your 30-second count by 2.

Try locating and taking the heart rate of a classmate at both the radial and carotid locations. Record your resting pulse counts in the spaces provided.

▷ Log on to **www.pearsonhighered.com/powers** to view demonstration videos of locating the radical and carotid pulses.

Carotid Pulse Count (self)	Heart Rate (bpm)	Radial Pulse Count (self)	Heart Rate (bpm)
15 seconds × 4		× 4	
30 seconds × 2		× 2	
60 seconds × 1		× 1	
Carotid Pulse Count (partner)	Heart Rate (bpm)	Radial Pulse Count (partner)	Heart Rate (bpm)
15 seconds × 4		× 4	
30 seconds × 2		× 2	
60 seconds × 1		× 1	

The target heart rate (THR) range is calculated in steps.

Step 1: Calculate your estimated maximal heart rate (HR_{max})

$$HR_{max} = 220 - age \underline{\qquad}$$

Step 2: Calculate your heart rate reserve (HRR) by subtracting your resting heart rate from your HR_{max} (use the 60-second count from above).

$$HRR = HR_{max} - resting\ heart\ rate$$
$$HRR = \underline{\qquad} - \underline{\qquad}$$
$$HRR = \underline{\qquad\qquad}$$

Step 3: Calculate 50% and 85% HRR (use decimal values)

Lower end of THR = 0.5 (HRR) = _____
Upper end of THR = 0.85 (HRR) = _____

Step 4: Add your resting heart rate back to these values

50% HRR + resting heart rate = _____

85% HRR + resting heart rate = _____

THR = _____ bpm to _____ bpm

1. Which of the resting pulses did you find easiest to locate on yourself?

   _____Carotid   _____ Radial

2. Which resting pulse was easiest to locate on your partner?

   _____Carotid   _____ Radial

3. Which of the two locations would you prefer to use when counting exercise heart rate?

   _____Carotid   _____ Radial

   Why? _____

NAME _____ DATE _____

Developing Your Personal Exercise Prescription

Using the boxes on pages 66–68 as models, develop your personal exercise program based on your current fitness level and goals. Record the appropriate information in the spaces provided below.

Week No.	Phase	Duration (min/day)	Intensity (% of HHR or RPE)	Frequency (days/week)	Exercise Mode	Comments
1						
2						
3						
4						
5						
6						
7						
8						
9						
10						
11						
12						
13						
14						
15						
16						

NAME _____ DATE _____

Determining Rate of Perceived Exertion

Rate of perceived exertion (RPE) was originally developed to correspond to heart rates. Adding a zero to the numerical rating produces the expected heart rate range for that rating. However, people perceive exertion differently, so ratings do not always match heart rate values. The important thing to learn is the RPE number that corresponds to your threshold of training heart rate and the RPE that represents the upper-limit heart rate of your target heart rate (THR) range. Typically, numerical RPE ratings for exercise in the THR zone will fall between 12 and 16. With practice, you can learn to make accurate ratings.

Use the following RPE scale to rate your exertion.

Scale	Verbal Rating
6	No exertion at all
7	Extremely light
8	
9	Very light
10	
11	Light
12	
13	Somewhat hard
14	
15	Hard (heavy)
16	
17	Very hard
18	
19	Extremely hard
20	Maximal exertion

Perform the following exercises:

1. Walk for 3 minutes at a brisk pace.

2. Jog for 3 minutes at a slow pace.

3. Jog for 3 minutes at a pace that will elevate your heart rate to your threshold level.

(continued)

After each exercise bout, take your heart rate. Also, rate the intensity of the exercise at the end of minute 3 using the RPE scale above. Record these values on the table that follows.

Next, perform a more intense 3-minute run that elevates your heart rate to the upper one-third of your THR zone. After the run, take your heart rate and give an RPE value.

Activity	Heart Rate (bpm)	Rating of Perceived Exertion
Walk		
Slow jog		
Faster jog (to reach training threshold)		
Intense run		

After you've completed your slow and faster jogs, answer the following questions:

1. Did you reach your heart rate training threshold with the walk or slow jog? ___ Yes ___ No

2. Was your RPE less than 12 for the walk or slow jog? ___ Yes ___ No

3. Was your RPE for the faster jog in the range of 12 to 16? ___ Yes ___ No

4. Did your heart rate reach the upper end of your THR for the run? ___ Yes ___ No

5. Was your RPE in the intense run in the range of 12 to 16? ___ Yes ___ No

6. Was your heart approximately 10 times your RPE? ___ Yes ___ No

7. With practice, do you think you could learn to use the RPE scale to assess your exercise intensity? _____

8. What are the limitations for using heart rate to assess your exercise intensity?

_____

_____

9. What are the limitations for using RPE to assess your exercise intensity?

_____

_____

Improving Muscular Strength and Endurance

4

true or false?

1. Women who lift weights will quickly develop "bulky" muscles.

2. Increasing muscle endurance will always increase muscle strength.

3. Muscle turns to fat if you don't use it regularly.

4. Weight lifters should take protein or other supplements to get bigger faster.

5. Strength training is important only when you are young.

Answers appear on the next page.

Can you imagine running the 26 continuous miles of a marathon or biking the 2241 miles in the Tour de France? Or would you consider competing in the Iron Man triathlon, in which you swim 2.4 miles, bike 112 miles, and then run 26.2 miles, all in less than 9 hours? These extraordinary feats of human performance are all possible because of the human body's great capacity for muscular strength and endurance. And although not everyone will compete in a bike race, marathon, or triathalon, improved muscular strength and endurance offers numerous everyday benefits for everyone.

In this chapter you'll learn about the everyday benefits of muscle strength and endurance, the anatomy and physiology behind them, how to assess your own level of muscle fitness, and how to develop an exercise plan to improve your strength and endurance.

The Need for Muscular Strength and Endurance in Daily Living

When you climb a flight of stairs or carry a heavy book bag across campus, you're relying on your muscular strength and endurance to perform the task without becoming exhausted. If you've ever worked in a job that required you to shuttle loaded trays of food among tables or move boxes from points A to B, you've relied on strength and endurance to earn your living. And if you play competitive or recreational sports, your skill level is determined in large part by the strength and reliability of your muscles. Whether we're aware of it or not, the strength and endurance of our muscles affects our physical performance numerous times every day.

Recall from Chapter 1 that muscular strength and endurance are related but are not the same thing. Muscular strength is the ability of a muscle to generate maximal force. In simple terms, muscular strength is the amount of weight that an individual can lift during one maximal effort. In contrast, muscular endurance is the ability to generate force over and over again. In general, increasing muscular strength by exercise training will also increase muscle endurance. However, training to improve muscular endurance does not significantly improve muscular strength.

Muscle strength and endurance can be increased and maintained with strength-training and endurance-training programs. In addition, regular strength training promotes numerous health benefits. For example, incidence of low back pain, a common problem in both men and women, can be reduced with the appropriate strengthening exercises for the lower back and abdominal muscles (1). Further, studies demonstrate that muscle-strengthening exercises may reduce the occurrence of joint and/or muscle injuries that occur during physical activity (2). Strength training can also delay the decrease in muscle strength experienced by sedentary older individuals (3) and may help prevent osteoporosis.

Another important benefit of strength training is that it increases **resting energy expenditure** in larger muscles. (4). Resting energy expenditure (also called *resting metabolic rate*) includes the energy required to drive the heart and respiratory muscles and to build

Answers

1. **FALSE** The male sex hormone testosterone affects muscle size. With the same amount of training, men will gain more muscle mass than women because they produce more testosterone.

2. **FALSE** The intensity and number of exercises you do to improve muscular endurance will not necessarily improve muscular strength.

3. **FALSE** Fat and muscle are two different types of tissue, and one cannot convert to the other. However, if you stop exercise and consume more calories than you expend, you may build up more fat tissue, and you will probably notice it in your physical appearance.

4. **FALSE** Buying supplements such as protein powders or pills is mostly a waste of your hard-earned funds. Although athletes do need slightly higher amounts of protein than less active people, their needs can be easily met through a healthy diet, so supplements are unnecessary.

5. **FALSE** Muscle strength and endurance are needed throughout the life span. Strength training for older individuals has been shown to help prevent falls and allow for independent living.

and maintain body tissues. An elevated metabolic rate allows the body to burn more calories throughout the day. Conversely, a lower metabolic rate burns fewer calories, thereby leading to weight gain.

How does strength training influence resting metabolic rate? One of the primary results of strength training is an increase in muscle mass in relation to body fat. An increase of 1 pound of muscle elevates resting metabolism by approximately 2–3%. This increase can be magnified with larger gains in muscle. For instance, a 5-pound increase in muscle mass results in a 10–15% increase in resting metabolic rate. Changes in resting metabolic rate of this magnitude can play an important role in helping you lose weight or maintaining desirable body composition throughout life. Although overall body weight may increase slightly as muscle mass increases, fat mass should decrease. Clothing may fit better, and self-image is likely to improve.

You now know that strength training will increase muscle mass. But how does this work, and how do muscles, in general work? We'll discuss this next.

Make sure you know...

> Muscular strength and endurance are important for numerous daily tasks. Strength training can reduce low back pain, reduce the incidence of exercise-related injuries, decrease the incidence of osteoporosis, and help maintain functional capacity that normally decreases with age.

> Muscular strength is the ability to generate maximal force, whereas muscular endurance is the ability to generate force over and over again.

> Strength training can improve a muscle's resting energy expenditure.

How Muscles Work: Structure and Function

There are about 600 skeletal muscles in the human body, and their primary function is to provide force for physical movement. When the muscles shorten or lengthen during a **muscle action,** they apply force to the bones, causing the body to move.

The skeletal muscles also are responsible for maintaining posture and help regulate body temperature through the mechanism of shivering (which results in heat production). Because all fitness activities require the use of skeletal muscles, anyone beginning a physical fitness program should understand basic muscle structure and function.

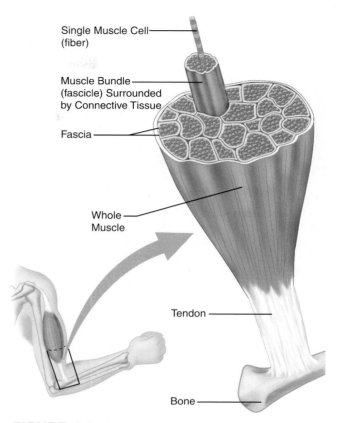

FIGURE 4.1
The structure of skeletal muscle.
Source: Johnson, M. *Human Biology,* 4th ed. San Francisco: Benjamin Cummings, 2008.

Muscle Structure

Skeletal muscle is a collection of long, thin cells called *fibers*. These fibers are surrounded by a dense layer of connective tissue called **fascia** that holds the individual fibers together and separates muscle from surrounding tissues (Figure 4.1).

Muscles are attached to bones by connective tissues known as **tendons.** Muscular action causes the tendons to pull on the bones, thereby causing movement. Muscles cannot push the bones; they can only

---

resting energy expenditure The amount of energy expended during all sedentary activities. Also called *resting metabolic rate.*

muscle action The shortening of a skeletal muscle (causing movement) or the lengthening of a skeletal muscle (resisting movement).

fascia A thin layer of connective tissue that surrounds the muscle.

tendon A fibrous connective tissue that attaches muscle to bone.

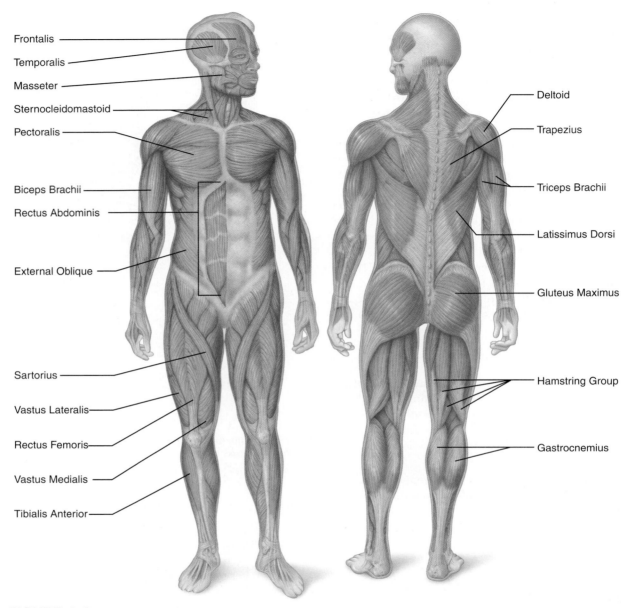

FIGURE 4.2
Major muscles of the human body.
Source: Johnson, M. *Human Biology,* 4th ed. San Francisco: Benjamin Cummings, 2008.

pull them. Many of the muscles involved in movement are illustrated in Figure 4.2.

Muscle Function

Muscle actions are regulated by electrical signals from motor nerves. Motor nerves originate in the spinal cord and send messages to individual muscles throughout the body. A motor nerve and an individual muscle fiber make contact at a neuromuscular junction (Figure 4.3). Note from the figure that each motor nerve branches

and then connects with numerous individual muscle fibers.

The motor nerve and all of the muscle fibers it controls comprise a **motor unit.** Motor units come in various sizes, depending on how many muscle fibers they contain. A motor nerve can innervate a few muscle fibers for fine motor control, such as blinking the eye, or it can innervate many muscle fibers for gross motor movement, such as kicking a ball.

A muscle action begins when a message to develop tension (called a nerve impulse) reaches the neuromus-

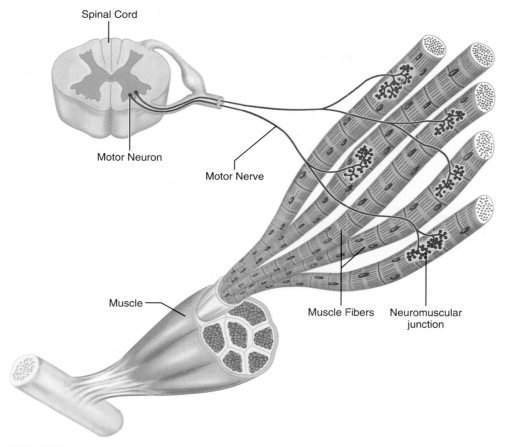

FIGURE 4.3
A motor unit. Two motor nerves from the central nervous system are shown innervating several muscle fibers. With one impulse from the motor nerve, all fibers respond.

cular junction. The arrival of the nerve impulse triggers the action process by permitting the interaction of contractile proteins in muscle. Just as the nerve impulse initiates the contractile process, the removal of the nerve signal from the muscle "turns it off." That is, when a motor nerve ceases to send signals to a muscle, the muscle action stops. Occasionally, however, an uncontrolled muscular action occurs, which results in a muscle cramp or a muscle twitch.

Muscle Exercise and Muscle Actions

Skeletal muscle exercise is classified into three major categories: **isotonic, isometric,** and **isokinetic.** Isotonic (also called *dynamic*) exercise results in movement of a body part at a joint. Most exercise or sports activities are isotonic. For example, lifting a dumbbell involves movement of the forearm and is therefore classified as an isotonic exercise.

An isometric (also called *static*) exercise requires the development of muscular tension but results in no movement of body parts. A classic example of isometric

exercise is pressing the palms of the hands together. Although there is tension within the muscles of the arms and chest, the arms do not move. Isometric exercises are an excellent way to develop strength during the early stages of an injury rehabilitation program.

Isokinetic exercises are performed at a constant velocity; that is, the speed of muscle shortening or lengthening is regulated at a fixed, controlled rate. This is generally accomplished by using a machine

motor unit A motor nerve and all of the muscle fibers it controls.

isotonic A type of exercise in which there is movement of a body part. Most exercise or sports skills are isotonic exercise. Also called *dynamic* exercise.

isometric A type of exercise in which muscular tension is developed but the body part does not move. Also called *static* exercise.

isokinetic A type of exercise that can include concentric or eccentric muscle actions performed at a constant speed using a specialized machine.

Concentric Action

Eccentric Action

FIGURE 4.4
Concentric and eccentric muscle actions in an isotonic exercise. The muscle shortens during a concentric action and lengthens during an eccentric action.
Source: Adapted from Powers, S., and E. Howley. *Exercise Physiology: Theory and Application to Fitness and Performance,* 7th ed. Copyright 2009. Reprinted by permission of McGraw-Hill Companies.

that provides an accommodating resistance throughout the full **range of motion.**

Muscle actions can similarly be classified as isometric, concentric, or eccentric, depending on the activity the muscle needs to perform. Like isometric exercise, isometric muscle actions are static and do not involve any joint movement. An isometric muscle action occurs during isometric exercises.

A **concentric muscle action** causes movement of the body part against resistance or gravity and occurs when the muscle shortens. Concentric muscle actions (also called *positive work*) can be performed during isotonic or isokinetic exercise. For example, the upward movement of the arm during a bicep curl (Figure 4.4, top) is an example of a concentric muscle action.

In contrast, **eccentric muscle actions** (also called *negative work*) control movement with resistance or gravity and occur when the muscle lengthens. The downward or lowering phase of the bicep curl is controlled as the biceps muscle lengthens (Figure 4.4, bottom). Here, the muscle is developing tension, but the force developed is not great enough to prevent the weight from being lowered.

Types of Muscle Fibers

There are three types of skeletal muscle fibers: slow-twitch, intermediate, and fast-twitch. These fiber types differ in their speeds of action and in fatigue resistance (5). Because most human muscles contain a mixture of

all three fiber types, it is helpful to understand each of them before beginning the strength-training process.

Slow-Twitch Fibers   As the name implies, **slow-twitch fibers** contract slowly and produce small amounts of force; however, these fibers are highly resistant to fatigue. Slow-twitch fibers appear red or darker in color because of the numerous capillaries that supply the fibers. They have the capacity to produce large quantities of adenosine triphosphate (ATP) aerobically, which makes them ideally suited for a low-intensity, prolonged exercise, such as walking or slow jogging. Because of their resistance to fatigue, most postural muscles are composed primarily of slow-twitch fibers.

Fast-Twitch Fibers   **Fast-twitch fibers** contract rapidly and generate great amounts of force, but fatigue quickly. These fibers have a low aerobic capacity and appear white because they are supplied by only a few capillaries. Fast-twitch fibers are well equipped to produce ATP anaerobically, but only for a short time. With their ability to shorten rapidly and produce large amounts of force, fast-twitch fibers are used during activities requiring rapid or forceful movement, such as jumping, sprinting, and weight lifting. In strenuous exercise, these fibers are most easily damaged and cause soreness.

Intermediate Fibers   **Intermediate fibers** have a combination of characteristics found in fast- and slow-twitch fibers. They contract rapidly, produce great force, and resist fatigue because they have a well-developed aerobic capacity. Intermediate fibers contract more quickly and produce more force than slow-twitch fibers, but they contract more slowly and produce less force than fast-twitch fibers. They are slightly redder in appearance than fast-twitch fibers but are not as red as the slow-twitch fibers. Table 4.1 summarizes the properties of all three fiber types.

You can see the differences in fiber types during your next chicken or turkey dinner. The dark meat of a chicken drumstick contains primarily slow-twitch fibers. Because these fibers are slow to fatigue, a living bird is able to walk around most of the day. The white meat in the chicken breast is composed of mostly fast-twitch fibers. Fast-twitch fibers allow the bird to fly, but only for short distances before fatiguing. The intermediate fibers found in the bird's wings exhibit the beneficial characteristics of each fiber type—they resist fatigue and generate high force.

Individual Variations in Fiber Type

People vary in the number of slow-twitch, intermediate, and fast-twitch fibers their muscles contain; however, the average nonathlete generally has equal num-

TABLE 4.1
Properties of Human Skeletal Muscle Fiber Types

	Fiber Type		
Property	Slow-Twitch	Intermediate	Fast-Twitch
Contraction speed	Slow	Intermediate	Fast
Resistance to fatigue	High	Intermediate	Low
Predominant energy system	Aerobic	Combination aerobic and anaerobic	Anaerobic
Force generation	Low	Intermediate	High
Color	Red	White (pink)	White
Best suited for	Endurance events (marathon)	Middle-distance events (5–10 K)	Fast events (100-m sprint)

bers of all three fiber types. Research has shown a relationship between muscle fiber type and athletic success. For example, champion endurance athletes, such as marathon runners, have a predominance of slow-twitch fibers. This finding is logical, because endurance sports require muscles with high fatigue resistance. In contrast, elite sprinters, such as 100-meter runners, have more fast-twitch fibers.

Muscle fiber type has also been suggested as a link to obesity and diabetes (6, 7). Individuals with a predominance of fast-twitch muscle fibers may be more susceptible to obesity and developing diabetes than those with a predominance of slow-twitch muscle fibers.

Some evidence has shown that fibers can be converted from one type to another. For example, endurance training has been shown to cause some fiber conversion between the intermediate- and fast-twitch fibers. However, there is limited evidence to support that fast- or intermediate-twitch fibers convert to slow-twitch fibers (8). This means that athletes that do well in short distances can stretch their careers by moving to intermediate distances, and athletes that do well at long distances can also move to the intermediate distances. But a long-distance athlete would not be able to switch to a short-distance event. Lance Armstrong, for example, started doing Iron Man for Kids triathlons when he was 13. He has had a great career as a long-distance bicyclist and has run several marathons.

Although endurance exercise training has been shown to cause some fiber conversion, the number and percentage of skeletal muscle fiber types are strongly influenced by genetics (5).

Recruitment of Muscle Fibers during Exercise

Many types of exercise use only a small fraction of the muscle fibers available in a muscle group. For example,

walking at a slow speed may use fewer than 30% of the muscle fibers in the legs. More intense types of exercise, however, require more force. To generate more force, a greater number of muscle fibers must be called into play. The process of involving more muscle fibers to produce increased muscular force is called **fiber recruitment.** Figure 4.5 illustrates the order in which muscle fibers are recruited as the intensity of exercise increases. Note that during low-intensity exercise, only slow-twitch fibers are used. As the exercise intensity increases, fibers are progressively recruited, from slow-twitch to intermediate fibers and finally to fast-twitch fibers. High-intensity activities, such as weight training, recruit large numbers of fast-twitch fibers.

range of motion The amount of movement possible at a joint.

concentric muscle action Action in which the muscle develops tension as it shortens against resistance and/or gravity. Also called *positive work.*

eccentric muscle action Action in which the muscle develops tension as it lengthens while controlling the movement with gravity. Also called *negative work.*

slow-twitch fibers Red muscle fibers that contract slowly and are highly resistant to fatigue. These fibers have the capacity to produce large quantities of ATP aerobically.

fast-twitch fibers White muscle fibers that contract rapidly but fatigue quickly. These fibers have a low aerobic capacity and produce ATP anaerobically.

intermediate fibers Muscle fibers with a combination of the characteristics of fast- and slow-twitch fibers. They contract rapidly and are fatigue resistant because they have a well-developed aerobic capacity.

fiber recruitment The process of involving more muscle fibers to increase muscular force.

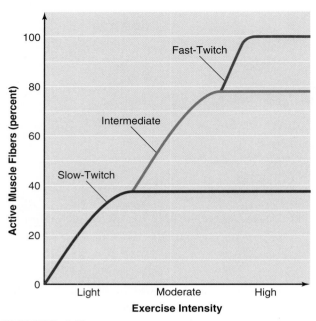

FIGURE 4.5

The relationship between exercise intensity and recruitment of muscle-fiber type.

Source: Adapted from Powers, S., and E. Howley. *Exercise Physiology: Theory and Application to Fitness and Performance*, 7th ed. Copyright 2009. Reprinted by permission of McGraw-Hill Companies.

Muscular Strength

Two physiological factors determine the amount of force that a muscle can generate: the size of the muscle and the number of fibers recruited during the contraction. Muscle size is the primary factor. The larger the muscle, the greater the force it can produce.

Although there is no difference in the chemical makeup of muscle in men and women, men tend to have more muscle mass and are therefore generally stronger. The larger muscle mass is due to higher levels of the hormone testosterone in men, which helps build muscle. The fact that testosterone promotes an increase in muscle size has led some athletes to use drugs in an attempt to improve muscular strength (see A Closer Look below).

The other significant factor that determines how much force is generated is the number of fibers recruited for a given movement. The more muscle fibers that are stimulated, the greater the total muscle force generated, because the force generated by individual fibers is additive (Figure 4.6).

Muscle fiber recruitment is regulated voluntarily through the nervous system. That is, we decide how much effort to put into a particular movement. For instance, when we choose to make a minimal effort to lift an object, we recruit only a few motor units, and the muscle develops limited force. However, if we decide to exert maximal effort to lift a heavy object, many muscle fibers are recruited, and a larger force is generated. Have you ever tried to open a locked door? If you didn't know the door was locked, your first attempt might involve minimal effort and few muscle fibers, because you hadn't anticipated having to use much force. However, once your first attempt didn't work, you might try again and recruit more muscle fibers to call upon more force to open the door. This process might continue until you either exerted enough force to yank the door open or gave up to go look for the key.

A CLOSER LOOK: ANABOLIC STEROID USE INCREASES MUSCLE SIZE BUT HAS SERIOUS SIDE EFFECTS

The abuse of *anabolic steroids* (synthetic forms of the hormone testosterone) and their precursors has mushroomed over the past several decades. The fierce competition in body building and other sports that require strength and power has driven both men and women to risk serious health consequences in the quest to develop large muscles.

The large doses of steroids needed to increase muscle mass produce several health risks. A partial list of the side effects caused by abusing steroids and

their precursors includes liver cancer, increased blood pressure, increased levels of "bad" cholesterol, severe depression, and prostate cancer. Prolonged use and high doses of steroids can be lethal.

One of the most popular chemical precursors to testosterone, androstenedione, is used to increase blood testosterone with the intent to increase strength, lean body mass, and sexual performance. However, research indicates that androstenedione does not significantly increase strength and/or lean body mass.

Another precursor to testosterone production in the body, dehydroepiandrosterone (DHEA), has also been used to increase testosterone in the body. DHEA is also advertised as a weight-loss and anti-aging supplement capable of improving libido, vitality, and immunity levels. However, the best evidence demonstrates that DHEA supplementation does not increase testosterone concentrations or increase strength in men, and it may have masculinizing effects in women.

Make sure you know...

> Skeletal muscle is composed of various types of fibers that are attached to bone by tendons.

> Skeletal muscle actions are regulated by signals coming from motor nerves. A motor unit consists of a motor nerve and all the muscle fibers it controls.

> Exercise can be isometric, isotonic, or isokinetic. Isometric actions do not result in movement, whereas isotonic actions move a body part.

> Isometric exercise involves isometric muscle actions. Isotonic and isokinetic exercises use concentric actions (muscle shortens) and eccentric actions (muscle lengthens).

> Slow-twitch muscle fibers shorten slowly but are fatigue resistant. Fast-twitch fibers shorten rapidly but fatigue rapidly. Intermediate fibers shorten quickly but fatigue slowly.

> The process of involving more muscle fibers to produce increased muscular force is called fiber recruitment.

> Two factors determine muscle force: the size of the muscle and the number of fibers recruited.

Evaluation of Muscular Strength and Endurance

Muscular strength can be assessed by the **one-repetition maximum (1 RM) test,** which measures the maximum amount of weight that can be lifted one time. Although the 1 RM test for muscular strength is widely accepted, it has been criticized as unsuitable for use by older individuals or highly deconditioned people (9). The major concern is the risk of injury. The 1 RM test should therefore be attempted only after several weeks of strength training, which will improve both skill and strength and will reduce the risk of injury. An older or sedentary individual would probably require 6 weeks of exercise training prior to the 1 RM test, whereas a physically active college-aged student could probably perform the 1 RM test after 1 to 2 weeks of training. See Laboratory 4.1 for a step-by-step walk-through of the 1 RM test.

To further reduce the possibility of injury during strength testing, researchers have also developed a method to estimate the 1 RM using a series of submaximal lifts. Although this method is slightly less accurate, it does reduce the risk of injury. You can read instructions for performing this test in Laboratory 4.2.

Muscular endurance is usually evaluated with two simple tests: the **push-up test** and either the **sit-up test** or **curl-up test.** Push-ups require endurance of

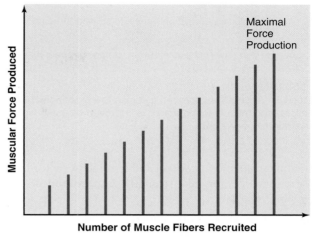

FIGURE 4.6
The relationship between recruitment of motor units and production of muscular force.

the shoulder, arm, and chest muscles, whereas sits-ups and curl-ups primarily require endurance of the abdominal muscles. To learn how to perform these tests and assess your own muscular endurance, turn to Laboratory 4.3 at the end of the chapter.

Make sure you know...

> The 1 RM test can be used to evaluate muscular strength.

> To reduce the possibility of injury, the estimated 1 RM test can be performed instead of the 1 RM test.

> The push-up and sit-up (or curl-up) tests are used to evaluate muscular endurance.

Principles for Designing a Strength and Endurance Program

In Chapter 2 we discussed the general principles for developing training programs to improve physical fitness. Before we discuss the specifics of how to develop a strength-training program, let's discuss how two

---

one-repetition maximum (1 RM) test Measurement of the maximum amount of weight that can be lifted one time.

push-up test A fitness test designed to evaluate endurance of shoulder and arm muscles.

sit-up test A test to evaluate abdominal and hip muscle endurance.

curl-up test A test to evaluate abdominal muscle endurance.

| High Resistance + Low Repetitions = Increased Strength |
| Low Resistance + High Repetitions = Increased Endurance |

FIGURE 4.7
Muscular strength is improved by using low repetitions/high weight, and muscular endurance is improved by using high repetitions/low weight.

training principles, overload and specificity, factor in the design of a muscular strength- and endurance-training program.

Progressive Resistance Exercise

The concept of **progressive resistance exercise (PRE)** is an application of the overload principle to strength and endurance exercise programs. If your goal is to develop strong biceps muscles, you must progressively increase the resistance that you lift. For example, you may begin your program using 10-pound dumbbells and perform one set of 8 repetitions 3 times a week. As this exercise becomes easier, you can progressively increase the workload by increasing the weight, increasing the number of sets up to 3, and/or increasing the number of repetitions up to 12.

Specificity of Training

The principle of **specificity of training** states that development of muscular strength and endurance is specific to both the muscle group that is exercised and the training intensity. Only those muscles that are trained will improve in strength and endurance. To improve the strength of the back muscles, for example, you need to train the specific muscles involved with movement of the lower back.

The intensity of training will determine whether the muscular adaptation is primarily an increase in strength or in endurance (Figure 4.7). High-intensity training (e.g., lifting heavy weights 6 to 8 times) increases muscular strength but yields only limited improvements in muscular endurance. Conversely, high-repetition, low-intensity training (e.g., lifting light weights 20–25 times or more) increases muscular endurance but yields only limited improvements in muscular strength.

Make sure you know...

> In the context of strength and endurance training, the PRE principle means you need to progressively increase the amount of resistance with which you train.

> The intensity of training determines whether you primarily increase muscular strength or endurance. High-intensity training will increase muscle strength and size; low-intensity training will increase muscular endurance.

Strength Training: How the Body Adapts

What physiological changes result from strength training? How quickly can you gain muscular strength? Do men and women differ in their responses to weight-training programs? Let's address these questions next.

Physiological Changes Due to Weight Training

You now know that programs designed to improve muscular strength can do so only by increasing muscular size and/or by increasing the number of muscle fibers recruited. Strength training alters both these factors (10). Research has shown that strength-training programs increase muscular strength first by altering fiber recruitment patterns, and then by increasing muscle size.

Increase in muscle size is due primarily to an increase in fiber size, called **hypertrophy** (10). Most research has shown that strength training has little effect on the formation of new muscle fibers, a process called **hyperplasia.** The role that hyperplasia plays in the increase in muscle size due to strength training remains controversial (11). Regardless, the increase in muscle size depends on diet, the muscle fiber type (fast-twitch fibers may hypertrophy more than slow-twitch fibers), blood levels of testosterone, and the type of training program.

Although strength training does not result in significant improvements in cardiorespiratory fitness (12), a regular weight-training program can provide positive changes in both body composition and flexibility. For most men and women, rigorous weight training results in an increase in muscle mass and in loss of body fat, both of which decrease the percentage of body fat.

Performing weight-training exercises over the full range of motion at a joint can improve flexibility (9). In fact, many diligent weight lifters have excellent flexibility. Therefore, the notion that weight lifting causes inflexibility is generally incorrect.

Rate of Strength Improvement with Weight Training

How rapidly does strength improvement occur? The answer depends on your initial strength level. Strength gains occur rapidly in untrained people, whereas gains are more gradual in individuals with relatively higher strength levels. In fact, for a novice lifter, strength gains can occur very quickly (13). These rapid strength gains tend to motivate the lifter to stick with a regular weight-training program.

Gender Differences in Response to Weight Training

Men and women do not differ in their initial responses to weight training programs (14). On a percentage basis, women gain strength as rapidly as men during the first 12 weeks of a strength-training program. However, as a result of long-term weight training, men generally exhibit a greater increase in muscle size than do women. The reason is that men have 20 to 30 times more testosterone than do women.

Make sure you know...

> Muscle size increases primarily because of hypertrophy (increase in size) of muscle fibers.

> Strength training promotes positive changes in both body composition and flexibility.

> The rate of improvement in weight training depends on initial strength level.

> Early in a weight-training program, women gain strength as fast as men.

Designing a Training Program for Increasing Muscle Strength

There are numerous approaches to designing weight-training programs. Any program that adheres to the basic principles described earlier will improve strength and endurance. However, the type of weight-training program that you develop for yourself depends on your goals and the types of equipment available to you. There are several other factors to consider in developing a weight-training program; we discuss those next.

Safety Concerns

Before beginning any weight-training program, you need to think about safety. Follow these safety guidelines when weight training:

- When using free weights (such as barbells), have spotters (helpers) help you perform the exercises. The purpose of a spotter is to help you complete a lift if you are unable to do it on your own. Using weight machines reduces the need for spotters.

- Be sure that the collars on the end of the bars of free weights are tightly secured to prevent the weights from falling off. Dropping weight plates on toes and feet can result in serious injuries. Again, many weight machines have safety features that reduce the risk of dropping weights.

- Warm up properly before doing any weight-lifting exercise. Stretching the intended muscles and lifting very light weight is a good way to start.

- Do not hold your breath during weight lifting. To prevent breath holding, follow this breathing pattern: Exhale while lifting the weight, and inhale while lowering it. Also, breathe through both your nose and mouth.

- Although debate continues as to whether high-speed weight lifting yields greater strength gains than slow-speed lifting, slow movements may reduce the risk of injury. A general rule of thumb is to lift the weight on the count of 2 and to lower the weight on the count of 4.

- Use light weights in the beginning so that you can maintain the proper form through the full range of motion in each exercise. This is particularly important when you are lifting free weights.

Types of Weight-Training Programs

Weight-training programs specifically designed to improve strength and programs designed to improve muscular endurance differ mainly in the number of repetitions and the amount of resistance (10). The combination of low repetition and high resistance appears to be the optimal training method to increase strength; moreover, this type of training improves muscular endurance as well. In contrast, weight training using high repetition and low resistance improves endurance but results in only small strength increases, particularly in less fit individuals.

As with types of weight-training exercise, weight-training programs can be divided into three general categories: isotonic, isometric, and isokinetic.

progressive resistance exercise (PRE) Application of the overload principle to strength and endurance exercise programs.

specificity of training The concept that the development of muscular strength and endurance, as well as cardiorespiratory endurance, is specific to both the muscle group exercised and the training intensity.

hypertrophy An increase in muscle fiber size.

hyperplasia An increase in the number of muscle fibers.

STEPS FOR
BEHAVIOR
CHANGE

Are you reluctant to strength train?

Answer the following questions to assess the barriers that prevent you from starting a strength-training program.

Y N

☐ ☐ I feel intimidated by other people in the strength-training facility.

☐ ☐ I cannot find time in my schedule to exercise.

☐ ☐ I do not know how to use the various machines or free weights.

☐ ☐ I do not know how to begin a strength-training program.

If you answered yes to more than one question, check out the following tips to help you break through the barriers.

TIPS TO EASE YOURSELF INTO A STRENGTH-TRAINING ROUTINE

☑ Fitness facilities cater to a wide range of clients, from beginners to professional body builders. Do your homework and find a facility that makes you feel welcome and comfortable.

☑ Make a commitment to set aside 30–60 minutes a day for training, and do not allow others to interfere with your personal time. Personal fitness does require a time commitment, but you are worth the investment.

☑ Take an orientation tour through a fitness facility to familiarize yourself with the machines and equipment. If you feel you need more individualized instruction, hire a personal trainer at the facility.

☑ Most facilities have fitness professionals that will assess your overall strength and suggest a starting program. The facility may also provide personal trainers for a reasonable hourly rate.

Isotonic Programs   Isotonic programs involve contracting a muscle against a movable load (usually a free weight or weights on a weight machine). The load is lifted on the up phase using concentric muscle actions and then lowered on the down phase using eccentric muscle actions. Isotonic programs are the most common type of weight-training program in use today.

Weight-training machines are ideal for the beginning exerciser because the weight is mounted to a cable or chain. If you were unable to complete a lift using a heavy weight and accidentally let go of the bar, the weights would slam down on the weight stack without injuring you or someone else. In addition, machines allow a single joint to be isolated and exercised.

Free weights are preferred by many serious weight lifters because they can be used to exercise multiple joints. For example, the squat exercise involves muscles at the hip, knee, and ankle, thus allowing three joints to be exercised during one movement.

Isometric Programs   An isometric strength-training program is based on the concept of contracting a muscle at a fixed angle against an immovable object,

using an isometric muscle action. Interest in strength training increased dramatically during the 1950s with the finding that maximal strength could be increased by contracting a muscle for 6 seconds at two-thirds of maximal tension once per day for 5 days per week. Although subsequent studies suggested that these claims were exaggerated, it is generally agreed that isometric training can increase muscular strength and endurance (15).

Two important aspects of isometric training make it different from isotonic training. First, in isometric training, the development of strength and endurance is specific to the joint angle at which the muscle group is trained (15). Therefore, if you use isometric techniques, you will need to perform isometric contractions at several different joint angles if you want to gain strength and endurance throughout a full range of motion. In contrast, because isotonic contractions generally involve the full range of joint motion, strength is developed over the full movement pattern.

Second, the static nature of isometric muscle actions can lead to breath holding (called a **Valsalva maneuver**), which can reduce blood flow to the brain and cause dizziness and fainting. In an individual at high risk for coronary disease, the maneuver could be extremely dangerous and should always be avoided. Remember: Continue to breathe during any type of isometric or isotonic exercise.

Isokinetic Programs   Recall that isokinetic exercise involves concentric or eccentric muscle actions performed at a constant speed (*isokinetic* refers to constant speed of movement). Isokinetic training is a relatively underused strength-training method, so limited research exists to describe its strength benefits compared with those of isometric and isotonic programs.

Isokinetic exercises require the use of machines that govern the speed of movement during muscle actions. The first isokinetic machines available were very expensive and were used primarily in clinical settings for injury rehabilitation. Recently, less expensive machines use a piston device (much like a shock absorber on a car) to limit the speed of movement throughout the range of the exercise.

Make sure you know...

> The greatest strength gains are made with a training program using low repetitions and high resistance, whereas the greatest improvement in endurance is made using high repetitions and low resistance.

> Isotonic programs include exercises with movable loads. Isometric training includes exercises in which a muscle contracts at a fixed angle against an immovable object. Isokinetic exercises involve machines that govern speed of movement during muscle contraction.

Exercise Prescription for Weight Training

We introduced in Chapter 2 the general concepts of the frequency, intensity, and duration (or time) of exercise required to improve physical fitness. Although these same concepts apply to improving muscular strength and endurance through weight training, the terminology used to monitor the intensity and duration of weight training is unique. For example, the intensity of weight training is measured not by heart rate but by the number of *repetition maximums*. Similarly, the duration of weight training is monitored not by actual time but by the number of sets performed. Let's discuss these two concepts briefly.

The intensity of exercise in both isotonic and isokinetic weight-training programs is measured by the repetition maximum (RM). Recall from earlier in the chapter that 1 RM is the maximal load that a muscle group can lift one time. Similarly, 6 RM is the maximal load that can be lifted six times. Therefore, the amount of weight lifted is greater when you perform a low

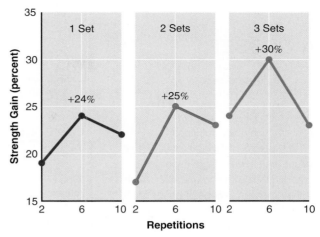

FIGURE 4.8

Strength gains from a resistance-training program consisting of various sets and repetitions. All programs were performed 3 days a week for 12 weeks. Note that the greatest strength gains (+30% improvement) were obtained using 3 sets of 6 reps per set.

Source: Adapted from Fox, E., R. Bowers, and M. Foss. *Fox's Physiological Basis of Exercise and Sports.* Copyright 1998, McGraw-Hill.

number of RM than a high number of RM; that is, the weight lifted while you perform 4 RM is greater than the weight lifted while you perform 15 RM.

The number of repetitions (reps) performed consecutively without resting is called a **set.** For example, if you lift 6 RM, 1 set = 6 reps. Because the amount of rest required between sets will vary among individuals depending on how fit they are, the duration of weight training is measured by the number of sets performed, not by actual time.

Although some experts disagree as to the optimum number of reps and sets required to improve strength and endurance, they do agree on some general guidelines. To improve strength, 3 sets of 6 reps for each exercise are generally recommended. Applying the concept of progressive resistance to a strength-training program involves increasing the amount of weight to be lifted a specific number of reps. For example, suppose that 3 sets of 6 reps were selected as your exercise prescription for increasing strength. As the training progresses and you become stronger, the amount of weight you lift must be increased. A good rule of thumb is that once you can perform 10 reps easily, you should increase the load to a level at which 6 reps are again maximal. Figure 4.8 illustrates the relationship between strength improvement and various combinations of reps and sets.

Valsalva maneuver   Breath holding during an intense muscle contraction; can reduce blood flow to the brain and cause dizziness and fainting.

set   The number of repetitions performed consecutively without resting.

A CLOSER LOOK: DO WEIGHT LIFTERS NEED LARGE AMOUNTS OF PROTEIN IN THEIR DIETS?

Although many nutritional supplement companies claim that weight lifters require large quantities of protein in their diets, organizations such as the American College of Sports Medicine (ACSM), American Dietetic Association (ADA), and Dietitians of Canada (DC) have concluded that athletes have only slightly higher protein requirements than nonathletes. These organizations have also found that most athletes consume protein far in excess of any increased protein requirement. Provided that sound nutrition principles are followed and energy intake is sufficient to maintain body weight, athletes require about 10–15% of their total caloric intake from protein and do not need to fortify their diets with expensive protein powders or amino acid supplements. The table at right illustrates the daily energy and protein requirements for the average endurance or strength athlete.

Daily Protein Requirement for a 154-lb Active Individual*

Type of Athlete	Energy (Calories per day)	Grams of Protein per lb Body Weight per Day[1]	Total Grams of Protein per Day	% of Daily Calories
Endurance	3800	0.55–0.64	84–98	9–10
Strength	3200	0.73–0.77	112–119	14–15

*Values assume a resting energy expenditure equivalent to 40 Kcal per kilogram (18 Kcal/lb) of body weight per day; a male runner who runs 10 miles per day at a pace of 6 minutes per mile with an energy expenditure for running of 0.11 Kcal per minute per pound of body weight; and an additional cost of 2.7 Kcal per pound body weight per day for heavy resistance training.
1. Data are from Campbell, B., R. Kreider, T. Ziegenfuss, P. La Bounty, M. Roberts, D. Burke, J. Landis, H. Lopez, and J. Antonio. International Society of Sports Nutrition position stand: Protein and exercise. *Journal of International Society of Sports Nutrition* 26(4):1–7, 2007.

A key point in Figure 4.8 is that programs involving 3 sets result in the greatest strength gains. The reason is that the third set requires the greatest effort and thus is the greatest overload for the muscle. Although it may seem that adding a fourth set would elicit even greater gains, most studies suggest that performing 4 or more sets results in overtraining and decreased benefits.

To improve muscular endurance, 4 to 6 sets of 18 to 20 reps for each exercise are recommended. Note that you can improve endurance by either increasing the number of reps progressively while maintaining the same load, or by increasing the amount of weight while maintaining the same number of reps. The advantage of the latter program is that it would also improve muscular strength.

Most research suggests that 2 to 3 days of exercise per week is optimal for strength gains (5). However, studies have also shown that once the desired level of strength has been achieved, one high-intensity training session per week is sufficient to maintain the new level of strength. Finally, although limited research exists regarding the optimal frequency of training to improve muscular endurance, 3 to 5 days per week appear adequate (13).

Make sure you know...

> Progressively overloading a muscle can be accomplished by changing the frequency, intensity, and or duration of the activity. Increasing the weight lifted will increase the intensity of the exercise. Increasing repetitions will increase the duration of the exercise.

> Exercising 2 to 3 days per week is optimal for strength gains; however, one high-intensity session per week is sufficient to maintain new strength levels; exercising 3 to 5 days per week is adequate to improve muscular endurance.

Starting and Maintaining a Weight-Training Program

As with any plan for behavior change, you should begin your weight-training program with both short- and long-term goals. Be sure to establish realistic short-term goals that you can reach in the first several weeks

TABLE 4.2
Suggested Isotonic Strength-Training Routine to Be Included in a Basic Fitness Program
The durations of the starter and slow progression phases will depend on your initial strength level.

Week	Phase	Frequency	Sets	Reps	Weight
1–3	Starter	2/week	2	15	15 RM
4–20	Slow progression	2–3/week	3	6	6 RM
20+	Maintenance	1–2/week	3	6	6 RM

Guidelines and Precautions to Follow Prior to Beginning a Strength-Training Program

- Warm up before beginning a workout. This involves 5 to 10 minutes of movement (calisthenics) using all major muscle groups.
- Start slowly. The first several training sessions should involve limited exercises and light weight!
- Use the proper lifting technique, as shown in the isotonic strength-training exercises in this chapter. Improper technique can lead to injury.
- Follow all safety rules (see the section on safety concerns on page 105).
- Always lift through the full range of motion. This not only develops strength throughout the full range of motion but also helps you maintain flexibility.

of training. Reaching these goals will help motivate you to continue training.

Developing an Individualized Exercise Prescription

An exercise prescription for strength training has three stages: the starter phase, the slow progression phase, and the maintenance phase.

The primary objective of the **starter phase** is to build strength gradually without developing undue muscular soreness or injury. You can accomplish this by starting your weight-training program slowly—beginning with light weights, a high number of repetitions, and only 1 set per exercise, gradually working up to 2 sets per exercise. The recommended frequency of training during this phase is twice per week. The duration of this phase varies from 1 to 3 weeks, depending on your initial strength fitness level. A sedentary person might spend 3 weeks in the starter phase, whereas a relatively well-trained person may spend only 1 to 2 weeks.

The **slow progression phase** may last 4 to 20 weeks, depending on your initial strength level and your long-term strength goal. The transition from the starter phase to the slow progression phase involves three changes in the exercise prescription: increasing the frequency of training from 2 to 3 days per week; increasing the amount of weight lifted (and decreasing the number of repetitions); and increasing the number of sets performed from 2 to 3 sets. The objective of the slow progression phase is to gradually increase muscular strength until you reach your desired level.

After reaching your strength goal, your long-term objective is to maintain this level of strength by entering the **maintenance phase** of the strength-training exercise prescription. Maintaining strength will require a lifelong weight-training effort. You will lose strength if you do not continue to exercise. The good news is that the effort required to maintain muscular strength is less than the initial effort needed to gain strength. Research has shown that as little as one workout per week is required to maintain strength (17).

Sample Exercise Prescription for Weight Training

As with training to improve cardiorespiratory fitness, the exercise prescription for improving muscular strength must be tailored to the individual. Before starting a program, review the guidelines and precautions listed in the box on this page.

Table 4.2 illustrates the stages of a suggested strength-training exercise prescription. When

starter phase The beginning phase of an exercise program. The goal of this phase is to build a base for further physical conditioning.

slow progression phase The second phase of an exercise program. The goal of this phase is to increase muscle strength beyond the starter phase.

maintenance phase The third phase of an exercise program. The goal of this phase is to maintain the increase in strength obtained during the first two phases.

TABLE 4.3
Total-Body Resistance-Training Program

Target Area	Muscles	Without Weights	With Weights
Arms	Biceps	Pull-up	Biceps curl
	Triceps	Push-up	Triceps extension
Chest	Pectoralis major	Push-up, dip	Fly, chest press, bench press
Upper back	Trapezius, rhomboids	Push-up	Upright row
Abdomen	Rectus abdominis, obliques	Curl-up, plank	Abdominal curl
Lower back	Latissimus dorsi	Pull-up	Lateral pulldown, back extension
Legs	Gluteus maximus	Lunge	Leg press
	Quadriceps	Lunge	Leg extension, leg press
	Hamstrings	Lunge	Hamstring curl
	Gastrocnemius, soleus	Heel raise	Calf raise

you reach the strength goals of the program, the maintenance phase begins. You will use the same routine as you used during the progression phase, but you'll need to perform the routine only once per week.

The isotonic strength-training program contains exercises that are designed to provide a whole-body workout. Although you can perform some exercises using either machines or free weights, keep in mind that safety and proper lifting techniques are especially important when using free weights.

Follow the exercise routines described and illustrated on the following pages, and develop your program using the guidelines provided in Table 4.2. This selection of exercises is designed to provide a comprehensive strength-training program that focuses on the major muscle groups. You can also use Table 4.3 to help you plan a program that works the total body. Be aware of which muscle groups are involved in an exercise to avoid overtraining any one muscle group. Note that it is not necessary to perform all exercises in one workout session; you can perform half of the exercises on one day and the remaining exercises on an alternate day.

Make sure you know...

> As you develop your strength-training program, divide it into three phases: a starter phase, a slow progression phase, and a maintenance phase.

Motivation to Maintain Strength Fitness

The problems associated with starting and maintaining a weight-training program are similar to those associated with cardiorespiratory training. You must find

time to train regularly, so good time management is critical.

Another key feature of any successful exercise program is that training must be fun. You can make weight training fun in a variety of ways. First, find an enjoyable place to work out. Locate a facility which contains the type of weights that you want to use and in which you feel comfortable and motivated. Second, develop a realistic weight-training routine. Designing a training routine that is too hard may be good for improving strength but does not increase your desire to train. Therefore, design a program that is challenging, but fun. Weight training is often more enjoyable with a partner. When looking for a workout buddy, ask a friend who is highly motivated to exercise and has strength abilities similar to yours.

Although the benefits of weight training are numerous, recent studies have shown that improved appearance, elevated self-esteem, and the overall feeling of well-being that result from regular weight training are the most important factors in motivating people to continue to train regularly. Looking your best and feeling good about yourself are excellent reasons to maintain a regular weight-training program. In addition, your elevated resting metabolic rate can help you burn calories more efficiently throughout the day, so even if you put on a few extra pounds of muscle mass, your clothes will fit better, and you will look better.

Some Isotonic Exercises for Increasing Muscular Strength*

EXERCISE 4.1 BICEPS CURL ▷

Purpose: To strengthen the **elbow flexor muscles** (biceps, brachialis, brachioradialis)

Position: Hold the grips with palms up and arms extended.

Movement: Curl up as far as possible and slowly return to the starting position.

EXERCISE 4.2 TRICEPS EXTENSION ▷

Purpose: To strengthen the muscles on the **back of the upper arm** (triceps)

Position: Sit upright with elbows bent.

Movement: With the little-finger side of the hand against the pad, fully extend the arms and then slowly return to the original position.

*Log on to **www.pearsonhighered.com/powers** to view demonstration videos of exercises marked with the ▷ icon.

Some Isotonic Exercises for Increasing Muscular Strength

EXERCISE 4.3   DUMBBELL FLY

Purpose: To strengthen the muscles of the **chest** (pectoralis major) and **shoulder** (anterior deltoid)

Position: Lie on an incline bench set at an angle between 45–60 degrees. Hold the dumbbells in front of your body with arms slightly flexed at the elbows.

Movement: Inhale, then lower the dumbbell until your elbows are at shoulder height. Raise the dumbbell while exhaling.

EXERCISE 4.4   UPRIGHT ROW

Purpose: To strengthen the muscles of the **upper back** (rhomboids, middle trapezius, posterior deltoid, latissimus dorsi)

Position: Stand with your weight equally distributed on both feet and bend legs slightly. Bend forward at the waist to a 45-degree angle with head up, looking straight ahead. Grasp the bar with an overhand grip and keep hands shoulder width apart.

Movement: Pull the bar to the chest on the count of 2. Lower the bar to the starting position on the count of 4.

Caution: Beginners and people with lower back problems should use very light weight or a dumbbell at first.

EXERCISE 4.5 LUNGE ▷

Purpose: To strengthen the muscles of the **hip** (gluteus maximus, hamstrings), **knee** (quadriceps), and **lower back** (erector spinae)

Position: Stand with your feet hip-width apart.

Movement: Lunge forward, putting all of the weight on your leading leg. Do not let the knee of your leading leg move in front of toes. Keep your knee in line with your ankle. Vary the stride length by taking a simple step forward to involve the quadriceps, or a large step forward to place more stress on the hamstrings and gluteals while stretching the quadriceps and hip flexors.

Some Isotonic Exercises for Increasing Muscular Strength

EXERCISE 4.6   LEG EXTENSION ▷

Purpose: To strengthen the muscles in the **front of the upper leg** (quadriceps [rectus femoris, vastus lateralis, vastus intermedius, vastus medialis])

Position: Sit in a nearly upright position and grasp the handles on the side of the machine. Position your legs so the pads of the machine are against the lower shin.

Movement: Extend the legs until they are completely straight and then slowly return to the starting position.

EXERCISE 4.7   HAMSTRING CURL ▷

Purpose: To strengthen the muscles on the **back of the upper leg** and **buttocks** (hamstrings [biceps femoris, semimembranosus, semitendinosis])

Position: In a seated position, extend legs so the pads of the machine are just below the calf muscles.

Movement: Curl the legs by pushing down on the pads to at least a 90-degree angle and then slowly return to the original position.

EXERCISE 4.8   ABDOMINAL CURL

Purpose: To strengthen the **abdominal muscles** (rectus abdominis, external oblique, internal oblique)

Position: Sit on the bench and place crossed arms on the padded armrest.

Movement: Bend forward until you feel the abdominals engage. Slowly return to starting position.

EXERCISE 4.9   BACK EXTENSION

Purpose: To strengthen the muscles of the **lower back** (erector spinae, quadratus lumborum)

Position: Sit with your upper back positioned against the back pads, and your feet flat on the platform. Push back against the pads until the spine is straight. Cross your arms over your chest and straighten your spine.

Movement: Press backward against the back pad and slowly extend at the hip, keeping your spine straight. Slowly return to the starting position, keeping the spine straight.

EXERCISES

115

Some Isotonic Exercises for Increasing Muscular Strength

EXERCISE 4.10   BENCH PRESS ▷

Purpose: To strengthen the muscles in the **chest**, the **front of the shoulders** (pectoralis major, anterior deltoid), and the **back of the upper arm** (triceps)

Position: Sit on the bench with the bench press hand grips level with your chest and your feet flat on the floor.

Caution: Do not arch your back while performing this exercise.

Movement: Grasp the bar handles and press outward until your arms are completely extended. Return slowly to the original position.

EXERCISE 4.11   PULLOVER

Purpose: To strengthen the muscles of the **chest** (pectoralis major) and **shoulder** (triceps, latissimus dorsi, teres major)

Position: Sit with your elbows against the padded ends of the movement arm and grasp the bar behind your head.

Movement: Press forward and down with your arms, pulling the bar overhead and down to your abdomen. Slowly return to the original position.

EXERCISE 4.12   DIP

Purpose: To strengthen the muscles of the **upper back, chest** (pectoralis major), and **shoulder** (triceps, deltoid)

Position: Stand in front of a platform or a box, facing forward. Place both hands on the platform behind you.

Movement: Dip down until the elbows are at 90-degree angles. Return to starting position.

EXERCISE 4.13   TOE RAISE

Purpose: To strengthen the **calf muscles** (gastrocnemius, soleus).

Position: Stand with your feet flat on the floor, or on the edge of a step.

Movement: Raise yourself up using the ankle joint only, and lower yourself back to starting position.

APPRECIATING
DIVERSITY STRENGTH TRAINING FOR OLDER ADULTS

According to the Centers for Disease Control and Prevention (CDC), about 1.9 million people aged 65 and older were treated in emergency rooms for injuries due to falls in 2004. Almost 15,000 people over age 65 died as a result of injuries sustained in falls. In an effort to combat the number and minimize the severity of the falls, the American Academy of Orthopedic Surgeons (AAOS) and the National Athletic Trainers Association (NATA) are teaming up to help older Americans avoid falls and reduce the severity of injuries when falls do occur. The two organizations have established guidelines that call for older adults to keep muscles and bones strong by strength training with weight-bearing and resistive exercise.

Weight-bearing exercises increase bone density and help prevent osteoporosis. Research has shown that resistance training can enhance muscle mass and function even in 90-year-old subjects. Seniors can increase their lean muscle mass, improve dynamic balance, and increase their strength by participating in a well–designed strength training program 2 or 3 days a week.

Sources: Centers for Disease Control and Prevention and The Merck Company Foundation. *The State of Aging and Health in America 2007.* Whitehouse Station, NJ: The Merck Company Foundation, 2007; Frontera, W. R., V. A. Hughes, R. A. Fielding, M. A. Fiatarone, W. J. Evans, and R. Roubenoff, Aging of skeletal muscle: A 12-yr longitudinal study. *Journal of Applied Physiology* 88: 1321–1326, 2000; McComas, A. J. *Skeletal Muscle: Form and Function*, 2nd ed. Champaign, IL: Human Kinetics, 2005.

Summary

1. Strength training can reduce low back pain, reduce the incidence of exercise-related injuries, decrease the incidence of osteoporosis, and help maintain functional capacity, which normally decreases with age.

2. Muscular strength is the ability of a muscle to generate maximal force. In simple terms, this refers to the amount of weight that an individual can lift during one maximal effort. Muscular endurance is the ability of a muscle to generate force over and over again. In general, increasing muscular strength by exercise training will also increase muscular endurance. In contrast, training to improve muscular endurance does not always result in improved muscular strength.

3. Skeletal muscle is composed of a collection of long thin cells (fibers). Muscles are attached to bone by thick connective tissue (tendons). Muscle actions result in the tendons pulling on bone, causing movement.

4. Muscle action is regulated by signals coming from motor nerves. Motor nerves originate in the spinal cord and branch out to individual muscles through-out the body. The motor nerve plus all of the muscle fibers it controls make up a motor unit.

5. Isotonic exercises result in movement of a body part. Isometric exercises involve developing tension within the muscle but result in no movement of body parts. Concentric muscle actions (positive work) involve muscle shortening. In contrast, eccentric muscle actions (negative contractions) involve muscle lengthening.

6. Human skeletal muscle can be classified into three major fiber types: slow-twitch, fast-twitch, and intermediate fibers. Slow-twitch fibers shorten slowly but are highly fatigue resistant. Fast-twitch fibers shorten rapidly but fatigue rapidly. Intermediate fibers possess a combination of the characteristics of fast- and slow-twitch fibers.

7. The process of involving more muscle fibers to produce increased muscular force is called fiber recruitment.

8. The percentages of slow-twitch, intermediate, and fast-twitch fibers vary among individuals. There is a relationship between predominant muscle fiber type and success in athletics. For example,

champion endurance athletes (e.g., marathon runners) have a high percentage of slow-twitch fibers.

9. Two primary physiological factors determine the amount of force that can be generated by a muscle: the size of the muscle and the number of fibers recruited.

10. Muscle size is increased primarily because of an increase in fiber size (hypertrophy).

11. The overload principle states that a muscle will increase in strength and/or endurance only when it works against a workload that is greater than normal. The concept of progressive resistance exercise (PRE) is the application of the overload principle to strength and endurance exercise programs.

12. A weight-training program using low repetitions and high resistance results in the greatest strength gains, whereas a weight-training program using high repetitions and low resistance results in the greatest improvement in muscular endurance.

13. Isotonic exercises involves contracting a muscle against a movable load (usually a free weight or weights on a weight machine). An isometric strength-training program is based on the concept of contracting a muscle at a fixed angle against an immovable object (using isometric muscle action). Isokinetic exercises require the use of machines that govern the speed of movement during muscle contraction throughout the range of motion.

14. To begin a strength-training program, divide the program into three phases: starter phase—2 to 3 weeks, with 2 workouts per week using 2 sets at 8 reps; slow progression phase—20 weeks, with 2 to 3 workouts per week using 3 sets at 6 reps; and maintenance phase—continues for life with 1 workout per week using 3 sets at 6 reps.

Study Questions

1. What type of muscle action occurs as the muscle lengthens and controls the movement with resistance and/or gravity?
   a. concentric action
   b. eccentric action
   c. isometric action

2. A slow-twitch muscle fiber
   a. contracts slowly and produces small amounts of force.
   b. contracts rapidly and generates great amounts of force.
   c. contracts rapidly, produces great force, and fatigues rapidly.
   d. fatigues rapidly and is ideal for short bursts of activity.

3. Muscular strength is defined as
   a. the ability of a muscle to generate force over and over again.
   b. the ability of a muscle to generate maximal force.
   c. the ability of a muscle to shorten as it moves a resistance.
   d. the ability of a muscle to increase in size.

4. Which of the following is a benefit of a regular strength training program?
   a. reduces the incidence of a back pain
   b. increases $\dot{V}O_2$max
   c. reduces the incidence of colds
   d. increases endurance exercise capacity

5. Which of the following should be the general rule to follow to increase strength in a weigh training program?
   a. high resistance — high repetitions
   b. low resistance — low repetitions
   c. low resistance — high repetitions
   d. high resistance — low repetitions

6. Define the following terms:
   hypertrophy
   hyperplasia
   isotonic exercise
   isometric exercise
   isokinetic exercise
   motor unit
   progressive resistance exercise
   static contraction
   Valsalva maneuver

7. List at least three reasons why training for strength and endurance is important.

8. List and discuss the characteristics of slow-twitch, fast-twitch, and intermediate skeletal muscle fibers.

9. Discuss the pattern of muscle fiber recruitment with increasing intensities of contraction.

10. Discuss the relationship of muscle fiber type to success in various types of athletic events.

11. What factors determine muscle strength?

12. What physiological changes result from strength training?

13. Describe the concept of progressive resistance exercise.

14. Discuss the concept of specificity of training.

15. Compare and contrast the differences in training to increase strength versus training to increase endurance.

16. Define the concept of 1 RM.

17. List the phases of a strength- and endurance-training program, and discuss how they differ.

18. Distinguish isometric, concentric, and eccentric muscle actions.

19. Describe each of the following types of exercise: isokinetic, isometric, and isotonic.

Suggested Reading

American College of Sports Medicine. The recommended quantity and quality of exercise for developing and maintaining cardiorespiratory and muscular fitness, and flexibility in healthy adults. *Medicine and Science in Sports and Exercise* 30:975–991, 1998.

Baechle, T. R., and R. Earle. *Essentials of Strength Training and Conditioning*, 3rd ed. Champaign, IL: Human Kinetics, 2008.

Bishop P. A., E. Jones, and A. K. Woods. Recovery from training: A brief review. *Journal of Strength and Conditioning Research* 22(3):1015–1024, 2008.

Blair, S. N., M. J. LaMonte, M. Z. Nichaman. The evolution of physical activity recommendations: How much is enough? *American Journal of Clinical Nutrition* 79(5):913S–920S, 2004.

Fleck, S. J., and W. J. Kraemer. *Designing Resistance Training Programs*. Champaign, IL: Human Kinetics, 2004.

Folland, J. P., and A. G. Williams. The adaptations to strength training: Morphological and neurological contributions to increased strength. *Sports Medicine* 37(2):145–168, 2007.

Galvão, D. A., and D. R. Taaffe. Single- vs. multiple-set resistance training: Recent developments in the controversy. *Journal of Strength and Conditioning Research* 18(3):660–667, 2004.

Hartman J. W., J. E. Tang, S. B. Wilkinson, M. A. Tarnopolsky, R. L. Lawrence, A. V. Fullerton, and S. M. Phillips. Consumption of fat-free fluid milk after resistance exercise promotes greater lean mass accretion than does consumption of soy or carbohydrate in young, novice, male weightlifters. *American Journal of Clinical Nutrition* 86(2):373–381, 2007.

Knuttgen, H. G. Strength training and aerobic exercise: Comparison and contrast. *Journal of Strength and Conditioning Research* 21(3):973–978, 2007.

Komi, P., ed. *Strength and Power in Sport: Olympic Encyclopaedia of Sports Medicine*, 2nd ed., Volume III. Malden, MA: Blackwell Science, Ltd., 2003.

Martel, G. F., S. M. Roth, F. M. Ivey, J. T. Lemmer, B. L. Tracy, D. E. Hurlbut, E. J. Metter, B. F. Hurley, and M.A. Rogers. Age and sex affect human muscle fibre adaptations to heavy-resistance strength training. *Experimental Physiology* 91(2):457–464, 2006.

Sandler, D. *Weight Training Fundamentals*. Champaign, IL: Human Kinetics, 2003.

Willardson, J. M. A brief review: Factors affecting the length of the rest interval between resistance exercise sets. *Journal of Strength and Conditioning Research* 20(4):978–984, 2006.

Zatsiorsky, V. M., and W. J. Kraemer. *Science and Practice of Strength Training*, 2nd ed. Champaign, IL: Human Kinetics, 2006.

For links to the organizations and websites listed below, visit The Total Fitness and Wellness Website at www.pearsonhighered.com/powers.

ACSM

Comprehensive website that provides equipment recommendations, how-to articles, book recommendations, and position statements about all aspects of health and fitness.

Women's Fitness

Provides basic information and programs, current articles, and exercises for beginner-level strength training.

WebMD

General information about exercise, fitness, wellness. Great articles, instructional information, and updates.

Meriter Fitness

Discusses injury prevention and treatment, weight training, flexibility, exercise prescriptions, and more.

Muscle Physiology

Includes in-depth discussions of how muscle works, as well as recent research articles from a world-renowned muscle physiology lab.

References

1. Kell R. T., and G. J. Asmundson. A comparison of two forms of periodized exercise rehabilitation programs in the management of chronic nonspecific low-back pain. *Journal of Strength and Conditioning Research* 23(2):513–523, 2009.

2. Buckwalter, J. A. Sports, joint injury, and posttraumatic osteoarthritis. *Journal of Orthopedics Sport and Physical Therapy* 33(10):578–588, 2003.

3. Seguin, R., and M. E. Nelson. The benefits of strength training for older adults. *American Journal of Preventive Medicine* 25(3 Suppl 2):141–149, 2003.

4. Winett, R. A., and R. N. Carpinelli. Potential health-related benefits of resistance training. *Preventive Medicine* 33(5):503–513, 2001.

5. Powers, S., and E. Howley. *Exercise Physiology: Theory and Application to Fitness and Performance*, 7th ed. New York: McGraw-Hill, 2009.

6. Oberbach A., Y. Bossenz, S. Lehmann, J. Niebauer, V. Adams, R. Paschke, M. R. Schön, M. Blüher, and K. Punkt. Altered fiber distribution and fiber-specific glycolytic and oxidative enzyme activity in skeletal muscle of patients with type 2 diabetes. *Diabetes Care* 29(4):895–900, 2006.

7. Karjalainen, J., H. Tikkanen, M. Hernelahti, and U. Kujala. Muscle fiber-type distribution predicts weight gain and unfavorable left ventricular geometry: A 19 year follow-up study. *BMC Cardiovascular Disorders* 10(6):1–8, 2006.

8. Wang, Y., C. Zhang, R. T. Yu, H. K. Cho, M. C. Nelson, C. R. Bayuga-Ocampo, J. Ham, H. Kang, and R. M. Evans. Regulation of muscle fiber type and running endurance by PPARδ. *PLoS Biology* 10: e294, 2004.

9. Monteiro, W. D., R. Simão, M. D. Polito, C. A. Santana, R. B. Chaves, E. Bezerra, and S. J. Fleck. Influence of strength training on adult women's flexibility. *Journal of Strength and Conditioning Research* 22(3):672–677, 2008.

10. Fleck, S. J., and W. J. Kraemer. *Designing Resistance Training Programs*. Champaign, IL: Human Kinetics, 2004.

11. Folland, J. P., and A. G. Williams. The adaptations to strength training : Morphological and neurological contributions to increased strength. *Sports Medicine* 37(2):145–168, 2007

12. Knuttgen, H. G. Strength training and aerobic exercise: Comparison and contrast. *Journal of Strength and Conditioning Research* 21(3):973–978, 2007.

13. American College of Sports Medicine. The recommended quantity and quality of exercise for developing and maintaining cardiorespiratory and muscular fitness, and flexibility in healthy adults. *Medicine and Science in Sports and Exercise* 30:975–991, 1998.

14. Hubal, M. J., S. R. Rubinstein, and P. M. Clarkson. Muscle function in men and women during maximal eccentric exercise. *Journal of Strength and Conditioning Research* 22(4):1332–1338, 2008.

15. Folland, J. P., K. Hawker, B. Leach, T. Little, and D. A. Jones. Strength training: Isometric training at a range of joint angles versus dynamic training. *Journal of Sports Sciences* 23(8):817–824, 2005.

16. Powers, S., and E. Howley. *Exercise Physiology: Theory and Application to Fitness and Performance*, 4th ed. Dubuque, IA: McGraw-Hill, 2003.

17. Gabriel, D. A., G. Kamen, and G. Frost. Neural adaptations to resistive exercise: Mechanisms and recommendations for training practices. *Sports Medicine* 36(2): 133–49, 2006.

Videos

Log on to www.pearsonhighered.com/powers to view these chapter-related videos.

Safety Tips: Dumbbells

Safety Tips: Resistance Bands

Safety Tips: Stability Balls

Biceps Curl (dumbbells)

Biceps Curl (resistance band)

Biceps Curl (machine)

Triceps Extension (dumbbells)

Triceps Extension (resistance band)

Triceps Extension (machine)

Dumbbell Fly

Fly (resistance band)

Chest Fly (machine)

Dumbbell Row

Upright Row (dumbbells)

Upright Row (resistance band)

Machine Row

Lunge

Walking Lunge

Two-Person Lunge (resistance band)

Leg Extension

Leg Curl (resistance band)

Leg Curl (stability ball)

Leg Curl (machine)

Abdominal Curl (stability ball)

Abdominal Curl (machine)

Back Extension

Back Extension (stability ball)

Bench/Chest Press (dumbbells)

Bench/Chest Press (resistance band)

Chest Press (machine)

Leg Press (resistance band)

Leg Press (machine)

Push-Ups

Modified Push-Ups

Plank (Push-Up Position)

Plank (Forearm Position)

NAME _____ DATE _____

Evaluating Muscular Strength: The 1 RM Test

The 1 RM test is used to measure muscular strength. You can use the following procedure to determine your 1 RM:

1. Begin with a 5- to 10-minute warm-up using the muscles to be tested.

2. For each muscle group, select an initial weight that you can lift without undue stress.

3. Gradually add weight until you reach the maximum weight that you can lift at one time. If you can lift the weight more than once, add additional weight until you reach a level of resistance such that you can perform only one repetition. Remember that a true 1 RM is the maximum amount of weight that you can lift one time.

 The seated chest press and the leg press are two common methods for the 1 RM test. The seated chest press measures upper body muscular strength, and the leg press measures muscular strength in the lower body.

The seated chest press can be used to evaluate upper-body muscular strength.
▷ View a demonstration video of this exercise at **www.pearsonhighered.com/powers**.

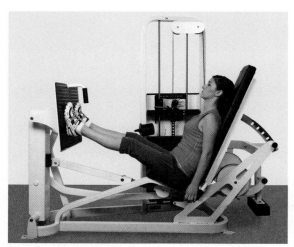

A leg press can be used to evaluate lower-body muscular strength.

▷ View a demonstration video of this exercise at **www.pearsonhighered.com/powers**.

Your muscle strength score is your percentage of body weight lifted in each exercise. To compute your strength score, divide your 1 RM weight in pounds by your body weight in pounds, and then multiply by 100. For example, suppose a 150-pound man has a bench press 1 RM of 180 pounds. This individual's muscle strength score for the bench press is computed as

$$\frac{1 \text{ RM weight}}{\text{body weight}} \times 100 = \text{muscle strength score}$$

Therefore,

$$\text{muscle strength score} = \frac{180 \text{ pounds}}{150 \text{ pounds}} \times 100 = 120$$

Table 4.4 and Table 4.5 on pages 125 and 126 list strength score norms for college-aged men and women for the seated chest press and leg press, respectively. According to Table 4.4, a muscle strength score of 120 on the seated chess press places a college-aged man in the "good" category.

In the spaces below, record your muscular strength score and fitness category for the 1 RM tests for the leg press and seated chess press.

Age: _____   Body weight: _____ lb

Date: _____

Exercise	1 RM (lb)	Muscular Strength	Fitness Category
Seated chest press			
Leg press			

Goal Setting

1. Based on your results, write a goal to maintain or improve your current fitness level. For example, if you scored "fair" on this test, your goal might be to improve your fitness level to a "good" rating. If your fitness level indicated a score of "excellent," your goal might be to maintain your current fitness status.

   Goal: _____

2. Write three strategies for how you intend to achieve the goal you wrote. For example, one strategy for improving your current fitness status might be to perform 1 set of 10 repetitions at 50% of your 1 RM, 3 times a week. To progressively overload the muscles, increase the number of sets, and increase the weight load by 5–10 lb.

   - _____
   _____

   - _____
   _____

   - _____
   _____

TABLE 4.4
Strength Score Norms for the Seated Chest Press
Locate your fitness level for upper body muscular strength using your seated chest press score.

Fitness Level	Age 20–29	Age 30–39	Age 40–49	Age 50–59	Age 60+
Men					
Superior	>148	>124	>110	>97	>89
Excellent	132–148	112–124	100–110	90–97	82–89
Good	114–131	98–111	88–99	79–89	72–81
Average	99–113	88–97	80–87	71–78	66–71
Poor	89–98	79–87	73–79	64–70	58–65
Very poor	<89	<79	<73	<64	<58
Women					
Superior	>90	>76	>71	>61	>64
Excellent	80–90	70–76	62–71	55–61	54–64
Good	70–79	60–69	54–61	48–54	47–53
Average	59–69	53–59	50–53	44–47	43–46
Poor	52–58	48–52	44–49	40–43	39–42
Very poor	<52	<48	<44	<40	<39

1 RM seated bench press with bench press weight ratio = weight pushed ÷ body weight × 100.

TABLE 4.5
Strength Score Norms for the Leg Press
Locate your fitness level for lower body muscular strength using your seated leg press score.

Fitness Level	Age 20–29	Age 30–39	Age 40–49	Age 50–59	Age 60+
Men					
Superior	>227	>207	>191	>179	>172
Excellent	213–227	193–207	182–191	171–179	162–172
Good	197–212	177–192	168–181	158–170	149–161
Average	183–196	165–176	157–167	146–157	138–148
Poor	164–182	153–164	145–156	133–145	126–137
Very poor	<164	<153	<145	<133	<126
Women					
Superior	>181	>160	>147	>136	>131
Excellent	168–181	147–160	137–147	125–136	118–131
Good	150–167	133–146	123–136	110–124	104–117
Average	137–149	121–132	113–122	99–109	93–103
Poor	123–136	110–120	103–112	89–98	86–92
Very poor	<123	<110	<103	<89	<86

1 RM seated leg press with leg press weight ratio = weight pushed ÷ body weight × 100.

NAME _____ DATE _____

Evaluating Muscular Strength: The Estimated 1 RM Test

You can use the following procedure to determine your estimated 1 RM for any particular lift (e.g., chest press):

1. First, perform a set of 10 repetitions using a light weight.

2. Next, add additional weight and perform another set of 10 repetitions.

3. Repeat this process until you reach a weight that you can lift only 10 times (called the 10 RM).

Be sure to have an experienced instructor supervise the process so that your 10 RM weight can be discovered in fewer than five trials. Rest about 5 minutes after each trial to recover.

After determining the 10 RM, you can use Table 4.6 on page 128 to estimate your 1 RM. For example, if your 10 RM for a particular lift is 100 pounds, then the estimate for the 1 RM would be about 135 pounds.

You can determine your muscle strength score from the estimated 1 RM using the same formula used for the 1 RM test. That is,

$$\text{muscle strength score} = \frac{1 \text{ RM weight}}{\text{body weight}} \times 100$$

Record your muscular strength scores below, and use Table 4.4 or Table 4.5 in Laboratory 4.1 to determine your fitness category.

Age: _____   Body weight: _____ lb

Date: _____

Exercise	1 RM (lb)	Muscular Strength	Fitness Category
Seated chest press			
Leg press press			

Goal Setting

1. Based on your results, write a goal to maintain or improve your current fitness level. For example, if your score was "fair" on this test, your goal might be to improve your fitness level to a "good" rating. If your fitness level indicated a score of "excellent," your goal might be to maintain your current fitness status.

    Goal: _____

2. Write three strategies for how you intend to achieve the goal you wrote. For example, one strategy for improving your current fitness status could be to perform 1 set of 10 repetitions at 50% of your 1 RM, 3 times a week. To progressively overload the muscles, increase the number of sets, and increase the weight load by 5–10 lb.

    • _____

    _____

- _____
  _____
  _____

- _____
  _____

Source: Roitman, J. (ed). *ACSM's Resource Manual for Guidelines for Exercise Testing and Prescription*. Philadelphia: Lippincott Williams & Wilkins, 2001.

TABLE 4.6
Estimating the 1 RM from the 10 RM

Estimated 1 RM (lb)	Lifted during 10 Repetitions (lb)	Estimated 1 RM (lb)	Lifted during 10 Repetitions (lb)
5.0	3.7	145.0	106.6
10.0	7.4	150.0	110.3
15.0	11.0	155.0	113.9
20.0	14.7	160.0	117.6
25.0	18.4	165.0	121.3
30.0	22.1	170.0	125.0
35.0	25.7	175.0	128.6
40.0	29.4	180.0	132.3
45.0	33.1	185.0	136.0
50.0	36.8	190.0	139.7
55.0	40.4	195.0	143.3
60.0	44.1	200.0	147.0
65.0	47.8	205.0	150.7
70.0	51.5	210.0	154.4
75.0	55.1	215.0	158.0
80.0	58.8	220.0	161.7
85.0	62.5	225.0	165.4
90.0	66.2	230.0	169.1
95.0	69.8	235.0	172.7
100.0	73.5	240.0	176.4
105.0	77.2	245.0	180.1
110.0	80.9	250.0	183.8
115.0	84.5	255.0	187.4
120.0	88.2	260.0	191.2
125.0	91.9	265.0	194.8
130.0	95.6	270.0	198.5
135.0	99.2	275.0	202.1
140.0	102.9		

Source: Axler, C., and S. McGill. Low back loads over a variety of abdominal exercises: Searching for the safest abdominal challenge. *Medicine and Science in Sports and Exercise* 29: 804–810, 1997.

NAME _____ DATE _____

Tracking Your Progress

Use the log below to chart your strength-training progress. Record the date, number of sets, reps, and the weight for each of the exercises listed in the left column.

Date				
Exercise	St/Rp/Wt*	St/Rp/Wt	St/Rp/Wt	St/Rp/Wt
Biceps curl (see Exercise 4.1)				
Triceps extension (see Exercise 4.2)				
Abdominal curl (see Exercise 4.8)				
Quadriceps extension (see Exercise 4.6)				
Hamstring curl (see Exercise 4.7)				
Bench press or chest press (see Exercise 4.10)				
Upright rows (see Exercise 4.4)				
Lunges (with or without weights) (see Exercise 4.5)				
Dumbbell fly (see Exercise 4.3)				

* St/Rp/Wt = Sets/Reps/Weight. *Example:* 2/6/80 = 2 sets of 6 reps each with 80 lb.

LABORATORY

NAME _____ DATE _____

Measuring Muscular Endurance: The Push-Up, Sit-Up, and Curl-Up Tests

The Standard Push-Up Test

Perform the standard push-up test as follows:

1. Position yourself on the ground in push-up position (Figure a). (Note that you can instead use the modified push-up position shown in Figures c and d.) Place your hands about shoulder width apart, and extend your leg in a straight line with your weight on your toes.

2. Lower your body until your chest is within 1 to 2 inches off the ground (Figure b), and raise yourself back to the up position. Be sure to keep your back straight and to lower your entire body as a unit.

3. Select a partner to count your push-ups and time your test (test duration is 60 seconds). Warm up with a few push-ups, and rest for 2 to 3 minutes after the warm-up to prepare for the test.

4. When your partner says "Go," start performing push-ups. Have your partner count your push-ups aloud, and ask him or her to let you know periodically how much time remains.

5. Record your score in the chart on page 133.

The standard push-up ▷ View a demonstration video at **www.pearsonhighered.com/powers**.

(a)

(b)

The modified push-up ▷ View a demonstration video at **www.pearsonhighered.com/powers**.

(c)

(d)

131

The Sit-up Test

You can perform the bent-knee sit-up test as follows:

1. Lie on your back with your arms crossed on your chest. Bend your knees so that they're approximately 90-degree angles, with your feet flat on the floor (Figure a).

2. Bring your chest up to touch your knees (Figure b), and then return to the original lying position. The entire movement counts as one full sit-up. Be sure to let your abdominal muscles do the work of the movement (avoid stress on your neck), and be careful not to hit your head on the floor when returning to the lying position. Performing the test on a mat is helpful.

3. Select a partner to count your sit-ups and hold your feet on the floor by grasping your ankles, and to time the test.

4. Warm up with a few sit-ups. Rest for 2 to 3 minutes after your warm-up before starting the test.

5. When you partner says "Go," start performing sit-ups and continue for 60 seconds. Have your partner count your sit-ups aloud, and ask him or her to let you know periodically how much time remains.

6. Record your score in the chart on page 133.

(a)

(b)

The Curl-Up Test

The curl-up differs from the sit-up in that the trunk is not raised more than 30 to 40 degrees above the floor. The advantages of curl-ups are that they use only the abdominal muscles (whereas the sit-up also involves the hip flexors), and they put less stress on the lower back than do the conventional sit-ups.

You can perform the curl-up test as follows:

1. Lie on your back with your legs shoulder-width apart, your knees bent 90 degrees, your arms straight at your sides, and your palms flat on the mat (Figure a).

2. Extend your arms so that your fingertips touch a strip of tape perpendicular to your body. A second strip of tape is located toward the feet and parallel to the first (10 centimeters apart).

3. Use the cadence provided on a metronome set to 50 beats per minute. Slowly curl up your upper spine until your fingers touch the second strip of tape. Then slowly return to the lying position with your head and shoulder blades touching the mat and your fingertips touching the first strip of tape. Breathe normally throughout, exhaling during the curling up stage.

4. Have your partner count the number of consecutive curl-ups you do in 1 minute, maintaining the metronome cadence and without pausing, to a maximum of 25, and record your score in the chart on page 133.

(a)

(b)

After you complete the regular push-up, sit-up, and curl-up tests, record your scores and fitness classifications (from Tables 4.7, 4.8, and 4.9 on pages 134 and 135.)

Age: _____

Date: _____

Number	Fitness Category
Push-ups (1 min):	
Sit-ups (1 min):	
Curl-ups (1 min):	

Goal Setting

1. Based on your results, write a goal to maintain or improve your current fitness level. For example, if your score was "fair" on this test, your goal might be to improve your fitness level to a "good" rating. If your fitness level indicated a score of "excellent," your goal might be to maintain your current fitness status.

   Goal: _____

2. Write three strategies for how you intend to achieve your goal. For example, a strategy for improving your current fitness status might be to perform 1 set of 10 push-ups (sit-ups or curl-ups), 3 times a week. To progressively overload the muscles, increase the number of sets to 2 and then 3.

   • _____
   _____
   • _____
   _____
   • _____
   _____

Curl-up test from Canadian Physical Activity, Fitness and Lifestyle Approach: CSEP-Health & Fitness Program's Appraisal & Counselling Strategy, Third Edition, © 2003. Reprinted with permission from the Canadian Society for Exercise Physiology.

TABLE 4.7
Norms for Muscular Endurance Using the Push-Up and Modified Push-Up Tests

Fitness Level	Age 20–29	Age 30–39	Age 40–49	Age 50–59	Age 60+
Men					
Superior	≥62	≥51	≥39	≥38	≥27
Excellent	47–61	39–51	30–39	25–38	23–27
Good	37–46	30–38	24–29	19–24	18–22
Fair	29–36	24–29	18–23	13–18	10–17
Poor	22–28	17–23	11–17	9–12	6–9
Very poor	≤21	≤16	≤10	≤8	≤5
Women (modified push-up)					
Superior	≥45	≥39	≥33	≥28	≥20
Excellent	36–44	31–38	24–32	21–27	15–19
Good	30–35	24–30	18–23	17–20	12–14
Fair	23–29	19–23	13–17	12–16	5–11
Poor	17–22	11–18	6–12	6–11	2–4
Very poor	≤16	≤10	≤5	≤5	≤1
Women (full push-up)					
Superior	≥42	≥39	≥20	Not available	Not available
Excellent	28–41	23–38	15–19	Not available	Not available
Good	21–27	15–22	13–14	Not available	Not available
Fair	15–20	11–14	9–12	Not available	Not available
Poor	10–14	8–10	6–8	Not available	Not available
Very poor	≤9	≤7	≤5	Not available	Not available

Source: Adapted with permission from the Cooper Institute, *Physical Fitness Assessments and Norms for Adults and Law Enforcement,* www.cooperinstitute.org.

TABLE 4.8
Norms for Muscular Endurance Using the Sit-Up Test

Fitness Level	Age 20–29	Age 30–39	Age 40–49	Age 50–59	Age 60+
Men					
Superior	>49	>45	>41	>35	>31
Excellent	44–49	40–45	35–41	29–35	25–31
Good	39–43	35–39	30–34	25–28	21–24
Average	35–38	31–34	27–29	22–24	17–20
Poor	25–35	22–30	17–26	13–21	9–16
Very poor	<25	<22	<17	<13	<9
Women					
Superior	>43	>39	>33	>27	>24
Excellent	37–43	33–39	27–33	22–27	18–24
Good	33–36	29–32	23–26	18–21	13–17
Average	29–32	25–28	19–22	14–17	10–12
Poor	18–28	13–24	7–18	5–13	3–9
Very poor	<18	<13	<7	<5	<3

Source: Norms are adapted from Golding, L. A., C. R. Myers, and W. E. Sinning. *Y's Way to Physical Fitness: The Complete Guide to Fitness Testing and Instruction,* 3rd ed. Champaign, IL: Human Kinetics, 1989.

TABLE 4.9
Norms for Muscular Endurance Using the Curl-Up Test

Fitness Level	Age 15–19	Age 20–29	Age 30–39	Age 40–49	Age 50–59	Age 60–69
Men						
Excellent	25	25	25	25	25	25
Very Good	23–24	21–24	18–24	18–24	17–24	16–24
Good	21–22	16–20	15–17	13–17	11–16	11–15
Fair	16–20	11–15	11–14	6–12	8–10	6–10
Needs Improvement	≤15	≤10	≤10	≤5	≤7	≤5
Women						
Excellent	25	25	25	25	25	25
Very Good	22–24	18–24	19–24	19–24	19–24	17–24
Good	17–21	14–17	10–18	11–18	10–18	8–16
Fair	12–16	5–13	6–9	4–10	6–9	3–7
Needs Improvement	≤11	≤4	≤5	≤3	≤5	≤2

Source: From "Canadian Physical Activity, Fitness and Lifestyle Approach: CSEP–Health and Fitness Program's Appraisal & Counseling Strategy," Third Edition © 2003. Reprinted with permission from the Canadian Society for Exercise Physiology.

NAME _____ DATE _____

Measuring Core Strength and Stability

Position a watch on the ground where you can easily see it.

1. Assume the basic press up position, with your elbows on the ground (see the figure below). Hold this position for 60 seconds.

2. Lift your right arm off the ground. Hold this position for 15 seconds.

3. Return your right arm to the ground, and lift your left arm off the ground.
   Hold this position for 15 seconds.

4. Return your left arm to the ground, and lift your right leg off the ground. Hold this position for 15 seconds.

5. Return your right leg to the ground, and lift your left leg off the ground. Hold this position for 15 seconds.

6. Lift your left leg and right arm off the ground. Hold this position for 15 seconds.

7. Return your left leg and right arm to the ground, and lift your right leg and left arm off the ground. Hold this position for 15 seconds.

8. Return to the basic press up position (elbows on the ground). Hold this position for 30 seconds.

Basic press up position
⊳ View a demonstration video of this exercise
at **www.pearsonhighered.com/powers**.

Analysis

Analysis of the result is by comparing it with the results of previous tests. It is expected that, with appropriate training between each test, the analysis would indicate an improvement.

If you were able to complete this test, you have good core strength. If you were unable to complete the test, then repeat the routine 3 or 4 times a week until you can.

Source: Modified from the Core Muscle Strength Test by Brian Mackenzie, www.brianmc.co.uk/coretest.htm. Used by permission of Brian Mackenzie.

LABORATORY

Goal Setting

1. Based on your results, write a goal to maintain or improve your current core strength and stability. For example, if you were able to hold the position for 60 seconds in step 1 but were unable to lift your right arm off the ground (step 2), your goal might be to work on completing step 2 and step 3. If you completed all steps, your goal could be to maintain your current core strength and stability.

   Goal: _____

2. Write three strategies for how you intend to achieve your goal. For example, an objective for improving your current fitness status might be to perform steps 3 and 4, 3 times a week. To progressively overload the muscles, increase to steps 5 and 6.

   - _____
   _____

   - _____
   _____

   - _____
   _____

Improving Flexibility

5

true or false?

1. Bouncing is the best way to stretch the muscles.

2. Stretching should always be done when the muscle is warm.

3. The purpose of stretching is to lengthen the ligaments that cross the joints.

4. For maximum results, you need to stretch to the point of pain.

5. Stretching the neck muscles throughout the day will help prevent neck aches.

Answers appear on the next page.

Abby is a 22-year-old college junior whose biology major requires a lot of paper writing. She finds herself at the library at least four nights a week, conducting hours of research about cell behavior and gene function. Often, by the time she looks up from her textbook, her eyes are blurry, and her neck aches. Abby's fitness instructor advised her to take periodic breaks during her study time and to stretch her neck muscles to alleviate the kink in her neck. Although she knows this is probably good advice, she hasn't tried it yet because she's not sure how to properly stretch her neck muscles, and she forgets to look it up when she has a chance. Hence, the stiffness in her neck continues.

What do you think is causing Abby's stiff neck? Do you think her instructor's advice to stretch her neck will help alleviate the problem? Do you know how to properly stretch your neck muscles? In this chapter we'll discuss what causes muscle tightness and how stretching can improve flexibility. We'll also discuss the proper way to do various stretches and to target specific areas of the body for improved flexibility.

The Need for Flexibility in Daily Living

Gymnasts and ice skaters are not the only people who need to maintain adequate **flexibility.** When you bend down to tie your shoes or reach up to pull a sweatshirt over your head, you're relying on your body's flexibility to perform these tasks. In fact, any movement that requires you to stretch, reach, or twist your body without pain or stiffness is possible because you enjoy a range of motion around your joints. Unfortunately, you may not appreciate the importance of flexibility as a fitness component until you experience an injury that keeps you from performing these routine movements.

People vary in their degrees of flexibility because of differences in body structure, and the range of motion of most joints can decline with disuse. Tightness of the muscle, tendon, and connective tissue surrounding a joint can limit your range of motion; however, this restriction can be eliminated through proper stretching.

Make sure you know...

> Flexibility is the range of motion of a joint, and it allows you to bend, twist, and reach without experiencing pain or stiffness.

> Stretching can alleviate tightness at a joint.

How Flexibility Works: Muscles, Joints, and Stretching

The range of motion around a joint is determined partly by the shapes and positions of the bones that make up the joint and partly by the composition and arrangement of muscles, tendons, and connective tissue around the joint (1, 2). Although the structure of the bones cannot be altered, the soft tissues can be lengthened to allow for greater range of motion.

Of course, there are some movements that you will not be able to do, no matter how much you stretch, without causing yourself harm. You can't bend your fingers backward, for example, or rotate your arm 360 degrees at the elbow. The reason is that you are limited in the range of motion at your joints by your body's anatomy. Let's take a closer look at how this works.

Answers

1. **FALSE** Bouncing can lead to a strained or torn muscle. For most people, slow static stretching will allow muscles to lengthen gradually.

2. **TRUE** A "cold" muscle is more reluctant to stretch than a warm muscle.

3. **FALSE** The purpose of stretching is to stretch muscle and tendon. Stretching the ligaments will cause injury and affect the stability of the joint.

4. **FALSE** Although stretching to the point of discomfort will help improve flexibility, a sharp pain during stretching can indicate that a ligament, muscle, or tendon has been torn.

5. **TRUE** Holding a muscle in one position for a long period of time, such as by staring at a computer screen for several hours, can result in muscle stiffness. Stretching can help alleviate this.

Structural Limitations to Movement

There are five primary anatomical factors that limit movement (Figure 5.1):

1. *The shape of the bones* determines the amount of movement possible at each joint. For example, because of the way they are structured, ball and socket joints, such as the shoulder and hip, have greater range of motion than hinge joints, such as the elbow and knee.

2. *A stiff muscle* will limit the range of motion at a joint; likewise, a warmed up muscle will be flexible and allow a greater range of motion.

3. *The connective tissue* within the joint capsule provides stability at the joint. **Ligaments,** for example, are positioned around the joint to prevent the bone ends from coming apart, as in a dislocation injury. They prevent movements that a normal, healthy joint is not supposed to do. **Cartilage** covers the ends of the bones and creates a better fit between the bones, which helps eliminate unnecessary movements.

4. *Tendons,* which connect muscle to bones and to connective tissue surrounding joints, are extensions of the muscle tissue. If the muscle is tight, the tendon will also be tight.

5. *Tight skin* can limit the range of motion at a joint.

Exercise aimed at improving flexibility does not change the structure of bone, but it alters the soft tissues (muscle, joint connective tissue, and tendons) that contribute to flexibility. Table 5.1 lists the resistance of the various soft tissues to total joint flexibility. Note that the structures associated with the joint capsule, muscles, and tendons provide most of the body's resistance to movement. Therefore, flexibility exercises must alter the resistance of one of these three to increase the range of motion around a joint. Stretching the muscle and tendon is desirable because these soft tissues can lengthen over time and improve flexibility. Stretching the ligaments in the joint capsule, in con-

FIGURE 5.1
A view of the knee joint and the anatomical structures that influence movement.

Source: Johnson, M., *Human Biology*, 4th ed. San Francisco: Benjamin Cummings, 2008, 114.

trast, is undesirable because it can lead to a loose joint that would be highly susceptible to injury.

Before we examine specific stretching exercises, let's find how stretching works.

Stretching and the Stretch Reflex

When a doctor taps you on the knee with a rubber hammer, your knee extends. This is a **stretch reflex** caused by the rapid stretching of the **muscle spindles**

TABLE 5.1
Soft-Tissue Resistance to Joint Movement

Structure	Limitation to Flexibility (% of total resistance)
Joint capsule	47
Muscle	41
Tendon	10
Skin	2

flexibility The ability to move joints freely through their full range of motion.

ligaments Connective tissue within the joint capsule that holds bones together.

cartilage A tough connective tissue that forms a pad on the end of long bones, such as the femur, tibia, and humerus. Cartilage acts as a shock absorber to cushion the weight of one bone on another and to provide protection from the friction due to joint movement.

stretch reflex Involuntary contraction of a muscle due to rapid stretching of that muscle.

muscle spindles The type of proprioceptor found within muscle.

Long/Strong Back Muscles

Lumbar Region of the Spine

Strong Abdominal Muscles

Long Hip Flexor Muscles

Long/Strong Hamstring Muscle

FIGURE 5.2
Strong abdominal and hip flexor muscles, balanced with strong back and hamstring muscles, help keep the spine and pelvis in neutral alignment, thereby lowering the risk of LBP.

within the quadriceps muscles that move the knee joint. Activating the stretch reflex is counterproductive to flexibility, because during the stretch the muscle shortens rather than lengthens. (Remember that the goal of stretching is to lengthen the muscle). Fortunately, you can avoid the stretch reflex if you stretch the muscles and tendons very slowly. In fact, if you hold a muscle stretch for several seconds, the muscle spindles allow the muscle being stretched to further relax and permit an even greater stretch (2, 3). Therefore, stretching exercises are most effective when they avoid promoting a stretch reflex.

Muscle spindles are one type of **proprioceptor,** specialized receptors in muscles and tendons that provide feedback to the brain about the position of the body parts. When you were learning to catch a ball, you had to look at the position of your arms and hands to make sure they were in line with the path of the ball. As your catching skills improved, you no longer had to look at the arm position to know that it was lined up with the ball. The proprioceptors in your muscles and tendons provided feedback to your brain about where the arm was positioned. The proprioceptors within the muscles are muscle spindles, and the proprioceptors within the tendons are **Golgi tendon organs.**

Make sure you know...

> The structural and physiological limits to flexibility are due to the characteristics of bone; muscle; connective tissue within the joint capsule, such as ligaments and cartilage; the tendons, which connect

muscle to bones and to connective tissue surrounding joints; and skin.

> If muscle spindles are stretched suddenly, they initiate a stretch reflex that causes the muscle to contract and shorten. However, if muscles are stretched slowly, the stretch reflex can be avoided.

> The proprioceptors (muscle spindles and Golgi tendon organs) monitor the muscles and tendons and report their positions to the brain.

Benefits of Flexibility

Although increased flexibility provides numerous benefits, including increased joint mobility, efficient body movement, and good posture (1, 3, 4), there is no research evidence to support the idea that it reduces the incidence of muscle injury during exercise. In fact, one critical review article suggests that stretching may contribute to injury (5). The only studies suggesting that stretching offers protection from muscle injury combined the stretching with a general warm-up.

However, improved flexibility does help keep your joints healthy and can prevent lower back pain. Let's look at these benefits more closely.

Keeping Joints Healthy

Joints will suffer from lack of movement if you do not regularly engage them. If a joint is not moved enough or has a limited range of motion, scar tissue can form that further restricts the joint motion and can be painful to the point that you may not be able to move the joint. The shoulder joint is particularly susceptible to this scar tissue formation. Mild stretching on a daily basis can prevent a joint from becoming immobile.

Joint mobility is also important for keeping the joint lubricated. Joints contain synovial fluid, which is needed to reduce friction and decrease wear and tear. Moving the joint helps circulate the synovial fluid, which in turn reduces the friction on the cartilage between the bones. Too much friction can damage cartilage, setting the stage for arthritis. Mild stretching can improve the mobility of the joint and promote normal wear on the cartilage covering the ends of the bones.

Stretching also directly affects the joints by reducing tension within the fibers of a muscle. When a muscle is stretched, these fibers are free to slide past one another, and the tension is literally worked out of the muscle. Reduced muscle tension reduces the tension exerted by the tendon as it crosses the joint. The force of the muscle exerted through the tendon on the bone can cause the bone ends of the joint to be pulled closer together, thus limiting the joint range of motion. In essence, stretching can have the same effects on muscle tension as a manual muscle massage, at a much lower cost.

Preventing Lower Back Pain

Another benefit of improved flexibility is that it can help prevent low back problems. Low back pain (LBP) is sometimes called a **hypokinetic disease,** that is, a disease associated with a lack of exercise. The weak abdominal muscles commonly seen in sedentary individuals and the lack of flexibility in the hip flexor muscles are two common causes of LBP.

The abdominal muscles play a significant role in keeping the pelvic girdle in a neutral alignment with the spine (Figure 5.2). When the abdominal muscles are weak, the pelvis tilts forward and creates an increased hyperextension (forward curve), called *lordosis*, in the lower back. The muscles that flex the hip can affect the pelvis in the same way; however, they pull the pelvis forward when they are tight. Stretching these muscles and strengthening the abdominal muscles are important to keep the pelvis in a neutral alignment.

In addition to the abdominal muscles and the hip flexor muscles, the hamstrings and the lower back muscles also attach to the posterior side of the pelvis and can affect its alignment. The hamstring muscles exert a downward pull on the pelvis, whereas the low back muscles exert an upward pull. Keeping all four muscle groups in balance helps keep the pelvis in a neutral alignment with the lumbar region of the spine and therefore diminishes the likelihood for LBP.

Up to 80% of people will experience LBP, and approximately 15% of Americans will be disabled by LBP in their lifetime (6). Men and women are affected equally by back pain, usually between the ages of 25 and 60. Most pain in the lower back goes away in a few days or weeks. Low back pain that lasts for longer than 6 months is considered chronic.

People who regularly carry heavy backpacks are at increased risk of lower back problems. In one study (7), curvature of the spine significantly increased as subjects wearing backpacks became fatigued. Interestingly, after the subjects rested for several minutes, both trunk and head angles were not significantly different from the fatigued condition. Although this study did not examine resulting back problems from the chronic wearing of a backpack, the findings certainly suggest that long-term backpack use can result in misalignment in the lower back.

The psychological, social, and physical costs of lower back pain are high, as are the economic costs. The medical, insurance, and business/industry costs are generally considered to be in the billions of dollars per year. Developing and maintaining healthy low back function requires a balance of flexibility, strength, and endurance.

Focus on the following stretches (shown later in this chapter) to help you maintain a healthy back: thigh stretch (Exercise 5.3), leg stretch (Exercise 5.4), hip and

Top Potential Contributors to Lower Back Pain

- *Poor low back lumbar flexibility.* Tight low back muscles exert an uneven pull on the pelvis, resulting in a hyperextended lumbar spine.
- *Poor hamstring flexibility.* Weak hamstring muscles allow the pelvis to tilt forward.
- *Poor hip flexor flexibility.* Tight hip flexors exert a forward and downward pull on the pelvis and lumbar vertebrae.
- *Poor strength and endurance of the forward and lateral abdominals.* Weak abdominal muscles allow the pelvis to tilt forward.
- *Poor flexibility and endurance of the back extensor muscles.* Back extensor muscles must have the endurance to exert a pull on the pelvis for the duration of exercise.

gluteal stretch (Exercise 5.7), lower back stretch (Exercise 5.8), and the trunk twister (Exercise 5.10). Leg pulls, sitting hamstring stretches, curl-ups, and knee-to-toe touches will also help. Also see Laboratory 5.3.

Make sure you know...

> Improved flexibility increases joint mobility and joint health, increases resistance to muscle injury, helps prevent low back problems, allows for efficient body movement, and improves posture and personal appearance.

> Flexibility of the hamstrings and lower back and strong abdominal muscles are important for a healthy back.

Evaluating Flexibility

Flexibility is joint specific. That is, you might be flexible in one joint but lack flexibility in another. You may also notice that you are more flexible on one side of your body than the other. This disparity is often due to the greater usage of the dominant side of the body.

proprioceptor Specialized receptor in muscle or tendon that provides feedback to the brain about the position of body parts.

Golgi tendon organ The type of proprioceptor found within tendons.

hypokinetic disease Disease associated with a lack of exercise.

Although no single test is representative of total body flexibility, measurements of trunk and shoulder flexibility are commonly evaluated. The **sit-and-reach test** measures the ability to flex the trunk, which means stretching the lower back muscles and the muscles in the back of the thigh (hamstrings). The figure in Laboratory 5.1 on page 163 illustrates the sit-and-reach test using a sit-and-reach box.

The **shoulder flexibility test** evaluates the range of motion at the shoulder. See Laboratory 5.1 at the end of the chapter for a walk-through of the sit-and-reach test and shoulder flexibility tests.

Once you complete the sit-and-reach test and the shoulder flexibility test, you will better understand how flexible or inflexible you are. Both active and inactive individuals are often classified as average or below average for trunk and shoulder flexibility. In fact, only individuals who regularly perform stretching exercises are likely to possess flexibility levels that exceed the average. Regardless of your current flexibility classification, your flexibility goal should be to reach a classification of above average (i.e., good, excellent, or superior).

Make sure you know...

> Flexibility measurements are joint specific.

> Two popular tests to evaluate flexibility are the sit-and-reach test and the shoulder flexibility test.

CONSIDER THIS!

Contrary to popular belief, weight lifting does not decrease flexibility. In fact, the use of proper form during weight lifting (lifting through the full range of motion) can actually increase flexibility.

kinds of stretching techniques are commonly used to increase flexibility: **dynamic stretching, ballistic stretching,** and **static stretching.** A fourth type of stretching called **proprioceptive neuromuscular facilitation (PNF)** is often used in rehabilitation settings (2, 8).

Dynamic stretching can be useful for athletes whose events involve quick changes of direction. The fluid, exaggerated movements in dynamic stretches mimic the movements that an athlete engages in during competition. Ballistic stretching, in contrast, involves rapid and forceful bouncing movements to stretch the muscles. The movements of ballistic stretching are more likely to cause injury, so exercises to warm up the muscles prior to stretching are helpful.

Ballistic stretches may be most beneficial to individuals involved in quick, explosive movements. With dynamic and ballistic stretching, the athlete trains the nervous system and the muscles to adapt to the movements that she routinely performs. However, for the average fitness enthusiast seeking to increase flexibility, ballistic movements may activate the stretch reflex, injuring muscles and tendons.

For this reason, ballistic stretching techniques are not usually incorporated into a nonathlete's fitness program.

Most people will benefit from incorporating static and proprioceptive neuromuscular facilitation techniques into their fitness program. We'll discuss these two types of stretching next.

Designing a Flexibility Training Program

Because flexibility training is a key part of any fitness program, you'll want to include stretching exercises in your fitness routine. As with designing programs for the other fitness components, your first step will be to set short- and long-term goals. Do you want to become more flexible in the shoulders, or is your aim more to improve your hamstring and low back flexibility? No matter what your goal, you will want to think about how you will get there before you begin your new flexibility training routine. Also consider keeping a record of your workouts and improvements to follow your progress and plan your future training schedule.

Once you've set your goals, you can consider the types of stretches to include in your program. Three

Static Stretching

Static stretching is extremely effective for improving flexibility (2, 4). Static stretching involves slowly lengthening a muscle to a point at which further movement is limited (slight discomfort is felt) and holding this position for a fixed period of time. Holding the stretch for 20 to 30 seconds, and repeating it 3 to 4 times, improves flexibility (4). Compared with ballistic stretching, the risk of injury to the muscle or tendon associated with static stretching is minimal. When performed during the cool-down period, static stretching may reduce the muscle stiffness associated with some exercise routines (2, 4).

You can perform static stretches at home, and you don't need any special equipment to do them. You can even do them while watching television or sitting at your computer. See Exercises 5.1 through 5.12 for examples of static stretches.

STEPS FOR BEHAVIOR CHANGE

Are you too stiff?

Answer the following questions to help determine whether you would benefit from increased flexibility.

Y N

☐ ☐ Do you often feel as though you have a stiff neck?

☐ ☐ Is your mobility impaired when you turn your head to the left or right?

☐ ☐ Do you have difficulty washing your own back?

☐ ☐ Does your lower back feel stiff when you sit at your desk for prolonged periods of time?

☐ ☐ Do your ankles and feet feel stiff when you get out of bed in the morning?

If you answered yes to more than one question, check out the following tips.

TIPS TO IMPROVE FLEXIBILITY

☑ If your neck feels stiff when you are working at your desk, perform 5 minutes of gentle neck stretches and shoulder rolls at the top of every hour.

☑ Next time you shower, let the warm water hit the back of your neck, shoulders, and upper back. Perform 10 shoulder rolls forward, 10 backward, and 10 neck tilts to the left and right while the shower spray is aimed at your neck and shoulders.

☑ To increase the flexibility in your shoulders, try holding a washcloth in your right hand as you reach behind your head. Grasp the washcloth with your left hand as you reach behind your back. Try pulling the washcloth up and down as you grasp it in both hands, increasing your range of motion with each up-and-down movement.

☑ If your low back is stiff after sitting for prolonged periods of time, try sitting on a physioball instead of a desk chair. The smaller muscles of the spine will be exercised as you balance on the physioball.

☑ Every morning when you wake up, sit on the edge of your bed and make 10 small and 10 large circles to the right and then to the left with your right foot. Switch and repeat circling motion with your left foot.

Proprioceptive Neuromuscular Facilitation

Proprioceptive neuromuscular facilitation (PNF) combines stretching with alternating contraction and relaxation of muscles. There are two common types of PNF stretching: *contract-relax (CR) stretching* and *contract-relax/antagonist contract (CRAC) stretching*. The CR stretch technique calls for first contracting the muscle to be stretched. Then, after the muscle is relaxed, it is slowly stretched. The CRAC method calls for the same contract-relax routine but adds to this the contraction of the **antagonist** muscle, the muscle on the opposite side of the joint. The purpose of contracting the antag-

sit-and-reach test A fitness test that measures the ability to flex the trunk.

shoulder flexibility test A fitness test that measures the ability of the shoulder muscles to move through their full range of motion.

dynamic stretching Stretching that involves moving the joints through the full range of motion to mimic a movement used in a sport or exercise.

ballistic stretching A type of stretch that involves sudden and forceful bouncing to stretch the muscles.

static stretching Stretching that slowly lengthens a muscle to a point where further movement is limited.

proprioceptive neuromuscular facilitation (PNF) A series of movements that combines stretching with alternating contraction and relaxation of muscles.

antagonist The muscle on the opposite side of the joint.

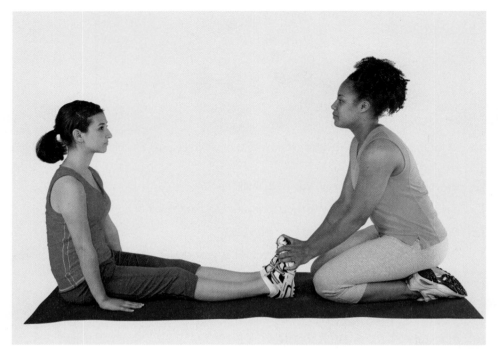

FIGURE 5.3
An example of a partner-assisted CRAC procedure for stretching the calf muscles. The exerciser contracts the calf muscles against resistance provided by the assistant. Then, unassisted, the exerciser contracts the shin (antagonist) muscles, thereby relaxing the calf muscles. Finally, while the exerciser continues contracting the shin muscles, the assistant stretches the calf muscles.

onist muscle is to promote a reflex relaxation of the muscle to be stretched.

How do PNF techniques compare with ballistic and static stretching? First, PNF has been shown to be safer and more effective in promoting flexibility than ballistic stretching (8). Further, studies have shown PNF programs to be equal to, or in some cases superior to, static stretching for improving flexibility (9).

Passive and Active Stretching

Some PNF stretches cannot be done alone — that is, they require a partner. The partner supplies resistance to the body part during the contraction of the antagonist muscles, thus preventing the body part from moving. This sequence of movements allows the muscle to relax more than in a static stretch, and greater range of motion can be achieved. The only drawback to this type of stretch is that the partner must provide resistance, which can be very tiring over a short period of time.

The following steps illustrate how a CRAC procedure can be done with a partner (Figure 5.3):

1. After the assistant moves the limb in the direction necessary to stretch the desired muscles to the point of tightness (where mild discomfort is felt), the exerciser isometrically contracts the muscle being stretched for 3 to 5 seconds and then relaxes it.

2. The exerciser then moves the limb in the opposite direction of the stretch by isometrically contracting the antagonist muscles. The exerciser holds this isometric contraction for approximately 5 seconds, during which time the muscles to be stretched relax. While the desired muscles are relaxed, the assistant may increase the stretch of the desired muscles.

3. The exerciser then isometrically contracts the antagonist muscles for another 5 seconds, which relaxes the desired muscles, and the assistant again stretches the desired muscles to the point of mild discomfort.

This cycle of three steps is repeated 3 to 5 times.

Some PNF stretches can also be done without a partner (Figure 5.4). Using a towel or other object to provide resistance can achieve the same benefits without fatiguing an assistant.

Applying the FIT Principle

So what are the best frequency, intensity, and time (duration) for your stretching routine (the FIT principle)? The answers vary according to your present level of flexibility, among other factors. However, a good rule of thumb is that the first week, or starter phase, of a stretching regimen should include one stretching session. During the next 4 weeks, or the slow progression phase, of the program, one stretching session should be added per week. Initially, the duration of each training session should be approximately 5 minutes and should increase gradually to 20 to 30 minutes following 6 to 12 weeks of stretching during the slow progression phase.

The physiological rationale for increasing the duration of stretching is that each stretch position is held for progressively longer durations as the program continues. For example, begin by holding each stretched position for 15 seconds, then add 5 seconds each week up to 30 seconds. Start by performing each of the exercises once (1 rep), and progress to 4 reps. The frequency and duration of a stretching exercise prescription should be 2 to 5 days per week for 10 to 30 minutes each day. Table 5.2 illustrates a sample exercise prescription for a flexibility program.

What about the intensity of stretching? In general, a limb should not be stretched beyond a position of mild discomfort. The intensity of stretching is increased by extending the stretch to the limits of your range of motion. Your range of motion will gradually increase as your flexibility improves during the training program.

To improve overall flexibility, all major muscle groups should be stretched. Just because you have good flexibility in the shoulders does not mean your flexibility will be good in the hamstrings. Exercises 5.1 through 5.12 illustrate the proper methods of performing 12 different stretching exercises. Integrate these exercises into the program outlined in Table 5.2.

These exercises are designed to be used in a regular program of stretching to increase flexibility. For safety reasons, all flexibility programs should consist of either PNF or static stretching exercises. The exercises presented involve the joints and major muscle groups for which range of motion tends to decrease with age and disuse. The exercises include both static and PNF movements and may require a partner. To avoid injury, be sure to follow the guidelines in the box on page 149.

Some stretches that were once thought to improve flexibility are now known to be potentially damaging to the musculoskeletal system. The photos starting on

FIGURE 5.4
You can use a towel to do some PNF stretches without a partner.

page 157 show some common exercises that may cause injury, and provide substitute exercises that help accomplish the same goals.

Make sure you know...

> Ballistic stretching involves sudden, forceful bouncing. Dynamic stretching involves moving the joints through a range of motion that is specific to a sport or activity. Static stretches involve stretching a

TABLE 5.2
Sample Flexibility Program Using the FIT Principle

Week	Phase	Duration of Stretch Hold	Repetitions	Frequency (times/wk)
1	Starter	15 sec	1	1
2	Slow progression	20 sec	2	2
3	Slow progression	25 sec	3	3
4	Slow progression	30 sec	4	3
5	Slow progression	30 sec	4	3–4
6	Slow progression	30 sec	4	4–5
7+	Maintenance	30 sec	4	4–5

A CLOSER LOOK

PILES—MORE THAN STRETCHING?

Pilates (pronounced Puh-**lah**-teez) is a widely used form of exercise among professional dancers, gymnasts, recreational exercisers, and rehabilitation specialists. It involves gentle, subtle stretching and contracting of muscles to produce very fluid, controlled movements that emphasize a mind–body interaction.

This body conditioning routine improves flexibility, strength, endurance and coordination without increasing muscle bulk. There are two forms of exercise in Pilates. The first form focuses on mat exercises that use your body weight as the resistance force. The other form involves using specialized machines to tone and strengthen the body. One piece of Pilates equipment, called the Reformer, consists of a moving carriage on a horizontal frame. There is a series of up to 100 exercises that can be performed on it without stopping.

Pilates emphasize the following basic principles:

- *Concentration*—The mind–body connection. This stresses that conscious control of movement enhances body awareness.
- *Control/precision*—It's not about intensity or multiple "reps"; it's more about proper form.
- *Centering*—A mental focus within the body calms the spirit, and a particular focus on the torso develops a strong core and enables the rest of the body

to function efficiently. All action initiates from the trunk and flows outward to the extremities.

- *Stabilizing*—Before you move, you have to be still. This helps provide a safe starting place for mobility.
- *Breathing*—Deep, coordinated, conscious diaphragmatic patterns of inhalation and exhalation initiate movement, help activate deep muscles, and keep you focused.

- *Alignment*—Proper alignment is key to good posture. You'll be aware of the position of your head and neck on the spine and pelvis, right down through the legs and toes.
- *Fluidity*—Smooth, continuous motion rather than jarring repetitions.
- *Integration*—Several different muscle groups are engaged simultaneously to control and support movement. All principles come together, making for a holistic mind–body workout.

muscle to the limit of movement and holding the stretch for an extended period of time. Proprioceptive neuromuscular facilitation (PNF) combines stretching with alternating contraction and relaxation of muscles to improve flexibility.

> Stretching exercises should be performed 2 to 5 days per week for 10 to 30 minutes each day.

> The intensity of a stretch is considered to be maximal where "mild discomfort" is felt.

> You can minimize your risk of injury during stretches by avoiding hazardous exercises and making sure to perform stretches correctly.

Avoiding Hazardous Exercises

To avoid injury during stretching exercises, follow these guidelines:

- Don't hold your breath. Try to breathe as normally as possible during the exercise.
- Do not fully extend the knee, neck, or back.
- Do not stretch muscles that are already stretched.
- Do not stretch to the point that joint pain occurs.
- Avoid stretching ligaments by avoiding unnatural movements at the joint.
- Use caution when having someone help you with passive stretches. Make sure you communicate about the end of the range of motion.
- Avoid forceful extension and flexion of the spine.

Motivation to Maintain Flexibility

Maintaining flexibility requires a commitment to performing regular stretching. Just as in other types of fitness training, good time management is critical if you are going to succeed. Set aside time for 3 to 5 stretching periods per week, and stick to your schedule. Remember that you can stretch almost anywhere, because you don't need special equipment. So take advantage of "windows" of free time in your day and plan stretching workouts.

You are not likely to maintain a lifetime stretching program if you do not enjoy your workouts. One suggestion for making stretching more fun is to perform stretching workouts while listening to music or during a television program you enjoy.

A CLOSER LOOK

WHEN MUSCLES CRAMP

A muscle cramp is one of the most common problems encountered in sports and exercise. For many years, the primary causes of muscle cramps were thought to be dehydration and/or electrolyte imbalances. Accordingly, drinking enough fluids and ensuring that the diet contains sufficient amounts of sodium (from table salt, for example) and potassium (e.g., from bananas) have long been encouraged as preventive measures. When muscles cramp, stretching and/or massage have been used to relieve the cramping until electrolyte balance can be restored.

More recent research, however, suggests that cramping may be due to abnormal spinal control of motor neuron activity, especially when a muscle contracts while shortened (8). For example, the cramping that often occurs in the calf muscles of recreational swimmers when their toes are pointed may occur because those calf muscles are contracting while they are shortened.

The most prevalent risk factors for cramps during exercise are muscle fatigue and poor stretching habits (failure to stretch regularly and long enough during each session). Other risk factors include older age, higher body mass index, and a family history of muscle cramps.

If cramping occurs, you should do the following:

- Passively stretch the muscle. Such stretching induces receptors that sense the stretch to initiate nerve impulses that inhibit muscle stimulation.

- Drink plenty of water to avoid dehydration or electrolyte imbalances. Sports drinks can help replenish glucose and electrolytes, but do not use salt tablets or drink fluids containing caffeine.

- Seek medical attention if multiple muscle groups are involved, because this could be a sign of more serious problems.

Although no strategies for preventing muscle cramping during exercise have been proven effective, regular stretching using PNF techniques, correcting muscle balance and posture, and proper training for the exercise activity involved may be beneficial.

Sample Flexibility Exercises*

EXERCISE 5.1   LOWER LEG STRETCH ▷

Purpose: To stretch the **calf** muscles (gastrocnemius, soleus) and the **Achilles' tendon**.

Position: Stand on the edge of a surface that is high enough to allow your heel to drop lower than your toes. Have a support nearby to hold for balance.

Movement: Rise up on your toes as far as possible for several seconds, then lower your heels as far as possible. Shift your body weight from one leg to the other for added stretch of the muscles.

Variation: Sit on the floor with leg outstretched, loop a towel under the ball of your foot, and gently pull your foot upward so that the top of the foot moves closer to your shin. Another variation (not pictured) is to sit on the floor with one leg outstretched, and the other leg flexed with the sole of your foot along the knee of your other leg. Reach down, grasp the toes of the outstretched leg, and gently pull the foot upward so that the top of the foot is moving closer to the shin.

*Log on to **www.pearsonhighered.com/powers** to view demonstration videos of exercises marked with the ▷ icon.

EXERCISE 5.2 SHIN STRETCH

Purpose: To stretch the muscles of the **shin** (tibialis anterior, extensor digitorum longus, extensor hallucis longus).

Position: Kneel on both knees, with your trunk rotated to one side and the hand on that side pressing down on your ankle.

Movement: While pressing down on your ankle, move your pelvis forward; hold for several seconds. Repeat on the other side.

EXERCISE 5.3 THIGH STRETCH

Purpose: To stretch the muscles in the front of the **thigh** (quadriceps) of the extended (rear) leg.

Position: Kneel on one knee, resting your rear shin and foot flat on the floor. Place both hands on the forward knee. *Note*: If you need more stability, you can place your hands on the floor on either side of the forward foot.

Movement: Slide your rear leg backward so that the knee is slightly behind your hips; then press your hips forward and down, and hold for several seconds. While stretching, maintain approximately a 90-degree angle at the knee of the front leg. Switch the positions of the legs to stretch the other thigh.

Sample Flexibility Exercises

EXERCISE 5.4 LEG STRETCH ▷

Purpose: To stretch the muscles on the **back of the hip** (gluteus maximus), the **back of the thigh** (hamstrings), and the **calf** (gastrocnemius and soleus).

Position: Lying on your back, bring one knee toward your chest, and grasp your toes with the hand on the same side. Place the opposite hand on the back of the leg just below the knee.

Movement: Pull your the knee toward your chest while pushing your heel toward the ceiling and pulling your toes toward your shin. Straighten your knee until you feel sufficient stretch in the muscles of the back of the leg, and hold for several seconds. Repeat for the other leg.

EXERCISE 5.5 MODIFIED HURDLER'S STRETCH ▷

Purpose: To stretch the **lower back muscles** (erector spinae) and muscles in the **back of the thigh** (hamstrings).

Position: Sit on a level surface with one leg out in front, bend the other knee, and place the sole of the foot alongside the knee of the outstretched leg.

Movement: Reach down, and grab the ankle of the outstretched leg. Keeping your head and trunk straight, lean your trunk forward, and attempt to touch your chest to your knee. Hold for several seconds. Return to the upright position, and alternate legs.

Variation: Grasp the toes of the extended leg, and pull your toes toward your shin while stretching. This will also stretch the calf muscles (gastrocnemius and soleus).

EXERCISE 5.6 INSIDE LEG STRETCH

Purpose: To stretch the muscles on the **inside of the thighs** (adductors and internal rotators).

Position: Sit with the bottoms of your feet together and place your hands just below your knees.

Movement: Try to raise your knees while pushing down with your hands and forearms. Then relax, and, using your hands, press your knees toward the floor; hold for several seconds.

EXERCISE 5.7 HIP AND GLUTEAL STRETCH

Purpose: To stretch the muscles at the **hip** (gluteals, tensor fasciae latae).

Position: Lie on your back, with one leg crossed over the other and both shoulders and both arms on the floor.

Movement: Grasp behind the knee of the leg that is not crossed over, and pull the thigh toward your chest. Hold for several seconds. Reverse the positions of the legs, and repeat the stretch.

EXERCISES

Sample Flexibility Exercises

EXERCISE 5.8 LOWER BACK STRETCH ▷

Purpose: To stretch the muscles of the **lower back** (erector spinae) and **buttocks** (gluteals).

Position: Lie on your back with your hips and knees bent, your feet flat on the floor, and your arms positioned along your sides.

Movement: First, arch your back, and lift your hips off the floor; hold for several seconds. Then relax and return to starting position. Place your hands behind your knees, and pull the knees to your chest. Hold for several seconds.

EXERCISE 5.9   SIDE STRETCH ▷

Purpose: To stretch the muscles of the **upper arm** (triceps) and **side of the trunk** (latissimus dorsi).

Position: Sit on the floor with your legs crossed.

Movement: Stretch one arm over your head while bending at your waist in the same direction. With the opposite arm, reach across your chest as far as possible; hold for several seconds. Do not rotate your trunk; try to stretch the muscle on the same side of the trunk as the overhead arm. Alternate arms to stretch the other side of the trunk.

EXERCISE 5.10   TRUNK TWISTER ▷

Purpose: To stretch the muscles of the **trunk** (obliques and latissimus dorsi) and **hip** (gluteus maximus).

Position: Sit with your left leg extended, your right leg bent and crossed over your left knee, and your right foot on the floor. Place your right hand on the floor behind your buttocks.

Movement: Placing your left arm on the right side of your right thigh, and your right hand on the floor, use your left arm to push against your right leg while twisting your trunk to the right; hold for several seconds. Then assume the starting position with your right leg extended, and stretch the opposite side of the body.

Sample Flexibility Exercises

EXERCISE 5.11 CHEST STRETCH ▷

Purpose: To stretch the muscles across the **chest** (pectoralis major) and **shoulder** (anterior deltoid and biceps).

Position: Stand in a doorway, and grasp the frame of the doorway at shoulder height.

Movement: Press forward on the frame for 5 seconds. Then relax, and shift your weight forward until you feel the stretch of muscles across your chest; hold for several seconds.

EXERCISE 5.12 NECK STRETCH ▷

Purpose: To stretch the muscles that rotate the **head** (sternocleidomastoid).

Position: After turning your head to one side, place your hand against your cheek with your fingers toward the ear, and your elbow pointing forward.

Movement: Try to turn your head and neck against the resistance of your hand; hold for a few seconds. Remove your hand and relax, then turn your head as far as possible in the same direction. Repeat the stretch, turning in the other direction.

Alternatives for Unsafe Exercises*

Purpose: To stretch the **lower back** and **buttocks**.

May Cause Injury:
KNEE PULL

This position places undue stress on the knee joint.

Try This Instead:
LEG PULL ▷

Lie on your back, and pull your knee toward your chest by pulling on the back of your leg just below the knee. Then extend the knee joint, and point the sole of your foot straight up. Continue to pull your leg toward your chest. Repeat several times with each leg.

Purpose: To strengthen the **upper leg** and stretch the **lower leg**.

May Cause Injury:
DEEP KNEE BEND

This movement hyperflexes the knee and "opens" the joint while stretching the ligaments.

Try This Instead:
LUNGE ▷

From a standing position, step forward with either foot and touch the opposite knee to the ground. Repeat with the opposite leg.

*Log on to **www.pearsonhighered.com/powers** to view demonstration videos of exercises marked with the ▷ icon.

EXERCISES

Alternatives for Unsafe Exercises

Purpose: To stretch the **lower back**, **buttocks**, and **hamstrings**.

May Cause Injury:
STANDING TOE TOUCH

This movement could damage the lower back.

Try This Instead:
SITTING HAMSTRING STRETCH

Sit at leg-length from a wall. With your foot on the wall and the other knee bent with the foot between the wall and your buttocks, bend forward, keeping your lower back straight. The bent knee can fall to the side.

Purpose: To strengthen the **abdominal muscles**.

May Cause Injury:
SIT-UP (HANDS BEHIND HEAD)

This movement could cause hyperflexion of the neck and strain the neck muscles.

Try This Instead:
CURL-UP

Lie on your back with your knees bent, and cross your arms over your chest. Using your abdominal muscles, curl up until the upper half of your back is off the floor, and then return to the starting position.

Purpose: To stretch the **neck muscles**.

May Cause Injury:
NECK CIRCLES

This movement hyperextends the neck, which can pinch arteries and nerves, as well as damage disks in the spine.

Try This Instead:
NECK STRETCHES ▶

Sit with your head and neck straight. Move your head down to flex your neck, and return your head upright. Then, slowly turn your head from side to side as far as possible; attempt to point your chin at each shoulder.

Purpose: To stretch and strengthen the **buttocks**.

May Cause Injury:
DONKEY KICK

When kicking the leg back, most people hyperextend the neck and/or back.

Try This Instead:
KNEE-TO-NOSE TOUCH

While on your hands and knees, lift one knee toward your nose and then extend that leg to the horizontal position. Alternate legs. Do not lift your leg higher than your hips, and keep your neck in line with your back.

Summary

1. Flexibility is the range of motion of a joint.
2. Improved flexibility results in the following benefits: increased joint mobility, prevention of low back problems, efficient body movement, and improved posture and personal appearance.
3. The five structural and physiological limits to flexibility are the shape of bone; muscle; connective tissue within the joint capsule; the tendons, which connect muscle to bones and to connective tissue that surrounds joints; and skin.
4. Proprioceptors are constantly monitoring the tension of the muscles and tendons and providing feedback to the brain. If muscle spindles are suddenly stretched, they respond by initiating a stretch reflex that causes the muscle to contract.

However, if the muscles and tendons are stretched slowly, the stretch reflex can be avoided.

5. Designing your flexibility program involves setting short-term and long-term goals and selecting stretches that will help you meet your goals. Static stretches involve stretching a muscle to the limit of movement and holding the stretch for an extended period of time. Dynamic stretches involve fluid, exaggerated movements designed to mimic the movements of a given sport or activity.
6. Proprioceptive neuromuscular facilitation (PNF) combines stretching with alternating contraction and relaxation of muscles to improve flexibility. Ballistic stretches may be appropriate for some athletes but are not safe for the general public.

Study Questions

1. Which of the following is not an anatomical factor that can limit movement at a joint?
   a. shape of the bones
   b. tight skin
   c. tight tendons
   d. length of the bone
2. Proprioceptors include which of the following?
   a. motor units
   b. Golgi organs
   c. muscle spindles
   d. a and b
   e. b and c
3. Static stretching is not advisable for nonathletes.
   a. True
   b. False
4. To avoid injury, most stretching should be done
   a. only at night.
   b. after the muscles have been warmed up.
   c. while watching television.
   d. to the point of pain.

5. Lower back pain is the result of
   a. weak abdominal muscles.
   b. weak hamstring muscles.
   c. hyperextension of the lower back.
   d. all of the above.
6. Define the following terms:
   flexibility
   range of motion
   cartilage
   ligament
   tendon
   proprioceptive neuromuscular facilitation
   antagonist
7. Describe the difference in function between ligaments and tendons.
8. Compare static and ballistic stretching.
9. List three primary reasons why maintaining flexibility is important.
10. List the factors that limit flexibility. Which factors place the greatest limitations on flexibility?
11. Briefly outline the exercise prescription to improve flexibility.
12. Describe why the stretch reflex should be avoided.

Suggested Reading

Blair, S. N., M. J. LaMonte, and M. Z. Nichaman. The evolution of physical activity recommendations: How much is enough? *American Journal of Clinical Nutrition* 79(5):913S–920S, 2004.

da Costa, B. R., and E. R. Vieira. Stretching to reduce work-related musculoskeletal disorders: A systematic review. *Journal of Rehabilitation Medicine* 40(5):321–328, 2008.

Guissard, N., and J. Duchateau. Neural aspects of muscle stretching. *Exercise and Sport Sciences Reviews* 34(4):154–158, 2006.

Herman, S. L., and D. T. Smith. Four-week dynamic stretching warm-up intervention elicits longer-term performance benefits. *Journal of Strength and Conditioning Research* 22(4):1286–1297, 2008.

Rubini, E. C., A. L. L. Costa, and P. S. C. Gomes. The effects of stretching on strength performance. *Sports Medicine* 37(3):213–224, 2007.

Small, K., L. McNaughton, and M. Matthews. A systematic review into the efficacy of static stretching as part of a warm-up for the prevention of exercise-related injury. *Research in Sports Medicine* 16(3):213–231, 2008.

Woods, K., P. Bishop, and E. Jones. Warm-up and stretching in the prevention of muscular injury. *Sports Medicine* 37(12):1089–1099, 2007.

For links to the organizations and websites listed below, visit The Total Fitness and Wellness Website at www.pearsonhighered.com/powers.

WebMD

General information about exercise, fitness, wellness. Great articles, instructional information, and updates.

ACSM

Comprehensive website of the American College of Sports Medicine. Provides information, articles, equipment recommendations, books, and position statements about all aspects of health and fitness.

Mayo Clinic

General information about fitness and wellness. Includes flexibility exercises for particular muscle groups, sports, and conditions.

References

1. Ylinen, J., T. Kankainen, H. Kautiainen, A. Rezasoltani, T. Kuukkanen, and A. Häkkinen. Effect of stretching on hamstring muscle compliance. *Journal of Rehabilitation Medicine* 41(1):80–84, 2009.

2. Guissard, N., and J. Duchateau. Effect of static stretch training on neural and mechanical properties of the human plantar-flexor muscles. *Muscle Nerve* 29(2): 248–255, 2004.

3. Sharman, M. J., A. G. Cresswell, and S. Riek. Proprioceptive neuromuscular facilitation stretching: Mechanisms and clinical implications. *Sports Medicine* 36(11):929–939, 2006.

4. American College of Sports Medicine. The recommended quantity and quality of exercise for developing and maintaining cardiorespiratory and muscular fitness, and flexibility in healthy adults. *Medicine and Science in Sports and Exercise* 30(6):975–991, 1998.

5. Small, K., L. McNaughton, and M. Matthews. A systematic review into the efficacy of static stretching as part of a warm-up for the prevention of exercise-related injury. *Research in Sports Medicine* 16(3):213–231, 2008.

6. Rubin, D. I. Epidemiology and risk factors for spine pain. *Neurologic Clinics* 25(2):353–371, 2007.

7. Orloff, H. A., and C. M. Rapp. The effects of load carriage on spinal curvature and posture. *Spine* 29(12): 1325–1329, 2004.

8. McAtee, R. *Facilitated Stretching*, 3rd ed. Champaign, IL: Human Kinetics, 2007.

9. Fasen, J. M., A. M. O'Connor, S. L. Schwartz, J. O. Watson, C. T. Plastaras, C. W. Garvan, C. Bulcao, S. C. Johnson, and V. Akuthota. A randomized controlled trial of hamstring stretching: Comparison of four techniques. *Journal of Strength and Conditioning Research* 23(2):660–667, 2009.

Videos

Log on to www.pearsonhighered.com/powers to view these chapter-related videos.

Calf Stretch

Shin Stretch

Hip Flexor Stretch

Low Back Knee-to-Chest Stretch

Modified Hurdler Stretch

Inner Thigh Butterfly Stretch

Outer Thigh Stretch

Back Bridge

Side Stretch

Torso Twist and Hip Stretch

Pectoral and Bicep Stretch

Head Turn and Head Tilt

Hamstrings Stretch (Seated)

Back Extension

Cat Stretch

NAME _____ DATE _____

Assessing Flexibility: Trunk Flexion (Sit-and-Reach) Test and the Shoulder Flexibility Test

The Sit-and-Reach Test

To perform the sit-and-reach test, start by sitting upright with your feet flat against a sit-and-reach box. Keeping your feet flat on the box and your legs straight, extend your hands as far forward as possible, and hold this position for 3 seconds. Repeat this procedure 3 times. Your score on the sit-and-reach test is the distance, measured in inches, between the edge of the sit-and-reach box closest to you and the tips of your fingers during the best of your three stretching efforts.

Note that you should warm up by stretching for a few minutes before you perform the test. To reduce the possibility of injury, avoid rapid or jerky movements during the test. It is often useful to have a partner help by holding your legs straight during the test and by measuring the distance. After completing the test, consult Table 5.3 on page 164 to locate your flexibility fitness category, and record your scores on the following page.

The sit-and-reach test.

The Shoulder Flexibility Test

To perform the shoulder flexibility test follow these steps. While standing, raise your right arm, and reach down your back as far as possible. At the same time, extend your left arm behind your back, and reach upward toward your right hand. The objective is to try to overlap your fingers as much as possible. Your score on the shoulder flexibility test is the distance, measured in inches, of finger overlap.

The shoulder flexibility test.

Measure the distance of finger overlap to the nearest inch. For example, an overlap of $\frac{3}{4}$ inch would be recorded as 1 inch. If your fingers fail to overlap, record this score as −1. Finally, if your fingertips barely touch, record this score as 0. After completing the test with the right hand up, repeat the test in the opposite direction (left hand up).

As with the sit-and-reach test, you should warm up with a few minutes of stretching prior to performing the shoulder flexibility test. Again, to prevent injury, avoid rapid or jerky movements during the test. After completion of the test, consult Table 5.4 on page 164 to locate your shoulder flexibility category, and record your scores on the following page.

Date: _____

Sit-and-reach score (inches): _____   Fitness category: _____

Shoulder flexibility (inches)

   Left side: _____   Fitness category: _____

   Right side: _____   Fitness category: _____

Goal Setting

1. Based on your results for the flexibility testing, write a goal to either improve or maintain your fitness category.

2. Write three objectives to help you achieve your goal.

   - _____
   - _____
   - _____

TABLE 5.3
Physical Fitness Norms for Trunk Flexion
Note that these norms are from the YMCA's sit-and-reach test. Units for the sit-and-reach are inches.

Age Group	Fitness Category Based on Sit and Reach		
	Excellent	Average	Poor
Men			
18–25	22	16	13
26–35	21	15	12
36–45	21	15	11
Women			
18–25	24	19	16
26–35	23	18	14
36–45	22	17	13

Source: Modified from Golding, L., ed. *YMCA Fitness Testing and Assessment Manual,* 4th edition. With permission of the YMCA of the USA, Chicago, IL. Copyright © 2000.

TABLE 5.4
Physical Fitness Norms for Shoulder Flexibility
Note that these norms are for both men and women of all ages. Units for the shoulder flexibility test score are inches and indicate the distance between the fingers of your right and left hands.

Right Hand up Score	Left Hand Up Score	Fitness Classification
<0	<0	Very poor
0	0	Poor
+1	+1	Average
+2	+2	Good
+3	+3	Excellent
+4	+4	Superior

Source: From Fox, El L., T. E. Kirby, and A. R. Fox. *Bases of Fitness.* Copyright © 1987. All rights reserved. Adapted by permission of Allyn and Bacon. Norms from Gretchell, B. *Physical Fitness: A Way of Life,* 5th ed. Needham Heights, MA: Allyn and Bacon, 1998.

NAME _____ DATE _____

Flexibility Progression Log

Use this log to record your progress in increasing flexibility in selected joints. Record the date, hold time, and sets for each of the exercises listed in the left column.

St/Hold = sets and hold time
Example: 2/30 = 2 sets held for 30 seconds each.

Date: _____

Exercise	St/Hold	St/Hold	St/Hold	St/Hold	St/Hold	St/Hold	St/Hold
Lower leg stretch (see Exercise 5.1)							
Shin stretch (see Exercise 5.2)							
Thigh stretch (see Exercise 5.3)							
Leg stretch (see Exercise 5.4)							
Modified hurdler's stretch (see Exercise 5.5)							
Inside leg stretch (see Exercise 5.6)							
Hip and gluteal stretch (see Exercise 5.7)							
Lower back stretch (see Exercise 5.8)							

LABORATORY

Exercise	St/Hold	St/Hold	St/Hold	St/Hold	St/Hold	St/Hold	St/Hold
Side stretch (see Exercise 5.9)							
Trunk twister (see Exercise 5.10)							
Chest stretch (see Exercise 5.11)							
Neck stretch (see Exercise 5.12)							

NAME _____ DATE _____

Stretching to Prevent or Reduce Lower Back Pain

Stretching exercises are important in maintaining a flexible and healthy back. Our daily activities often result in overuse and tightening of back muscles. Chronic overuse and straining can cause significant back pain and increase your risk for back injury.

In this lab, you will learn exercises to stretch the lower muscles of your back to help in maintaining flexibility. Performing these stretches will help prevent back pain and may help reduce back aches.

▷ Log on to **www.pearsonhighered.com/powers** to view demonstration videos of these stretches.

Back Extension — Prone

1. Lie on your stomach.
2. Prop yourself up on your elbows, extending your back.
3. Start straightening your elbows, further extending your back.
4. Continue straightening your elbows until you feel a gentle stretch.
5. Hold for 15 seconds.
6. Return to the starting position.
7. Repeat 10 more times.

Cat Stretch

1. Get down on the floor on your hands and knees.
2. Push your back up toward the ceiling (like a cat arching its back).
3. Continue arching until you feel a gentle stretch in your back.
4. Hold for 15 seconds.
5. Return to the starting position.
6. Repeat 10 more times.

The Pelvic Tilt

1. Lie on your back, with your knees bent and feet flat on the floor.
2. Exhale, and press the small of your back against the floor.
3. Hold for 15 seconds.
4. Return to the starting position.
5. Repeat 10 more times.

Body Composition

true or false?

1. An overweight person can be fit.

2. Over half of the U.S. adult population is overweight or obese.

3. Body mass index (BMI) is the best way to estimate body composition.

4. Moderate weight loss in an obese person can reduce the risk for heart disease and diabetes.

5. Being underweight can increase the risk for certain health problems.

Answers appear on the next page.

Josh is a 19-year-old college sophomore who is a sprinter on his school's track team. His training routine involves track workouts and short-distance runs 5 days a week, and weight lifting 3 days a week. At 5 feet, 10 inches and 190 pounds, Josh is solid and hefty and considers himself to be in pretty good shape. Jason, meanwhile, is his 20-year-old roommate who makes it to the gym once in a while but spends most of his free time studying in the student lounge or meeting with friends at a favorite local hangout. Jason is also 5 feet 10 inches and weighs in at 168 pounds, which is about 15 pounds more than he weighed when he graduated from high school 2 years ago.

Would you be surprised to learn that Josh's higher weight is healthier than Jason's lower one? In this chapter, we will find out how to assess your level of body fat, how much body fat is considered healthy, and the health benefits and problems associated with having too much or too little body fat.

What Is Body Composition and What Does It Tell Us?

Body composition refers to the relative amounts of fat and fat-free tissues (e.g., bone, muscle, and inter-

nal organs) in the body. When body composition is assessed, it is typically expressed as a percentage of fat in the body. So, if a person has 20% body fat, 20% of his body weight is fat mass, and the remaining 80% of his body weight is fat-free or lean body mass. A high percentage of body fat is associated with an increased risk of heart disease, diabetes, and other conditions, whereas too low a percentage is also associated with health problems, such as malnutrition and osteoporosis.

Measuring percentage of body fat can help determine whether a person is at a healthy weight, **overweight,** or **obese.** Someone who is overweight has a body fat percentage above the recommended level that is considered to be "healthy." The "overweight" classification is based on research examining the relationship between body fatness and rates of disease. A person classified as obese has a very high percentage of body fat, generally over 25% for men and over 30% for women (1–5).

Make sure you know...

> Body composition refers to the relative amounts of fat and fat-free mass in the body and is generally reported in terms of the percentage of fat in the body.

> Measuring percentage body fat can help determine whether someone is overweight or obese.

Answers

1. TRUE Research has shown that individuals who are overweight, but active or fit, have lower risk for heart disease than both low-active, low-fit overweight individuals and low-active, low-fit normal-weight individuals.

2. TRUE It is estimated that approximately 65% of U.S. adults are overweight or obese.

3. FALSE BMI can provide information about whether a person is at a healthy weight, and BMI is related to body fat percentage. However, there are limitations for BMI in assessing body fat percentage, because it can overestimate body fat for muscular individuals.

4. TRUE A weight loss of as little as 5–10% can reduce the risk of heart disease and diabetes in overweight and obese individuals.

5. TRUE The relationship between weight and health follows what is referred to as a J-shaped curve. Although disease risk is greater for obese individuals, people at the lowest end of range are also at increased risk for disease.

How Is Body Composition Related to Health?

You need to consider percentage of body fat when determining a healthy body weight because a person can be "overweight" (i.e., based on height/weight charts) without being over-fat. Consider an athlete who is very muscular, like Josh. The athlete might weigh the same or even more than an individual who is clearly overweight because of a high percentage of body fat. The opposite is also true. A person can be over-fat, like Jason, without being considered "overweight." A sedentary person who appears to be at a healthy weight based on height and weight charts might have a percentage of body fat that is considered unhealthy or even obese.

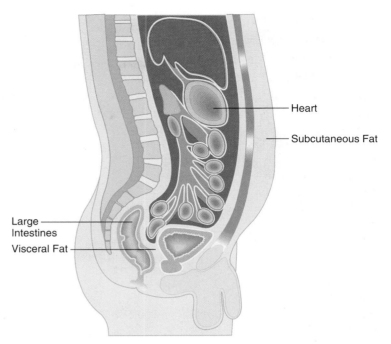

FIGURE 6.1
Storage fat can be visceral or subcutaneous. Visceral fat is stored around the organs; subcutaneous fat is stored between the skin and muscle layers.

We Need Some Fat

Although we worry about having too much body fat, a certain amount is necessary. **Essential fat** is necessary for body functions such as facilitating nerve impulses. Some locations of this fat include nerves, the heart, mammary glands, and liver. Men have approximately 3% of their body weight as essential fat, and women—who carry more fat in their breasts, uterus, and other sex-specific sites—have approximately 12%.

The fat we have in addition to the essential fat, called **storage fat,** is contained within **adipose tissue** in the body. This fat may be **visceral fat,** which means it is located around internal organs, or **subcutaneous fat,** which is located just below the skin (Figure 6.1).

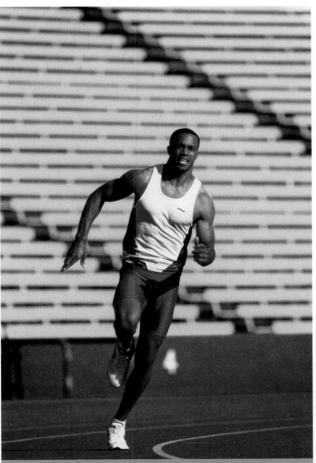

Some muscular athletes can be "overweight" without being over-fat.

body composition The relative amounts of fat and fat-free mass in the body.

overweight A weight above the recommended level for health.

obese An excessive amount of fat in the body; typically above 25% for men and 30% for women.

essential fat Body fat that is necessary for physiological functioning.

storage fat Excess fat reserves stored in the body's adipose tissue.

adipose tissue Tissue where fat is stored in the body.

visceral fat Fat stored in the abdomen and around the organs.

subcutaneous fat Fat stored just beneath the skin.

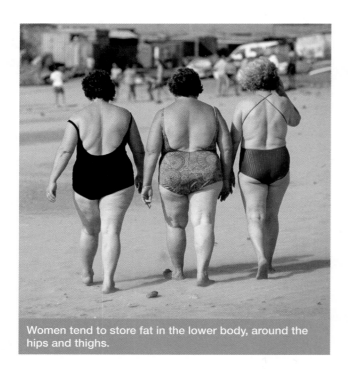

Women tend to store fat in the lower body, around the hips and thighs.

Men tend to store fat in the upper body, around the abdomen.

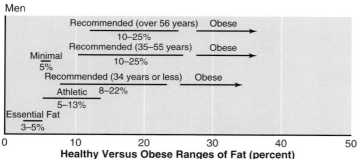

Healthy Versus Obese Ranges of Fat (percent)

FIGURE 6.2

Recommended levels of body fat for men and women according to age. Note the differences for athletes and the general population.

Source: American College of Sports Medicine. *Resource Manual for Guidelines of Exercise Testing and Prescription*, 5th ed. Philadelphia: Lippincott Williams & Wilkins, 2006, p. 204.

Storage fat provides energy for activity, insulates the body to retain heat, and protects against trauma to the body.

In general a healthy percentage body fat for men can range from 8–22%, and for women, from 20–35% (1). However, many fitness experts recommend levels at the lower end of these ranges for young adults, 12–15% and 22–25% for men and women, respectively (1). For most people, a body fat percentage outside these ranges indicates an unhealthy body weight. However, athletes or very active individuals might have lower values. Some athletic men have as little as 5–13% fat, and athletic women can have as little as 12–22% (1). Keep in mind that these values are not recommended for the general population and that you can be healthy if your body fat percentage falls within the earlier mentioned ranges. See Figure 6.2 for ranges according to sex and age.

It is not just *how much* body fat a person carries that can greatly affect his risk for several chronic diseases; *where* he carries it also matters. Fat cells are unequally distributed throughout the body, and the distribution of body fat is determined largely by genetics. We inherit specific fat storage traits that determine the regional distribution of fat. For example, many men have a high number of fat cells in the upper body and as a result store more fat within the abdominal area (e.g., around the waist). This is referred to the **android pattern** of obesity. In contrast, women tend to carry more fat cells in the waist, hips, and thighs of the lower body. This is called

APPRECIATING
DIVERSITY THE SEARCH FOR OBESITY-RELATED GENES

Even though obese individuals are found in every segment of the U.S. population, certain subsets of Americans experience the greatest prevalence of obesity. For example, compared to the U.S. population as a whole, the risk of becoming obese is greatest among Mexican American women, African American women, some Native Americans (for example, Pima Indians), and children from low-income families. The high prevalence of obesity in these populations places individuals in those groups at the greatest risk of developing obesity-related diseases.

Research efforts to understand the roles of genetics in the high prevalence of obesity in these populations are expanding. One large investigation, called the Heritage Family Study, is searching for the genes responsible for both obesity and weight loss. Results from this and other genetics studies are expected to provide important information for developing programs that can prevent and treat obesity in high-risk populations.

Source: Changnon, Y. C., et al. Genomic scan for genes affecting body composition before and after training in Caucasians from HERITAGE. *Journal of Applied Physiology* 90:1777–1787, 2001.

the **gynoid pattern** of obesity. People who carry body fat primarily in the abdominal or waist area are at greater risk for developing heart disease and diabetes than are those who store body fat in the hips or lower part of the body (6, 7).

Mental and Physical Health Benefits of a Healthy Weight

Maintaining a healthy weight is important for physical health, and it is also associated with certain aspects of mental health. People who are overweight or obese are more likely to have poor body image and low self-esteem compared to people of normal weight. An unhealthy body image and poor self-esteem are associated with poor health behavior choices and increased risk for physical and mental health problems, such as depression and increased anxiety (8, 9). Maintaining a healthy body weight will make physical activity and everyday activities easier. Individuals who maintain a healthy body weight have a lower risk for developing major chronic conditions such as cardiovascular disease, type 2 diabetes, and certain types of cancers. Cardiovascular disease and all-cause death rates are also lower in people at their recommended body weights compared to overweight and obese individuals (10–11).

CONSIDER THIS!

On average, college students gain 4–15 pounds during their first year of college.

Overweight and Obesity in the United States

Obesity is often defined as a fat percentage body greater than 25% for men and greater than 30% for women. Current estimates for the United States suggest that over 72 million people meet the criteria for obesity (12). Obesity is a major health problem in the United States, and numerous diseases have been linked to being too fat. Because of a strong link between obesity and disease, the National Institutes of Health has estimated that obesity directly contributes to 15–20% of the deaths in the United States (13).

The burden of obesity also has had a significant effect on health care costs. An estimated 9.1% of medical costs, or about $80 billion, were attributed to overweight- and obesity-related health problems in 1998, and estimates had reached almost $100 billion

android pattern A pattern of fat distribution characterized by fat stored in the abdominal region; more common in men.

gynoid pattern A pattern of fat distribution characterized by fat stored in the hips and thighs; more common in women.

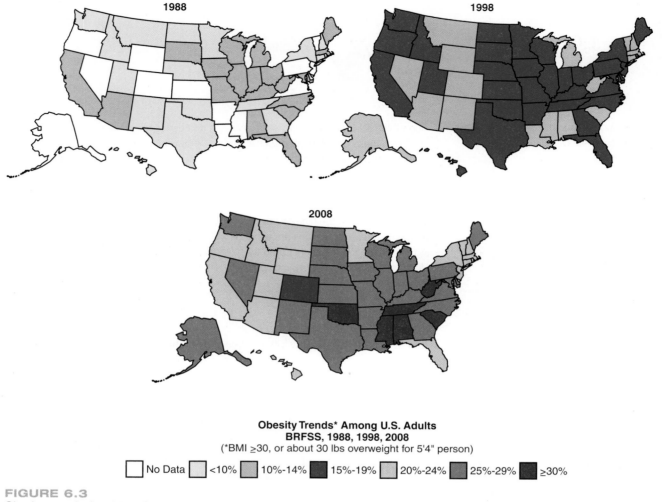

Obesity Trends* Among U.S. Adults
BRFSS, 1988, 1998, 2008
(*BMI ≥30, or about 30 lbs overweight for 5'4" person)

☐ No Data   ☐ <10%   ☐ 10%-14%   ■ 15%-19%   ☐ 20%-24%   ☐ 25%-29%   ■ ≥30%

FIGURE 6.3

Obesity rates in the United States increased dramatically in the 20 years between 1988 and 2008.

Source: Centers for Disease Control and Prevention, "U.S. Obesity Trends: 1985–2008, Obesity Trend Maps," www.cdc.gov/nccdphp/dnpa/obesity.

dollars by 2002 (14). However, total health care costs are an estimated $117 billion in the United States for the direct *and* indirect costs of overweight and obesity (15).

News sources frequently report that the obesity rates in America are the highest in the world and continue to climb. The reports are based on studies indicating that the number of obese or overweight people in the United States has increased by 40% in the last few decades (16). In 1980, 46% of Americans were obese or overweight; by 2000, the number had increased to 66%. You can see the changes in obesity across the United States from 1988 to 2008 in Figure 6.3. Despite the sounding of the alarm, recent studies reveal that the increase of obesity has mostly leveled off since 1999, and obesity prevalence has not risen significantly since 2003 (13). This is the good news. The bad news is that 66% of all Americans are either obese or overweight, and there is no evidence of a decrease

in the rate of obesity among adults or children (13, 17). Therefore, obesity continues to be a major threat to wellness in the United States.

Why are so many Americans obese? There is no single answer. Obesity is related to both genetic traits and lifestyle (18, 19). These influences will be discussed more in Chapter 8. Many individuals, such as Jason (introduced at the beginning of the chapter), who put on 15 pounds over 3 years, experience **creeping obesity** by gradually adding fat over a period of time.

This type of weight gain is usually attributed to poor diet (including increased food intake) and a gradual decline in physical activity (20). The woman in Figure 6.4 is gaining one-half pound of fat per month (6 pounds per year), and after five years, she will have gained 30 pounds! The weight gain is so gradual that it typically does not become a concern until years later, when the total weight is more noticeable.

Body Weight (pounds)

130   136   142   148   154

2008   2009   2010   2011   2012
Year

FIGURE 6.4
The concept of creeping obesity.

Chronic Conditions Associated with Overweight and Obesity

Obesity increases the risk of developing at least 26 diseases. Heart disease, colon cancer, hypertension (high blood pressure), kidney disease, arthritis, and diabetes are among the most serious (12, 13, 20).

Heart Disease   Heart disease (also called *cardiovascular disease,* or *CVD*) is the leading cause of death in the United States for both men and women. Obesity is considered a major independent risk factor for coronary heart disease, which happens to be the leading cause of heart attacks. Obesity has been shown to increase the risk of heart attack by 60–80% (21).

Hypertension (high blood pressure) is more common among overweight and obese individuals. However, on a positive note, blood pressure is usually reduced with weight loss. Obesity is linked to elevated cholesterol levels and unhealthy blood lipid profiles. As with hypertension, the cholesterol profile typically improves with weight loss. High blood pressure and cholesterol levels are also independent risk factors for

coronary heart disease, so the combination of obesity with these risk factors poses a significantly greater risk for a heart attack. Heart disease will be discussed in much greater detail in Chapter 9.

Diabetes   **Diabetes** is a metabolic disorder characterized by high blood glucose levels that affects over 18 million people. Chronic elevation of blood glucose is associated with increased incidence of heart disease, kidney disease, nerve dysfunction, and eye damage. In fact, diabetes is one of the leading causes of death and disability in the United States, and its incidence is increasing.

There is a strong relationship between the onset of type 2 diabetes and body fatness; over 80% of people with type 2 diabetes are obese. Type 2 diabetes has

creeping obesity A slow increase in body weight and percentage of body fat over several years.

diabetes A metabolic disorder characterized by high blood glucose levels that is associated with increased risk for heart disease, kidney disease, nerve dysfunction, and eye damage.

traditionally been referred to as *adult-onset diabetes* because its risk increases after age 45. However, this type of diabetes is largely associated with behavioral factors, such as poor dietary habits, physical inactivity, and obesity. As obesity among young people has increased, so has the incidence of type 2 diabetes among adolescents and young adults.

Type 2 diabetes is also known as non–insulin-dependent diabetes, because insulin is not always required as treatment. In type 2 diabetes, the body can produce insulin, but there is a reduced ability of insulin to transport glucose from the blood to the cells. This problem, called *decreased insulin sensitivity*, results in elevated blood glucose levels. People can have decreased insulin sensitivity but not have blood glucose levels high enough to be diagnosed with diabetes. In this case, a person has *pre-diabetes*, which is also more common among obese individuals. As with heart disease, weight loss can significantly reduce the risk of diabetes and help manage diabetes. In fact, research has indicated that modest weight loss of 5–10% can reduce the risk of heart disease and type 2 diabetes (22, 23).

Other Conditions Obesity is a risk factor for some of the most prevalent types of cancers, including breast, prostate, and colon cancer. Overweight and obese individuals are at higher risk for joint problems and osteoarthritis. Sleep apnea, a condition in which a person stops breathing for brief periods while sleeping, and gallbladder disease are more common among obese individuals. Additionally, obese women are more likely to experience menstrual abnormalities, difficulty conceiving, and complications during pregnancy than women of normal weight.

Health Effects of Underweight

Although the current rates of overweight and obesity among U.S. adults indicate there is an obesity epidemic, a small percentage of people in the country suffers from health problems associated with being underweight. As with overweight, underweight can be determined by measuring height, weight, and body fat

CONSIDER THIS!

Sedentary adults are over 2.5 times more likely to experience significant weight gain over 10 years compared to those who report that they exercise vigorously 2 or more times per week.

percentage. However, just as with determining overweight and obesity, it is best to use a measure of body composition to determine whether one is underweight. Getting close to or below the level of essential body fat is an indicator that an individual might be too thin.

Health problems associated with being underweight are typically related to malnutrition, because the person is likely not eating enough to get all the necessary nutrients. Severe and prolonged malnutrition can result in a loss of muscle mass and strength. Further, underweight individuals are at increased risk for osteoporosis, and under-

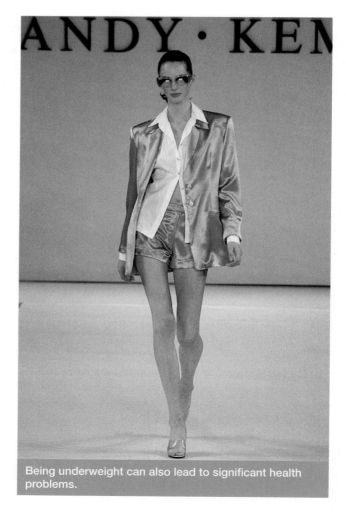

Being underweight can also lead to significant health problems.

STEPS FOR
BEHAVIOR CHANGE

Are you at risk for developing diabetes?

Does your body composition, or other factors, put you at increased risk for developing diabetes? To find out whether you are at increased risk, respond true or false to the following statements.

T   F

☐ ☐   I have a BMI that puts me in the overweight or obese category.

☐ ☐   I am under 65 years of age AND I get little or no exercise.

☐ ☐   I have a sister or brother with diabetes.

☐ ☐   I have a parent with diabetes.

☐ ☐   I am a woman who has had a baby weighing more than 9 pounds at birth.

In general, the more "true" answers you have, the higher your risk.

TIPS TO REDUCE YOUR RISK OF DIABETES

☑ Determine whether you are overweight, and if so, lose weight. If you have a BMI above the healthy range, get a body composition assessment to determine your level of fat. If your percentage of body fat is above the healthy range, talk to your instructor or a health educator at your campus health center about setting goals and preparing a plan for weight loss.

☑ Get more exercise. Be more active most days of the week. See Chapter 1 for tips to change your health behavior.

☑ Incorporate more fresh fruits and vegetables and whole grains into your diet, and cut back on the salt and high-fat foods.

☑ See your health care provider. A lot of people have diabetes and pre-diabetes without knowing it.

Source: American Diabetes Association. Diabetes risk test. www.diabetes.org.

---

weight women are at increased risk for menstrual abnormalities that can lead to infertility. People with eating disorders, such as anorexia nervosa and bulimia, can experience many other health problems. Heart problems, digestive disorders, kidney damage, anemia, lethargy, muscle weakness, dry skin, and poor immune function are some of the common problems associated with anorexia nervosa or bulimia nervosa.

Eating disorders are complex conditions that involve much more than just being underweight. We will discuss these conditions in greater detail in Chapter 8.

Make sure you know...

> Overweight refers to a weight above the recommended level, and obesity refers to a high percentage of body fat.

> A certain amount of fat is needed for normal physiological functioning, and excess storage fat is associated with increased risk for numerous conditions.

> Physical and mental health are affected by unhealthy levels of body fat.

> Rates of obesity in the United States are high and contribute significantly to health care costs.

> The amount and distribution of excess storage fat can lead to increased risk of illness and death associated with heart disease and diabetes.

> Having too little body fat can lead to significant health problems.

A CLOSER LOOK

CAN YOU BE FIT AND FAT?

Although overweight and obesity are associated with numerous unhealthy conditions, and people should always strive for a healthy body weight, it is possible to be fit and overweight. Think about watching your favorite football team. Do all the players look thin and healthy? Probably not. However, because of their intense workouts even those players with the seemingly unhealthy looking physiques can still be healthy.

Multiple research studies have found that overweight individuals can be healthy if they are physically active or fit. The strongest evidence comes from longitudinal studies conducted at the Cooper Clinic in Dallas, Texas. Researchers examined heart disease and death risk

and overall death rates in men and women. Death risk was 1.5 times greater for low-fit participants compared to highly fit participants across both normal and overweight BMI classifications. Those with the highest fitness levels and the lowest BMIs had the lowest risk for disease and death. However, overweight highly fit men and women had lower risk for death than their overweight low-fit counterparts and than low-fit weight men and women of normal weight. Others have found reduced risk for heart disease and death in active and fit overweight and obese individuals.

These findings support the fact that efforts to incorporate regular physical activity into one's lifestyle are not in vain,

because active overweight individuals do enjoy the benefits of lower risk of heart disease. People who are inactive but at a recommended weight still should consider a regular exercise program to minimize their risk of chronic disease.

Sources: Lohman, T., et al. Body fat measurement goes high-tech: Not all are created equal. *ACSM'S Health and Fitness Journal* 1(1):30–35, 1997; Lee, C. D., S. N. Blair, and A. S. Jackson. Cardiorespiratory fitness, body composition, and all-cause cardiovascular disease mortality in men. *American Journal of Clinical Nutrition* 69:373–380, 1999; Lee, C. D., A. S. Jackson, and S. N. Blair. U.S. weight guidelines: Is it also important to consider cardiorespiratory fitness? *International Journal of Obesity and Related Metabolic Disorders* 22 (suppl 2):S2–S7, 1998; Church, T., and S. N. Blair. Does physical activity ameliorate the health hazards of obesity? *British Journal of Sports Medicine* 43:80–81, 2009.

Assessing Body Composition

Several field and laboratory methods for assessing body composition have been developed. Field methods require little equipment and can be easily administered at a fitness center or gym to determine weight status or body composition. The laboratory measures are used more frequently in research or medical settings. Each measure has strengths and limitations.

Field Methods

Several quick and inexpensive field techniques are used to evaluate body composition and the risk for disease (24–26). The procedures discussed in this section have been validated and can provide good estimates of your level of body fat or level of disease risk.

Body Mass Index One of the easiest techniques used to determine whether someone is overweight or obese is the **body mass index (BMI).** The BMI is

simply the ratio of the body weight (in kilograms; kg) divided by height (in meters squared; m²):

$$BMI = weight\ (kg) \div height\ (m)^2$$
(*Note*: 1 kg = 2.2 lb, and 1 m = 39.25 in.)

For example, for an individual who weighs 64.5 kg and is 1.72 m tall, the BMI would be computed as follows:

$$64.5\ kg/(1.72\ m)^2 = 64.5 \div 2.96 = 21.8\ kg/m^2$$

The concept behind the BMI is that individuals with low percentage of body fat will have a low BMI. For example, men and women with a BMI of less than 25 kg/m², respectively, are classified as having optimal body fat (Table 6.1). In contrast, men and women with a BMI of greater than 30 kg/m² are considered obese. Additionally, research has indicated that individuals classified as overweight or obese according to BMI are at increased risk for cardiovascular disease and death.

BMI is a simple and inexpensive method for determining your weight status, but it has limitations. For example, BMI does not give you a direct measure of fat percentage. In fact, in some cases the method can over- or underestimate body fatness. An individual with

TABLE 6.1
Ranges and Classification for BMI and Waist Circumference

	BMI	Disease Risk* Relative to Normal Weight and Waist Circumference	
		Men, ≤102 cm Women, ≤88 cm	Men, >102 cm Women, >88 cm
Underweight	<18.5	—	—
Normal	18.5–24.9	—	—
Overweight	25.0–29.9	Increased	High
Obesity			
Class I	30.0–34.9	High	Very high
Class II	35.0–39.9	Very high	Very high
Class III	≥40	Extremely high	Extremely high

*Disease risk for type 2 diabetes, hypertension, and cardiovascular disease. Dashes (—) indicate that no additional risk at these levels of BMI was assigned. Increased waist circumference can also be a marker for increased risk even in persons of normal weight.

Source: Modified from American College of Sports Medicine. *ACSM's Guidelines for Exercise Testing and Prescription,* 7th ed. Philadelphia: Lippincott Williams & Wilkins, 2006, p. 58.

a low percentage of body fat but a high level of muscularity would typically have a relatively high BMI, which would incorrectly suggest a high percentage of body fat. If you calculate BMI values for Josh and Jason, for example, you might be surprised to learn that, based on BMI guidelines, Josh is "overweight" and Jason is in the normal-weight category.

BMI is best used to obtain an initial estimate of whether one's weight is at a healthy level. You should follow up a BMI calculation with a measure of body fat percentage, especially if you feel you are at a healthy weight and your BMI indicates otherwise.

Skinfold Assessment   Because more than 50% of body fat is subcutaneous fat that lies just beneath the skin, a **skinfold test** can be used to estimate a person's overall body fatness (20, 27). In a skinfold test, subcutaneous fat is measured using an instrument called a skinfold caliper. To be accurate, skinfold tests to estimate body fat for both men and women require at least three skinfold measurement sites (20). The anatomical sites to be measured in men (abdominal, chest, thigh skinfolds) and in women (suprailium, triceps, and thigh skinfolds) are illustrated in Laboratory 6.1. Note that for standardization, all measurements should be made on the right side of the body.

Skinfold measurements to determine body fat are reliable but generally have a ± 3–4% margin of error (27, 28). Using calibrated metal calipers (instead of plastic) and having a skilled technician do the test are two ways to increase accuracy. If you are having a skinfold measure taken, it is very important that you follow

the instructions given by the fitness professional to ensure the most accurate readings.

Skinfold assessment is an easy measure to obtain and can provide good estimates when done properly. However, it is not necessarily a good measure to assess body composition for very obese individuals, because it is often difficult to obtain accurate readings. Inaccurate estimates can be misleading and discouraging and can interfere with setting an appropriate goal weight. Bioelectrical impedance (discussed later in this chapter) may be preferred for obese individuals.

Waist Measurement and Waist-to-Hip Ratio   Waist measurements and the **waist-to-hip ratio** can be used to determine the risk of disease associated with high body fat. These techniques do not provide an estimate of body fat percentage. However, they are excellent indicators of whether the body fat distribution is unhealthy. Waist measurements greater or equal to 40 inches (102 cm) for men and 35 inches (88 cm) for women are considered high risk and

body mass index (BMI) A ratio of body weight (kg) divided by height squared (m²) used to determine whether a person is at a healthy body weight; BMI is related to the percentage of body fat.

skinfold test A field test used to estimate body composition; representative samples of subcutaneous fat are measured using calipers to estimate the overall level of body fat.

waist-to-hip ratio A ratio of the waist and hip circumferences used to determine the risk for disease associated with the android pattern of obesity.

indicate the android pattern of obesity. You can better evaluate your risk according to waist measurement by also considering your BMI (see Table 6.1). A high waist measurement alone might not indicate increased risk. For example, a high waist measurement for someone who is tall might be proportional to his height, and the level of BMI and body fat might be well within the healthy ranges.

Another way to estimate disease risk according to body fat distribution is the waist-to-hip ratio. An individual with a large fat deposit in the abdominal region would have a high waist-to-hip ratio and would have a higher risk of disease than someone with a lower waist-to-hip ratio.

Both waist and hip circumference measurements should be made while the person is standing, using a nonelastic tape. It is important that the person not wear bulky clothing during the measurement, because it could alter the measurements. During measurements, the tape should be placed snugly around the body but should not press into the skin. Record your measurements to the nearest millimeter or sixteenth of an inch. The specific procedure is detailed in Laboratory 6.1.

Laboratory Measures

Body fat measurements performed in a laboratory are considered the gold standard for assessing body composition. However, these techniques require expensive specialized equipment and are often not readily available to the general public. The methods are usually used by researchers or clinicians to determine body fat percentage in research participants or patients.

Dual Energy X-Ray Absorptiometry   **Dual energy X-ray absorptiometry (DXA)** involves taking a low radiation X-ray scan (involving considerably less radiation than a typical X-ray scan) of the entire body to obtain estimates of body fat percentage. In this procedure, the person lies still on a table while an X-ray arm passes over the body. The scan typically requires about 15 minutes to complete.

The advantage of using DXA is that it provides a measure of total body fat as well as a measure of regional fat distribution. It can also be used to assess bone density as it relates to osteoporosis and osteoporosis risk. However, the technique is generally not used outside research or clinical settings. The equipment is expensive, and because it uses an X ray only trained professionals can perform the scan. Therefore, most people will not have the opportunity to have this assessment.

Hydrostatic Weighing   **Hydrostatic weighing,** also called underwater weighing, is a technique that involves weighing the individual both on land and in a tank of water to determine body volume and body density. Lean mass has a higher density than water, whereas fat mass is less dense than water. The more muscular person will weigh more under water. Because fat tends to float, the person with more fat will weigh less under water. After the two weights are obtained, they are used to calculate percentage of body fat.

Underwater weighing is very time-consuming and requires expensive equipment. Additionally, this measure typically does not appeal to most individuals, because it involves wearing a bathing suit and being completely submerged underwater. Thus, this procedure is rarely employed to assess body composition in collegiate physical fitness courses.

Air Displacement   **Air displacement** is a fairly new method used to assess body composition and is similar in principle to hydrostatic weighing. Instead of being submerged in water, the individual is seated in a chamber (the Bod Pod®). Computerized sensors are used to estimate the amount of air that is displaced when the participant is in the chamber. From knowing the amount of air that is displaced, body volume and then body fat can be calculated. Estimates of body fat percentage from air displacement are similar to measures from hydrostatic weighing.

Air displacement is less time-consuming than underwater weighing; however, the equipment is expensive, so this technique is not available in fitness centers. Air displacement is more commonly used in research settings, and as a newer measure it needs more assessment in a variety of populations (e.g., athletes, older adults, ethnic minorities) to determine overall accuracy.

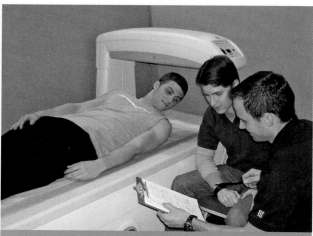

The DXA scan is considered the gold standard for measuring body composition.

Hydrostatic weighing involves being weighed while submerged in a tank of water.

The Bod Pod® uses air displacement to measure body composition.

Bioelectrical Impedance Analysis

Bioelectrical impedance analysis (BIA) is a procedure used in fitness centers as well as in research laboratories. With commercially available BIA monitors, the person either stands on sensors of a scale-like piece of equipment or holds sensors between both hands. In the laboratory, the participant lies on a table with surface electrodes placed at the hand and foot. Then, a very low level electrical current (too low to be felt) is passed through the body between the electrodes or sensors. Because lean tissue contains more water, it is a good conductor of the current. Fat tissue, in contrast, contains less water and impedes the flow of the current. Body fat is estimated according to the resistance to the flow of the current.

BIA is typically an acceptable measure to most people. However, the commercially available monitors do not provide a total body measure, and estimates can be less accurate because a smaller area is assessed and the reading may be influenced by regional fat distribution. The total body measure used in laboratory and re-

search settings is noninvasive and easy to administer, but its accuracy and reliability have been questioned. A significant source of error is a failure to follow instructions. If you were to have a BIA performed, the fitness professional or lab technician would give you very explicit instructions in regard to exercise, voiding, eating, and drinking prior to the assessment. The in-

dual energy X-ray absorptiometry (DXA) A technique for assessing body composition using a low radiation X ray; it is typically used in research or clinical settings and is considered a gold-standard measure.

hydrostatic weighing A method of determining body composition that involves weighing an individual on land and in a tank of water.

air displacement A technique used to assess body composition by estimating body volume based on air displaced when a person sits in a chamber.

bioelectrical impedance analysis (BIA) A method of assessing body composition by running a low-level electrical current through the body.

structions address factors that affect your level of hydration, which is crucial for an accurate measurement. Failure to comply with the pre-assessment instructions can significantly impair the accuracy of the reading.

Make sure you know...

> There are several laboratory and field methods used to assess body composition and weight status.

> BMI, skinfold, and waist-to-hip ratio are the most common assessments for general use in fitness courses and fitness centers.

> Laboratory assessments such as DXA, hydrostatic weighing, air displacement, and BIA provide very good estimates of body composition, but most are not practical for commercial use because of their cost.

Using Body Composition to Determine Your Ideal Body Weight

The fitness categories presented for body composition differ from those for the other components of health-related physical fitness. Whereas "superior" was the highest fitness level for cardiorespiratory, strength, and muscular endurance fitness, the classification of "optimal" is the highest standard for body composition. Any category other than "optimal" is considered unsatisfactory for health-related fitness. Therefore, your goal should be to reach and maintain an optimal body composition.

Research suggests that a range of 8%–22% body fat is an optimal health and fitness goal for men, and the optimal range for women is 20%–35% (1). These ranges provide little risk of disease associated with body fatness and permit individual differences in physical activity patterns and diet.

Once we have calculated our body fat percentage and know the optimal range of body fat, how can we determine the desired range of body weight? A typical 20-year-old man who has 30% body fat and weighs 185 pounds can calculate his optimal range of body weight in two simple steps:

Step 1. Compute fat-free weight—that is, the amount of total body weight contained in bones, organs, and muscles:

Total body weight − fat weight = fat-free weight
$$100\% - 30\% = 70\%$$

This means that 70% of total body weight is fat-free weight. Therefore, the fat-free weight for this student is

$$70\% \times 185 \text{ lb} = 129.5 \text{ lb}$$

Step 2. Calculate the optimal weight (which for men is 8–22% of total body weight): The formula to compute optimum body weight is

Optimum weight
$$= \text{fat-free weight} \div (1 - \text{optimal \% fat})$$

Note that fat percentage should be expressed as a decimal. Thus, for 8% body fat,

$$\text{Optimum weight} = 129.5 \div (1 - 0.08)$$
$$= 140.8 \text{ pounds}$$

For 22% body fat,

$$\text{Optimum weight} = 129.5 \div (1 - 0.22)$$
$$= 166 \text{ pounds}$$

Basically, we assume that this man will maintain his lean body mass and lose fat. So, his 129.5 pounds of lean mass will be 78–92% of his new optimal body weight to achieve a healthy body composition. Hence, the optimal body weight for this individual is between 140.8 and 166.0 pounds. Laboratory 6.2 provides the opportunity to compute your optimal body weight using both body fat percentage and body mass index.

Make sure you know...

> Healthy body weight should be determined based on the optimal level of body fat for your age, height, and sex.

> Ideal weight can be easily calculated if you know your percentage of body fat.

Behavior Change: Set Goals and Get Regular Assessments

You will learn about weight management in Chapter 8, but here we want to briefly discuss the importance of getting regular body composition assessments as you attempt to lose or gain weight. When we calculated the goal weight based on the optimal level of body fat, we assumed only fat weight was lost. However, a person

experiencing weight loss may also lose water weight and possibly lose lean mass. Incorporating regular aerobic and resistance exercise along with a healthy diet will maximize the amount of fat that is lost and maintain more lean mass.

As the body changes with weight loss or gain, the weights that were originally calculated might not correspond exactly with the desired body fat percentage. In the example above, the individual might lose 7 pounds and be in the optimal range if he also increased lean mass. Additionally, regular assessments will help you determine whether the weight you are losing is fat and not lean mass. Therefore, it is important to have regular body composition assessments as you are trying to reach a new goal weight. It is important to get the same type of test when you get follow-up assessments. If possible, it also is recommended that the same person perform the assessment. These factors will reduce error of the measurement. The frequency of the assessments will depend on your goal.

Make sure you know...

> You should have regular body composition assessments when trying to lose or gain weight to ensure the healthiest changes.

> Follow-up assessments should be made with the same measure as the original assessment.

Summary

1. Body composition refers to the relative amounts of fat and fat-free tissue in the body. Fat in the body can be essential fat or storage fat. A healthy body weight should be based on the recommended amount of body fat.

2. Body composition is an important component of health-related physical fitness because a high percentage of body fat is associated with an increased risk for numerous diseases. The distribution of fat also affects disease risk associated with overweight and obesity. A very low percentage of body fat is also associated with increased risk for disease.

3. Common field techniques for assessing body fat and healthy weight are skinfold measurements, BMI assessment, and examination of the waist-to-hip ratio.

4. Laboratory techniques for estimating body fat are most commonly used in research and clinical settings. DXA is considered the gold-standard measure for estimating body fat.

5. You can calculate your healthy weight range by knowing your desired percentage of body fat or BMI. You should have regular body composition assessments when trying to lose or gain weight.

Study Questions

1. How much essential fat do the average man and woman carry?
   a. 25% and 30%
   b. 3% and 12%
   c. 10% and 20%
   d. 5% and 18%

2. Which of the following is not a potential health consequence of being overweight or obese?
   a. low self-esteem
   b. gallbladder disease
   c. osteoarthritis
   d. anemia

3. Storing excess fat in the hips and thighs puts an individual at greater risk for heart disease and diabetes than storing excess fat in the abdomen.
   a. true
   b. false

4. Which technique is used to assess disease risk status associated with the regional fat distribution?
   a. waist-to-hip ratio
   b. skinfold test
   c. underwater weighing
   d. bioelectrical impedance analysis

5. For disease risk and health standards, a BMI of _____ kg/m² is considered obese.
   a. 27
   b. 25
   c. 30
   d. 45

6. Which of the following is a common field measure for assessing body composition?
   a. waist measurement
   b. skinfold test
   c. hydrostatic weighing
   d. DXA

7. Which is not a potential health consequence of being underweight or having an eating disorder?
   a. malnutrition
   b. menstrual abnormalities
   c. digestive disorders
   d. type 1 diabetes

8. A person classified as normal weight based on a BMI in the healthy range can be over-fat.
   a. true
   b. false

9. Discuss the different types of field measurement techniques for assessing body composition. Discuss the strengths and limitations of each.

10. Discuss potential health consequences of not maintaining a healthy body composition.

11. Define overweight and obesity. What is the public health impact of overweight and obesity in the United States?

Suggested Reading

Church, T., and S. N. Blair. Does physical activity ameliorate the health hazards of obesity? *British Journal of Sports Medicine* 43:80–81, 2009.

Donnelly, J., S. Blair, J. Jakicic, M. Manore, J. Rankin, and B. Smith. American College of Sports Medicine Position Stand. Appropriate physical activity intervention strategies for weight loss and prevention of weight gain for adults. *Medicine and Science in Sports and Exercise* 41:459–471, 2009.

Heyward, V. H., and D. R. Wagner *Applied Body Composition Assessment*, 2nd ed. Champaign, IL: Human Kinetics, 2004.

Nelson, T. F., S. L. Gortmaker, S. V. Subramanian, L. Cheung, and H. Wechsler. Disparities in overweight and obesity among US college students. *American Journal of Health Behavior* 31(4):363–73, 2007.

Smith, S. C., and D. Haslem. Abdominal obesity, waist circumference and cardio-metabolic risk: Awareness among primary care physicians, the general population and patients at risk—the Shape of the Nations survey. *Current Medical Research and Opinion* 23(1):29–47, 2007.

Waisted: Abdominal obesity and your health. *Harvard Men's Health Watch* 13:1–6, 2009.

For links to the organizations and websites listed below, visit The Total Fitness and Wellness Website at www.pearsonhighered.com/powers.

ACSM
Provides information about all aspects of health and fitness.

American Diabetes Association
Provides diabetes information, including exercise and diet guidelines to reduce your risk.

American Heart Association
Contains information about a variety of topics related to heart disease and stroke, including exercise and diet tips to reduce your risk.

References

1. Kaminsky L. A., (ed.). *ACSM'S Resource Manual for Guidelines for Exercise Testing and Prescription*. Philadelphia: Lippincott, Williams and Wilkins, 2006.

2. Bjorntorp, P., and B. Brodoff, eds. *Obesity*. Philadelphia: Lippincott, Williams and Wilkins, 1992.

3. Perri, M., A. Nezu, and B. Viegener. *Improving the Long-Term Management and Treatment of Obesity*. New York: John Wiley and Sons, 1992.

4. Stefanik, M. Exercise and weight control. In *Exercise and Sport Science Reviews*, J. Holloszy, ed. Baltimore: Williams and Wilkins, 1993.

5. Stunkard, A., and T. Wadden, eds. *Obesity: Theory and Therapy*. New York: Raven Press, 1993.

6. Atkinson, R. Treatment of obesity. *Nutritional Reviews* 50:338–345, 1992.

7. Bouchard, C., R. Shepherd, T. Stephens, J. Sutton, and B. McPherson, eds. *Exercise, Fitness, and Health: A Consensus of Current Knowledge*. Champaign, IL: Human Kinetics, 1990.

8. Cohen T., and M. Esther. Depressed mood and concern with weight and shape in normal women. *International Journal of Eating Disorders* 14:223–227, 1993.

9. Kirkcaldy, B. D., M. Eysenck, A. F. Furnham, and G. Siefen. Gender, anxiety, and self-image. *Personality and Individual Differences* 24:677–684, 1998.

10. Mokdad, A. H., M. K. Serdula, W. H. Dietz, B. A. Bowman, J. S. Marks, and J. P. Koplan, Prevalence of obesity, diabetes, and obesity-related health risk factors, 2001. *Journal of the American Medical Association* 289:76–79, 2003.

11. McGinnis, J. M., and W. H. Foege. Actual cases of death in the United States. *Journal of the American Medical Association* 270:2207–2212, 1993.

12. Ogden, C., M. Carroll, M. McDowell, and K. Flegal. *Obesity Among Adults in the United States—No Statistically Significant Change Since 2003–2004*. NCHS data brief no 1. Hyattsville, MD: National Center for Health Statistics, 2007.

13. Van Itallie, T. Health implications of overweight and obesity in the United States. *Annals of Internal Medicine* 103:983–988, 1985.

14. Finkelstein, E. A., I. C. Fiebelkorn, and G. Wang. National medical spending attributable to overweight and obesity: How much, and who's paying? *Health Affairs* W3:219–226, 2003.

15. Weight Control Information Network, National Institute of Diabetes and Digestive and Kidney Diseases, National Institutes of Health, http://win.niddk.nih.gov/statistics

16. Stein, C., and G. Colditz. The epidemic of obesity. *Journal of Clinical Endocrinology and Metabolism* 89:2522–2525, 2004.

17. Hedley, A., C. Ogden, C. Johnson, M. Carroll, L. Curtin, and K. Flegal. Prevalence of overweight and obesity among US children, adolescents, and adults, 1999–2002. *Journal of the American Medical Association* 16:2847–2850, 2004.

18. Bouchard, C., A. Tremblay, J. Despres, et al. The response to long-term overfeeding in identical twins. *New England Journal of Medicine* 322:1477–1482, 1990.

19. Stunkard, A., T. Sorensen, C. Hanis, et al. An adoption study of human obesity. *New England Journal of Medicine* 314:193–198, 1986.

20. Williams, M. *Lifetime Fitness and Wellness*. Dubuque, IA: William C. Brown, 1996.

21. Health implications of obesity: National Institutes of Health consensus development conference. *Annals of Internal Medicine* 103:977–1077, 1985.

22. Diabetes Prevention Research Group. Impact of intensive lifestyle and Metformin therapy on cardiovascular disease risk factors in the diabetes prevention program. *Diabetes Care* 28:888–894, 2005.

23. Wing, R. R., E. Venditti, J. M. Jakicic, B. A. Polley, and W. Lang. Lifestyle intervention in overweight individuals with a family history of diabetes. *Diabetes Care* 21:350–359, 1998.

24. Howley, E., and D. Franks. *Health Fitness Instructor's Handbook*, 4th ed. Champaign, IL: Human Kinetics, 2003.

25. DiGirolamo, M. Body composition—roundtable. *Physician and Sports Medicine* (March):144–162, 1986.

26. Van Itallie, T. Topography of body fat: Relationship to risk of cardiovascular and other diseases. In *Anthropometric Standardization Reference Manual*, T. Lohman et al., eds. Champaign, IL: Human Kinetics, 1988.

27. Stunkard, A., and T. Wadden, eds. *Obesity: Theory and Therapy*. New York: Raven Press, 1993.

28. Powers, S., and E. Howley. *Exercise Physiology: Theory and Application to Fitness and Performance*, 7th ed. New York: McGraw-Hill, 2009.

29. Jackson, A., and M. Pollock. Practical assessment of body composition. *Physician and Sports Medicine* 13:76–90, 1985.

30. Racette, S. B, S. S. Deusinger, M. J Strube, G. R. Highstein, and R. H. Deusinger. Weight changes, exercise, and dietary patterns during freshman and sophomore years of college. *Journal of American College Health* 53:245–251, 2005.

31. Anderson, D. A., J. R. Shapiro, and J. D. Lundgren. The freshman year of college as a critical period for weight gain: An initial evaluation. *Eating Behaviors* 4:363–367, 2003.

32. Levitsky, D. A., C. A. Halbmaier, and G. Mrdjenovic. The freshman weight gain: A model for the study of the epidemic of obesity. *International Journal of Obesity* 28:1435–1442, 2004.

33. Haapanen N., S. Miilunpalo, M. Pasanen, P. Oja, and I. Vuori. Association between leisure time physical activity and 10-year body mass change among working-aged men and women. *International Journal of Obesity and Related Metabolic Disorders* 21:288–296, 1997.

34. Church, T., and S. N. Blair. Does physical activity ameliorate the health hazards of obesity? *British Journal of Sports Medicine* 43:80–81, 2009.

NAME _____ DATE _____

Assessing Body Composition

Equipment

Tape measure, skinfold caliper, scale

Directions

Complete the assessments described below as directed by your instructor. Then, record your body composition data and weight classifications for BMI, waist circumference, waist-to-hip ratio, skinfold, and/or other measures in the spaces below.

BMI

Weight (kg)   _____

Height (m²)   _____

BMI   _____

Classification (see Table 6.1 on page 179):

_____   Underweight

_____   Normal

_____   Overweight

_____   Obese

Skinfold Test

Directions for taking skinfold measurements are on the next page.

Sum of 3 skinfolds (mm)   _____
Percent body fat _____
Classification:

_____   Underweight

_____   Normal

_____   Overweight

_____   Obese

Skinfold Measurement Sites

Men

Abdomen

Chest

Thigh

Women

Suprailium

Triceps

Thigh

To perform skinfold measurements:

- Hold the skinfold between your thumb and index finger.
- Slowly release the tension on the skinfold calipers to pinch the skinfold within $\frac{1}{2}$ inch of your fingers.
- Hold the skinfold, and fully release the tension on the calipers.
- Read the number (the skinfold thickness in millimeters) from the gauge.
- Release the skinfold, and allow the tissue to relax.
- Measure the skinfold thickness at each site.
- Repeat three times, and average the measurements.
- Total the measurements, and use Tables 6.2 and 6.3 on pages 189 and 190 to determine the percent body fat.
- Enter your data in the spaces on page 187

TABLE 6.2
Percent Fat Estimate for Women
Sum of Triceps, Suprailium, and Thigh Skinfolds

Sum of Skinfolds (mm)	Age								
	Under 22	23–27	28–32	33–37	38–42	43–47	48–52	53–57	Over 57
23–25	9.7	9.9	10.2	10.4	10.7	10.9	11.2	11.4	11.7
26–28	11.0	11.2	11.5	11.7	12.0	12.3	12.5	12.7	13.0
29–31	12.3	12.5	12.8	13.0	13.3	13.5	13.8	14.0	14.3
32–34	13.6	13.8	14.0	14.3	14.5	14.8	15.0	15.3	15.5
35–37	14.8	15.0	15.3	15.5	15.8	16.0	16.3	16.5	16.8
38–40	16.0	16.3	16.5	16.7	17.0	17.2	17.5	17.7	18.0
41–43	17.2	17.4	17.7	17.9	18.2	18.4	18.7	18.9	19.2
44–46	18.3	18.6	18.8	19.1	19.3	19.6	19.8	20.1	20.3
47–49	19.5	19.7	20.0	20.2	20.5	20.7	21.0	21.2	21.5
50–52	20.6	20.8	21.1	21.3	21.6	21.8	22.1	22.3	22.6
53–55	21.7	21.9	22.1	22.4	22.6	22.9	23.1	23.4	23.6
56–58	22.7	23.0	23.2	23.4	23.7	23.9	24.2	24.4	24.7
59–61	23.7	24.0	24.2	24.5	24.7	25.0	25.2	25.5	25.7
62–64	24.7	25.0	25.2	25.5	25.7	26.0	26.7	26.4	26.7
65–67	25.7	25.9	26.2	26.4	26.7	26.9	27.2	27.4	27.7
68–70	26.6	26.9	27.1	27.4	27.6	27.9	28.1	28.4	28.6
71–73	27.5	27.8	28.0	28.3	28.5	28.8	29.0	29.3	29.5
74–76	28.4	28.7	28.9	29.2	29.4	29.7	29.9	30.2	30.4
77–79	29.3	29.5	29.8	30.0	30.3	30.5	30.8	31.0	31.3
80–82	30.1	30.4	30.6	30.9	31.1	31.4	31.6	31.9	32.1
83–85	30.9	31.2	31.4	31.7	31.9	32.2	32.4	32.7	32.9
86–88	31.7	32.0	32.2	32.5	32.7	32.9	33.2	33.4	33.7
89–91	32.5	32.7	33.0	33.2	33.5	33.7	33.9	34.2	34.4
92–94	33.2	33.4	33.7	33.9	34.2	34.4	34.7	34.9	35.2
95–97	33.9	34.1	34.4	34.6	34.9	35.1	35.4	35.6	35.9
98–100	34.6	34.8	35.1	35.3	35.5	35.8	36.0	36.3	36.5
101–103	35.3	35.4	35.7	35.9	36.2	36.4	36.7	36.9	37.2
104–106	35.8	36.1	36.3	36.6	36.8	37.1	37.3	37.5	37.8
107–109	36.4	36.7	36.9	37.1	37.4	37.6	37.9	38.1	38.4
110–112	37.0	37.2	37.5	37.7	38.0	38.2	38.5	38.7	38.9
113–115	37.5	37.8	38.0	38.2	38.5	38.7	39.0	39.2	39.5
116–118	38.0	38.3	38.5	38.8	39.0	39.3	39.5	39.7	40.0
119–121	38.5	38.7	39.0	39.2	39.5	39.7	40.0	40.2	40.5
122–124	39.0	39.2	39.4	39.7	39.9	40.2	40.4	40.7	40.9
125–127	39.4	39.6	39.9	40.1	40.4	40.6	40.9	41.1	41.4
128–130	39.8	40.0	40.3	40.5	40.8	41.0	41.3	41.5	41.8

Source: Jackson, A. S., and M. L. Pollock, 1985. Practical assessment of body composition. *The Physician and Sportsmedicine* 13(5):76–90, Tables 6 & 7, pp. 86, 87. Copyright © 2005. The McGraw-Hill Companies. All rights reserved. Reprinted with permission from The McGraw-Hill Companies.

Percent Fat Estimate for Men
Sum of Chest, Abdomen, and Thigh Skinfolds

Sum of Skinfolds (mm)	Age								
	Under 22	23–27	28–32	33–37	38–42	43–47	48–52	53–57	Over 57
8–10	1.3	1.8	2.3	2.9	3.4	3.9	4.5	5.0	5.5
11–13	2.2	2.8	3.3	3.9	4.4	4.9	5.5	6.0	6.5
14–16	3.2	3.8	4.3	4.8	5.4	5.9	6.4	7.0	7.5
17–19	4.2	4.7	5.3	5.8	6.3	6.9	7.4	8.0	8.5
20–22	5.1	5.7	6.2	6.8	7.3	7.9	8.4	8.9	9.5
23–25	6.1	6.6	7.2	7.7	8.3	8.8	9.4	9.9	10.5
26–28	7.0	7.6	8.1	8.7	9.2	9.8	10.3	10.9	11.4
29–31	8.0	8.5	9.1	9.6	10.2	10.7	11.3	11.8	12.4
32–34	8.9	9.4	10.0	10.5	11.1	11.6	12.2	12.8	13.3
35–37	9.8	10.4	10.9	11.5	12.0	12.6	13.1	13.7	14.3
38–40	10.7	11.3	11.8	12.4	12.9	13.5	14.1	14.6	15.2
41–43	11.6	12.2	12.7	13.3	13.8	14.4	15.0	15.5	16.1
44–46	12.5	13.1	13.6	14.2	14.7	15.3	15.9	16.4	17.0
47–49	13.4	13.9	14.5	15.1	15.6	16.2	16.8	17.3	17.9
50–52	14.3	14.8	15.4	15.9	16.5	17.1	17.6	18.2	18.8
53–55	15.1	15.7	16.2	16.8	17.4	17.9	18.5	19.1	19.7
56–58	16.0	16.5	17.1	17.7	18.2	18.8	19.4	20.0	20.5
59–61	16.9	17.4	17.9	18.5	19.1	19.7	20.2	20.8	21.4
62–64	17.6	18.2	18.8	19.4	19.9	20.5	21.1	21.7	22.2
65–67	18.5	19.0	19.6	20.2	20.8	21.3	21.9	22.5	23.1
68–70	19.3	19.9	20.4	21.0	21.6	22.2	22.7	23.3	23.9
71–73	20.1	20.7	21.2	21.8	22.4	23.0	23.6	24.1	24.7
74–76	20.9	21.5	22.0	22.6	23.2	23.8	24.4	25.0	25.5
77–79	21.7	22.2	22.8	23.4	24.0	24.6	25.2	25.8	26.3
80–82	22.4	23.0	23.6	24.2	24.8	25.4	25.9	26.5	27.1
83–85	23.2	23.8	24.4	25.0	25.5	26.1	26.7	27.3	27.9
86–88	24.0	24.5	25.1	25.7	26.3	26.9	27.5	28.1	28.7
89–91	24.7	25.3	25.9	26.5	27.1	27.6	28.2	28.8	29.4
92–94	25.4	26.0	26.6	27.2	27.8	28.4	29.0	29.6	30.2
95–97	26.1	26.7	27.3	27.9	28.5	29.1	29.7	30.3	30.9
98–100	26.9	27.4	28.0	28.6	29.2	29.8	30.4	31.0	31.6
101–103	27.5	28.1	28.7	29.3	29.9	30.5	31.1	31.7	32.3
104–106	28.2	28.8	29.4	30.0	30.6	31.2	31.8	32.4	33.0
107–109	28.9	29.5	30.1	30.7	31.3	31.9	32.5	33.1	33.7
110–112	29.6	30.2	30.8	31.4	32.0	32.6	33.2	33.8	34.4
113–115	30.2	30.8	31.4	32.0	32.6	33.2	33.8	34.5	35.1
116–118	30.9	31.5	32.1	32.7	33.3	33.9	34.5	35.1	35.7
119–121	31.5	32.1	32.7	33.3	33.9	34.5	35.1	35.7	36.4
122–124	32.1	32.7	33.3	33.9	34.5	35.1	35.8	36.4	37.0
125–127	32.7	33.3	33.9	34.5	35.1	35.8	36.4	37.0	37.6

Source: Jackson, A. S., and M. L. Pollock, 1985. Practical assessment of body composition. *The Physician and Sportsmedicine* 13(5):76–90, Tables 6 & 7, pp. 86, 87. Copyright © 2005. The McGraw-Hill Companies. All rights reserved. Reprinted with permission from The McGraw-Hill Companies.

Waist Circumference and Waist-to-Hip Ratio

(a)   (b)

To perform waist-to-hip circumference measurements.

- Perform the waist measurement first.
- Place the tape at the level of the navel (a), and make your measurement at the end of a normal breath.
- For the hip measurement, place the tape around the maxmum circumference of the buttocks (b).
- Divide the waist circumference by the hip circumference to determine the waist-to-hip ratio.
- Use Table 6.4 on page 192 to determine the waist-to-hip ratio rating.
- Use Table 6.1 on page 179 to determine your waist measurement rating.
- Enter your data in the spaces below.

Waist measurement _____

Hip measurement   _____

Waist-to-hip ratio   _____

TABLE 6.4
Waist-to-Hip Circumference Ratio Standards for Men and Women

	Age	Low	Moderate	High	Very High
			Risk		
Men	20–29	<0.83	0.83–0.88	0.89–0.94	>0.94
	30–39	<0.84	0.84–0.91	0.92–0.96	>0.96
	40–49	<0.88	0.88–0.95	0.96–1.00	>1.00
	50–59	<0.90	0.90–0.96	0.97–1.02	>1.02
	60–69	<0.91	0.91–0.98	0.99–1.03	>1.03
Women	20–29	<0.71	0.71–0.77	0.78–0.82	>0.82
	30–39	<0.72	0.72–0.78	0.79–0.84	>0.84
	40–49	<0.73	0.73–0.79	0.80–0.87	>0.87
	50–59	<0.74	0.74–0.81	0.82–0.88	>0.88
	60–69	<0.76	0.76–0.83	0.84–0.90	>0.90

Source: Reprinted with permission from Heyward, V. H., and L. M. Stolarczyk. *Applied Body Composition Assessment*. Champaign, IL: Human Kinetics, 1996, p. 82.

Classification

_____ Low risk   _____ Low risk

_____ Moderate risk   _____ Moderate risk

_____ High risk   _____ High risk

_____ Very high risk   _____ Very high risk

Other Measure: _____

Percent body fat _____

Classification:

_____ Underweight

_____ Normal

_____ Overweight

_____ Obese

Questions

1. Are your classifications for each assessment similar? If not, why do you think there are discrepancies?

   _____

   _____

2. Which assessment did you feel was most accurate for you, and why?

   _____

   _____

NAME _____ DATE _____

Determining a Healthy Body Weight

Equipment

Results from Laboratory 6.1 and a calculator

Directions

If your results from Laboratory 6.1 indicate that you need to lose or gain weight, you should calculate your goal body weight needed to achieve an optimal level of body fat or optimal BMI. Keep in mind that not everyone will need to lose or gain weight. If your weight is within the recommended levels and you are happy with your current body composition, weight maintenance should be your goal.

Part I

		Example:	
Current weight	_____	*Current weight*	*176*
Current percent fat	_____	*Current percent fat*	*38*
Current BMI	_____	*Current BMI*	*29.3**
Goal percent fat	_____	*Goal percent fat*	*25–30†*
Goal BMI	_____	*Goal BMI*	*20–25 kg/m²*

Step 1: Calculate % of fat-free mass.

1 − _____ (current percent fat ‡) = _____ (% fat-free mass)

Example: 1 − (0.38) = 0.62

Step 2: Calculate fat-free weight.

_____ (% fat-free mass ‡) × _____ (current body weight) = _____ (fat-free weight)

Example: 0.62 × 176 = 109.12

Step 3: Calculate optimal weight, lower and upper ends of the range.

_____ (optimal weight) = _____ (fat-free weight) /(1 − _____ [optimal percent fat ‡])
Repeat for the upper end of the range.

Example: 109.12 ÷ (1 − 0.25) = 145.5
109.12 ÷ (1 − 0.30) = 155.9
Example optimal range = 146 to 156 pounds

Your optimal range: _____ to _____

---

*We used a height of 65 inches.
†We selected values within the recommended healthy range. You can use the whole range, or you can use part of the range, as we did. The important thing to remember is that your goal should be within the recommended levels for your age and activity level.
‡ Expressed as a decimal.

Step 4: Calculate BMI based on your optimal weight range.

_____ to _____

Example:
1 m = 39.25 in., 1 lb = 2.2 kg
65 in. ÷ 39.25 = 1.65 m
146 lb ÷ 2.2 = 66.2 kg
$66.2 ÷ 1.65^2 = 24.3$ kg/m^2
156 lb ÷ 2.2 = 70.7 kg
$70.7 ÷ 165^2 = 25.9$ kg/m^2
BMI: 24.3 to 25.9 kg/m^2

Part 2

Repeat the calculations for determining a healthy goal weight, using BMI.

$$\text{goal weight (kg)} = \text{desired BMI} \times \text{height (m}^2)$$

Repeat for the upper end of the range

_____ to _____

Questions

1. Do the BMI values in part 1 of the lab place you in the recommended range? If not, why not?

   _____

   _____

2. Are there any differences between the BMI values from parts 1 and 2? If so, why?

   _____

   _____

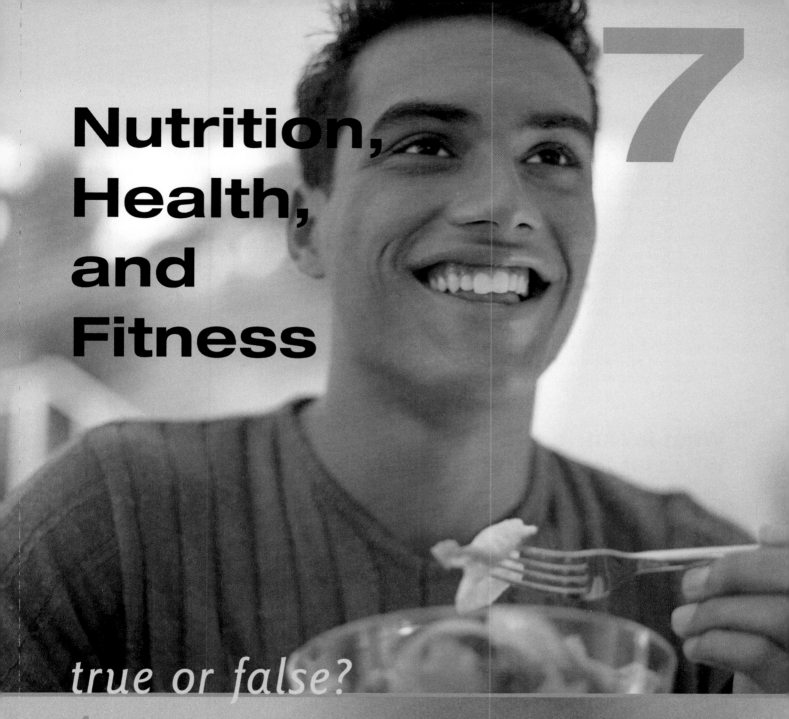

Nutrition, Health, and Fitness

7

true or false?

1. People in the U.S. don't eat enough protein.
2. Carbohydrates cause weight gain.
3. Most people need vitamin supplements.
4. All foods contain antioxidants.
5. Whole foods are more healthy than processed foods.

Answers appear on the next page.

When you sit down to lunch at your campus cafeteria, do you think to yourself, "Wow, this looks like a great plate of protein, carbohydrate, and phytochemicals"? Or are you more likely to appreciate the hamburger, french fries, and ketchup on your tray? You probably don't often consider the nutrient components of food or how they ultimately drive your body to function. However, understanding these nutrients, and the processes that break them down to make them available for use, can help you appreciate their importance to health and help you improve your food choices.

In this chapter, we'll find out how your body uses the food you eat. We'll discuss the classes of nutrients and their functions, the fundamental concepts of good nutrition, and guidelines for a healthy diet. We also explore how exercise training can modify nutritional requirements.

What Is Nutrition and Why Is it Important?

Nutrition is the study of food and the way the body uses it to produce energy and build and repair itself. It involves understanding the relationship between food and health or disease. Good nutrition means a diet that supplies all of the essential nutrients required to maintain a healthy body. Consuming too much or too little of any of the essential nutrients will eventually lead to health problems. In the past, it was dietary deficiencies of nutrients that caused health problems for many peo-

ple; for example, insufficient intake of vitamin C can lead to scurvy, and insufficient iron intake can lead to a form of anemia—both of which were once prevalent in much of the world's population (and are still common in the developing world). Although these conditions still exist today, excess consumption of calories, and the overweight and obesity that result from it, are greater causes of health problems in the United States.

Diets that are too high in calories, sugar, fats, and/or sodium have been linked to diseases and conditions such as cardiovascular disease, cancer, obesity, and diabetes. These conditions are the leading killers in the United States (1). According to the U.S. Department of Health and Human Services, over half of all deaths are associated with health problems linked to poor nutrition (2). The good news is that analyzing and modifying your diet can help prevent many of these nutrition-related diseases. A basic understanding of nutrition is therefore important for everyone.

What Are Nutrients?

Nutrients are the basic substances in foods that your body uses to maintain health. They can be divided into two categories: macronutrients and micronutrients. The **macronutrients** (carbohydrates, fats, and proteins) are needed in greater amounts and primarily build and maintain body tissues and provide energy for daily activities. **Micronutrients** (vitamins and minerals) are needed in much smaller amounts by your body, but they are essential for numerous processes, including regulating cell functions. The final class of nutrient is water, which is so important for body function that you can't survive more than a few days without it.

Macronutrients

Macronutrients provide the energy, in the form of **kilocalories** (more commonly called *calories*), that your body needs daily to function. Carbohydrates and protein provide 4 calories per gram, and fat provides 9 calories per gram. Under normal conditions, carbohydrates and fats are the primary fuels the body uses to produce energy. The primary role of protein is to build and repair tissues. However, when carbohydrate is in short supply or the body is under stress, protein can be used for energy. A well-balanced diet is composed of approximately 58% carbohydrates (including complex carbohydrates and simple sugars), 30% fat, and 12% protein (Figure 7.1).

Table 7.1 lists some major food sources of carbohydrates, proteins, and fats.

Carbohydrates
Whole grains, pasta, fruits, and vegetables are excellent sources of **carbohydrates,** the main source of fuel for your brain. Carbohydrates are especially important during many types of physical activity, because they are a key energy source for muscular contraction. However, not all carbohydrates are created equal—simple carbohydrates (or sugars) are easier for the body to break down and use for energy, and complex carbohydrates (starch and fiber) can be used for energy but also serve other purposes.

Types of Carbohydrates
Simple carbohydrates consist of chains of one or two simple sugars. **Glucose** is the most noteworthy of the simple sugars because it is the only sugar molecule that can be used directly by the body. To be used for fuel, all other carbohydrates must first be converted to glucose. The body stores glucose in the form of **glycogen** in skeletal muscles and the liver. Glucose that is not immediately used for energy or stored as glycogen will be stored as fat for future energy use. The central nervous system uses glucose almost exclusively for its energy needs. If you don't consume

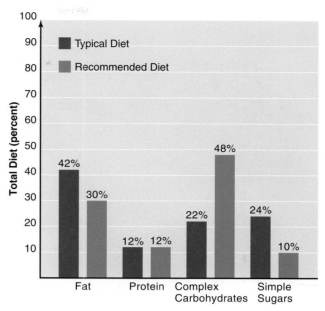

FIGURE 7.1

The recommended nutritionally balanced diet compared with the typical U.S. diet. The average American consumes too much fat and simple sugar, and too few complex carbohydrates.

Source: Block, G. Junk foods account for 30% of caloric intake. *Journal of Food Composition and Analysis* 17:439–447, 2004.

enough carbohydrates in food, your body has to make glucose from protein. This is undesirable because it results in the breakdown of body protein for use as fuel. Dietary carbohydrates are important not only as a direct fuel source, but also for their protein-sparing effect.

nutrition The study of food and the way the body uses it to produce energy and build or repair body tissues.

nutrients Substances in food that are necessary for good health.

macronutrients Carbohydrates, fats, and proteins, which are necessary for building and maintaining body tissues and providing energy for daily activities.

micronutrients Vitamins and minerals. Micronutrients are involved in many body processes, including regulating cell function.

kilocalorie The unit of measure used to quantify food energy or the energy expended by the body. Technically, a kilocalorie is the amount of energy necessary to raise the temperature of 1 gram of water 1°C. The terms *kilocalorie* and *calorie* are often used interchangeably.

carbohydrate A macronutrient that is a key energy source for muscular contraction.

glucose A simple carbohydrate (sugar) that can be used directly by the body. All other carbohydrates must be converted to glucose before being used for fuel.

glycogen The storage form of glucose in the liver and skeletal muscles.

TABLE 7.1
Food Sources of the Macronutrients

Carbohydrate (4 calories/ gram)	Protein (4 calories/ gram)	Fat (9 calories/ gram)
Grains	Meats	Butter
Fruits	Fish	Margarine
Vegetables	Poultry	Oils
Concentrated sweets	Eggs	Shortening
Bread	Milk	Cream
Beans/peas	Beans	
	Rice	

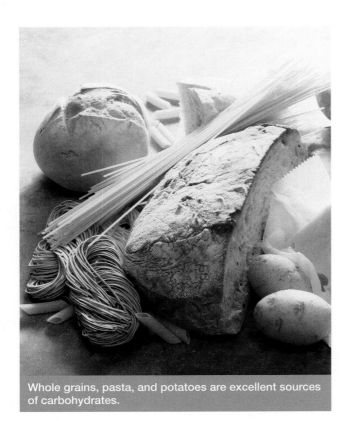
Whole grains, pasta, and potatoes are excellent sources of carbohydrates.

There are several other simple sugars found in foods, including fructose, galactose, lactose, maltose, and sucrose. Fructose is found primarily in fruit, and galactose and lactose are found in milk and dairy products. Maltose is found in some grains, and sucrose, commonly known as table sugar, is the white, granular product used for household baking.

Complex carbohydrates come in the forms of starch and fiber. **Starches** are long chains of glucose units and are often used for that sudden burst of energy we need during physical activity. **Fiber** is a stringy, nondigestible carbohydrate found in plants. Because fiber is nondigestible, it is not a fuel source. However, it is important in helping prevent some chronic diseases.

The Importance of Fiber Dietary fiber provides bulk in the intestinal tract. This bulk aids in the formation and elimination of food waste products, thus reducing the time necessary for wastes to move through the digestive system and lowering the risk of colon cancer. Dietary fiber is also thought to be a factor in reducing the risk for coronary heart disease and breast cancer and in controlling blood sugar in individuals with diabetes (3). Some types of fiber bind with cholesterol in the digestive tract and prevent its absorption into the blood, thereby reducing blood cholesterol levels.

Fiber can be classified according to its viscosity (its thickness when mixed with digestive juices in the in-

testines). **Soluble fiber** is more viscous than **insoluble fiber** and is usually found in oats, barley, beans, peas, and citrus fruits. Insoluble fiber is typically concentrated in whole wheat and vegetables. A higher viscosity slows transit in the intestines, allowing nutrients to be absorbed more readily. This helps in regulating glucose levels, appetite, and the reabsorption of bile acids. The primary health benefit of insoluble fiber is its water-binding capacity, which quickens transit time in the large intestine. A faster transit time also helps with regularity of bowel movements and reduces the risk of colon cancer (4).

You should eat a minimum of 25 grams of fiber a day; however, be aware that excessive amounts of fiber in the diet can cause intestinal discomfort and decreased absorption of calcium and iron into the blood (3). Your best bet for getting plenty of fiber is to eat adequate amounts of whole grains, legumes, fruits, and vegetables (including the skins) every day. You'll also want to drink plenty of fluid to prevent constipation.

Carbohydrates in Foods Some foods, such as pasta, potatoes, and bread, are famous for containing high amounts of carbohydrates, but there are numerous other foods that can also contribute to your daily carbohydrate needs. Fruits and honey provide fructose. Dairy foods contain lactose. Sucrose is found in table sugar, including some of the packets you may use to sweeten your coffee or tea. Starch is plentiful in potatoes, corn, bread, and rice, and fiber is found in all

TABLE 7.2
Types of Carbohydrates and Their Sources

Simple Carbohydrates	Source(s)
Fructose	Fruits: apples, pears, citrus, and so on
	Honey
Galactose	Breast milk, vegetables
Glucose	Made by the body
Lactose (galactose + glucose)	Milk products
Maltose (glucose + glucose)	Barley
Sucrose (fructose + glucose)	Table sugar

Complex Carbohydrates	Source(s)
Starch	Potatoes, rice, bread
Fiber	Fruits and vegetables, including apples, oranges, pears, celery, and broccoli; whole grains

TABLE 7.3
Fatty Acids, Food Sources, and Effects on Blood Cholesterol Levels

Type of Fatty Acid	Primary Sources	State at Room Temperature	Effect on Cholesterol
Monounsaturated	Canola* and olive oils; foods made from and prepared in them	Liquid	Lowers LDL; no effect on HDL
Polyunsaturated†	Soybean, safflower, corn, and cottonseed oils; foods made from and prepared in them	Liquid	Lowers both LDL and HDL
Saturated	Animal fat from red meat, whole milk, and butter; also, coconut and palm oils	Solid	Raises LDL and total cholesterol
Trans	Partially hydrogenated vegetable oils used in cooking, margarine, shortening, baked and fried foods, and snack foods	Semisolid	Raises LDL and total cholesterol

*Many nutritionists consider canola oil the most healthful vegetable oil because it's low in saturated fat, high in monounsaturated fat, and has a moderate level of omega-3 polyunsaturated fat.
†Contains the omega-3 and omega-6 essential fatty acids that the human body can't make on its own.
Source: Fats: The good, the bad, the trans. *Health News,* July 25, 1999, pp. 1–2. Massachusetts Medical Society, Published by Englander Communication, LLC, an affiliate of Behavior Publications, Inc.

plant-derived foods. See Table 7.2 for examples of food sources for different types of carbohydrates.

Fats and Lipids   **Fats** (technically known as triglycerides) are actually one type in a larger class of substances called **lipids.** Fats are the most common type of lipid found in foods and in your body. Once consumed, they are broken down and used to produce energy to power muscle contractions during exercise. Fat is an efficient storage form for energy, because at 9 calories per gram, it holds more than twice the energy of either carbohydrate or protein.

Excess fat in the diet is stored in fat cells located under the skin and around internal organs. In addition to fat you take in from foods, your body forms fat from excess carbohydrate and protein in the diet.

Although fat is often avoided by people who want to lose weight, you would never want to eliminate it from your diet. Dietary fat is the only source of linoleic and linolenic acids, the two fatty acids that are essential for normal growth and healthy skin. Fat also protects internal organs and assists in absorbing, transporting, and storing the fat-soluble vitamins A, D, E, and K.

Types of Fats   Triglycerides are made up of three **fatty acids** (essentially, chains of carbon and hydrogen atoms) attached to a glycerol backbone. Depending on their structure, fatty acids are classified as monounsaturated, polyunsaturated, saturated, or trans (Table 7.3).

Unsaturated fatty acids include monounsaturated and polyunsaturated fatty acids. They are found in plants (including nuts, seeds, grains, and vegetable oils) and are liquid at room temperature. Unsaturated fats, which contain mostly unsaturated fatty acids, are

thought to be the most heart healthy because of their effect on blood cholesterol levels (we'll discuss cholesterol later in the chapter).

One type of polyunsaturated fatty acid, called **omega-3 fatty acid,** is reported to lower both blood cholesterol and triglycerides. This fatty acid is found primarily in fish, especially fresh or frozen mackerel, herring, tuna, and salmon. Some researchers have argued that one or two servings per week of fish

complex carbohydrates Long chains of sugar units linked together to form starch or fiber.

starches Long chains of glucose units; commonly found in foods such as corn, grains, and potatoes.

fiber A stringy, nondigestible complex carbohydrate found in whole grains, vegetables, and fruits.

soluble fiber Viscous fiber found in oats, barley, peas, and citrus fruits.

insoluble fiber Type of fiber found in whole wheat and vegetables.

fats (triglycerides) The form of lipid that is broken down in the body and used to produce energy to power muscle contractions during exercise.

lipids A group of insoluble compounds that include fats and cholesterol.

fatty acids The basic structural unit of triglycerides; they are important nutritionally not only because of their energy content, but also because they play a role in cardiovascular disease.

unsaturated fatty acid A type of fatty acid that comes primarily from plant sources and is liquid at room temperature.

omega-3 fatty acid A type of unsaturated fatty acid that lowers both blood cholesterol and triglycerides and is found abundantly in some fish.

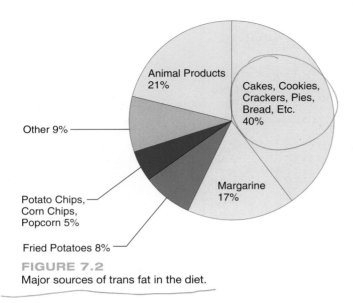

FIGURE 7.2
Major sources of trans fat in the diet.

containing omega-3 fatty acids reduces the risk of heart disease (5). However, some people, in particular pregnant women and children, may need to limit their consumption of these fish because of the possibility of methylmercury contamination (see the Appreciating Diversity box below).

Saturated fatty acids are solid at room temperature. They generally come from animal sources (meat and dairy products), but some (coconut oil, for example), come from plant sources. Saturated fatty acids increase blood levels of cholesterol. High cholesterol levels, in turn, promote the buildup of fatty plaque in

the coronary arteries, which can eventually lead to heart disease (Chapter 9).

Trans fatty acids, found primarily in baked and fried foods, but also naturally in some animal foods (Figure 7.2), tend to raise total cholesterol in the blood. For this reason, they are considered to be heart-unhealthy. The U.S. Food and Drug Administration (FDA) recommends limiting the amount of trans fat in the diet—and even requires that food manufacturers list trans fat on food labels—to help consumers avoid products that contain it. Some U.S. cities, including New York and Philadelphia, have banned or greatly restricted the use of trans fats in restaurants. As more is learned about the effects of trans fats on health, food manufacturers and restaurateurs are likely to phase it out of their products.

Other Types of Lipids   In addition to fat, there are two other forms of lipids: **phospholipids** and **sterols.** Phospholipids are important components of cell membranes and play a key role in emulsification. The most common sterol, **cholesterol,** is an important component of cells and is used to manufacture certain types of hormones, including some male and female sex hormones.

Lipoproteins are combinations of protein, triglycerides, and cholesterol. Although lipoproteins exist in several forms, the two primary types are low-density lipoproteins (LDL cholesterol) and high-density lipoproteins (HDL cholesterol). LDL, or "bad," cholesterol consists of a limited amount of protein and triglycerides but contains large amounts of cholesterol. It is associated with promoting fatty plaque buildup in the arteries

APPRECIATING
DIVERSITY SHOULD PREGNANT WOMEN EAT FISH?

Seafood can be an important part of a healthy diet during pregnancy. Fish is low in fat and a great source of high-quality protein and other nutrients. However, some fish may contain a form of mercury that could harm the nervous system of a developing fetus. Pregnant women need to know the types of fish that carry the highest risk of containing methylmercury and other contaminants so that they can avoid or reduce their intake of these fish during pregnancy.

Methylmercury is a toxin produced from the inorganic mercury that gets into water after the burning of wastes and

fossil fuels. It enters the food chain when fish and other aquatic organisms acquire it from the water. When larger fish eat smaller fish, the methylmercury from the smaller fish will accumulate in the larger fish's body. Thus older, larger fish have higher concentrations of methylmercury in their bodies than smaller, younger fish. Some of the highest levels of methylmercury are found in large predatory fish, such as shark, swordfish, king mackerel, and tilefish, so pregnant women should avoid these species. However, eating less than 12 ounces per week of other species, such as shellfish, canned fish,

small ocean fish, or farm-raised fish, can safely provide protein and other nutrients.

In addition to the wild or farmed fish found in the local grocery store, pregnant women also need to be aware of the risks for contamination of locally caught fish. The U.S. Environmental Protection Agency (EPA) provides current advice on consuming fish from your local freshwater lakes and streams. You can also contact your state or local health department for specific consumption recommendations about fish caught or sold in your area.

of the heart, which is the primary cause of heart disease. In contrast, HDL, or "good," cholesterol is primarily composed of protein, has limited amounts of cholesterol, and is associated with a low risk of heart disease. We discuss HDL and LDL cholesterol again in Chapter 9.

Fats and Lipids in Foods   You can find "good" fats, including the two essential fatty acids, in fish, seeds, nuts, and vegetable oils. Unhealthy, saturated fats are in fatty meats, butter, lard, fried foods, and many baked items. These items should be avoided or eaten only in limited amounts.

Dietary cholesterol is present in many foods from animal sources, including meats, shellfish, and dairy products. Although your body needs some cholesterol for normal function, you actually don't need to consume cholesterol from foods, because your body can make all that it needs. In fact, diets high in saturated fats cause the body to produce more than normal amounts of cholesterol.

Proteins   The primary role of protein is to serve as the structural unit to build and repair body tissues, including muscle and connective tissue. Proteins are also important for the synthesis of enzymes, hormones, and antibodies. These compounds regulate body metabolism and provide protection from disease.

As mentioned earlier, proteins are not usually a major fuel source. However, if your dietary intake of carbohydrates is too low (such as during a diet or fast), proteins can be converted to glucose and used as fuel. If you consume adequate amounts of carbohydrates, excess calories from dietary protein are stored in adipose tissue as an energy reserve.

The Structure of Proteins   The basic structural units of proteins are called **amino acids.** There are 20 different amino acids, and they can be linked in various combinations to create different proteins with unique functions. Some are **essential amino acids,** meaning that the body cannot make them and they must be consumed in the diet. Others are **nonessential amino acids,** meaning that the body can synthesize them in adequate amounts. There are 9 essential amino acids, and 11 nonessential amino acids.

Protein in Foods   **Complete proteins** contain all of the essential amino acids and are present only in animal foods and soy products. **Incomplete proteins** are missing one or more of the essential amino acids and are present in numerous vegetable sources. Vegetarians, who avoid animal foods, must be careful to eat a variety of foods so that they consume all of the essential amino acids.

Calculating Your Protein Needs	Example (Adult Female)
1. Determine your body weight	1. An adult female weighs 110 pounds.
2. Convert pounds (lb) to kilograms (kg) by dividing number of pounds by 2.2	2. 110 / 2.2 lb/kg = 50 kg
3. Multiply by 0.8 (adult females) or 0.9 (adult males) to get an RDA in grams/day	3. 50 kg × 0.8 g/kg = 40 g
	A 110 pound female needs to consume 40 grams of protein per day.

FIGURE 7.3
Estimated daily protein needs for adults. You can calculate the number of grams of protein you should consume daily.

Because of its role in building body tissue, protein is particularly important during periods of rapid growth, such as adolescence. Adolescents need to take in more than 12% of their calories from protein (the recommended amount for adults). For adolescents, the recommended dietary allowance (RDA) for proteins is 1 gram per kilogram of body weight (3). The recommendation decreases to 0.8 g/kg in women and 0.9 g/kg in men at the end of adolescence (Figure 7.3).

saturated fatty acid A type of fatty acid that comes primarily from animal sources and is solid at room temperature.

trans fatty acid A type of fatty acid that increases cholesterol in the blood and is a major contributor to heart disease.

phospholipid A type of lipid that contains phosphorus and is an important component of cell membranes.

sterol A type of lipid that does not contain fatty acids; cholesterol is the most commonly known sterol.

cholesterol A type of lipid that is necessary for cell and hormone synthesis. Found naturally in animal foods, but made in adequate amounts in the body.

lipoproteins Combinations of protein, triglycerides, and cholesterol in the blood that are important because of their role in influencing the risk of heart disease.

amino acids The building blocks of protein. There are 20 different amino acids that can be linked in various combinations to create different proteins.

essential amino acids The nine amino acids that cannot be manufactured by the body and must therefore be consumed in the diet.

nonessential amino acids Eleven amino acids that the body can make and are therefore not necessary in the diet.

complete proteins Proteins containing all the essential amino acids; found only in soy and animal foods (meats and dairy products).

incomplete proteins Proteins that are missing one or more of the essential amino acids; found in plant sources such as nuts and legumes.

TABLE 7.4
Selected Vitamins: Food Sources, Functions, and Deficiency and Toxicity Symptoms

Vitamin	Selected Food Sources	Selected Functions	Deficiency Symptoms	Toxicity Symptoms
Fat-soluble				
A	Liver, spinach, carrots, sweet potatoes; other orange and green leafy vegetables	Necessary for vision, bone growth, fertility	Night blindness, impaired immunity, infertility	Birth defects, loss of appetite, blurred vision, hair loss, liver damage
D	Fortified milk; produced in the skin with sunlight	Regulates blood calcium levels; bone health; cell differentiation	Rickets in children, bone weakness and increased fractures in adults	Hypercalcemia, calcium deposits in kidney and liver
E	Vegetable oils, whole grains, nuts, seeds	Antioxidant; improves absorption of vitamin A	Anemia, impaired nerve transmission, muscle weakness	Inhibited blood clotting
K	Green leafy vegetables; cabbage, cauliflower	Helps with blood clotting	Reduced ability to form blood clots	No known symptoms
Water-soluble				
Thiamin (B$_1$)	Whole grains, organ meat, lean pork	Coenzyme in carbohydrate metabolism and some amino acid metabolism	Beriberi, weight loss, confusion, muscle weakness	No known symptoms
Riboflavin (B$_2$)	Dairy products, enriched breads and cereals, lean meats, poultry, fish	Coenzyme; helps maintain mucous membranes	Sore throat, swelling of the tongue, anemia	No known symptoms
Niacin (B$_3$)	Eggs, poultry, fish, milk, whole grains, nuts, enriched breads and cereals	Coenzymes in carbohydrate and fatty acid metabolism; plays role in DNA replication and repair and cell differentiation	Pellagra, rash, vomiting, constipation or diarrhea	Flushing, liver damage, glucose intolerance, blurred vision
Vitamin B$_6$	Eggs, poultry, fish, whole grains, liver, kidney, pork	Coenzyme involved in amino acid and carbohydrate metabolism; synthesis of blood cells	Dermatitis, anemia, convulsions	Skin lesions
Vitamin B$_{12}$	Meat, fish, poultry, fortified cereals	Coenzyme that assists with blood formation and nervous system function	Pernicious anemia, pale skin, fatigue, shortness of breath, dementia	No known symptoms
Folate	Green leafy vegetables, yeast, oranges, whole grains, legumes	Coenzyme involved in DNA synthesis and amino acid metabolism	Macrocytic anemia, weakness and fatigue, headache, neural tube defects in developing fetus	Masks symptoms of vitamin B$_{12}$ deficiency; neurological damage
Vitamin C	Citrus fruits, peppers, spinach, strawberries, tomatoes, potatoes	Antioxidant; assists with collagen synthesis; enhances immune function; enhances iron absorption	Scurvy, bleeding gums and joints, loose teeth, depression, anemia	Nausea and diarrhea, nosebleeds, abdominal cramps

Source: Adapted from Thompson, J., and M. Manore. *Nutrition: An Applied Approach,* 2nd ed. San Francisco: Benjamin Cummings, 2009.

Because the average person in industrialized countries consumes more than enough protein, the nutritional problem associated with protein intake is one of excess. Protein foods from animal sources are often high in fat (and high in calories), which can lead to an increased risk of heart disease, cancer, and obesity.

Micronutrients

Micronutrients include **vitamins** and **minerals.** Though needed in smaller amounts, micronutrients are as important to body function as macronutrients and are required to sustain life. Although they do not supply energy, they are essential to the breakdown and use of the macronutrients.

Vitamins   Vitamins play a key role in many bodily functions, including the regulation of growth and metabolism. Some vitamins are soluble in water; others are soluble in fat. Water-soluble vitamins include the B vitamins and vitamin C. These vitamins are generally not stored in the body and can be eliminated by the kidneys. Vitamins A, D, E, and K are fat soluble. They are stored in body fat and can therefore accumulate to toxic levels. Table 7.4 lists some functions and dietary sources of both water-soluble and fat-soluble vitamins.

In addition to their essential roles in body processes, some vitamins and minerals may also protect against tissue damage (3, 6). This has important implications for individuals engaged in an exercise program. This potential new role for micronutrients is discussed later in this chapter.

Minerals   Minerals are chemical elements such as sodium and calcium that are required by the body for normal function. Like vitamins, minerals play important roles in regulating key body functions, such as the conduction of nerve impulses, muscular contraction, enzyme function, and maintenance of water balance. Minerals serve a structural function as well; calcium, phosphorus, and fluoride all are important components in bones and teeth.

Three minerals that play important roles in the body are calcium, iron, and sodium. Calcium is important in bone formation. A deficiency of calcium contributes to the development of the bone disease called **osteoporosis.** A deficiency of dietary iron may lead to iron-deficiency **anemia,** which results in chronic fatigue. High sodium intake has been associated with hypertension, a major risk factor for heart disease.

Table 7.5 summarizes several key minerals and their functions.

Vitamin and Minerals in Foods   Though a few vitamins, including A, D and K, can be made in the body, most must be consumed in foods. If you're eating

Water is a key ingredient in a healthy diet.

a balanced diet with plenty of fresh fruits, vegetables, and whole grains, and some lean meat and poultry, you're likely getting all of the vitamins and minerals that you need. (See Tables 7.4 and 7.5 for specific food sources for these and other vitamins and minerals). In general, the more brightly colored the fruit or vegetable, the higher its vitamin and mineral content. Note that some water-soluble vitamins can be destroyed during cooking or processing, so minimal cooking (such as by steaming, rather than boiling) and eating fresh rather than canned produce will provide higher amounts of micronutrients.

---

vitamins Micronutrients that play a key role in many body functions, including the regulation of growth and metabolism. They are classified according to whether they are soluble in water or fat.

minerals Chemical elements (e.g., sodium and calcium) that are required by the body in small amounts for normal functioning.

osteoporosis Bone disease in which mineral content of bone is reduced and the bone is weakened and at increased risk of fracture.

anemia Deficiency of red blood cells and/or hemoglobin that results in decreased oxygen-carrying capacity of the blood.

TABLE 7.5
Selected Minerals: Food Sources, Functions, and Deficiency and Toxicity Symptoms

Mineral	Selected Food Sources	Selected Functions	Deficiency Symptoms	Toxicity Symptoms
Major Minerals				
Calcium	Milk and milk products; sardines; dark green, leafy vegetables; fortified orange juice	Builds bones and teeth; helps maintain acid-base balance; maintains normal nerve transmission	Osteoporosis, bone fractures, convulsions and muscle spasms, heart failure	Can interfere with the absorption of iron, zinc, and magnesium; shock, fatigue, kidney failure
Phosphorus	Meat, poultry, fish, eggs, milk, soft drinks	Maintains fluid balance; plays a role in bone formation	Muscle weakness or damage, bone pain, dizziness	Muscle spasms, convulsions, low blood calcium levels
Magnesium	Grains, legumes, nuts (especially almonds and cashews), seeds, soybeans	Essential component of bone tissue; bone growth; supports muscle contraction and blood clotting	Hypomagnesemia, resulting in low blood calcium levels, muscle cramps, spasms, or seizures; chronic diseases such as heart disease, high blood pressure, and osteoporosis	Diarrhea, nausea, abdominal cramps
Potassium	Potatoes, bananas, tomato juice, orange juice	Regulates muscle contraction and transmission of nerve impulses; maintains blood pressure	Muscle weakness, paralysis, confusion	Muscle weakness, irregular heartbeat, vomiting
Sodium	Salt, soy sauce, fast foods and processed foods	Maintains acid-base balance; assists with nerve transmission and muscle contraction	Muscle cramps, dizziness, fatigue, nausea, vomiting, mental confusion	Water retention; high blood pressure; may increase loss of calcium in urine
Trace Minerals				
Iron	Meat and poultry; green, leafy vegetables; fortified grain products	Assists with oxygen transport in blood and muscle; conenzyme for energy metabolism	Anemia, fatigue, depressed immune function, impaired memory	Nausea, vomiting, diarrhea, dizziness, rapid heart beat, death
Zinc	Whole grains, meat, liver, seafood	Coenzyme for hemoglobin production; plays role in cell replication, protein synthesis	Growth retardation, diarrhea, delayed sexual maturation, hair loss	Intestinal pain, nausea, vomiting, loss of appetite, diarrhea; headache, depressed immune function
Iodine	Iodized salt, seafood, processed foods	Synthesis of thyroid hormones; temperature regulation	Goiter (enlargement of the thyroid gland), hypothyroidism; deficiency during pregnancy can cause birth defects	Goiter
Fluoride	Fluoridated water, tea, fish	Maintains health of bones and teeth	Dental caries and tooth decay; lower bone density	Teeth fluorosis (staining and pitting of the teeth); skeletal fluorisis
Selenium	Organ meats, such as liver and kidney; pork; seafood	Antioxidant; immune function; assists in production of thyroid hormone	Keshan disease, impaired immune function, infertility, muscle pain	Brittle hair, skin rashes, weakness, cirrhosis of the liver

Source: Adapted from Thompson, J., and M. Manore. *Nutrition: An Applied Approach,* 2nd ed. San Francisco: Benjamin Cummings, 2009.

Water

Water makes up approximately 60–70% of your body, and it is important for everything from temperature regulation, digestion, absorption, and blood formation to waste elimination. Water is especially important for physically active people. A person engaged in heavy exercise in a hot, humid environment can lose 1 to 3 liters of water per hour through sweating (7). Losing as little as 5% of body water causes fatigue, weakness, and the inability to concentrate; losing more than 15% can be fatal. Chapter 11 provides guidelines for maintaining proper hydration during exercise training.

You should consume 8–10 cups of water per day through foods and beverages. Drinking water throughout your day will help you meet this goal, as will eating food with high water content, such as fruits and vegetables. People who experience excess sweating, diarrhea, or vomiting or who donate blood may have higher water requirements. Figure 7.4 compares the sources of water intake and output in the average person.

Make sure you know...

> Nutrition is the study of food and its relationship to health and disease.

> Carbohydrates, fat, and protein are the three calorie-containing macronutrients. A well-balanced diet is composed of approximately 58% complex carbohydrates, 30% fat, and 12% protein.

> The kilocalorie is a unit of measure for the energy in food or the energy expended by the body. The kilocalorie is more commonly referred to as the calorie.

> Carbohydrates are the primary source of fuel for the body. Glucose is the most important of the simple carbohydrates, and all other simple and complex carbohydrates must be converted to glucose before being used by the body. Starch and fiber are complex carbohydrates.

> Fats are the most common form of lipid in foods and in the body. All excess calories consumed in the diet will eventually be converted to fat for storage. Dietary cholesterol and trans fat are heart-unhealthy, and you should limit or avoid your consumption of foods containing them.

> Proteins are made up of amino acids, and are the key structural unit for building and repairing cells. All amino acids either are made by the body (nonessential amino acids) or must be consumed in the diet (essential amino acids).

> Vitamins serve many important functions in the body, including facilitating metabolism. The B

Daily Water Balance in the Body

8–10 cups

Metabolism 10%
Foods 30%
Beverages 60%

Sweat 8%
Feces 4%
Insensible Losses via Skin and Lungs 28%
Urine 60%

Daily Intake **Daily Output**

FIGURE 7.4
The amount of water you consume in food and beverages and produce during metabolism is about equal to the amount you excrete in urine, sweat, and feces and through exhalation and insensible water loss.

vitamins and vitamin C are water soluble and are not generally stored by the body. Vitamins A, D, E and K are fat soluble and can be stored in the body.

> Minerals are chemical elements in foods that, like vitamins, play important roles in many body functions. The mineral calcium is important for bone health; iron is important for healthy blood, and too much sodium can have a negative effect on heart health.

> Approximately 60–70% of body weight is water. You should consume 8–10 cups of water from foods and beverages each day.

What Are the Guidelines for a Healthy Diet?

Nutrition may seem like a complex subject, but the basics of consuming a healthy diet are fairly simple: Balance the calories, eat a variety of foods, and consume less-healthy foods only in moderation. Additionally, everyone should strive to be physically active.

To make these points more clear, and to provide specific guidance in these areas, several national health agencies have suggested guidelines for healthy diets. For instance, the United States Department of Agriculture (USDA) released its latest version of the *Dietary Guidelines for Americans* in 2005 (the next update is due in late 2010). Among its key points of advice:

• Consume adequate nutrients within energy needs: Choose foods that limit the intake of saturated and trans fats, cholesterol, added sugars, salt, and alcohol.

- Balance energy intake with energy expended.
- Engage in regular physical activity.
- Consume sufficient amounts of fruits, vegetables, and whole grains while staying within energy needs.
- Consume less than 10% of energy intake from saturated fats and less than 300 mg per day of cholesterol; consume as little trans fat as possible.
- Choose fiber-rich fruits, vegetables, and whole grains often; choose and prepare foods and beverages with little added sugars or caloric sweeteners.
- Consume less than 1 tsp of salt per day.
- If you choose to drink alcohol, do so only in moderation.
- Take proper food safety precautions.

Let's explore some of these guidelines in more depth and discuss additional tools you can use, including MyPyramid, to plan a healthy diet.

Eat More Fruits, Vegetables, and Whole Grains

Choosing unprocessed foods that are modest in calories and low in fat and sodium is the best way to create a healthy diet. This means doing much of your grocery store shopping in the produce aisle (and perhaps stopping by the meat or seafood counter) and buying whole-grain bread and cereal products. When you eat out with friends or dine with your family, try to keep your portions of fatty meats and high-sugar desserts small, and load up on the undressed fruits and vegetables. Similarly, when you're in need of a midmorning or late afternoon snack, reach for a banana, whole-grain crackers, or air-popped popcorn rather than a bag of chips or chocolate bar.

Once you've adopted these healthy eating strategies, you're likely to see the benefits quickly. You will have more energy and feel less lethargic in the afternoon, and you may even lose weight. Over the long term, you will have a lower risk for many chronic diseases and conditions.

CONSIDER THIS!

The average American consumes more than 80 pounds of table sugar and 45 pounds of high fructose corn syrup each year.

Watch Your Intake of Calories, Sugar, Alcohol, Fat, and Sodium

With the rise in rates of overweight and obesity in the United States, it's clear that the balance of "calories in" versus "calories out" has become an issue for many individuals. Several factors are increasing calorie consumption. For example, one factor is that people consume a lot of simple sugar, often in the form of sucrose (table sugar) or high fructose corn syrup (a commercial sweetener). The problem with simple sugars is that they often contain many calories but few micronutrients (which is why they're called "empty calories"). An estimated half of the dietary carbohydrate intake of the average U.S. citizen is in the form of simple sugars (3). Sucrose and high fructose corn syrup are used to make cakes, candies, and ice cream, as well as to sweeten beverages, cereals, and other foods.

The amount of sugar in sweets adds a tremendous amount of calories to the diet. This leads to obesity, which contributes to many health problems (e.g., diabetes). Sugar in sweets also leads to tooth decay. Although brushing your teeth after eating sweets can prevent this problem, it will not solve the other problems of overconsumption of sugar. One way to trim your sucrose intake is to use sugar substitutes instead of sugar to sweeten some foods or beverages. Artificial sweeteners such as saccharin (Sweet'N Low), aspartame (Equal), or sucralose (Splenda) add sweetness with little or no calories.

Alcohol, if consumed in excess, is another source of empty calories that can undermine an otherwise healthy diet. Chronic alcohol consumption also tends to deplete the body's stores of some vitamins, possibly leading to severe deficiencies. Drinking too much alcohol can displace other, healthier foods in the diet by making you too full to eat or causing you to forget to eat. Finally, alcohol significantly increases your risk of accidents and injury. When it comes to drinking alcohol, the best plan is to avoid it or, if you do drink, to do so only in moderation.

Another factor behind the rise in overweight and obesity in the United States is the high amount of fat in many people's diets. Foods high in fat not only tend to

Guidelines for Cutting Fat from Your Diet

- Choose low-fat or nonfat foods over full-fat foods.

- For baking and sautéing, use vegetable oils, such as olive oil, that do not raise cholesterol levels.

- Choose only lean meats, fish, and poultry. Always remove the skin before eating, and bake or broil meats whenever possible. Drain off all oils from meats after cooking.

- Avoid cold cuts and processed meats (e.g., bacon, sausage, hot dogs). Beware of meat products that claim to be "95% fat-free," because they may still have a high fat content.

- Select nonfat dairy products whenever possible. Part-skim-milk cheeses such as mozzarella, farmer's, and ricotta are the best choices.

- Use broth, wine, vinegar, or low-calorie salad dressing to flavor foods during cooking rather than butter, margarine, oils, sour cream, or mayonnaise.

- Offset a high-fat breakfast with a low-fat lunch or dinner.

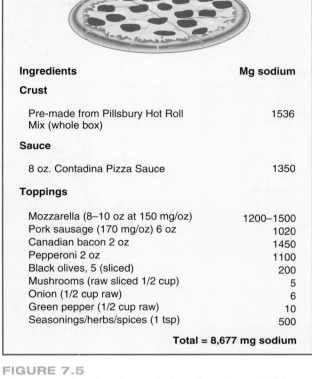

Ingredients	Mg sodium
Crust	
Pre-made from Pillsbury Hot Roll Mix (whole box)	1536
Sauce	
8 oz. Contadina Pizza Sauce	1350
Toppings	
Mozzarella (8–10 oz at 150 mg/oz)	1200–1500
Pork sausage (170 mg/oz) 6 oz	1020
Canadian bacon 2 oz	1450
Pepperoni 2 oz	1100
Black olives, 5 (sliced)	200
Mushrooms (raw sliced 1/2 cup)	5
Onion (1/2 cup raw)	6
Green pepper (1/2 cup raw)	10
Seasonings/herbs/spices (1 tsp)	500
Total = 8,677 mg sodium	

FIGURE 7.5
The amount of sodium in a typical medium pizza with "the works" will probably surprise you. Even if you eat only two slices, you are still likely consuming more than a 1000 mg of sodium! Note though, that cutting back on the meat toppings and loading up on the veggies will significantly lower the sodium.

be rich in cholesterol, but also contain over twice as many calories per gram than carbohydrate or protein (9 calories/gram versus 4 calories/gram). Limiting fat in the diet helps limit calories and also reduces the risk of heart disease. Both saturated and unsaturated fats are linked to heart disease, obesity, and certain cancers. The box on this page provides guidelines to help you cut your dietary fat intake.

Eating less dietary cholesterol will help lower your blood cholesterol, which will in turn lower your risk of heart disease. Research has shown that a 1% reduction in dietary cholesterol results in a 2% reduction in risk (Chapter 9). Additionally, many foods that are high in cholesterol are also high in fat (and therefore, calories).

Although salt (sodium chloride) is a necessary micronutrient, the body's daily requirement is small (less than 1/4 of a teaspoon). For very active people who perspire a great deal, this need may increase to over 1 1/2 teaspoons per day. However, most people consume much more sodium than they need, and this increased intake

CONSIDER THIS!

The average American consumes between 3 and 10 teaspoons of salt per day.

is putting them at increased risk for high blood pressure (hypertension). You might be surprised just how much salt is in many of your foods. For example, Figure 7.5 illustrates the "hidden" salt in an average pizza.

As mentioned, consuming too much sodium can be a complicating factor for people with high blood pressure. In countries where salt is not added to foods, either during cooking or at the table, high blood pressure is virtually unknown (8). Even if you don't already have high blood pressure, you should limit salt in your diet to only the minimal daily requirements.

Anatomy of MyPyramid

One Size Doesn't Fit All

USDA's new MyPyramid symbolizes a personalized approach to healthy eating and physical activity. The symbol has been designed to be simple. It has been developed to remind consumers to make healthy food choices and to be active every day. The different parts of the symbol are described below.

Activity
Activity is represented by the steps and the person climbing them, as a reminder of the importance of daily physical activity.

Moderation
Moderation is represented by the narrowing of each food group from bottom to top. The wider base stands for foods with little or no solid fats or added sugars. These should be selected more often.

Personalization
Personalization is shown by the person on the steps, the slogan, and the URL. Find the kinds and amounts of food to eat each day at MyPyramid.gov.

Proportionality
Proportionality is shown by the different widths of the food group bands. The widths suggest how much food a person should choose from each group. The widths are just a general guide, not exact proportions.

Variety
Variety is symbolized by the 6 color bands representing the 5 food groups of the Pyramid and oils. Foods from all groups are needed each day for good health.

Gradual Improvement
Gradual improvement is encouraged by the slogan. It suggests that individuals can benefit from taking small steps to improve their diet and lifestyle each day.

MyPyramid.gov
STEPS TO A HEALTHIER YOU

GRAINS | VEGETABLES | FRUITS | OILS | MILK | MEAT & BEANS

FIGURE 7.6
The USDA's MyPyramid food guidance system reminds you to eat a varied diet with lots of nutrient dense foods and to incorporate physical activity into your daily routine.
Source: www.mypyramid.gov.

Use the Recommended Dietary Allowances, MyPyramid, and Food Labels to Plan Healthy Meals

The National Academy of Science has established guidelines concerning the quantities of each micronutrient required to meet the minimum needs of most individuals (9). These Recommended Dietary Allowances (RDAs) are listed in Table 7.6 on pages 210–211. See also the Closer Look box on page 213 for an explanation of other important guidelines, in particular the Dietary Reference Intakes (DRIs).

Once you know the recommended daily allowances for nutrients, the key question is how to choose foods to meet these goals.

MyPyramid is the latest visual guide to eating healthy developed by the USDA. Its shape, colored bands, and other graphic elements emphasize several key aspects of planning a healthy diet. (See Figure 7.6 for a walk-through of the graphic elements of MyPyramid). For instance, you should strive to eat a wide variety of "nutrient-dense" foods—that is, foods with high nutrient content per calorie—from each of the food groups, rather than "empty-calorie" foods.

Another tool that the consumer can use when making food choices is the food label that's required on almost all packaged foods (Figure 7.7). Among the important information contained on the label is the number of calories contained per serving, a list of ingredients found in the food (listed in order of the amount contained), the amount of sodium and fat per serving, and the percent **Daily Values** of total fat, carbohydrate, and protein.

Now that we have presented the guidelines for a healthy diet, let's put these principles into practice and construct a day's healthy diet. As we discuss the steps for choosing the right foods, refer to Table 7.7 on page 214, which presents a sample of a healthful 1-day diet for a college-aged woman weighing 110 pounds and with light daily activities. Her projected daily caloric need is approximately 1690 calories. For your use of this diet plan, adjust the quantities accordingly.

Breakfast   A healthy breakfast might include a grapefruit, whole-grain cereal, low-fat milk, and a banana. This meal would provide two fruits, one bread/cereal, and one dairy product to start the day. The breakfast is low in fat, cholesterol, and sodium. A large part of her daily protein need is met, as well as over 40% of her calcium and iron needs. The fruits alone provide almost all of the recommended vitamin A and C intake for the day.

Snack   A morning snack adds some energy and helps to suppress the appetite before lunch. You might choose a second dairy product for the day (in this example, low-fat yogurt) that provides 130 calories of energy and lots of calcium.

Lunch   For lunch, a turkey sandwich (made with low-sodium turkey) on whole-wheat bread and a handful of baby carrots will provide one serving of meat, two more servings of breads/cereals, and one vegetable. This lunch provides a low-calorie meal with lots of protein, vitamin A, and iron.

Snack   A piece of cheese pizza as an afternoon snack will add a third dairy and fourth bread/cereal serving. Be careful in ordering pizza, because some toppings (meats and additional cheese) can add lots of fat, sodium, and calories to your diet. In contrast, vegetable toppings such as peppers, onions, and mushrooms can provide valuable nutrients without the fat, sodium, and calories.

Dinner   You might finish the day by adding a second serving of meat and two more vegetables, to make a total of five. A peach for dessert will provide lots of vitamin A. Salmon contains protein and plenty of heart-healthy omega-3 fatty acids. Broccoli adds vitamins A and C and calcium. Lima beans add vitamin A and iron.

Watch for Special Dietary Considerations

Some people have special dietary considerations that affect their needs for certain nutrients. Strict vegetari-

Sample Label for Macaroni and Cheese

FIGURE 7.7

The Nutrition Facts Label can help you select foods that are low in fat, cholesterol, sodium, and calories and that are adequate in protein, vitamins A and C, iron, and calcium. The percent Daily Value (DV) helps you determine how good a source a food is for a given nutrient. In general, foods with less than 5% of the DV are considered low in a nutrient, whereas those with more than 20% of the DV are considered high in that nutrient.

Source: U.S. Department of Agriculture, *Dietary Guidelines for Americans 2000*. Washington, DC: U.S. Government Printing Office.

ans, for example, need to monitor their intake of protein, calcium, and some vitamins, and children and pregnant women need to be sure to consume enough iron to help with growth. Let's take a look at some of these nutrient considerations.

(text continues on page 212)

Daily Values standard values for nutrient needs, used as a reference on food labels. The Daily Values may not exactly reflect the true nutrient needs for all people.

TABLE 7.6
Recommended Dietary Allowances of Micronutrients

Life Stage Group	Calcium (mg/d)	Phosphorus (mg/d)	Magnesium (mg/d)	Iron (mg/d)	Zinc (mg/d)	Selenium (µg/d)	Iodine (µg/d)	Copper (µg/d)	Manganese (mg/d)	Fluoride (mg/d)	Chromium (µg/d)	Molybdenum (µg/d)
Infants												
0–6 mo	210*	100*	30*	0.27*	2*	15*	110*	200*	0.003*	0.01*	0.2*	2*
7–12 mo	270*	275*	75*	11	3	20*	130*	220*	0.6*	0.5*	5.5*	3*
Children												
1–3 y	500*	460	80	7	3	20	90	340	1.2*	0.7*	11*	17
4–8 y	800*	500	130	10	5	30	90	440	1.5*	1*	15*	22
Males												
9–13 y	1300*	1250	240	8	8	40	120	700	1.9*	2*	25*	34
14–18 y	1300*	1250	410	11	11	55	150	890	2.2*	3*	35*	43
19–30 y	1000*	700	400	8	11	55	150	900	2.3*	4*	35*	45
31–50 y	1000*	700	420	8	11	55	150	900	2.3*	4*	35*	45
51–70 y	1200*	700	420	8	11	55	150	900	2.3*	4*	30*	45
>70 y	1200*	700	420	8	11	55	150	900	2.3*	4*	30*	45
Females												
9–13 y	1300*	1250	240	8	8	40	120	700	1.6*	2*	21*	34
14–18 y	1300*	1250	360	15	9	55	150	890	1.6*	3*	24*	43
19–30 y	1000*	700	310	18	8	55	150	900	1.8*	3*	25*	45
31–50 y	1000*	700	320	18	8	55	150	900	1.8*	3*	20*	45
51–70 y	1200*	700	320	8	8	55	150	900	1.8*	3*	20*	45
>70 y	1200*	700	320	8	8	55	150	900	1.8*	3*	20*	45
Pregnancy												
≤18 y	1300*	1250	400	27	12	60	220	1000	2.0*	3*	29*	50
19–30 y	1000*	700	350	27	11	60	220	1000	2.0*	3*	30*	50
31–50 y	1000*	700	360	27	11	60	220	1000	2.0*	3*	30*	50
Lactation												
≤18 y	1300*	1250	360	10	13	70	290	1300	2.6*	3*	44*	50
19–30 y	1000*	700	310	9	12	70	290	1300	2.6*	3*	45*	50
31–50 y	1000*	700	320	9	12	70	290	1300	2.6*	3*	45*	50

TABLE 7.6   (CONTINUED)

	Vitamins													
Life Stage Group	Vitamin A (µg/d)[a]	Vitamin D (µg/d)[b]	Vitamin E (mg/d)[c]	Vitamin K (µg/d)	Thiamin (mg/d)	Riboflavin (mg/d)	Niacin (mg/d)[d]	Pantothenic Acid (mg/d)	Biotin (µg/d)	Vitamin B$_6$ (mg/d)	Folate (µg/d)[e]	Vitamin B$_{12}$ (µg/d)	Vitamin C (mg/d)	Choline (mg/d)
Infants														
0–6 mo	400*	5*	4*	2.0*	0.2*	0.3*	2*	1.7*	5*	0.1*	65*	0.4*	40*	125*
7–12 mo	500*	5*	5*	2.5*	0.3*	0.4*	4*	1.8*	6*	0.3*	80*	0.5*	50*	150*
Children														
1–3 y	300	5*	6	30*	0.5	0.5	6	2*	8*	0.5	150	0.9	15	200*
4–8 y	400	5*	7	55*	0.6	0.6	8	3*	12*	0.6	200	1.2	25	250*
Males														
9–13 y	600	5*	11	60*	0.9	0.9	12	4*	20*	1.0	300	1.8	45	375*
14–18 y	900	5*	15	75*	1.2	1.3	16	5*	25*	1.3	400	2.4	75	550*
19–30 y	900	5*	15	120*	1.2	1.3	16	5*	30*	1.3	400	2.4	90	550*
31–50 y	900	5*	15	120*	1.2	1.3	16	5*	30*	1.3	400	2.4	90	550*
51–70 y	900	10*	15	120*	1.2	1.3	16	5*	30*	1.7	400	2.4	90	550*
>70 y	900	15*	15	120*	1.2	1.3	16	5*	30*	1.7	400	2.4	90	550*
Females														
9–13 y	600	5*	11	60*	0.9	0.9	12	4*	20*	1.0	300	1.8	45	375*
14–18 y	700	5*	15	75*	1.0	1.0	14	5*	25*	1.2	400	2.4	65	400*
19–30 y	700	5*	15	90*	1.1	1.1	14	5*	30*	1.3	400	2.4	75	425*
31–50 y	700	5*	15	90*	1.1	1.1	14	5*	30*	1.3	400	2.4	75	425*
51–70 y	700	10*	15	90*	1.1	1.1	14	5*	30*	1.5	400	2.4	75	425*
>70 y	700	15*	15	90*	1.1	1.1	14	5*	30*	1.5	400	2.4	75	425*
Pregnancy														
≤18 y	750	5*	15	75*	1.4	1.4	18	6*	30*	1.9	600	2.6	80	450*
19–30 y	770	5*	15	90*	1.4	1.4	18	6*	30*	1.9	600	2.6	85	450*
31–50 y	770	5*	15	90*	1.4	1.4	18	6*	30*	1.9	600	2.6	85	450*
Lactation														
≤18 y	1200	5*	19	75*	1.4	1.4	17	7*	35*	2.0	500	2.8	115	550*
19–30 y	1300	5*	19	90*	1.4	1.4	17	7*	35*	2.0	500	2.8	120	550*
31–50 y	1300	5*	19	90*	1.4	1.4	17	7*	35*	2.0	500	2.8	120	550*

Source: Reprinted with permission from the National Academies Press. Copyright 1997, 1998, 2000, 2001, 2005 by the National Academy of Sciences. These reports may be accessed via www.nap.edu.

Note: This table is adapted from the DRI reports; see www.nap.edu. It lists Recommended Dietary Allowances (RDAs), with Adequate Intakes (AIs) indicated by an asterisk (*). RDAs and AIs may both be used as goals for individual intake. RDAs are set to meet the needs of almost all (97 percent to 98 percent) individuals in a group. For healthy breastfed infants, the AI is the mean intake. The AI for other life stage and gender groups is believed to cover the needs of all individuals in the group, but lack of data prevents being able to specify with confidence the percentage of individuals covered by this intake.

[a]Given as retinal activity equivalents (RAE).

[b]Also known as calciferol. The DRI values are based on the absence of adequate exposure to sunlight.

[c]Also known as α-tocopherol.

[d]Given as niacin equivalents (NIE), except for infants 0–6 months, which are expressed as preformed niacin.

[e]Given as dietary folate equivalents (DFE).

STEPS FOR
BEHAVIOR
CHANGE

Do you consume too much sugar?

Take the quiz below to find out whether there is too much sugar in your diet.

Y N

☐ ☑ Do you consume a bowl of sweetened breakfast cereal more than two mornings a week?

☑ ☐ Do you sweeten your tea or coffee with packets of white or brown sugar?

☐ ☑ Is a morning donut or muffin or an afternoon cookie part of your regular routine?

☐ ☑ Do you eat candy more than twice a week?

☐ ☑ Do you consume more than one can or bottle of soda on most days of the week?

If you answered yes to to more than two of these questions, your diet could use an upgrade.

TIPS TO CUT DOWN ON SUGAR

☑ Know how to spot sugar. When you see terms such as *sucrose, glucose, maltose, dextrose, fructose,* or *high fructose corn syrup* on the ingredients list, beware. These are all forms of sugar. If sugar or its "pseudos" are in the first three ingredients on a label, avoid the product. It has a high sugar content by weight.

☑ Try a noncalorie sugar substitute, such as Sweet'N Low, NutraSweet, or Splenda in your tea or coffee, or flavor your tea with lemon instead of sugar.

☑ Start your morning with a piece of whole-grain toast or a fresh bowl of fruit, instead of a sugar-sweetened cereal or muffin. If you have to have cereal, opt for whole-grain granola or raisin bran, rather than sugar-sweetened puffed cereal.

☑ Eat graham crackers, yogurt, fresh fruits, air-popped popcorn, and other healthy substitutes for high-sugar sweets when you need a snack.

Source: Adapted from Boyle, M., and G. Zyla. *Personal Nutrition.* St. Paul, MN: West Publishers, 1991.

Vitamins: B$_{12}$, D, and Folate   Though most people will not need vitamin supplements if they are eating a healthy diet, people who have increased nutrient needs or special circumstances may benefit from enriched or fortified foods, a multivitamin, or other vitamin supplement. For example, strict vegetarians (vegans), who eat no animal foods, need to be sure to get enough vitamin B$_{12}$ (which is found primarily in animal products) through fortified foods, such as breakfast cereals, or by taking a supplement. Vegetarians who do not get 15 to 30 minutes of exposure to sunlight every few days may also need to take a vitamin D supplement.

Pregnant women need to be sure to consume enough folic acid, usually through a supplement, to reduce the risk of birth defects in their growing babies. And some older individuals, who may have depressed appetites or may not be able to cook or consume meals easily, may be advised to take a multivitamin to ensure that they meet their needs.

Other individuals also might benefit from vitamin supplementation:

- People with chronic illnesses that depress the appetite or the absorption of nutrients
- People on medications that affect appetite or digestion
- Athletes engaged in a rigorous training program
- Lactating women
- Individuals on prolonged low-calorie diets.

Minerals: Iron and Calcium   Iron is an essential component of red blood cells, which carry oxygen

A CLOSER LOOK

DIETARY REFERENCE INTAKES

Recommended Dietary Allowances (also known as RDAs) are the daily amounts of the different food nutrients the National Academy of Sciences deems adequate for healthy individuals. However, even today, RDAs for some nutrients are not known. Thus, the Academy has issued additional indices to guide people in monitoring their diets. They refer to these indices as Dietary Reference Intakes (DRIs).

The 2005 DRIs are divided into four categories, each of which addresses a different nutritional issue:

1. *Recommended Dietary Allowance (RDA).* The RDAs are the amount of nutrient that will meet the needs of almost every healthy person in a specific age and gender group. Also, the latest RDAs are meant to reduce disease risk, not just prevent deficiency.

2. *Adequate Intake (AI).* This value is used when the RDA is not known because the scientific data aren't strong enough to produce a specific recommendation, yet there is enough evidence to give a general guideline. Thus, the AI is an "educated guess" at what the RDA would be if it were known.

3. *Estimated Average Requirement (EAR).* This is a value that is esti-mated to satisfy the needs of 50% of people in a given age group. It is primarily used to establish the RDA. In addition, it is used for evaluating and planning the diets of large groups of people (such as the army), not individuals.

4. *Tolerable Upper Intake Level (UL).* This is the maximal amount that a person can take without risking "adverse health effects." Anything above this amount might result in toxicity. In most cases, this number refers to the total intake of the nutri-ent—from food, fortified foods, and nutritional supplements.

The latest guidelines group the nutrients according to their functional properties. The following list shows the groups, the year of the latest update, and the nutrients in each.

- **Dietary Reference Intakes (DRIs) for Calcium, Phosphorus, Magnesium, Vitamin D, and Fluoride (1997).** These nutrients have key roles in developing and maintaining bone and other calci-fied tissues in the body.

- **DRIs for Energy, Carbohydrate, Fiber, Fat, Fatty Acids, Cholesterol, Protein, and Amino Acids (Macronutrients) (2005).** These macronutrients provide energy.

- **DRIs for Thiamin, Riboflavin, Niacin, Vitamin B$_6$, Folate, Vitamin B$_{12}$, Pan-tothenic Acid, Biotin, and Choline (1998).** These water-soluble vitamins are involved with energy metabolism and processes of macronutrient break-down.

- **DRIs for Vitamin C, Vitamin E, Sele-nium and Carotenoids (2000).** These micronutrients have been shown to have antioxidant properties and to play important roles in combating various chronic diseases.

- **DRIs for Vitamin A, Vitamin K, Ar-senic, Boron, Chromium, Copper, Io-dine, Iron, Manganese, Molybdenum, Nickel, Silicon, Vanadium, and Zinc (2001):** These micronutrients have been shown to have important roles in combating various chronic diseases.

- **DRIs for Water, Potassium, Sodium, Chloride and Sulfate (2004).** These nutrients are important in maintaining fluid balance in the body.

- **DRIs: Proposed Definition of Dietary Fiber (2001).** Fiber has been shown to be important in regulating digestive tract function and preventing intestinal cancers.

Source: National Academy of Sciences. *Dietary Reference Intakes: Applications in Dietary Assess-ment.* Washington, DC: National Academy Press, 2005.

to all our tissues for energy production. An iron defi-ciency can result in decreased oxygen transport to tis-sues and thus an energy crisis. Getting enough iron can be a problem for women who are menstruating, preg-nant, or nursing. Indeed, only half of all women of child-bearing age get the necessary 15 mg of iron per day (3). Five percent suffer from iron-deficiency ane-mia. Although these individuals should not take iron supplements unless their physician prescribes them (because the body excretes very little iron, there is a potential for toxicity if too much is consumed), they

can modify their diets to ensure getting the RDA of iron. The following dietary modifications can help meet this requirement:

- Eat legumes, fresh fruits, whole-grain cereals, and broccoli, all of which are high in iron.
- Also eat foods high in vitamin C, which helps iron absorption.
- Eat lean red meats high in iron at least two or three times per week.
- Eat iron-rich organ meats, such as liver, once or twice per month.

TABLE 7.7
Sample Diet for a College-Aged Female Weighing 110 Pounds, Assuming Light Daily Activities

	kcal	Fat (g)	Cholesterol (mg)	Sodium (mg)	Carbohydrate (g)	Protein (g)	Vitamin A (RE)*	Vitamin C (mg)	Calcium (mg)
Breakfast									
1/2 grapefruit	38	0.1	0	0	10.7	0.8	2	41.3	14
Whole-grain cereal (1 cup)	127	0	0	244	33	3	0	0	16
Low-fat milk (1 cup)	225	2.6	10	121	42	9	20	1.4	314
1 banana	105	1	0	1	27	1	93	10	7
Snack									
Low-fat yogurt (1 cup)	130	2.6	10	121	44	9	20	1.4	314
Lunch									
Turkey sandwich: whole-wheat bread with mustard	191	3.7	9	784	25	9.4	0	0	78
Baby carrots (10)	36	1	0	35	8	1	1972	8	23
Snack									
1 slice pizza with Parmesan cheese	145	3	8	336	21	8	382	1	117
Dinner									
Broiled salmon (1/2 fillet)	180	5	83	107	0	32	169	0	21
Mushrooms (1/2 cup)	20	0	0	2	4	2	0	3	5
Whole-wheat dinner rolls (2)	150	2	0	272	27	4	0	0	60
Broccoli (3 spears)	26	0	0	25	5	3	1434	87	45
Lima beans (1/2 cup)	90	0	0	15	21	6	332	9	29
Peach (1)	37	0	0	0	10	1	465	6	4
Totals	1500	21	120	2065	247.4	88.2	4907	169.1	883
RDA	1690	<30%	<300	<3000	>58%	40	700	75	1000
% of RDA	89	14	40	68	72	220	953	225	88

*RE = retinol equivalents.

• Don't drink tea with your meals; it interferes with iron absorption.

Another mineral, calcium, is the most abundant mineral in the body and is essential for building bones and teeth, as well as for normal nerve and muscle function. Adequate calcium is especially important for pregnant or nursing women. There is some evidence that calcium may help prevent colon cancer (3).

The most recent RDAs call for a significant increase in calcium intake for both sexes beginning at age 9. Children between 9 and 18 years of age should consume a 1300 mg of calcium each day. Adequate calcium intake during those years may be a crucial factor in preventing osteoporosis in later years, which strikes one in two women and one in five men over the age of 50 (10). Adults over age 18 should consume 1000 mg of calcium per day.

A CLOSER LOOK

WHAT IS THE GLYCEMIC INDEX AND WHEN IS IT HELPFUL?

Low-carbohydrate diets are based on the notion that some carbohydrate-rich foods cause a dramatic increase in blood insulin levels that results in increased storage of fat and a decrease in blood glucose that increases appetite. The diets are based on the **glycemic index** (GI) of foods, a measure of the effect a given food will have on the amount of glucose in the blood after the food is eaten. The concept is that eating foods with a low glycemic index results in less glucose fluctuation in the blood after a meal, which in turn stabilizes insulin levels and appetite. The typical reference for the GI is pure glucose, which has a GI of 100.

The GI of a food is not always easy to predict. Although some foods that contain simple sugars, such as candy, will logically have a higher GI, some foods with natural sugar, such as an apple (which is high in fructose) will have a lower GI. Additionally, the way the food is prepared and its fat and fiber content can affect its GI ranking. Instant mashed potatoes, white bread, and white rice have higher GIs than oat bran or kidney beans.

The glycemic index can be useful for some individuals, such as people with diabetes, to help them avoid fluctuations in blood glucose levels. In general, if you want to eat foods with lower, rather than higher, GIs, follow these guidelines:

- Eat breakfast cereals made of oats, barley, and bran.
- Eat dense, chewy breads made with whole seeds, not white bread.

- Eat fewer potatoes, but more al dente pasta.
- Choose basmati rather than white rice.
- Enjoy all types of vegetables.
- Eat plenty of salad vegetables with vinaigrette dressing.
- Balance a meal containing high-GI foods with extra low-GI foods.
- Add food acids (such as citrus fruits) to help slow stomach emptying and reduce the glycemic response.
- Eat fewer sugary foods, such as cookies, cakes, candy, and soft drinks.

Glycemic Index Range		
	Range	**Example Foods**
Low GI	0–55	Apples, oranges, bananas
Medium GI	56–69	White rice, ice cream
High GI	70–100	White bread, crispy rice cereal

The following recommendations can help you get the calcium you need:

- Add low-fat or nonfat dairy products to your diet.
- Choose other calcium-rich alternatives, such as canned fish (with the bones, packed in water), turnip and mustard greens, and broccoli.
- Eat foods rich in vitamin C to boost absorption of calcium.
- Use an acidic dressing, made with citrus juices or vinegar, to enhance calcium absorption from salad greens.
- Add a supplement if you can't get enough calcium in the foods you like. However, beware of supplements made with dolomite or bone meal, because they may be contaminated with lead.

Make sure you know...

> The basic guidelines for a healthy diet are to eat adequate amounts of fruits, vegetables, and whole grains and to watch your intake of calories, sugar, alcohol, fat and sodium. If you choose to drink alcohol, do so only in moderation.

> Recommended dietary allowances (RDAs), Dietary Reference Intakes (DRIs), and the USDA's MyPyramid are tools you can use to plan a healthy diet. You can use food labels to choose foods that are low in calories, fat, sodium, and sugar.

> Some people, including children, pregnant and lactating women, and strict vegetarians, may have special nutrient needs and may therefore benefit from choosing enriched or fortified foods and/or taking a vitamin or mineral supplement.

glycemic index A ranking system for carbohydrates based on a food's effect on blood glucose levels.

STEPS FOR BEHAVIOR CHANGE

Are you a fast food junkie?

Although eating at fast-food restaurants is generally not a healthy habit, there are choices you can make to improve your diet. Take the following quiz to assess your current behavior.

Y   N

- ☐ ☑ Do you typically order the largest size on the menu?

- ☐ ☑ Do you always order a burger or fried fish or fried chicken sandwich?

- ☐ ☑ Do you always get french fries as a side?

- ☐ ☑ Is soda your "default" beverage for washing down your meal?

- ☐ ☑ Are your fast-food sandwiches and salads typically loaded up with mayonnaise, creamy dressings, or other high-fat sauces?

If you answered yes to more than two of these questions, you're probably consuming major amounts of fat and calories with every fast-food meal. Fortunately, there's a lot you can do to improve the nutritional quality of your next fast-food meal, without forgoing the drive-through altogether.

TIPS FOR THE NEXT TIME YOU'RE AT THE FAST-FOOD COUNTER

☑ Order the small-sized items. Don't "supersize" your meal. Consider these numbers: Depending on the restaurant, a double cheeseburger may contain 600–700 calories, 30–40 grams fat, 120–140 mg cholesterol, and 1000–1200 mg sodium! You'll be surprised how satisfied you'll be with just a single burger and small order of fries, and you'll save yourself a ton of calories.

☑ Forgo the sauces and creamy salad dressing. A typical tablespoon of tartar sauce contains about 20 grams of fat and 220 mg of sodium, and a tablespoon of mayonnaise will add 100 calories and 11 grams of fat to your sandwich. Ordering you sandwich without the mayo is an easy way to cut a quick 100 calories.

☑ Order grilled meat instead of fried. Breaded chicken typically contains double the amount of fat as a broiled piece.

☑ Choose healthier sides: Try ordering a small salad instead of french fries, or a fruit cup rather than an apple pie for dessert.

☑ Skip the soda or milkshake. Drink water, nonfat milk, or 100% juice with your meal. Cutting back your regular soda intake is one of the fastest ways to cut down on the calories (not to mention the sugar).

How Does Nutrition Affect Physical Fitness?

Think about the last radio, TV, or online ad you saw for a nutrition-related product. Do you remember what was said about the product, and did you question whether it was true? The reality is that much of what you see and hear in such advertisements is not based on sound research and, in some cases, is entirely made up. Often, successful athletes endorse various nutri-tional products and convince the public that a particular food or beverage is responsible for their success. Even though most of the claims made in commercial endorsements are not supported by research, the claims often become accepted as fact.

The truth is, there are no miracle foods to improve physical fitness or exercise performance. In the sections that follow we discuss the specific nutritional needs of individuals in a regular exercise program.

Influence of Exercise Intensity on Fuel Use
Both intensity and duration of exercise will govern which fuel
predominates during an exercise session. The following table
illustrates how intensity affects fuel use during endurance-type
exercises.

Exercise Intensity	Fuel Used by Muscle
Less than 30% $\dot{V}O_2$max	Mainly fat stores
40–60% $\dot{V}O_2$max	Fat and carbohydrate equally
75% $\dot{V}O_2$max	Mainly carbohydrate
Greater than 80% $\dot{V}O_2$max	Nearly 100% carbohydrate

FIGURE 7.8
The importance of a high-carbohydrate diet during exercise training. With a low-carbohydrate diet (solid line), glucose stored in muscles as glycogen is depleted by daily training sessions. If a high-carbohydrate diet is consumed (dashed line), muscle glycogen levels are maintained at near normal levels.

Source: David C. Nieman, *Exercise Testing and Prescription: A Health Related Approach.* Copyright © 2003. Reprinted by permission of the McGraw-Hill Companies.

Carbohydrates Are Used for Energy during Exercise

You need more fuel during exercise than when you're sedentary. Recall that carbohydrates and fats are the primary fuels used to provide energy for exercise. Because even very lean people have a large amount of energy stored as fat, lack of fat for fuel is not a problem during exercise. In contrast, the carbohydrate stores in the liver and muscles can reach critically low levels during intense or prolonged exercise (7) (Figure 7.8).

Because carbohydrates play a critical role in providing energy during exercise, some exercise scientists have suggested that people participating in daily exercise programs should increase the complex carbohydrates in their diet from 58–70% of the total calories consumed (fat intake is then reduced to 18% of total caloric intake) (7). If exercise is intense, carbohydrates can be depleted from the liver and muscles, resulting in fatigue. The intensity of the exercise determines whether carbohydrates or fat is the predominant source of energy production (7, 11) (Table 7.8).

In most cases, the energy you use during your workout comes from energy stored from meals eaten the previous day. Hence, products such as sports drinks and gels may not be as useful for energy during exercise as they are marketed to be. In fact, sugared sports drinks can cause a rapid rise in blood glucose, which promotes hormonal changes that reduce blood glucose to levels below normal and results in feelings of fatigue (7).

Increasing the percentage of complex carbohydrates in the diet and maintaining sufficient caloric intake can ensure that an adequate supply of energy from carbohydrates is stored in the muscles and the liver to meet the needs of a rigorous exercise training program.

Protein Needs Can Be Met with a Healthy Diet

Many bodybuilders consume large quantities of protein in supplements, in addition to the protein they take in through their normal diet, because they think this will promote muscular growth. Unfortunately, they're drinking those shakes and eating those bars largely in vain, because research has shown that a normal, well-balanced diet meets the protein requirements of most bodybuilders (12, 13). The increased caloric needs of someone in a strength-training program should come from additional amounts of nutrient-dense foods and not simply from additional protein. This strategy supplies not only the extra macronutrients, but also the micronutrients necessary for energy production.

High Vitamin Intake Does Not Improve Performance

Some vitamin manufacturers have argued that megadoses of vitamins can improve exercise performance. This belief is based on the notion that exercise in-

Products such as sports gels and drinks are sometimes used by athletes during competition. Usually, these are unnecessary. Use caution when using them, and make sure they are appropriate for your situation.

creases the need for energy and, because vitamins are necessary for the breakdown of foods for energy, an extra load of vitamins should be helpful. There is no evidence to support this claim (14). The energy supplied for muscle contraction is not enhanced by vitamin supplements. In fact, megadoses of vitamins may interfere with the delicate balance of other micronutrients and can be toxic as well (3). For example, excess vitamin A can cause damage to the nervous system, cleft palate, and eye problems in unborn babies.

Antioxidants Help Prevent Oxidative Damage

Antioxidants are vitamins and micronutrients that protect cells by preventing a process called *oxidation*. (Oxidation is the same process that causes iron to rust over time. In fact, you can think of oxidation in the body as something like rusting from the inside.) Antioxidants work by combining with, and neutralizing, **free radicals** before they can damage cells. Excess production of free radicals has been implicated in cancer, lung disease, heart disease, and even the aging process (15). Therefore, increasing the level of antioxidants may be beneficial to health. Several micronutrients, including vitamins A, E, and C, beta-carotene, zinc, and selenium, have been identified as potent antioxidants.

Recent research suggests that the increased muscle metabolism associated with exercise may increase free radical production (16). Several studies have shown that this increase in free radicals may contribute to fatigue and perhaps even muscle damage.

Preliminary studies have indicated that antioxidants, primarily vitamin E, play a positive role in neutralizing exercise-produced free radicals. In fact, recent reports have demonstrated a reduction in muscle damage following administration of antioxidants (16). Several researchers have suggested that an additional 400 IU of vitamin E be consumed daily to protect against free radical damage. However, you should consult a nutritionist before consuming more than the RDA of fat-soluble vitamins. Remember: Fat-soluble vitamins are stored in the body, and their accumulation may lead to toxicity.

Make sure you know...

> The amount of carbohydrate and fat used as fuel during exercise will vary according to the intensity of the exercise.

> The extra energy needed for strength training should not come solely from increased protein intake.

> Excess vitamin intake does not improve exercise performance.

> Antioxidants help prevent free radicals from damaging cells. To date, vitamins A, E, and C, beta-carotene, zinc, and selenium have been identified as potent antioxidants.

Do Supplements Provide an Edge for Health and Performance?

As previously mentioned, athletes aren't the only ones who may consider taking supplements. Many less-active individuals also use (or consider using) vitamins, minerals, herbs, enzymes, amino acids, or other compounds in pill, powder, or tablet form to improve health and wellness. Over the past decade, the use of nutritional and pharmaceutical supplements has become common in the United States. The search for a speedy path to health, wellness, and fitness led Americans to spend almost $20.3 billion on nutritional supplements in 2005 (1). This has led the U.S. government to look closely at how this industry is regulated. In the following sections we examine how supplements are regulated and which ones might have the potential to be beneficial.

The Role of Supplements in a Healthy Diet

The FDA estimates that more than 25,000 products are available as dietary supplements. There is no scientific evidence to validate most of the claims that supplements improve health or exercise performance. You can view some of the more popular supplements cur-

DO PHYTOCHEMICALS PROTECT AGAINST DISEASE?

Besides nutrients, plant foods—legumes, vegetables, fruits, and whole grains—contain a whole other "crop" of chemicals called phytochemicals (*phyto* means "plant"). These substances, which plants produce naturally to protect themselves against viruses, bacteria, and fungi, may help protect us from diseases as well.

Phytochemicals include hundreds of naturally occurring substances, including carotenoids, flavonoids, indoles, isoflavones, capsaicin, and protease inhibitors. And just as occurs with vitamins and minerals, different plant foods contain different kinds and amounts of phytochemicals.

Certain phytochemicals appear to protect against some cancers, heart disease, and other chronic health conditions. Until more is known, the nutrition bottom line still applies: Eat a wide variety of fruits, vegetables, legumes, and whole grains, and count on food, not diet supplements, to get the nutrients your body needs. That way, you'll reap the potential benefits of the many phytochemicals found in all kinds of plant foods.

Source: Heber, D. Vegetables, fruits and phytoestrogens in the prevention of diseases. *Journal of Postgraduate Medicine* 50(2):145–149, 2004.

---

rently marketed for improving health and enhancing exercise performance in Table 7.9.

Our knowledge of the relationship between diet and disease points out the importance of consuming adequate amounts of nutrients while avoiding dietary excesses. However, not much is known about newly discovered, unclassified, and naturally occurring micronutrient components of food and their effects on health and disease. For example, several studies have identified numerous plant compounds, called phytochemicals, that—when ingested by humans in small amounts—may protect against a variety of diseases. We still don't know whether the large amounts of phytochemicals typically present in supplements are safe or effective. (See the Closer Look box above). Given our current incomplete knowledge, eating a wide variety of foods and avoiding excesses from dietary supplements are the best ways to obtain adequate amounts of beneficial food components.

Regulation of Supplements

Dietary supplements are not regulated in the same way that foods and prescription and over-the-counter drugs are regulated. The difference is that foods and drugs are tested and approved by governmental agencies (such as the FDA), whereas supplements are not. Manufacturers, not the government, are responsible for the safety of supplements. Supplement manufacturers are not required to get FDA approval before they market their products, and the FDA does not test supplements. Rather, the FDA trusts the manufacturers to ensure that the products are safe and effective.

However, the claims made on supplement labels are regulated. Supplement manufacturers are allowed to claim effects on the "structure or function" of the body but are not allowed to make claims concerning the treatment, prevention, cure, or diagnosis of disease. The FDA instituted the "structure/function rule" in 2000 to distinguish disease claims from structure/function claims. Disease claims require evidence of safety and benefits to be demonstrated to the FDA prior to marketing, and structure/function claims do not. The rule prohibits both express disease claims (such as, "prevents heart disease") and implied disease claims (such as, "prevents bone fragility in postmenopausal women") without prior FDA review. However, the rule permits health-maintenance claims (such as, "maintains healthy bones"), other claims not related to disease (such as, "for muscle enhancement"), and claims for the relief of common minor symptoms associated with life stages (such as, "for common symptoms of PMS").

Since its release, the rule has been modified both to expand the number of acceptable structure/function claims and to narrow the definition of *disease* to disallow structure/function claims pertaining to aging, pregnancy, menopause, and adolescence. Supplement manufacturers are required to keep on file substantiation of any structure/function claims they make. However, the FDA neither examines nor substantiates the legitimacy of this documentation. Manufacturers must also include on their labels a disclaimer stating that their dietary supplements are not drugs and received no FDA

antioxidants Molecules that neutralize free radicals, thereby preventing them from causing damage to cells.

free radicals Oxygen molecules that can potentially damage cells.

TABLE 7.9
Comparison of Dietary Supplements

Supplement	Origin	Benefits Claimed	Evidence of Effectiveness
Androstenedione	Made by the body as part of testosterone production	Enhances the production of testosterone and causes an increase in muscle mass.	Evidence suggests that it does not increase testosterone, and it may increase female hormones in men.
Antioxidants	Produced by cells to protect against free radical production. Some vitamins, minerals, and other chemicals in foods also have antioxidant properties.	Buffer free radical damage, which could help prevent fatigue and/or muscle damage during exercise. Also, could help protect against some diseases.	No evidence to suggest enhancement of exercise performance. Some evidence to suggest a benefit in preventing damage to tissues. Growing evidence to suggest benefits in fighting many conditions such as cancer, heart and lung disease, and aging.
Caffeine	Compound found in coffee, cola, candy, stimulants, weight-loss products.	Used to increase muscle fiber activation to increase strength, or to increase fat metabolism and endurance.	Increases endurance in events lasting greater than 20 minutes. No consistent effects on strength.
Carbohydrates	Component of most food. Usually found as a dietary supplement in the form of beverages or bars.	Increase in stored glucose in muscle and liver and increase in endurance.	Improves endurance in events longer than 90–120 minutes. Also helps restore glucose after exercise.
L-carnitine	Made by the body and ingested in meat products.	Increases transport of fat in cells, reduces lactate accumulation.	Carnitine is in adequate supply in the cells, and additional amounts provide no benefit before, during, or after exercise.
Chromium picolinate	Chromium is a trace element found in several foods; picolinate is added to supplements to aid absorption.	Helps insulin action and is thought to aid glucose metabolism, blood fats, and have anabolic effects.	No good evidence for any benefits. *Side effects: Stomach upset, anemia, genetic damage, kidney damage.*
Coenzyme Q-10	Made by the body as a component of the biochemical pathway that makes adenosine triphosphate (ATP).	Enhances ATP production.	No evidence suggests a benefit during or after exercise.
Creatine	Made by the body and also found in meat products.	Decreases fatigue in short, intense exercise. Increases muscle size and strength.	Increases endurance in short, intense exercise. Causes water gain in muscle but not increases in strength.
Echinacea	Herbal supplement.	Reduces duration of colds, boosts immune system, heals wounds.	Some evidence suggests it may be beneficial for these conditions. *Side effects: Uncommon, but possible GI upset, chills, nausea.*
Ginkgo biloba	Extracts of dried leaves of *Ginkgo* plant.	Used for antioxidant properties and to improve blood flow and memory.	Does have antioxidant properties that may be beneficial in improving blood flow, improving neural function, and reducing production of stress hormones. *Side effects: nausea, headache, dizziness, skin rash, hemorrhage if used with blood thinners.*
St. John's wort	Plant extract.	Used to treat depression and external wounds, burns, and muscle aches.	Some evidence suggests that it is beneficial for treating these conditions.

CONSUMER
CORNER
DETECTING SUPPLEMENT FRAUD

Most of the dietary supplements on the market today are useless. These products often do nothing more than cheat consumers out of their money or steer them away from products that have been proven useful. Some supplement products may do more harm than good.

How can you avoid being scammed by the maker of a worthless supplement? Marketers have sophisticated ways of making their products attractive to potential buyers, but you can protect yourself by learning about marketing ploys. Beware of the following techniques, claims, or catch-phrases:

- **The product "does it all."** Be suspicious of any supplement that claims to have multiple benefits. No one product is likely to be capable of so great a range of effectiveness.

- **The product is supported by personal testimonials.** Testimonials are often simply stories that have been passed from person to person, and sometimes they are completely made up. Because testimonials are difficult to prove, they may be a "tip" to the possibility of fraud.

- **The product provides a "quick fix."** Be skeptical of products that claim to produce immediate results. Among the tip-offs are ambiguous language such as, "Provides relief in days," or "You'll feel energized immediately." Unscrupulous marketers use such phrases to protect themselves against any subsequent legal action.

- **The product is "natural."** The term *natural* suggests that the product is safer than conventional treatments. However, any product—whether synthetic or natural—that is potent enough to produce a significant physiological effect is potent enough to cause side effects.

- **The product is "a new, time-tested treatment."** A product is usually one or the other, but be suspicious of any product that claims to be both a breakthrough and a decades-old treatment. If a product that claims to be an "innovation" or a "new discovery" were really so revolutionary, it would be widely reported in the media and prescribed by health professionals, not featured in obscure ads.

- **Your "satisfaction is guaranteed."** Money-back guarantees are often empty promises. The makers of this claim know most people won't go to all the trouble involved in trying to get a refund of only $9.95 or so.

- **The product's ads contain meaningless medical jargon.** The use of scientific-sounding terms such as "aerobic enzyme booster" may seem impressive and may even contain an element of truth, but these terms likely cover up a lack of scientific data concerning the product.

Always ask yourself, Does this claim seem too good to be true? If it does, then the product is probably a fraud. If you're still not sure, talk to your doctor or other health professional. The Better Business Bureau or your state attorney general's office can tell you whether other consumers have lodged complaints about a product or its marketers. If a product is promoted as being helpful for a specific condition, check with the appropriate professional group—for example, consult the American Heart Association about products that claim some effectiveness concerning heart disease.

approval before marketing. Additionally, manufacturers must notify the FDA of a product claim within 30 days of marketing it. All this means that the consumer is ultimately responsible for determining whether a given supplement is needed or safe. See the Consumer Corner box.

Make sure you know...

> Supplements should never replace foods as major sources of dietary nutrients.

> Supplements are not tested or approved by the FDA or other governmental body. However, the FDA does mandate that the only claims that can be made about supplements must relate to effects on "structure or function" of the body. Manufacturers are allowed to make no label claims about the effects of a supplement on disease.

> Because dietary supplements are poorly regulated, consumers should be cautious when choosing and using such supplements.

Washing fresh produce under running tap water will help you avoid foodborne illness.

Topics in Food Safety and Technology

The quality of your food choices and an adequate (but not too high) calorie intake are two aspects of a healthy diet. Ensuring the foods you eat are safe and free from contamination is another component of eating well. Let's discuss the specifics of food safety and technology next.

Foodborne Illness

If a food carries a disease-causing microorganism, such as a bacterium, consuming the food can potentially make you sick. According to the Institute of Food Technologists, approximately 80 million cases of foodborne bacterial disease occur each year. These illnesses produce nausea, vomiting, and diarrhea from 12 hours to 5 days after infection (17). The severity of the illness depends on the microorganism ingested and the victim's overall health. Foodborne infections can be fatal in children, people with compromised immune systems, or other people in ill health.

Two types of foodborne illness that you may have heard about are *Salmonella* contamination and botulism. The *Salmonella* bacterium is usually found in raw or undercooked chicken and eggs and in processed meats. The relatively uncommon but sometimes fatal botulism usually results from improper home-canning procedures. A particular strain of the *Escherichia coli* bacterium, O157:H7, is sometimes found in contaminated raw or undercooked ground beef and can lead to bloody diarrhea, among other symptoms.

To reduce your risk of contracting foodborne illness, follow these guidelines:

- Select foods that appear clean and fresh.
- Wash produce thoroughly with running water; use a vegetable brush on firm fruits and vegetables.
- Drink only pasteurized milk and juices.
- Don't eat raw eggs.
- When storing perishable foods for future consumption, keep them cold or frozen to prevent bacterial growth.
- Cook all meat products, such as chicken, pork, and ground beef, thoroughly. When dining out, order meats well done.
- Cook all shellfish thoroughly; steaming them open may not be sufficient.
- Avoid raw fish; it may contain parasitic roundworms. Keep fish frozen, and cook until well done.
- Use separate sets of cutting boards and utensils (e.g., knives) for meat and produce; chopping raw meat and vegetables with the same knife, without washing it thoroughly first, can lead to crosscontamination.
- Wash utensils, plates, cutting boards, knives, blenders, and other cooking equipment with soap and very hot water after each use.

See the Closer Look box on the next page for more about minimizing your risk for foodborne illness.

Food Additives

Food additives are used by manufacturers for a variety of reasons: to improve nutritional quality, as a preservative to maintain freshness and/or increase shelf life, to improve taste or color, or otherwise to make it more appealing. Among the most commonly used additives are sugar, salt, and corn syrup. Other additives, such as monosodium glutamate (MSG) and sulfites, may cause a reaction in people who are particularly sensitive to them. Nitrites, which are found in bacon, sausages, lunch meats, and other processed foods, may also form

A CLOSER LOOK: KEEP HOT FOODS HOT AND COLD FOODS COLD TO AVOID FOODBORNE ILLNESS

Whether from restaurants, super-markets, or quick-service estab-lishments, take-out foods have become a part of our way of life. But to avoid food-borne illnesses, you must keep these foods at the appropriate temperature. The next time you order take-out or bring a hot or cold food to a party or family function, keep the following recommen-dations in mind.

FOR HOT FOODS

- Keep hot foods above 140°F. You can cover food with foil (to keep it moist) and keep it warm—140°F or above—in the oven (check the food's tempera-ture with a meat thermometer). Using a slow cooker is another option for some foods. It's best to eat food within 2 hours of preparation.

- If the food won't be eaten for more than 2 hours, refrigerate it in shallow, covered containers. Before serving, re-heat it in an oven to 165°F or until it's hot and steaming. If you prefer, reheat food in a microwave oven—cover and rotate—and then let it stand for 2 min-utes to ensure thorough, even heating.

FOR COLD FOODS

- Keep cold foods at 40°F or below.

- If cold foods are not eaten right away, refrigerate them as soon as possible.

- Discard any foods kept at room tem-perature for more than 2 hours. If con-ditions are warmer than 90°F, toss the food after only 1 hour.

- Transport and store cold foods in chilled, insulated coolers.

- If you're going to put out a deli platter, keep it on a bowl of ice.

Source: USDA Food Safety and Inspection Ser-vice. *Cooking for Groups: A Volunteer's Guide to Food Safety*. Item #604H, Pueblo, CO 81009.

cancer-causing agents (nitrosamines) in the body. If you think you are sensitive to a particular food additive, read labels carefully and avoid foods that contain additives to which you are likely to have a reaction.

Antibiotics, Hormones, and Organically Grown Foods

As consumers become more aware of the quality of the foods they eat, they are buying increasing quantities of **organic** foods. *Organic*, in this context, refers to foods that are grown without the use of pesticides, hormones, antibiotics, or chemical fertilizers. Currently, the United States, the European Union, Japan, and many other countries require producers to obtain certifica-tion to market food as organic.

Livestock animals raised on factory farms are often treated with high doses of antibiotics to ward off poten-tial infections. Though there is little evidence to sup-port the view, some people are concerned that eating meat or drinking milk from these animals could lead to the development of antibiotic-resistant bacteria in humans.

Farmers also often use hormones in animals to in-crease production of meat and milk. Most notably, a form of growth hormone, bovine somatotropin, has been used to increase milk production in dairy cows.

Some people fear that hormones in food may cause health problems, such as cancer, in humans. Many su-permarkets are restricting the sale of milk produced with the aid of hormone supplements.

Should you buy organic foods? This is a decision you have to make for yourself. However, be aware that there is no research to support that organic foods are nutritionally superior to nonorganic foods, and organic foods tend to be more expensive than their nonorganic counterparts.

Irradiated and Bioengineered Foods

Irradiation is sometimes used to kill microorganisms in foods and prolong the shelf life of the food (17). In fact, irradiated food can be stored for years in sealed containers at room temperature without spoiling. In addition, irradiation can delay the sprouting of vegeta-bles such as potatoes and onions and delay the ripening

organic Plant or animal foods that are grown without the use of pesticides, chemical fertilizers, antibiotics, or hormones.

irradiation The use of radiation (high-energy waves or particles, including radioactivity and X rays) to kill microorganisms that grow on or in food.

of fruits such as bananas, tomatoes, and avocados. This can result in significant cost savings.

Are these irradiated foods safe to eat? Currently, all research indicates that the foods are safe and nutritional content is maintained, but only limited data exist (17). Irradiated foods must carry a seal of approval to inform consumers that they have been treated.

Another practice that has become more controversial is the use of bioengineered foods. Bioengineering involves inserting the genes from one plant or animal species into another plant or animal's DNA to achieve a desired trait. Food crops such as corn and tomatoes have been bioengineered to improve yields, pest resistance, and longevity (which improves the crops' ability to be shipped long distances). Although the benefits of bioengineering can be great, the practice is considered unproven, and possibly unsafe, in some countries.

Make sure you know...

> Proper food storage and preparation are the keys to preventing foodborne illness. Select foods that appear clean and fresh; keep foods cold or frozen to prevent bacteria from growing; clean fresh fruits, vegetables, and meats thoroughly; cook all meats thoroughly; order meats well done when dining out.

> The use of the word *organic* on food labels is strictly regulated; organic foods are grown without the use of pesticides and other chemicals.

> Irradiation and bioengineering are two forms of food technology that are used to enhance food safety and increase yields and pest resistance. Despite all indications that they are safe, both techniques remain somewhat controversial.

Summary

1. Nutrition is the study of food and its relationship to health and disease. In industrialized countries, the current primary problem in nutrition is overeating.

2. A well-balanced diet is composed of approximately 58% complex carbohydrates, 30% fat, and 12% protein. The macronutrients provide the energy (kilocalories, or calories) necessary for bodily functions. The calorie is a unit of measure of the energy value of food or the energy required for physical activity.

3. Carbohydrate is a primary fuel used by the body to provide energy. Simple carbohydrates, or sugars, include glucose, fructose, sucrose, galactose, lactose, and maltose. The complex carbohydrates consist of starches and fiber. Starches are composed of chains of glucose. Fiber is a nondigestible but essential form of complex carbohydrates contained in whole grains, vegetables, and fruits. Fiber is important in regulating digestion and forming waste products.

4. Fat is an efficient storage form for energy, because each gram contains over twice the energy of carbohydrates or protein. Fat can be derived from dietary sources or formed from excess carbohydrates and protein consumed in the diet.

5. Fats are a type of lipid. Most of the fat found in foods and in your body is in the form of triglycerides. Triglycerides consist of three fatty acids attached to a glycerol backbone. Fatty acids are classified as either saturated or unsaturated, depending on their chemical structures. Cholesterol is another

form of lipid. Blood cholesterol levels can affect your risk of heart disease.

6. The primary role of protein is to serve as the structural unit for building and repairing cells in all tissues of the body. Protein consists of amino acids made by the body (11 nonessential amino acids) and those available only through dietary sources (9 essential amino acids). If you consume inadequate amounts of carbohydrates or fat, protein can be broken down and used for energy.

7. Vitamins serve many important functions in the body, including regulation of growth and metabolism. The B-complex vitamins and vitamin C are water soluble and, for the most part, cannot be stored in the body. The fat-soluble vitamins A, D, E, and K can be stored in the body.

8. Minerals are inorganic chemical elements that serve many important roles in regulating body functions.

9. Approximately 60–70% of the body is water. Water is involved in all vital processes in the body and is particularly important for physically active individuals. You need to consume 8–10 cups of water in food and beverages daily.

10. A healthy diet consists of adequate amounts of fruits, vegetables, whole grains, and lean meats and dairy products, with limited amounts of sugar, fat, and sodium. You should balance the calories you consume with the calories you expend, and if you drink alcohol, do so only in moderation. You can

use the RDAs, DRIs, MyPyramid, and food labels to help you choose healthy foods.

11. The intensity of exercise dictates the relative proportions of fat and carbohydrates that are used as fuel during exercise. In general, the lower the intensity of exercise, the more fat is used as a fuel. Conversely, the greater the intensity of exercise, the more carbohydrates are used as a fuel.

12. Antioxidants are nutrients that prevent free radicals from damaging cells. Vitamins E and C, beta-carotene, zinc, and selenium have been identified as antioxidants.

13. Most people can consume adequate nutrients through a healthy diet and do not need to take supplements. However, pregnant women, strict vegetarians, older adults, and some others, may benefit from a dietary supplement.

14. The key to preventing foodborne illness is to prepare, store, and cook foods properly. Select foods that appear clean and fresh; keep foods cold or frozen to prevent bacteria from growing; thoroughly clean fresh fruits, vegetables, and meats; cook all meats thoroughly, and order well-done meats when dining out.

Study Questions

1. What is the primary role of carbohydrates in the diet?
   a. build tissue
   b. provide energy
   c. form hormones
   d. form enzymes

2. The primary role of protein in the diet is to
   a. provide energy
   b. provide hydration
   c. build tissues
   d. regulate hormones.

3. Water is important for
   a. providing energy.
   b. building bones.
   c. forming blood.
   d. building protein.

4. What approximate percentages of carbohydrates, fat, and protein in the diet are recommended daily?
   a. 60, 20, 20
   b. 58, 22, 20
   c. 40, 20, 40
   d. 58, 30, 12

5. Which of the following may protect the body's cells against damage during normal and elevated metabolism?
   a. proteins
   b. hormones
   c. antioxidants
   d. antibiotics

6. List the major food sources of dietary carbohydrates.

7. List the various subcategories of carbohydrates.

8. Define *triglyceride*, and discuss its use in the body.

9. Distinguish between saturated and unsaturated fatty acids.

10. What are omega-3 fatty acids?

11. What is the difference between essential and nonessential amino acids?

12. What are the classes of vitamins, and what role do vitamins play in body function?

13. Outline the role that minerals play in body function.

14. How many calories are contained in 1 gram of carbohydrate, fat, and protein, respectively?

15. Discuss the special need for carbohydrates in an individual who is engaging in an exercise training program.

16. Discuss the special need for protein for an individual who is engaging in an exercise training program.

17. Discuss the impact of the following on heart disease:
    high-density lipoproteins (HDL cholesterol)
    low-density lipoproteins (LDL cholesterol)

18. Discuss the structure/function rule pertaining to dietary supplements.

Suggested Reading

Block, G. Junk foods account for 30% of caloric intake. *Journal of Food Composition and Analysis* 17:439–447, 2004.

Heber, D. Vegetables, fruits and phytoestrogens in the prevention of diseases. *Journal of Postgraduate Medicine* 50(2):145–149, 2004.

Kant, A. K. Dietary patterns and health outcomes. *Journal of the American Dietetic Association* 104(4):615–635, 2004.

Maughan, R. J., D. S. King, and T. Lea. Dietary supplements. *Journal of Sports Sciences* 22(1):95–113, 2004.

Position of the American Dietetic Association, Dietitians of Canada, and the American College of Sports Medicine: Nutrition and athletic performance. *Journal of the American Dietetic Association* 100(12):1543–1556, 2000.

Spriet, L. L., and M. J. Gibala. Nutritional strategies to influence adaptations to training. *Journal of Sports Sciences*. 22(1):127–141, 2004.

Srinath, R. K., and M. B. Katan. Diet, nutrition and the prevention of hypertension and cardiovascular diseases. *Public Health and Nutrition* 7(1A):167–186, 2004.

Thompson, J., and M. Manore. *Nutrition: An Applied Approach*. San Francisco: Benjamin Cummings, 2005.

Willett, W. C., and M. J. Stampfer. Rebuilding the food pyramid. In *Annual Editions: Nutrition 2004/2005*. Dubuque, IA: McGraw-Hill, 2004, pp. 11–16.

Wood, O. B., and C. M. Bruhn. Position of American Dietetic Association: Food irradiation. *Journal of the American Dietetic Association* 100(2):246–253, 2000.

For links to the organizations and websites listed below, visit The Total Fitness and Wellness Website at www.pearsonhighered.com/powers.

Center for Food Safety and Applied Nutrition
Home page for the FDA office of supplement regulation. Great information on food safety and supplements.

The Food and Nutrition Board
Part of the National Academy of Sciences, whose mission is to establish principles and guidelines of adequate dietary intake.

MedlinePlus Health Information: Vitamin and Mineral Supplements
A service of the National Library of Medicine, National Institutes of Health, that provides information on health topics, including vitamin and mineral supplements.

FDA Dietary Supplement Questions and Answers
Provides information about what dietary supplements are and how they are regulated, including the labeling and claims that can be made for supplements.

Nutrition.gov
A federal resource that provides easy access to all online federal government information on nutrition.

MedlinePlus
Contains a wealth of up-to-date, quality nutrition information from the world's largest medical library, the National Library of Medicine at the National Institutes of Health.

Food and Drug Administration
In the summer of 2001, the FDA began publishing a quarterly newsletter titled *Dietary Supplement and Food Labeling Electronic Newsletter*. The newsletter's goal is to provide key information and updates about regulatory actions related to food labeling, nutrition, and dietary supplements, as well as educational materials and important announcements. To subscribe to the letter, visit the link.

Nutrition Café
Contains several intriguing nutritional games, including one in which you build a meal from the menu and then get nutritional information about your selections.

FoodSafety
Gateway to government food safety information. Includes news and safety alerts, consumer advice, national food safety programs, and foodborne pathogens.

Ask the Dietician
Presents sound nutritional advice on many diet-related questions. Includes an excellent "Health Body Calculator" for formulating diet and exercise programs.

USDA Center for Nutrition Policy and Promotion
Provides governmental guidelines for diets.

USDA Food Safety Publications
Contains articles about all aspects of safety in food preparation, storage, and handling.

Fast Food Finder
Enables you to search for desired fast food (by restaurant or food) and find nutritional information.

Veggies Unite! On-line guide to vegetarianism
Includes recipes, books, articles, and discussions.

American Dietetic Association
Presents nutritional resources, FAQs, links, and more.

Crunch Your Numbers
When it comes to health, everything really does add up. So here are 34 fun, easy-to-use calculators. Learn your ideal weight, determine your protein needs, assess your heart rate, determine how many calories your favorite sport will burn, and more.

References

1. Nutrition Business Journal, *NBJ's Supplement Business Report 2005*, http://Nbj.stores.yahoo.Net/Nbsupbusrep2.html.

2. Mokdad, A. H., J. S. Marks, D. F. Stroup, and J. L. Gerberding. Actual causes of death in the United States, 2000. *Journal of the American Medical Association* 291(10):1238–1245, 2004.

3. Wardlaw, G. M., J. Hampl, and R. DiSilvestro. *Perspectives in Nutrition*, 7th ed. Columbus, OH; McGraw-Hill, 2007.

4. Jenkins, D., C. Kendall, and V. Vuksan. Viscous fibers, health claims, and strategies to reduce cardiovascular disease risk. *American Journal of Clinical Nutrition* 71(2):401–402, 2000.

5. Tucker, K. L. Dietary intake and coronary heart disease: A variety of nutrients and phytochemicals are important. *Current Treatment Options in Cardiovascular Medicine* 6(4):291–302, 2004.

6. Dragsted, L. O., A. Pedersen, A. Hermetter, S. Basu, M. Hansen, G. R. Haren, M. Kall, V. Breinholt, J. J. Castenmiller, J. Stagsted, J. Jakobsen, L. Skibsted, S. E. Rasmussen, S. Loft, and B. Sandstrom. The 6-a-day study: Effects of fruit and vegetables on markers of oxidative stress and antioxidant defense in healthy non-smokers. *American Journal of Clinical Nutrition* 79(6):1060–72, 2004.

7. Powers, S., and E. Howley. *Exercise Physiology: Theory and Application to Fitness and Performance*, 7th ed. New York: McGraw-Hill, 2009.

8. Karppanen, H., and E. Mervaala. Sodium intake and hypertension. *Progress in Cardiovascular Disease* 49(2):59–75, 2006.

9. Food and Nutrition Information Center, U.S. Department of Agriculture. Dietary Reference Intakes (DRI) and Recommended Dietary Allowances (RDA), www.nal.usda.gov/fnic.

10. Keen, R. Osteoporosis: Strategies for prevention and management. *Best Practice and Research Clinical Rheumatology* 21(1):109–122, 2007.

11. Jones, N. L., and K. J. Killian. Exercise limitation in health and disease. *New England Journal of Medicine* 343(9):632–641, 2000.

12. Tipton, K. D., and R. R. Wolfe. Exercise, protein metabolism, and muscle growth. *International Journal of Sport Nutrition and Exercise Metabolism* 11(1):109–132, 2001.

13. Lemon. P. W., J. M. Berardi, and E. E. Noreen. The role of protein and amino acid supplements in the athlete's diet: Does type or timing of ingestion matter? *Current Sports Medicine Reports* 1(4):214–221, 2002.

14. Lukaski, H. C. Vitamin and mineral status: Effects on physical performance. *Nutrition* 20(7–8):632–644, 2004.

15. Young, I. S., and J. V. Woodside. Antioxidants in health and disease. *Journal of Clinical Pathology* 54(3):176–186, 2001.

16. Powers, S. K., K. C. DeRuisseau, J. Quindry, and K. L. Hamilton. Dietary antioxidants and exercise. *Journal of Sports Sciences* 22(1):81–94, 2004.

17. Food Safety Policy, Science, and Risk Assessment: Strengthening the Connection: Workshop Proceedings (2001), Institute of Medicine, Washington, DC: National Academy Press, 2001.

Videos

Log on to www.pearsonhighered.com/powers to view these chapter-related videos.

Nutrition

You Are What You Eat

Going Green

NAME _____ DATE _____

Analyzing Your Diet

The purpose of this exercise is to analyze your eating habits during a 3-day period. For a 3-day period (two weekdays and one weekend day), eat the foods that typically constitute your normal diet. At the end of each day, record on the following chart the foods you ate that day and the amounts of the listed nutrients contained in each. You can use the food labels on your foods to obtain the nutrient values, or refer to the Appendix at the end of this text (you can also use a diet analysis software program, if you have access to one.)

Total the values for each nutrient at the bottom of the chart. Transfer the total to the next chart. At the end of the 3-day period, total the daily values and divide by 3 to get the average dietary intake for each of the nutrients analyzed.

Compare your average intake for each of the nutrients with those recommended at the bottom of the page for your sex and age group. (Remember that this analysis is only as representative of your normal diet as the foods you eat over the 3-day period). Then, answer the following questions:

1. How did you do on calories? Are you taking in more or fewer calories than you should be for your sex, age, and activity level?

   _____

2. Was your fat, sodium, and cholesterol intake higher than it should be?

   _____

3. What nutrients did you eat in inadequate amounts?

   _____

4. What are three substitutions you could have made that would improve the quality of your diet?

   _____

Recommended Dietary Allowances*

- Kcal total (total daily energy expenditure) equals body weight multiplied by kcal per pound per day:

  _____ × _____ = _____

  body weight in lb   kcal per lb per day   **kcal total (total daily**
             (from Table 8.1)   **energy expenditure)**

- Kcal from fat should be no more than 30% of total calories per day:

  _____ × _____ = _____

  30% (0.3)   kcal per day   **recommended MAXIMUM kcal from fat**

- Protein intake should be 12% of total calories per day, or 0.8 to 0.9 gram per kilogram (0.36 g per pound) of body weight. (Pregnant women should add 15 g, and lactating women should add 20 g):

  _____ × _____ = _____

  0.36 g   body weight in lb   **recommended protein intake**

- Carbohydrate intake should be approximately 58% of total calories per day:

  _____ × _____ = _____

  58% (0.58)   kcal per day   **recommended carbohydrate intake**

Fat <30% of diet; fiber ~30% of diet; saturated fat <10% of diet; cholesterol <300 mg.; sodium <3000 mg

*See Table 7.6 on pages 210 and 211 for vitamin and mineral RDA values.

LABORATORY

Daily Nutrient Intake

Name: _____ Date: _____

Foods	Amount	kcal (total)	kcal from fat	Protein (gm)	Carb. (gm)	Fiber (gm)	Fat (gm)	Fat % (kcal)	Sat. Fat (gm)	Chol. (mg)	Sodium (mg)	Vit. A (I.U.)	Vit. C (mg)	Calcium (mg)	Iron (mg)	Vit. B₁ (mg)	Vit. B₂ (mg)	Niacin (mg)
Totals																		

Look in your Behavior Change Log Book for an additional 3-day nutrient intake log.

Three-Day Nutrient Summary

Name: _____

Date: _____

Day	kcal (Total)	kcal from Fat	Protein (gm)	Carb. (gm)	Fiber (gm)	Fat (gm)	Fat % (kcal)	Sat. Fat (gm)	Chol. (mg)	Sodium (mg)	Vit. A (IU)	Vit. C (mg)	Calcium (mg)	Iron (mg)	Vit. B$_1$ (mg)	Vit. B$_2$ (mg)	Niacin (mg)
One																	
Two																	
Three																	
Totals																	
Average																	

NAME _____ DATE _____

Setting Goals for a Healthy Diet

What are your three worst dietary habits?

1. _____

2. _____

3. _____

Check the appropriate boxes in the table below to indicate the changes that you think you need to make to improve your diet.

	Increase	Decrease	Keep the Same
Calories			
Carbohydrates			
Fat			
Protein			
Vitamins			
Minerals			

Based on your selections above, list two short-term and two long-term goals for improving your diet:

Short-term goal 1

_____

Short-term goal 2

_____

Long-term goal 1

_____

Long-term goal 2

_____

NAME _____ DATE _____

Planning a New Diet

The purpose of this exercise is to plan a new diet using the principles outlined in this chapter. After completing Laboratory 7.1, you should have a general idea of how your diet may need modification. Follow the example given in Table 7.7 on page 214 and the discussion in the text to choose foods to build a new diet that meets the recommended dietary goals presented in this chapter. Fill in the chart on the following page with the requested information obtained from this book's appendix or from package labels. Use the totals for each column and the RDA for each nutrient in Laboratory 7.1 or Table 7.6 on pages 210 and 211 to determine your percentage of RDA for each nutrient.

	kcal (g)	Protein (g)	Sat. Fat (g)	Chol. (mg)	Sod. (mg)	Carb. (g)	Vit. A (IU)	Vit. C (mg)	Ca (mg)	Iron (mg)	GI
Breakfast											
Lunch											
Dinner											
Totals											
RDA	*	<30%†	<10%	<300	3000	>58%	1000	60	1200	12	‡
% of RDA											

*See Chapter 8 for determination of kcal requirements.

†Protein intake should be 0.8 g/kg of body weight (0.36 g/lb). Pregnant women should add 15 g, and lactating women should add 20 g.

‡For a complete list of the glycemixc index of various foods, visit www.glycemicindex.com

NAME _____ DATE _____

Assessing Nutritional Habits

Read the following scenarios and select which option applies to you. Score your answers according to the instructions at the end.

1. You don't have time to make dinner, so you run out to get "fast food." What do you get?

   a. grilled chicken breast sandwich

   b. supersized burger

2. You go to a movie, find yourself hungry, and cannot resist a snack. Which do you buy?

   a. unbuttered popcorn

   b. candy

3. You're late for work and realize you forgot breakfast. You decide to stop and grab something to eat. What do you pick up?

   a. a banana

   b. a sausage biscuit

4. You decide to go out for a nice dinner at an Italian restaurant. What do you order?

   a. spaghetti with red sauce

   b. five-cheese lasagna

5. It's 3:00 PM, and you didn't have much lunch and need an afternoon snack. What do you reach for?

   a. an apple

   b. M&Ms

6. You stop for ice cream. Which do you pick?

   a. a fruit sorbet

   b. regular ice cream

7. What kind of dessert would you normally choose to eat?

   a. a bowl of mixed berries with a sprinkling of sugar

   b. chocolate cake with frosting

8. What do you use to stir fry vegetables?

   a. olive oil

   b. margarine

9. Which of the following salty snacks would you prefer?

   a. pretzels

   b. potato chips

10. You want cereal for breakfast. Which would you choose?

    a. whole-grain flakes

    b. peanut butter puffs

Interpretation

If you answered "b" to any of the above questions, you chose foods that are high in calories, fat, or sugar. Follow the advice in this chapter and in the MyPyramid food guidance system to improve your food choices.

Exercise, Diet, and Weight Control

8

true or false?

1. The key to weight loss is to not eat snacks.

2. Low-carbohydrate diets are the only ones that really work.

3. Your genes determine whether you'll be obese.

4. A successful weight management program involves both diet and exercise.

5. Anorexia nervosa occurs only in women.

Answers appear on the next page.

illions of people in the United States are overweight. In fact, according to the Centers for Disease Control and Prevention, the prevalence of overweight and obesity has increased sharply for both adults and children. Obesity represents a global epidemic and is now one of the leading causes of illness worldwide (1). Being overweight has been shown to be a risk factor for health problems such as diabetes, gallbladder disease, high blood pressure, high cholesterol, heart disease, and even some cancers. As a result of this connection between health and increased body weight, more people are trying to lose weight, and an estimated 43% of overweight women and 28% of overweight men attempt to lose weight each year (2).

This epidemic in overweight and obesity has given birth to a multi-billion-dollar weight-loss industry in the United States. Consumers spend about $30 billion per year on diet sodas, appetite suppressants, diet books, commercial diets, and medically supervised diets in an attempt to lose weight or prevent weight gain. In addition, the number of individuals seeking gastric bypass surgery increased from 10,000 in 1996 to more than 178,000 in 2006 (3). Many commercial weight-loss programs advertise that they are highly successful. Unfortunately, research has found that with no other treatment, only 5% of individuals maintain the weight loss for 5 years after completing the program (2). The good news is that long-term weight loss is achievable, and many people do successfully alter their diet and lifestyle habits to achieve a healthy weight. The key is to recognize that short-term diets and gimmicks work only temporarily and that the only solution for long-term weight loss is to retool one's eating and physical activity patterns.

In this chapter, we will discuss the principles of determining an ideal body weight for health and fitness;

how to use a combination of diet, exercise, and behavior modification to successfully reduce body fat; and the principles involved in maintaining a desirable body weight throughout life. Finally, we will look at the symptoms and health effects of several disordered eating patterns. We begin by revisiting the concept of optimal body weight, which you read about in Chapter 6.

What Is Your Optimal Body Weight?

Before you can decide whether you should implement a weight-loss program, you need to find out whether you're currently at an optimal body weight. Recall from Chapter 6 that in general, optimal body fat for health and fitness in men ranges from 10–20%, whereas the optimal range of body fat for women ranges from 15–25% (4). These ranges allow for individual differences in physical activity and appearance and are associated with limited risk of the diseases linked to body fatness. How can you compute your desired range of body weight? The calculation can be done in two simple steps; the first step is to calculate your fat-free weight. Consider the following example of a male college student who has 25% body fat and weighs 185 pounds.

> **Step 1:** Compute fat-free weight—that is, the amount of total body weight contained in bones, organs, and muscles:
>
> % total body weight − % fat weight = % fat–free weight
> $$100\% - 25\% = 75\%$$
>
> This means that 75% (or 0.75, expressed as a decimal) of total body weight is fat-free weight. Therefore, the fat-free weight for this student is
> $$0.75 \times 185 \text{ pounds} = 138.8 \text{ pounds}$$

Step 2: Calculate the optimal weight (which for men is 10–20% of total body weight). The formula to compute optimum body weight is

Optimum weight = fat–free weight ÷ (1 − optimal % fat)

Note that % fat should again be expressed as a decimal. Thus, for 10% body fat,

Optimum weight = 138.8 ÷ (1 − 0.10) = 154.2 pounds

For 20% body fat,

Optimum weight = 138.8 ÷ (1 − 0.20) = 173.5 pounds

Hence, the optimal body weight for this individual is between 154.2 and 173.5 pounds. See Laboratory 8.1 to compute your optimal body weight, using both percentage of body fat and body mass index (from Chapter 6).

Make sure you know...

> The ranges of optimal body fat for health and fitness are 10–20% for men and 15–25% for women.
> You can calculate your optimal body weight using your percent body fat and current body weight.

What Factors Can Affect Weight Management?

In most obese people, being overfat is a result of a complex interaction between internal and external (environmental) factors. Internal factors include genetics and hormonal secretions. External factors such as diet, exercise, and social settings also directly affect weight management. Let's examine these two sets of influences more closely.

Genetic Factors and Hormones

There are a few rare conditions, including Prader-Willi syndrome and Bardet-Biedl syndrome, that account for extreme obesity in about 1% of the population. These two conditions are genetic disorders and are present at birth (5). Other physiological causes of obesity may be related to the release of hormones, especially leptin and ghrelin, and much current research focuses on this area.

The hormone **leptin** appears to depress appetite by acting on areas of the brain that control hunger (6). Researchers working on the connection between hormones and obesity found that obese mice had very low levels of leptin, and when injected with leptin, the mice became lean. Leptin was believed to be the cure-all for the obesity epidemic until it was later discovered that many obese people produce abnormally high levels of leptin. Further research has focused on how leptin works with other hormones such as insulin (a hormone manufactured by the pancreas). Researchers aren't sure how leptin and insulin interact, but it provides an intriguing area of further study.

Another hormone called **ghrelin** promotes feelings of hunger. High levels of ghrelin trigger nerve signals running from the gut to the brain, causing the hunger signal to turn on and keep ringing. Research has been conducted to determine how to suppress ghrelin production, whereas other studies have focused on the effects of exercise on ghrelin production. Although there have been no reported changes in ghrelin production following aerobic exercise, there is some evidence that moderate-intensity resistance training may suppress ghrelin production, thus reducing appetite (7). Gastric bypass surgery has also been shown to suppress ghrelin levels (8).

Hormonal influences on ghrelin have also revealed that leptin and insulin work together to lower the production levels of ghrelin. In addition, certain types of food affect the production of ghrelin. Foods rich in fat are less effective in suppressing the production of ghrelin than foods containing proteins or sugars (2). These discoveries about the hormones that affect hunger and appetite have led researchers to believe that a cure for obesity in humans may be attainable.

Environmental Factors

Environmental factors still remain the primary focus for many health care professionals in treating overweight and obese individuals. Diet and exercise are the two major factors that can be controlled and modified in fighting the obesity epidemic. What you eat, and how much you eat, as well as how much you exercise, are very much within your control.

Understanding what triggers our eating habits may be an important first step in weight management. For some people, eating has become a response to emotional stressors, both good and bad. On the one hand, think about how your family celebrates an accomplishment, such as graduation from college, or a milestone, such as a birthday or anniversary. These positive stressors bring people together to celebrate, and food is often at the center of that celebration. On the other hand, when dealing with negative feelings such as depression, loneliness, or boredom, some people turn to food for comfort. Eating habits become ingrained as part of our family practices and may be difficult to change.

leptin A hormone that appears to depress appetite.
ghrelin A hormone that contributes to feelings of hunger.

STEPS FOR
BEHAVIOR
CHANGE

What triggers your eating?

Take the following quiz to help assess some of the cues that cause you to eat.

Y   N

☐   ☐   I need to have a snack and a beverage nearby when I study.

☐   ☐   I cannot watch television or sit through a movie without a snack in my hand.

☐   ☐   I would order the small portion at a fast-food restaurant, but I get more for my money if I order the largest size possible.

☐   ☐   Leaving food on my plate is wasteful.

☐   ☐   I like to have a beverage in my cupholder when I'm driving.

If you answered yes to more than one of these questions, you're likely eating out of habit or because of your environment. This behavior could lead to weight gain.

TIPS TO CURB YOUR CALORIE CONSUMPTION

☑ Drink water while studying instead of soda, and if you get hungry, stop for a break and go get a piece of fruit for a snack.

☑ Visit friends or go for a walk in the evening instead of watching television. You'll eat less and work in some physical activity.

☑ Order only small sandwiches and fries when eating fast food, or, better yet, order no fries and a side salad instead.

☑ Despite what our families may have taught us, clearing your plate is probably leading to your eating long after you're full. Next time you sit down for a home-cooked meal, try grabbing smaller portions to begin with, then go back for seconds only if you're really still hungry.

☑ Opt for a reusable water bottle in your car, and use that to stay hydrated during road trips. The calories in sodas and sugar-and-milk-laden coffee drinks will quickly add up.

Eating habits have also changed as fast-food restaurants have proliferated throughout the country. The convenience of these food outlets has made it easy to "grab" a quick sandwich and eat it en route to work, play, or the next event. Convenience, cost, and portion size have made fast-food restaurants a likely culprit in the obesity epidemic. The restaurant industry overall has increased portion sizes to give customers more for their money. As portion sizes increase, so do the waistlines of the customers. In fact, serving sizes have increased to the point that the average person does not realize what a normal serving size should be. In the end, most people underestimate the amount of food they eat. Paying attention to how much and what we consume is an important first step in weight management.

Do you know what situations or events affect your eating habits? See the Steps for Behavior Change box above and the box on the next page to identify some of your food triggers.

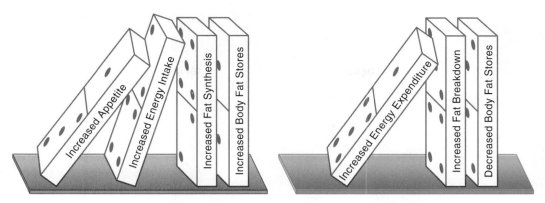

FIGURE 8.1
Numerous factors compound to lead to weight gain or weight loss.

The Concept of Energy Balance

Simply stated, body fat stores are regulated by two factors: the rate at which fat is synthesized and stored, and the rate at which energy is expended and fat is metabolized (broken down). In general, fat stores increase when energy intake ("calories in") exceeds energy expenditure ("calories out") and decrease when energy expenditure exceeds energy intake. This concept can be simplified into the phrase "calories in versus calories out." If you take in more calories than you expend, you will gain weight, and if you expend more calories than you consume, you will lose weight. You can see in Figure 8.1 that an increase in energy intake

(calories) in response to increased appetite leads to increases in fat synthesis and storage. In contrast, fat stores are reduced when fat is broken down for use as a source of energy for the body.

If you want to maintain a constant body weight, your food energy intake (expressed in calories) must equal your energy expenditure; that is, you must be in **energy balance** (Figure 8.2). Healthy weight-loss

Energy Expenditure = Energy Intake

FIGURE 8.2
The concept of energy balance. To maintain body weight, the number of calories you consume must equal the number of calories you expend. An imbalance on either side of the scale will result in a change in body weight.

Social and Environmental Factors That May Contribute to Overeating

- *Activities*. You may find a correlation between specific types of activities, such as watching TV and eating snacks.

- *Emotional behavior before or during eating*. For instance, many people overeat when they are depressed or under stress.

- *Location of meals*. Do you eat your meals in front of the television? Do you associate specific rooms with snacking?

- *Time of day and level of hunger*. Do you eat at specific times of the day? Do you eat even if you are not hungry?

- *People involved*. Are specific people associated with periods of overeating?

energy balance The state of consuming a number of calories that is equal to the number expended. Over the long term, energy balance results in maintenance of a constant body weight.

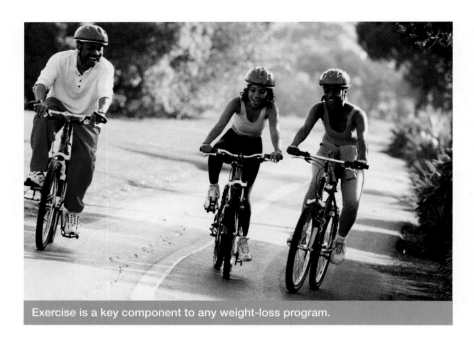
Exercise is a key component to any weight-loss program.

programs include both a reduction in caloric intake and an increase in caloric expenditure achieved through exercise (4, 9, 10).

Estimating your daily energy expenditure is a key factor in planning a weight-loss program and adjusting the energy balance equation. The daily expenditure of energy involves both the resting metabolic rate and exercise metabolic rate.

Resting metabolic rate (RMR) is the amount of energy expended during all sedentary activities. That is, RMR includes the energy required to maintain necessary bodily functions (called the basal metabolic rate) plus the additional energy required to perform such activities as sitting, reading, typing, and digesting food. The RMR is an important component of the energy balance equation because it represents approximately 90% of the total daily energy expenditure in sedentary individuals (11).

Resting metabolic rate is influenced by several factors, including age, gender, and the amount of lean body mass that an individual possesses. For example, resting metabolic rate (expressed per pound of body weight) is generally higher in growing children than in adults. Moreover, resting metabolic rate declines with age, and men have a higher resting metabolic rate than women. Finally, resting metabolic rate is elevated in people with a low percentage of body fat and a high percentage of lean mass. The physiological explanation for this is that the energy required to maintain muscle tissue is greater than the energy required to maintain fat tissue (4).

Exercise metabolic rate (EMR) represents the energy expenditure during any form of exercise (walking, climbing steps, weight lifting, and so on). In seden-

tary individuals, EMR constitutes only 10% of the total daily energy expenditure. By comparison, EMR can account for 20–40% of the total daily energy expenditure in active individuals (11). For example, during heavy exercise, EMR may be 10–20 times greater than RMR (4). Therefore, increased daily exercise increases the EMR and is a key factor in weight control programs.

One of the simplest ways to estimate your daily caloric expenditure is to determine your activity level and use it to calculate the average number of calories you expend in a 24-hour period (Table 8.1). For example, the estimated daily caloric expenditure for a moderately active college-aged woman who weighs 120 pounds is calculated by multiplying 120 (her body weight in pounds) by 15 (the calories she expends per pound per day):

$$\text{Daily caloric expenditure} = 120 \text{ pounds} \times 15 \text{ calories/pound/day}$$

$$= 1800 \text{ calories/day}$$

If this woman takes in an average of 2000 calories per day in her meals and snacks, those extra 200 calories put her on the road to weight gain. Do this same calculation for your own daily caloric expenditure. Do you think your daily expenditure is equal to or higher than the amount of calories you take in per day? If you need to lose weight, what activities could you add to your routine to increase your daily caloric expenditure?

Now that you know the basic physiological and environmental factors that affect weight management and understand the concept of energy balance, let's discuss the strategies that can lead to safe and effective weight loss.

Make sure you know...

> Physiological (internal) factors that contribute to overweight and obesity include genetics and hormonal excretions; external factors that affect weight management include diet, exercise, and social settings.

> To maintain a constant body weight, your food energy (caloric) intake must equal your caloric expenditure; that is, you must maintain a state of energy balance. Consuming more calories than you expend results in weight gain, and consuming fewer calories than you expend results in weight loss.

TABLE 8.1

Estimating Daily Caloric Expenditure

To compute your estimated daily caloric expenditure, multiply your body weight in pounds by the calories per pound that corresponds to your activity level.

Activity Level	Description	Calories per Pound of Body Weight Expended during 24-Hour Period
1 Very sedentary	Restricted movement, such as a patient confined to a house	13
2 Sedentary	Light work or office job	14
3 Moderate activity	Some daily activity and weekend recreation	15
4 Very physically active	Vigorous activity at least 3–4 times/week	16
5 Competitive athlete	Daily activity in high energy sport	17–18

> Daily energy expenditure can be estimated by considering both your resting metabolic rate and your exercise caloric expenditure.

Designing a Successful Weight-Loss Program

The basic strategy for successful weight loss is to expend more calories than you consume and to make changes to your diet and lifestyle that you will be able to maintain over the long term. The maximum recommended rate for weight loss is 1 to 2 pounds per week. Diets resulting in a weight loss of more than 2 pounds per week are associated with a significant loss of lean body mass (i.e., muscle and body organs).

The energy deficit required to lose 1 pound per week is approximately 3500 calories. Therefore, a negative energy balance of 500 calories per day would theoretically result in a loss of 1 pound of fat per week (3500 calories per week ÷ 7 days per week = 500 calories per day).

The rate of loss during the first several days of dieting will be greater than later in the dieting period. At the onset of a diet, you lose not only fat, but also carbohydrate and water stores, which also results in some weight loss (4). Further, you may also lose some lean tissue, such as muscle, during the beginning of any diet; therefore, you will lose more than 1 pound during the first 3500-calorie deficit. However, as the diet continues, you will lose weight at a slower rate. Don't be discouraged if weight loss levels off after the first week. The weight you lose later will come primarily from fat stores, and sticking with your weight-loss plan for several weeks will result in a significant fat loss.

To lose weight and keep it off, you need to implement four basic steps:

1. Establish a realistic goal for weight loss.
2. Assess your diet, and determine how you can modify it to reduce your caloric intake while still consuming all the nutrients you need for health.
3. Decide which physical activities you will begin doing to raise your daily caloric expenditure and increase (or maintain) muscle mass.
4. Modify your diet and lifestyle to lose the weight you want to lose and prevent future weight gain.

Let's take a closer look at what's involved in each of these steps.

Set a Realistic Goal for Weight Loss

The first step in setting a realistic weight loss goal is to decide where your percentage of body fat should fall within the optimal healthy range (10–20% for men, 15–25% for women). Many people who are beginning a comprehensive weight-loss program set a long-term weight loss goal that will place them in the middle of the optimal weight range (15% body fat for men, 20% body fat for women). After choosing your long-term goal, it is also useful to establish short-term weight-loss

resting metabolic rate (RMR) The amount of energy expended during all sedentary activities.

exercise metabolic rate (EMR) The amount of energy expended during any form of exercise.

goals—usually expressed in the number of pounds lost per week. Keep in mind that 1–2 pounds per week is a realistic weight-loss goal. Establishing a goal of losing 5 pounds in a week is not realistic and will set you up for failure.

If your goal is to lose 1 pound per week, you must establish how you will achieve that. For example, "I will lose 1 pound by walking 20 minutes each day and limiting my soda consumption to one, 8-ounce glass a day."

Remember, setting realistic goals is an important first step in weight management. Using the optimal healthy range for percent body fat as your guide is healthier and much more realistic than aiming for a tiny dress size or waist measurement. See Laboratory 8.3 for a worksheet you can use to help set your long-term and short-term goals.

CONSIDER THIS!

Approximately 90% of fat loss occurs in the body regions with the highest fat storage, generally the thighs and hips in women, and the abdominal region in men. In other words, you cannot spot-reduce fat stores.

Assess and Modify Your Diet

Another key to losing weight successfully is to recognize the healthy and less healthy dietary choices you're making on a daily basis. If you're eating fast food regularly, you may be consuming too many high-fat, high-calorie foods that are impeding your ability to lose weight. Similarly, if you can't remember the last time you ate a fresh fruit or vegetable, you may be getting too few nutrients and other healthy substances. A balanced, healthy diet can naturally lead to weight loss, and once you know the areas of your diet that could be improved, you can work on making changes that are likely to help you lose weight.

Most people tend to underestimate the amount of food they consume. Keeping a food diary for as few as 2–3 days can make

TABLE 8.2
Popular Diet Plans

Diet	Description/ Examples	Recommended?	Comments
Low-carbohydrate	High in protein (meat, beans, animal products) and may also be high in fat. Examples: Atkins diet, Zone diet, and Sugar-Busters	No	Typically high in fat and cholesterol. Initial weight loss is attributed to water loss. Success in keeping weight off over time is minimal because of tendency to return to regular eating habits.
Low-calorie liquid diet	Prepackaged liquid meal replacement plans Example: Slim-Fast	No	Although nutritionally balanced, these diets are typically monotonous and unsatisfying.
Very-low-calorie diet	Provides 300–600 calories per day	No	Nutritionally unbalanced and unsafe for long-term use.
Balanced low-calorie diet	Typically involves reduction in calorie intake by 500–1000 calories per day. Example: diet that follows the recommendations in the MyPyramid food guidance system	Yes	Can be nutritionally balanced and safe for long-term use. Safely allows 1–2 pounds of weight loss per week.

A CLOSER LOOK FACTS AND MYTHS ABOUT LOW-FAT AND LOW-CARB DIETS

Most people are aware that eating foods high in fat can be detrimental to the waistline, so they search for foods that are labeled "low-fat" or "fat-free." This is an important first step in reducing fat intake; however, it does not always lead to weight loss. Consumers should read beyond the fat calories and be aware that many of these "reduced-fat" products may actually be higher in total calories than their alternatives. Eating less fat should not result in eating more calories, because this will be detrimental to weight loss.

Proponents of low-carbohydrate diets argue that these diets have two major advantages over conventional diet plans. First, eating high-carbohydrate foods promotes the use of carbohydrates as fuel and reduces the rate of fat metabolism. This argument is supported experimentally, and the physiology to explain this claim is that consuming high-carbohydrate foods promotes an increase in the hormone insulin. High insulin levels are counterproductive to weight loss because insulin stimulates both fat storage and a reduction in the use of fat as a body fuel (4, 22).

The second argument in favor of low-carbohydrate diets is that high-carbohydrate foods are less satiating than foods containing high levels of proteins or fats (25). Therefore, low-carbohydrate diets may promote satiety, reduce overall caloric intake, and assist in achieving a negative caloric balance. Although evidence exists to support this argument, low-carbohydrate diets do not suppress appetite in all people.

Low-carbohydrate diets are sometimes promoted as diets on which "you never feel hungry" and "you will lose weight fast." Both claims can be misleading. As previously stated, not everyone loses appetite while on a low-carbohydrate diet. Further, the initial weight loss seen in many low-carbohydrate diets is likely temporary, because it is due to water loss rather than to fat loss. The body will regain the water after the person resumes a normal diet, thereby voiding the initial weight loss (4).

Some low-carbohydrate diets have been associated with health problems, such as high blood cholesterol, hypo–glycemia, and other metabolic disorders. These observations suggest that low-carbohydrate diets can be dangerous. The evidence is somewhat contradictory: Some low-carbohydrate (and high-fat diets) have been shown to lead to high blood cholesterol, but one study reveals that a low-carbohydrate diet with relatively low fat does not elevate blood cholesterol levels or promote cardio-vascular risk factors (23). Nonetheless, the safety and effectiveness of a low-carbohydrate/high-protein diet needs further long-term study before firm recommendations can be made (4).

See Table 8.2 for examples of other popular weight-loss diets. Note that the only recommended solution for long-term weight loss is a balanced, low-calorie diet combined with daily physical exercise.

you aware of the food choices you are making and allow you to see where you can make changes in the future.

If you are considering a diet for the purpose of losing weight, you should be aware of the following: the diets promoted in books and on websites to promote weight loss often do not provide balanced nutrition (see the Closer Look boxes above and on page 248, and Table 8.2, for more on several specific types of weight-loss diets). When you are assessing new diets, a general rule of thumb is to avoid fad diets that promise fast and easy weight loss. If you have concerns about the safety or effectiveness of a published diet, you can either contact your local branch of the American Dietetic Association for information or approach a dietitian at a hospital or college. By learning the basic nutrition principles contained in this chapter and in Chapter 7, you should be able to critically evaluate most diet plans.

Any safe and nutritionally sound diet should adhere to the following guidelines (12–14).

- The diet should be low in calories but provide all the essential nutrients the body requires. It should be balanced with foods that provide adequate vitamins and minerals on a daily basis.
- The diet should be low in fat (less than 30% of total calories) and high in complex carbohydrates.
- The diet should promote a variety of foods to appeal to your tastes and to prevent hunger between meals, as well as to keep you from getting bored.
- The diet should be compatible with your lifestyle, and the foods should be easily obtainable.

A CLOSER LOOK
FREQUENTLY ASKED QUESTIONS ABOUT WEIGHT-LOSS DIETS

WHAT IS A "FAD DIET"?

A diet is considered a "fad" if it gains fame but then fades in popularity when consumers realize that the diet does not perform as advertised. Numerous "fad" diets currently exist, and these diets come and go. Examples such as the Abs Diet, which purports to reduce stomach fat and claims that dieters will lose as much as 12 pounds in 2 weeks, and the grapefruit diet, which calls for eating only grapefruit, at the least will be ineffective and at worst may cause health problems. The fact is, there are no magical diets to lose weight. Remember, any diet plan that claims to spot-reduce or allow you to lose weight without exercising and/or reducing caloric intake will not result in the loss of body fat.

WHAT IS THE "GLYCEMIC INDEX" OF FOODS?

The "glycemic index" is a measure of how much insulin is released when a particular type of food is consumed. Foods that produce the highest release of insulin are assigned a high glycemic index. Because insulin release promotes fat storage in the body, proponents of low-carbohydrate diets argue that people should avoid foods with a high glycemic index. Most whole-grain foods, fruits, and vegetables have a low glycemic index, whereas foods such as white rice, potatoes, and pasta have a high glycemic index.

WHAT ARE HIGH-PROTEIN DIETS, AND DO THEY DIFFER FROM LOW-CARBOHYDRATE DIETS?

High-protein diets are essentially low-carbohydrate diets that emphasize consuming protein in unrestricted amounts. A health concern associated with high-protein diets is that people on them often consume large quantities of red meat, eggs, and cheese. Therefore, high-protein diets may also be high-fat diets. A high-fat diet can result in elevated blood levels of cholesterol and therefore increase the risk of cardiovascular disease. Moreover, a high fat-diet has been associated with an increased risk of certain cancers. For this reason, the World Cancer Research Fund discourages the use of any high-protein diet.

CAN CALORIC RESTRICTION SLOW AGING AND INCREASE LONGEVITY?

This practice involves consuming a balanced diet but restricting your caloric intake by approximately 20 to 40 percent below the level of energy consumed in a freely chosen diet. This practice has been shown to extend life span in a variety of animal species including rats, mice, and worms. However, whether prolonged caloric restriction increases life span or reduces the rate of aging in humans is unknown.

WHAT ROLE DO DIETARY CALCIUM AND DAIRY PRODUCTS PLAY IN WEIGHT MANAGEMENT?

New evidence suggests that dietary calcium from dairy products may play an important role in weight management. The proposed mechanism relates to the fact that calcium plays a key role in fat metabolism and fat storage. Specifically, a diet high in calcium from dairy products has been shown to promote fat metabolism, inhibit fat synthesis, and, therefore, increase the loss of body fat. These concepts have been confirmed by epidemiological data and clinical studies indicating that diets high in dairy products (more than 3 servings per day) accelerate fat loss compared with diets low in dairy products. Although these results are promising, additional studies are required to confirm that increasing calcium intake by consuming dairy products is a useful adjunct to a weight-loss program.

Sources: Heilbronn, L., and E. Ravussin. Calorie restriction and aging: Review of the literature and implications for studies in humans. *American Journal of Clinical Nutrition* 78:361–369, 2003; Zemel, M. B. Role of calcium and dairy products in energy partitioning and weight management. *American Journal of Clinical Nutrition* 79:9075–9125, 2004.

• The diet should be a lifelong diet; that is, it should be one that you can follow for the long term. This type of diet greatly increases your chances of keeping weight off once you've lost it.

In addition to these diet guidelines, here are some helpful reminders (some of which were covered in Chapter 7) for planning a healthy, balanced diet:

• Avoid high-calorie, low-nutrient foods such as those high in sugar (e.g., candy bars, cookies, soft drinks, and alcohol). Instead, select low-calorie, nutrient-dense foods such as fruits, vegetables, and whole-grain breads.

• Reduce the amount of saturated fat in your diet, and avoid trans fats (which are sometimes found in processed foods and baked goods). High-fat foods are high in calories, and eating too much saturated fat can also increase your risk for heart disease. For example, eat less butter, and choose lean meats such as lean cuts of beef, chicken, and fish. Avoid fried foods; choose nonfat or low-fat dairy products, such as milk, yogurt, and cottage cheese.

- Select fresh fruits and vegetables whenever possible, and avoid fruits that are canned in heavy syrup.

- Limit salt intake. Use herbs and other seasonings instead of salt to flavor foods.

- Drink fewer alcoholic beverages. Alcoholic beverages are low in nutrients and high in calories.

- Eat to satisfy hunger, not boredom or other emotional situations. Remember that a negative energy balance of 500 calories per day will result in a weight loss of approximately 1 pound per week. The key to maintaining a caloric deficit of 500 calories per day is careful planning of meals and accurate calorie counting.

Plan Your Physical Activity

Physical activity and exercise play a key role in weight loss for several reasons (15, 16). Increased physical activity elevates your daily caloric expenditure and therefore helps you expend more calories, and regular cardiorespiratory exercise improves the ability of skeletal muscles to burn fat as energy. Regular resistance exercise (such as weight training) can also reduce the loss of muscle that occurs during dieting. This is important because your primary goal during weight loss is to lose fat, not muscle mass. Finally, increasing your muscle mass (as through weight training) increases resting metabolic rate, which further aids in weight loss (17).

What type of exercise is best for losing weight? You should perform both cardiorespiratory training (i.e., running, cycling, swimming, and so on) and strength training while dieting. (See the Closer Look box on page 250.) The combination of these two types of training will maintain cardiorespiratory fitness and reduce muscle loss.

How much exercise must you perform during a weight-loss program? In general, exercise sessions designed to promote weight loss should expend more than 250 calories. Further, the negative caloric balance should be shared equally by exercise and diet. For instance, an individual who wishes to achieve a 500 calorie per day deficit should increase energy expenditure (exercise) by 250 calories per day and decrease caloric intake by 250 calories.

Although intensity of exercise is an important factor in improving cardiorespiratory fitness, it is the total

Alcohol contributes calories to the diet, so people trying to lose weight should restrict the amount of alcohol they consume or avoid it altogether.

amounts of energy expended and fat burned that are important in weight loss. Some authors have argued that low-intensity prolonged exercise (such as walking 1–2 miles a day) is better than short-term high-intensity exercise (e.g., sprinting 50 yards) in burning fat calories and promoting weight loss (18). However, evidence clearly demonstrates that both high- and low-intensity exercise can promote fat loss (4). Nonetheless, for the sedentary or obese individual, low-intensity exercise is the best choice because it can be performed for longer time periods and increases the ability of skeletal muscle to metabolize fat for energy (see the Appreciating Diversity box on page 250) (11, 15).

To determine your caloric expenditure (per minute) during an activity, simply multiply your body weight in kilograms (2.2 pounds = 1 kilogram) by the calories burned per minute, per kilogram (see Table 8.3 for the calories burned per minute of some common activities) and by the exercise time. For example, suppose a 70-kilogram (kg) individual plays 20 minutes of handball. How many calories did he or she expend

A CLOSER LOOK WHAT INTENSITY OF AEROBIC EXERCISE IS BEST FOR BURNING FAT?

Many people assume that the intensity of aerobic exercise (running, cycling, and so on) must be maintained at a low level if fat is to be burned as fuel. It is true that fat is a primary fuel source during low-intensity exercise. But as the figure in this box shows, the total amount of fat burned during exercise varies with the intensity of exercise, and for a given exercise duration, more total fat is metabolized during moderate-intensity exercise. Therefore, moderate-intensity exercise (that is, approximately 50% $\dot{V}O_2$max) is typically the optimal intensity of exercise for burning the most fat during an endurance exercise workout.

Source: Coyle, E. Fat metabolism during exercise. *Sports Science Exchange* (Gatorade Sports Science Institute) 8:6, 1995.

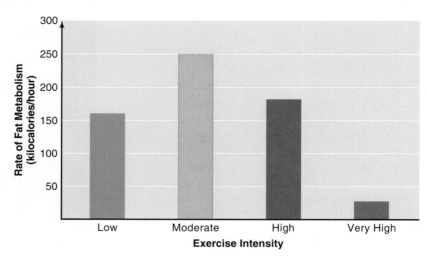

The rates of fat metabolism at low-intensity (20% $\dot{V}O_2$max), moderate-intensity (50% $\dot{V}O_2$max), high-intensity (80% $\dot{V}O_2$max), and very high intensity (100% $\dot{V}O_2$max) exercise. Although this figure is not intended to reveal any "ideal" exercise intensity for all individuals, it indicates that moderate-intensity exercise is often optimal for maximizing the amount of fat metabolized during exercise.

APPRECIATING DIVERSITY EXERCISE PRESCRIPTIONS FOR OBESE INDIVIDUALS

Although it is well established that exercise is an important factor in promoting weight loss, exercise prescriptions for obese individuals require special attention. For example, obese individuals may be limited by the following conditions: heat intolerance, shortness of breath during heavy exercise, lack of flexibility, frequent musculoskeletal injuries, hypertension, and a lack of balance during weight-bearing activities such as walking or running.

Exercise programs for obese individuals should emphasize activities that can be sustained for long periods of time (30 minutes or more), such as walking, swimming, water exercise, or bicycling. Further, obese people should avoid exercise in a hot or humid environment. The initial goal of the exercise program should not be to improve cardiovascular fitness, but rather to increase voluntary energy expenditure and to establish a regular exercise routine. Therefore, the beginning exercise intensity should be below the typical target heart rate range for improving cardiorespiratory fitness, and the initial duration of exercise should be short (about 5–10 min/day) to reduce the risk of soreness and injury. The duration can be gradually increased in 1-minute increments to achieve an energy expenditure

of approximately 300 kcal per workout. As the musculoskeletal system adapts to the exercise regimen, the intensity, too, can gradually be increased.

Sources: Fransen, M. Dietary weight loss and exercise for obese adults with knee osteoarthritis: Modest weight loss targets, mild exercise, modest effects. *Arthritis and Rheumatology* 50(5):1366–1369, 2004; Jakicic, J. M. Exercise in the treatment of obesity. *Endocrinology and Metabolic Clinics of North America* 32(4):967–980, 2003; and American College of Sports Medicine. Position stand: The recommended quantity and quality of exercise for developing and maintaining cardiorespiratory and muscular fitness, and flexibility in healthy adults. *Medicine and Science in Sports and Exercise* 30:975–991, 1998.

TABLE 8.3
Calories Expended during Selected Activities

Activity	Calories/Minute/Kilogram	Calories/Minute *	METs†
Bowling	0.0471	3.2	2.7
Golf	0.0559	3.8	3.2
Walking (17 min per mile)	0.0794	5.4	4.5
Tennis (doubles)	0.0882	6.0	5.1
Cycling (6.4 min per mile)	0.0985	6.7	5.6
Tennis (singles)	0.1029	7.0	5.8
Canoeing (15 min per mile)	0.1029	7.0	5.8
Swimming (50 yards per min)	0.1333	9.1	7.6
Running (10 min per mile)	0.1471	10.0	8.0
Cycling (5 min per mile)	0.1559	10.6	8.5
Handball (singles)	0.1603	10.9	9.1
Running (8 min per mile)	0.1856	12.6	10.0
Running (6 min mile)	0.2350	16.0	12.8

* These values are for a 150-lb (68-kg) person.
† 1 MET equals your resting metabolic rate.

Source: From Bud Getchell, *Physical Fitness: A Way of Life*, 5th ed. Copyright © 1998. Reprinted by permission of Pearson Education, Inc.

during the time of play? The total estimated caloric expenditure is computed as follows:

$$\text{Caloric expenditure} = 70 \text{ kg} \times 0.1603 \text{ calories/kg/min} \times 20 \text{ min} = 224 \text{ calories}$$

If your exercise routine involves using fitness equipment such as stationary bicycles, treadmills, or ellipticals, the machine will probably provide a summary of caloric expenditure at the end of your exercise bout.

Focus on Behavior Modification

Research demonstrates that behavior modification plays a key role in both achieving short-term weight loss and maintaining weight loss over the long term (12, 13). Many behaviors are learned and can therefore be modified. For example, many people eat popcorn and candy when they attend a movie at the theater. Similarly, a nightly television habit is often accompanied by snacking on chips, sodas, and other high-calorie, low-nutrition items. The fact that these behaviors are learned means that they can also be unlearned. In regard to weight control, behavior modification is used primarily to reduce or (ideally) eliminate social or environmental stimuli that promote overeating.

The first step in a diet-related behavior modification program is to identify those social or environmental factors that promote overeating. This can be done by keeping a written record of daily activities for 1 or 2 weeks to identify factors associated with consumption of high-calorie meals. Refer to the box on page 243 for common social and environmental factors that may contribute to your overeating. How many of these factors occur in your food diary?

After identifying the behaviors that contribute to weight gain, you can design a program to modify those behaviors. The following weight control techniques may make weight loss easier (14, 23).

- *Make a personal commitment to losing weight.* This is the first step toward behavior modification and weight loss. Establishing realistic short-term and long-term weight loss goals helps you maintain a lifelong commitment to weight management.

- *Develop healthy low-calorie eating patterns.* Avoid eating when you are not hungry. Learn to eat slowly and only while sitting at the table. Finally, keep food quantities to the minimum amount within your caloric guidelines.

- *Avoid social settings where you are likely to overeat.* If you go to parties where high-calorie foods are served, don't show up hungry. Eat a low-calorie meal before going.

- *Exercise daily.* Regular exercise that uses large-muscle groups can play an important role in increasing your daily caloric expenditure and can therefore assist in weight loss and weight management.

- *Reward yourself for successful weight loss with non-food rewards.* Positive feedback is an important part of behavior modification, and it doesn't have to relate to food to be effective. For example, after reaching your first short-term weight-loss goal, do something you like to do but don't get to do often, such as buying a new item of clothing or going to the movies.

- *Think positively.* Positive thinking promotes confidence and maintains the enthusiasm necessary for a lifetime of successful weight management.

Make sure you know...

> A safe rate of weight loss is 1 to 2 pounds per week; this equals approximately 3500 fewer calories consumed per week, or 500 fewer calories per day.

> There are four basic steps to designing a successful weight loss program: set realistic goals, assess and modify your diet, plan regular exercise, and modify your behavior.

Exercise and Diet Programs to Gain Weight

Thus far, this chapter has focused on how to lose body fat. However, some people may have the opposite problem—being underweight—and they may need to implement a program to gain weight. You can achieve weight gain by creating a positive energy balance, that is, by taking in more calories than you expend. When increasing body weight, however, you'll want to aim to increase muscle mass, rather than fat mass, for the sake of your health. Let's discuss how to do this.

The key to gaining muscle mass is a program of rigorous weight training combined with the increase in caloric intake needed to meet the increased energy expenditure and energy required to synthesize muscle. Exercise programs designed to improve muscular strength and size are discussed in Chapter 4 and are not addressed here. Here we focus on the dietary adjustments needed to optimize gains in muscle mass. Again, to gain muscle mass, you need to create a small positive caloric balance to provide the energy required to synthesize new muscle protein. Nonetheless, before we provide dietary guidelines, let's discuss how much energy is expended during weight training and how much energy is required to promote muscle growth.

Energy expenditure during routine weight training is surprisingly small. For instance, a 70-kg man performing a 30-minute weight workout probably burns fewer than 70 calories (14). The reason for this low caloric expenditure is that during 30 minutes in the weight room, the average person spends only 8 to 10 minutes lifting weights; much time is spent in recovery periods between sets.

Current estimates are that approximately 2500 calories are needed to synthesize one pound of muscle mass, of which about 400 calories (100 grams) must be protein (14). To compute the additional calories required to produce an increase in muscle mass, you must first estimate your rate of muscular growth. This is difficult because the rate of muscular growth during weight training varies among people. Although relatively large muscle mass gains are possible in some individuals, studies have shown that most men and women rarely gain more than 0.25 pound of muscle per week during a 20-week weight training program (3 days per week, 30 minutes per day). If we assume that the average muscle gain is 0.25 pound per week and that 2500 calories are required to synthesize one pound of muscle, a positive caloric balance of fewer than 100 calories per day is needed to promote muscle growth (0.25 pound per week × 2500 calories per pound = 625 calories per week; therefore, 625 calories per week ÷ 7 days per week = 90 calories per day).

You can use the MyPyramid food guidance system presented in Chapter 7 to increase your caloric intake. This will ensure that your diet meets the criteria for healthful living and provides adequate protein for building muscle. Be sure to avoid high-fat foods, and limit your positive caloric balance to approximately 90 calories per day. Increasing your positive caloric balance above this level will not promote a faster rate of muscular growth but will increase body fat. Finally, if you discontinue your weight-training program, be sure to lower your caloric intake to match your daily energy expenditure.

Make sure you know...

> Gaining weight can be achieved by creating a positive caloric balance. Before deciding to gain body fat, you should consider whether your current body composition is within your desired range.

> Gaining muscle mass can be achieved by combining exercise with proper nutrition.

Lifetime Weight Management

Weight loss and weight management are not short-term events. Maintaining a healthy body weight over the long term requires adherence to several healthy diet and exercise guidelines. If you diet and exercise for a while to lose weight but then slip into unhealthy habits of overeating or being too sedentary once the weight has come off, you will likely undo your efforts. And you may even gain more weight than you initially lost. This is the reason that short-term, fad diets are typically unsuccessful.

The key factors in long-term weight management are a positive attitude, regular exercise, and a personal commitment to maintaining a desired body composition. Like many other facets of personal or professional life, weight control has its ups and downs. Be prepared for occasional setbacks. For instance, many people gain weight during holiday periods. If this happens to you, avoid self-criticism, quickly reestablish your personal commitment to a short-term weight loss goal, and develop a new diet and exercise plan to lose the undesired fat. Remember, you can lose any amount of weight you've gained by applying the principles discussed in this chapter.

Finally, we cannot overemphasize the importance of family and friends in lifetime weight management. Their encouragement and support can help you maintain healthy long-term eating habits and sustain a commitment to exercise. Losing weight is much easier if the people close to you try to help you achieve your goals rather than tempt you into unhealthy behaviors. Encourage others to join you as you exercise. Your friends and family members may need a little encouragement to get started, but you may be the role model that they need to make the change. Children are especially susceptible to live the life that you model.

Extreme Measures for Weight Loss

Most people can attain a healthy body weight through diet and exercise, but for some extremely obese individuals, these may not be enough. In such cases, surgical procedures or prescription medications may be recommended by a health care provider.

Surgery

According to the American Society for Bariatric Surgery, surgical procedures may be recommended for weight loss in severely obese individuals. The surgery is considered a last resort in weight reduction for individuals who have tried and failed at losing weight and whose obesity poses a serious health risk. Weight-loss surgery is of two types: restrictive procedures and malabsorptive procedures. Restrictive procedures, such as gastric banding, work by decreasing the amount of food consumed at one time. The reduced stomach capacity, along with behavioral changes, can result in lower

Weatherman Al Roker is one individual who underwent gastric bypass surgery and lost more than 100 pounds. Such weight-loss measures are appropriate only for people with extreme obesity.

caloric intake and consistent weight loss. Malabsorptive procedures alter digestion by bypassing the small intestine, thus limiting the absorption of calories. The most common bariatric surgery is a combination of restrictive and malabsorptive procedures. The combination helps patients lose weight quickly and continue to lose weight for 18–24 months after the surgery (19).

Prescription Medications

Unlike diet pills, which are typically ineffective (Table 8.4), prescription medications such as orlistat and Meridia have been scientifically shown to help some people achieve weight loss. Orlistat (also called Xenical) works by preventing about one-third of ingested fat from being absorbed in the digestive tract. The undigested fat is eliminated in bowel movement; hence, one side effect may be an oily stool. Orlistat is the only FDA-approved weight-loss drug that acts to block fat absorption.

The prescription drug Meridia suppresses appetite by increasing serotonin levels in the brain. Meridia and Xenical are the only two weight-loss medications approved for longer term use in significantly obese people; however, their safety and effectiveness have not been established for use beyond 1 year.

TABLE 8.4
Myths and Facts about Weight Loss

Weight-Loss Myth	The Facts
Diet pills really work.	Most over-the-counter diet pills contain caffeine and other mild stimulants. Unfortunately, none of these products has been scientifically shown to assist in achieving safe and permanent weight loss. One study of individuals using commercially available diet pills reported that fewer than 3% lost weight and retained weight-loss longer than 12 months.
You can spot-reduce body fat.	There is no scientific evidence to show that exercising a specific area of the body promotes fat loss in that area (23). Rather, evidence suggests that when a caloric deficit exists, fat will be lost from areas where the most fat is stored (23).
Eating before bedtime causes weight gain.	Although eating a late-night meal or snack might not be a good dietary habit, this practice does not result in a greater weight gain than consuming the same meal at another time during the day. The total daily caloric intake determines fat gain, not the timing of the meal.
Cellulite is a special form of fat.	Although many people believe that cellulite is different from other body fat, this is not true. Cellulite is just plain fat, not a special type of fat. The "dimpled" appearance comes from accumulation of fat into small clusters beneath the skin. Many products, from special creams and lotions to massage appliances, are advertised as helping reduce cellulite, but no scientific evidence exists to support these claims. The only way to lose fat is to reduce calorie intake and increase exercise. Weight training helps tighten the skin over the muscle and eliminates space between the skin and muscle for fat pockets.
Saunas, steambaths, and rubber suits can aid in weight loss.	These methods do result in body water loss due to sweating. However, the weight is regained as soon as body water is restored to normal levels. Using saunas or steambaths and exercising while wearing a rubber suit may increase body temperature well above normal, which puts additional stress on the heart and circulatory system and could increase the risk of cardiac problems for older individuals or anyone with heart problems.

What Is Disordered Eating?

Although attaining a healthy body weight is a highly desirable goal, for some people the social pressures to be thin and/or muscular can lead to a negative body image and an unhealthy relationship with food. Women may feel like they need to emulate the often unattainably thin figures of popular actresses and models, or men may wish to achieve the bulked-up look of professional athletes, in the pursuit of a more "perfect" body. When these desires lead to unhealthy behaviors, such as bouts of self-starvation, binging, and/or purging, the individual may develop a pattern of disordered eating.

Three common conditions of disordered eating that affect young adults are anorexia nervosa, bulimia nervosa, and binge eating. Let's discuss the symptoms and health consequences of these conditions.

Anorexia Nervosa

Anorexia nervosa is an eating disorder in which the individual severely limits caloric intake, resulting in an eventual state of starvation. As the condition advances, the individual becomes emaciated. The psychological cause of anorexia nervosa is unclear, but it seems to be linked to an unfounded fear of fatness that may be related to familial or societal pressures to be thin (14).

Although the condition occurs in both men and women, rates of anorexia nervosa are particularly high among adolescent girls, and as many as 1 of every 100 adolescent girls may suffer from this condition. Anorexia nervosa affects approximately 1% of the female adolescent population, with an average age of onset between 14 and 18 years (20, 21). Upper-middle-class young women who are extremely self-critical have the highest probability of developing anorexia nervosa.

People suffering from anorexia nervosa may use a variety of techniques to remain thin, including starvation, excessive exercise, and laxatives. The effects of anorexia nervosa include excessive weight loss, cessation of menstruation, and, in extreme cases, death. Because the condition is a serious mental and physical disorder, medical treatment by a team of professionals (physician, psychologist, nutritionist) is needed to correct the problem. Treatment may require years of psychological counseling and nutritional guidance.

The first step in seeking treatment for anorexia nervosa is recognizing that a problem exists. The following common symptoms may indicate that someone is exhibiting anorexia nervosa:

- An intense fear of gaining weight or becoming obese
- The feeling that one is fat even at normal or below-normal body fatness because of a highly distorted body image
- In women, the absence of three or more menstrual cycles
- The possible development of odd behaviors concerning food; for example, preparing elaborate meals for others but only a few low-calorie foods for one's own consumption

CONSIDER THIS!

The average "female" store mannequin is 6 feet tall and has a 23-inch waist, whereas the average woman is 5 feet, 4 inches tall and has a 30-inch waist.

Bulimia Nervosa

About 50% of people with anorexia nervosa eventually suffer **bulimia nervosa,** which is characterized by cycles of binging and purging. People with bulimia nervosa may repeatedly ingest large quantities of food and then force themselves to vomit to prevent weight gain. The frequent vomiting associated with bulimia nervosa may result in damage to the teeth and the esophagus due to exposure to stomach acids. Like anorexia nervosa, bulimia nervosa is most common in young women, has a psychological origin, and requires professional treatment when diagnosed. Bulimia affects approximately 1–3% of adolescents in the United States. The illness usually begins in late adolescence or early adult life (21).

People with bulimia nervosa may look "normal" and be of normal weight. However, even when their bodies are slender, their stomachs may protrude because they have been stretched by frequent eating binges. Other common symptoms of bulimia nervosa include the following:

- Recurrent binge eating
- A lack of control over eating behavior
- Regular self-induced vomiting and/or use of diuretics or laxatives
- Strict fasting or use of vigorous exercise to prevent weight gain
- Averaging two or more binge eating episodes per week during a 2- to 3-month period
- Excessive concern with body shape and weight

Binge Eating Disorder

A disordered eating pattern that has recently begun to attract attention from the medical community is **binge eating disorder,** a condition in which an individual consumes mass quantities of food but, unlike people

People with anorexia nervosa restrict their caloric intake to the point of starvation.

anorexia nervosa An eating disorder in which a person severely restricts caloric intake because of an intense fear of gaining weight.

bulimia nervosa An eating disorder that involves overeating (called *binge eating*) followed by vomiting (called *purging*).

binge eating disorder The compulsive need to gorge on food without purging.

with bulimia nervosa, does not purge after binging. The person may feel embarrassed and ashamed about gorging and resolve to stop doing it, but the compulsion continues. The end result of consuming large quantities of food is that the person gains weight. The cause of binge eating is unknown, and only a very small percentage of overweight and obese individuals engage in binge eating.

Although maintaining an optimal body composition is a primary health goal, eating disorders are not appropriate means of weight loss. If you or any of your friends exhibit one or more of the symptoms cited here, please seek professional advice and treatment.

Make sure you know...

> Eating disorders such as anorexia nervosa, bulimia nervosa, and binge eating disorder involve patterns of severe calorie restriction, binging, and/or purging and can result in severe physical symptoms and possibly death.

Summary

1. Factors that can affect weight management include genetic, dietary, and lifestyle factors. Genetic disorders cause extreme obesity in about 1% of the population. For the rest, however, research supports that environmental and lifestyle factors are more likely to affect body weight than genetics.

2. Energy balance is achieved when the number of calories you take in through food and beverages equals the number of calories you expend through physical activity and normal body processes.

3. Total daily energy expenditure is the sum of resting metabolic rate and exercise metabolic rate.

4. Losing 1 to 2 pounds per week is considered a safe rate of weight loss. Body fat will be lost first in the areas of the body that store the most fat, such as the thighs and hips in women, and the abdominal region in men.

5. The four basic components of a comprehensive weight-control program are setting realistic goals for weight loss, assessing and modifying your diet, planning physical activity, and modifying your behaviors that contribute to weight gain.

6. Weight-loss goals should include both short-term and long-term goals.

7. People seeking to gain weight need to take in more calories than they expend. They should seek to gain muscle mass rather than fat by engaging in an appropriate strength-training program.

8. The eating disorders anorexia nervosa, bulimia nervosa, and binge eating disorder are serious medical conditions that require professional treatment.

Study Questions

1. The optimal percentage of body fat for men and women is
   a. 5–15% for men and 10–20% for women.
   b. 10–20% for men and 15–25% for women.
   c. 15–25% for men and 20–30% for women.
   d. 20–30% for men and 25–35% for women.

2. Hormones that play a role in appetite include which of the following?
   a. insulin
   b. ghrelin
   c. leptin
   d. estrogen
   e. both (a) and (d) are correct
   f. both (b) and (c) are correct

3. Identify the true statement regarding energy balance:
   a. Caloric intake should equal caloric expenditure.
   b. Weight gain occurs when caloric intake exceeds caloric expenditure.
   c. Weight loss occurs when caloric expenditure exceeds caloric intake.
   d. All of the above statements are true.

4. The two forms of exercise that are most beneficial in helping you lose and maintain weight are

   a. flexibility and Pilates training.

   b. yoga and anaerobic exercise.

   c. strength training and cardiorespiratory endurance training.

   d. Exercise is not helpful for weight loss.

5. Disordered eating includes all of the following except

   a. anorexia nervosa.

   b. bulimia nervosa.

   c. binge eating.

   d. using MyPyramid to plan a healthy diet.

6. What is optimal body weight, and how is optimal body weight calculated?

7. Explain the roles of resting metabolic rate and exercise metabolic rate in determining total caloric expenditure. Which is more important in total daily caloric expenditure in a sedentary individual?

8. Outline a simple method for computing your daily caloric expenditure. Give an example.

9. List the four major components of a weight-loss program.

10. Discuss the role of behavior modification in weight loss.

11. Compare and contrast the symptoms of anorexia nervosa, bulimia nervosa, and binge eating disorder.

12. Define the following terms:

   energy balance

   resting metabolic rate

   fad diet

13. Compare exercise metabolic rate with resting metabolic rate.

Suggested Reading

Donnelly, J., S. Blair, J. Jakicic, M. Manore, J. Rankin, and B. Smith. Appropriate physical activity intervention strategies for weight loss and prevention of weight regain for adults. (ACSM Position Stand). *Medicine and Science in Sports and Exercise* 41:459–471, 2009.

Gardner, C., A. Kiazand, S. Alhassan, S. Kim, R. Stafford, R. Balise, H. Kraemer, and A. King. Comparison of the Atkins, Zone, Ornish, and LEARN diets for change in weight and related risk factors among overweight premenopausal women: The A TO Z weight loss study: A randomized trial. *Journal of the American Medical Association* 297:969–977, 2007.

Martins, C., L. Morgan, and H. Truby. A review of the effects of exercise on appetite regulation: An obesity perspective. *International Journal of Obesity* 32:1337–1347, 2008.

Powers, S., and E. Howley. *Exercise Physiology: Theory and Application to Fitness and Performance*, 7th ed. New York: McGraw-Hill, 2009.

Sherer, E., and J. Sherer. Examining the most popular weight loss diets: How effective are they? *Journal of the American Academy of Physician Assistants* 21:31–34, 2008.

Volpe, S. L. Popular weight reduction diets. *Journal of Cardiovascular Nursing* 21:34–39, 2006.

For links to the organizations and websites listed below, visit The Total Fitness and Wellness Website at www.pearsonhighered.com/powers.

American Dietetic Association

Contains articles about nutrition and fad diets.

MyPyramid.gov

Walks you through the advice illustrated in the MyPyramid food guidance system.

References

1. Kopelman, P. G. Obesity as a medical problem. *Nature* 404:635–643, 2000.

2. Serdula, M. K., A. H. Mokdad, D. F. Williamson, D. A. Galuska, J. M. Mendlein, and G. W. Heath. Prevalence of attempting weight loss and strategies for controlling weight. *Journal of the American Medical Association* 282:1353–1358, 1999.

3. American Society for Metabolic and Bariatric Surgery. News Release: Bariatric Surgical Society Takes on New Name, New Mission and New Surgery. August 22, 2007. www.asbs.org/Newsite07/resources/press_release_8202007.pdf.

4. Powers, S., and E. Howley. *Exercise Physiology: Theory and Application to Fitness and Performance*, 7th ed. New York: McGraw-Hill, 2009.

5. Raloff, J. Still hungry? Fattening revelations—and new mysteries—about the hunger hormone. *Science News Online* 167: April 2, 2005.

6. Frubeck, G., J. Gomez-Amrosi, F. Muruzabal, and M. Burrell. The adipocyte: A model for integration of endocrine and metabolic signaling in energy metabolism regulation. *American Journal of Physiology* 280: E827–E847, 2001.

7. Kraemer, R. R., and V. D. Castracane. Exercise and humoral mediators of peripheral energy balance: Ghrelin and adiponectin. *Experimental Biology and Medicine* 232:184–194, 2007.

8. Cummings, D. E., D. S. Weigle, R. S. Frayo, P. A. Breen, M. K., Ma, E. P. Dellinger, and J. Q. Purnell. Plasma ghrelin levels after diet-induced weight loss or gastric bypass surgery. *New England Journal of Medicine* 346:1623–1630, 2002.

9. Bailey, J., R. Barker, and R. Beauchene. Age-related changes in rat adipose tissue cellularity are altered by dietary restriction and exercise. *Journal of Nutrition* 123:52–58, 1993.

10. Blair, S. Evidence for success of exercise in weight loss control. *Annals of Internal Medicine* 119:702–706, 1993.

11. Poehlman, E. A review: Exercise and its influence on resting energy metabolism in man. *Medicine and Science in Sports and Exercise* 21:515–525, 1989.

12. Bjorntorp, P., and B. Brodoff, eds. *Obesity*. Philadelphia: Lippincott, 1992.

13. Perri, M., A. Nezu, and B. Viegener. *Improving the Long-term Management and Treatment of Obesity*. New York: John Wiley and Sons, 1992.

14. Williams, M. *Lifetime Fitness and Wellness*. Dubuque, IA: Wm. C. Brown, 1996.

15. Ross, R., J. Freeman, and I. Janssen. Exercise alone is an effective strategy for reducing obesity and related co-morbidities. *Exercise and Sport Sciences Reviews* 28(4):165–170, 2000.

16. Jakicic, J. et al. Appropriate intervention strategies for weight loss and prevention of weight regain for adults.

(ACSM Position Stand). *Medicine and Science in Sports and Exercise* 33:2145–2156, 2001.

17. Broeder, C., K. Burrhus, L. Svanevik, and J. Wilmore. The effects of either high intensity resistance or endurance training on resting metabolic rate. *American Journal of Clinical Nutrition* 55:802–810, 1992.

18. Romijn, J., E. Coyle, L. Sidossis, et al. Regulation of endogenous fat and carbohydrate metabolism in relation to exercise and duration. *American Journal of Physiology* 265:E380–E391, 1993.

19. Weight-control Information Network. Gastrointestinal surgery for severe obesity. NIH Publication no. 04-4006. December 2004. http://win.niddk.nih.gov/publications/gastric.htm.

20. American Psychiatric Association. APA Expert Opinion: Pauline S. Powers, MD. http:/healthyminds.org/expertopinion9.cfm. Accessed July 2007.

21. Office on Women's Health, U.S. Department of Health and Human Services. Eating disorders. February 2000. www.4woman.gov.owh/pub/factsheets/eatingdisorders.pdf.

22. Johnson, R., M. Segal, Y. Sautin, T. Nakagawa, D. Feig, D. Kang, M. Gersh, S. Benner, and L. Sanchez-Lozada. Potential role of sugar (fructose) in the epidemic of hypertension, obesity and the metabolic syndrome, diabetes, kidney disease, and cardiovascular disease. *American Journal of Clinical Nutrition* 86:899–906, 2007.

23. Gardner, C., A. Kiazand, S. Alhassan, S. Kim, R. Stafford, R. Balise, H. Kraemer, and A. King. Comparison of the Atkins, Zone, Ornish, and LEARN diets for change in weight and related risk factors among overweight premenopausal women: The A TO Z weight loss study: A randomized trial. *Journal of the American Medical Association* 297:969–977, 2007.

Videos

Log on to www.pearsonhighered.com/powers to view these chapter-related videos.

Managing Your Weight
Food Diary Diet

NAME _____ DATE _____

Determining Ideal Body Weight Using Percent Body Fat and the Body Mass Index

There are several different ways to compute an ideal body weight. In Chapter 6 we discussed body fat percentage (estimated from skinfold measurements). Method A of this laboratory enables you to compute and record your ideal body weight using that method. Method B enables you to calculate and record your ideal body weight using the body mass index (BMI) procedure (Chapter 6). Choose one of these techniques, and complete the appropriate section.

Method A: Computing Ideal Body Weight Using Percent Body Fat

Step 1: Calculate fat-free weight

100% − your percent body fat estimated from skinfold measurement = _____ % fat free weight.

Therefore,

_____ % fat–free weight expressed as a decimal × _____ your body weight in pounds

= _____ pounds of fat–free weight.

Step 2: Calculate optimal weight

Remember: Optimal body fat ranges are 10–20% for men and 15–25% for women.

Optimal weight = fat–free weight ÷ (1.00 − optimal %fat), with optimal %fat expressed as a decimal. Therefore, the low and high optimal weight ranges for your gender are as follows:

For low %fat: Optimal weight _____ pounds
For high %fat: Optimal weight _____ pounds

Method B: Computing Ideal Body Weight Using Body Mass Index (BMI)

The BMI uses the metric system. Therefore, you must express your weight in kilograms (1 kilogram = 2.2 pounds) and your height in meters (1 inch = 0.0254 meter).

Step 1: Compute your BMI

BMI = body weight (kg) ÷ (height in meters)^2
Your BMI = _____

Step 2: Calculate your ideal body weight based on BMI*

The ideal BMI is 21.9 to 22.4 for men and 21.3 to 22.1 for women. The formula for computing ideal body weight using BMI is

$$\text{Ideal body weight (kilograms)} = \text{Desired BMI} \times (\text{height in meters})^2$$

Consider the following example as an illustration of the computation of ideal body weight. A man who weighs 60 kilograms and is 1.5 meters tall computes his BMI to be 26.7. His ideal BMI is between 21.9 and 22.4; therefore, his ideal body weight range is as follows:

Low end range: $21.9 \times 2.25 = 49.3$ kilograms
High end of range: $22.4 \times 2.2550.4$ kilograms

Now complete this calculation using your values for BMI.

My ideal body weight range using the BMI method is _____ to _____ kilograms.

*Note: BMI may not be a good method to determine ideal body weight for a highly muscled individual.

Estimating Daily Caloric Expenditure and the Caloric Deficit Required to Lose 1 Pound of Fat per Week

Part A: Estimating Your Daily Caloric Expenditure

Using Table 8.1, compute your estimated daily caloric expenditure.

Estimated daily caloric expenditure = _____ calories/day.

Note: For you to maintain current body weight, your caloric intake should equal your daily caloric expenditure.

Part B: Calculating Caloric Intake Required to Promote 1 Pound Per Week of Weight Loss

Recall that 1 pound of fat contains approximately 3500 calories. Therefore, a negative caloric balance of 500 calories per day will result in a weight loss of 1 pound per week. Use the following formula to compute your daily caloric intake to result in a daily caloric deficit of 500 calories.

Estimated daily caloric expenditure − 500 calories (deficit) = Daily caloric intake

needed to produce a 500−calorie deficit

In the space provided, compute your daily caloric intake needed to produce 1 pound per week of weight loss.

_____ (estimated caloric expenditure)
− 500 (caloric deficit)
= _____ (target daily caloric intake)

Note: To increase body weight by 1–2 pounds per week, increase daily caloric intake by 90–180 calories per day.

NAME _____   DATE _____

Weight-Loss Goals and Progress Report

In the spaces provided, record your short-term and long-term weight-loss goals. Then keep a record of your progress on the chart.

Ideal body weight (range): _____

Short-term weight loss goal: ____1–2____ (pounds/week)

Long-term weight loss goal: _____ pounds

Week No.	Body Weight	Date	Weight Loss
1			
2			
3			
4			
5			
6			
7			
8			
9			
10			
11			
12			
13			
14			
15			

NAME _____ DATE _____

Assessing Body Image

Respond to the questions below to assess your body image.

1. Where do you get your ideas about the "ideal body"? If more than one applies, how do they rank?

   a. TV/movies _____

   b. friends (including boyfriends and girlfriends) _____

   c. parents and family _____

   d. professional athletes _____

2. What other sources contribute to your image of the "ideal body"?

   _____

   _____

   Fill in the blanks to complete the following statements about your body image. Use extra paper if needed.

3. The thing I like most about my body is

   _____

   _____

4. The thing I like least about my body is

   _____

   _____

5. When I eat a big meal, I feel

   _____

   _____

6. When I look in the mirror, I see

   _____

   _____

7. I like/dislike (circle one) shopping for clothes because

   _____

   _____

8. I feel self-conscious when

   _____

   _____

9. Compared to others, I feel my body is

   _____

   _____

LABORATORY

10. In the presence of someone I find attractive, I feel

_____

_____

11. I feel that my appearance is

_____

_____

12. One word to describe my body is

_____

Interpretation

Now review your answers to the previous questions and think about whether they are positive or negative. To improve a negative body image, keep the following strategies in mind:

- Focus on good physical health. Engage in physical activities that you enjoy.
- Remember that your self-worth is not dependent on how you look.
- Avoid chronic, restrained dieting.
- Recognize that there is much more to you than your body. Think about the qualities that you like best about yourself, and be sure to appreciate them.

NAME _____ DATE _____

What Triggers Your Eating?

There are many things that cause us to eat. Usually, just by identifying the triggers that cause you to eat, you can develop a strategy to counter those habits. Use the questions below to determine your motivation for eating. For each statement, check yes or no.

Emotional Triggers

Yes   No

___   ___   I cannot lose weight and keep it off.

___   ___   My eating is out of control.

___   ___   Even if I'm not hungry, I eat.

___   ___   I eat when I am stressed or upset.

___   ___   Food gives me great pleasure and I use it as a reward.

___   ___   Eating is usually on my mind.

___   ___   My eating causes problems with weight management.

___   ___   I go on eating "binges" or find myself eating constantly.

___   ___   My eating habits cause me embarrassment.

___   ___   I use food to help me cope with feelings.

Social Triggers

Yes   No

___   ___   I eat whenever others around me are eating.

___   ___   If anyone offers food, I take it.

___   ___   Whenever I am in a stressful social situation, I want to eat.

___   ___   Whenever I am in a relaxed social situation, I want to eat.

___   ___   I eat more in a social setting than I do at home.

___   ___   I eat less when others are around to see me.

___   ___   In a social setting, the amount of food I eat depends on the group of people.

___   ___   I eat different foods in a social setting than I do at home.

Environmental Triggers

Yes   No

___   ___   I eat more at restaurants than I do at home.

___   ___   I eat less at restaurants than I do at home.

___   ___   If I smell or see food I can't resist the urge to eat.

___   ___   If I walk by a restaurant or bakery I can't resist the urge to eat.

___   ___   I like to eat while reading or watching TV.

___   ___   I find food comforting in different environmental conditions, such as on a rainy day or in cold weather.

___   ___   I find food comforting when I am in unfamiliar surroundings.

___   ___   If I am outdoors, I feel like I can eat more.

Interpretation

Insignificant influence: If you answered yes to one question within a section or fewer than six questions total, weight management is probably relatively easy for you.

Some influence: If you answered yes to two questions within a section or six to nine questions total, there are issues complicating your weight management. It might help to talk with a health care professional while developing a weight management plan.

Significant influence: If you answered yes to three questions within a section or 10–13 questions total, there are several issues affecting your weight management plan. Speaking with a health care professional or counselor can help you deal with issues that trigger your eating.

Severe influence: If you answered yes to four or more questions within a section or 14 or more questions total, there are many issues that complicate your weight management. Counseling and speaking with a health care professional will help you to develop a weight-management plan.

Preventing Cardiovascular Disease

9

true or false?

1. Smoking has no effect on heart health.

2. As long as you consume no more than 5 teaspoons of salt per day, you don't have to worry about its effect on your blood pressure.

3. Cardiovascular disease is caused primarily by inherited factors, so there's not much you can do to prevent it.

4. A sedentary lifestyle contributes to the likelihood of developing heart disease.

5. Before the age of 50, men are more likely to die of a heart attack than women.

Answers appear on the next page.

Have you ever known someone who's been the victim of a heart attack or stroke? If so, perhaps you're familiar with the symptoms that occur during a heart attack or with the weeks and months of rehabilitation necessary for stroke survivors to return to a "normal" life. Every year, more than 900,000 people die from these two conditions, and another 1.9 million people are permanently injured. Although genetics plays a role in cardiovascular disease in some people, most people can reduce their risk by adopting healthy diet and lifestyle habits. In this chapter, we'll explore the particulars of cardiovascular disease. We'll also focus on lifestyle changes (e.g., exercise and diet) that can reduce your risk of cardiovascular diseases.

What Is Cardiovascular Disease and How Prevalent Is It?

Cardiovascular disease (CVD) is a major health problem around the world, but its greatest incidence occurs in industrialized countries, and the United States has one of the world's highest CVD death rates (1). Although it is impossible to place a dollar value on human life, the economic cost of cardiovascular disease in the United States is great (Figure 9.1). Estimates of lost wages, medical expenses, and other related costs exceeded $475 billion in 2009 (2). Developing a national strategy to reduce the risk of cardiovascular disease is a major heath priority. Let's begin our discussion with an overview of cardiovascular disease in the United States.

Cardiovascular Disease in the United States

Although public awareness is currently more focused on diseases such as cancer and AIDS, cardiovascular disease remains the number-one cause of death in the United States, accounting for nearly one of every two deaths. More than 80 million adults have one or more forms of CVD, and over 1 million people die annually from cardiovascular disorders (1). CVD is the leading cause of death in men between the ages of 35 and 44, and its incidence among women is rising (1).

Types of Cardiovascular Disease

There are hundreds of diseases that can impair normal cardiovascular function. The four most common are arteriosclerosis, coronary heart disease, stroke, and hypertension. Let's look at each of these in more depth.

Arteriosclerosis **Arteriosclerosis** is a group of diseases characterized by a narrowing, or "hardening," of the arteries. The end result of any form of arteriosclerosis is a progressive blockage of the artery, which eventually impedes blood flow to vital organs. **Atherosclerosis** is a special type of arteriosclerosis that results in arterial blockage due to buildup of a fatty deposit inside the blood vessel (Figure 9.2). This plaque deposit is typically composed of cholesterol, cellular debris, fibrin (a clotting material in the blood), and calcium. Atherosclerosis is a progressive disease that begins in childhood, and symptoms appear later in life. The disease occurs in varying degrees, with some arteries exhibiting little blockage and others exhibiting major obstruction. Development of severe atherosclerosis within arteries that supply blood to the heart is the cause of almost all heart attacks.

Answers

1. FALSE Smoking is a major risk factor for the development of cardiovascular disease.

2. FALSE For salt-sensitive people, consuming high levels of salt (which contains sodium) may increase blood pressure.

3. FALSE Heredity is only one of several major risk factors for heart disease. There are several other major risk factors you can modify by changing your behavior (e.g., stop smoking; be more active).

4. TRUE Inactivity is a major risk factor for developing heart disease.

5. TRUE Throughout their younger years, men are at greater risk of dying of a heart attack than women. However, after age 65, the risk of dying from heart disease increases markedly in women.

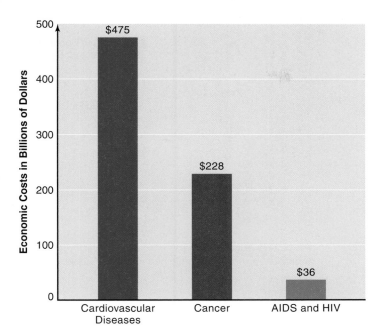

FIGURE 9.1

Comparison of the economic costs of cardiovascular diseases with cancer (second leading killer) and AIDS/HIV in the United States. Economic costs include both health care costs and loss of wages.

Source: Heart disease and stroke statistics—2009 update. *Circulation* 119:e21–e181, 2009.

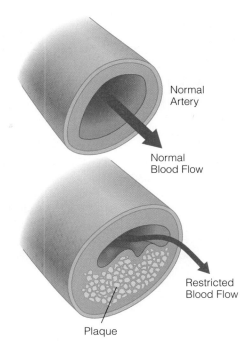

FIGURE 9.2

As plaque builds up in an artery, blood flow is restricted.

Source: From Joan Salge Blake, *Nutrition & You,* p. 152. Copyright © 2008 by Pearson Education, Inc. publishing as Benjamin Cummings. Reprinted by permission.

Coronary Heart Disease **Coronary heart disease (CHD)** is the result of atherosclerotic plaque blocking one or more blood vessels that supply the heart. When a major coronary artery becomes more than 75% blocked, the restriction of blood flow to the heart muscle causes chest pain. This type of chest pain, called *angina pectoris*, occurs most frequently during exercise or emotional stress, when the heart rate increases and the heart works harder than normal (3). The elevated heart work requires an increase in blood flow to the heart muscle to provide both oxygen and nutrients. Blockage of coronary blood vessels by atherosclerotic plaque prevents the necessary increase in blood flow to the heart, and pain results.

If coronary arteries are severely blocked, a blood clot can form around the layer of plaque. If the resulting blockage completely impedes blood flow to the heart, a **heart attack** can occur (Figure 9.3). A heart attack results in the death of heart muscle cells in the left ventricle, and the severity of the heart attack is judged by how many heart muscle cells are damaged (24). A "mild" heart attack may damage only a small portion of the heart, whereas a "major" heart attack may destroy a large number of heart muscle cells. Because the number of heart muscle cells destroyed during a heart attack determines the patient's chances of

recovery, recognizing the symptoms of a heart attack and getting prompt medical attention are crucial (see the Closer Look box, page 273).

Stroke Each year, an estimated 795,000 Americans suffer a **stroke** (1), during which the blood supply to the brain is reduced for a prolonged period of time. A common cause of stroke is blockage (due to atherosclerosis) of arteries leading to the brain (Figure 9.4). However, strokes can also occur when a blood vessel in the brain ruptures and disturbs normal blood flow to that region of the brain.

cardiovascular disease (CVD) Any disease that affects the heart or blood vessels.

arteriosclerosis A group of diseases characterized by a narrowing, or "hardening," of the arteries.

atherosclerosis A special type of arteriosclerosis that results in arterial blockage due to buildup of a fatty deposit (called *atherosclerotic plaque*) inside the blood vessel.

coronary heart disease (CHD) Also called *coronary artery disease*; the result of atherosclerotic plaque blocking one or more coronary arteries (the blood vessels that supply the heart).

heart attack Stoppage of blood flow to the heart resulting in the death of heart cells; also called *myocardial infarction*.

stroke Brain damage that occurs when the blood supply to the brain is reduced for a prolonged period of time.

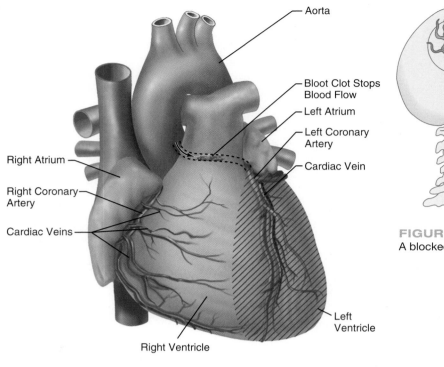

Aorta

Bloot Clot Stops Blood Flow

Left Atrium

Left Coronary Artery

Cardiac Vein

Right Atrium

Right Coronary Artery

Cardiac Veins

Left Ventricle

Right Ventricle

Indicates Area of Heart Damaged during Heart Attack

FIGURE 9.3

If the coronary arteries become blocked, the lack of oxygen due to restricted blood flow will lead to damaged muscle tissue.

Source: Michael D. Johnson, *Human Biology: Concepts and Current Issues*, 4th ed., p. 172. Copyright © 2008 Pearson Education, Inc. publishing as Benjamin Cummings. Reprinted by permission.

Area of Brain Damage Due to Reduced Blood Flow

Blot Clot Stops Blood Flow

FIGURE 9.4

A blocked artery in the brain can result in a stroke.

Similar to a heart attack, which results in death of heart cells, a stroke results in death of brain cells. The severity of the stroke may vary from slight to severe, depending on the location and the number of brain cells damaged. Minor strokes may involve a loss of memory, speech problems, disturbed vision, and/or mild paralysis in the extremities. Severe strokes may result in major paralysis or death.

Hypertension **Hypertension** is abnormally high blood pressure. Your blood pressure is the force blood exerts against the artery walls. When the heart contracts, blood pressure increases, and it decreases when the heart relaxes. Blood pressure is measured in millimeters of mercury (mm Hg) and is expressed with two numbers: the systolic blood pressure (pressure when your heart contracts) and the diastolic

CONSIDER THIS!

40% of heart attack victims die within the first hour.

blood pressure (pressure when your heart relaxes). Normal systolic blood pressure is typically 120 mm Hg, and normal diastolic is 80 mm Hg. Clinically, hypertension is defined as a resting blood pressure over 140 mm Hg systolic or 90 mm Hg diastolic (3).

Your blood pressure will increase during periods of exertion, such as during exercise. This increase in blood pressure is short term and does not cause damage. However, longer-term, acute hypertension can be a significant health problem. High blood pressure increases the workload on the heart, which may eventually damage the heart muscle's ability to pump blood effectively throughout the body (3). High blood pressure may also damage the lining of arteries, resulting in atherosclerosis and therefore increasing the risk of CHD and stroke (3).

Several factors can increase your risk of hypertension, including lack of exercise, a high-salt diet, obesity, chronic stress, family history of hypertension, gender (men have a greater risk than women), and race (blacks have a greater risk than whites). Note that you can control some of these factors, but cannot control others (more on this later in the chapter).

The prevalence of hypertension in the United States is remarkably high (Figure 9.5). The American Heart Association estimates that approximately one of

A CLOSER LOOK

DURING A HEART ATTACK, EVERY SECOND COUNTS

I f you ever witness someone having a heart attack, or have one yourself, recognizing the symptoms and taking appropriate emergency action could mean the difference between life and death.

Here are the common signs of a heart attack (3):

- Mild to moderate pain in the chest that may spread to the shoulders, neck, or arms

- Uncomfortable pressure or sensation of fullness in the chest

- Severe pain in the chest

- Dizziness, fainting, sweating, nausea, or shortness of breath

Note that not all of these symptoms occur in every heart attack. Therefore, if you or someone you're with experiences any one of these symptoms for 2 minutes or more, call the emergency medical service or get to the nearest hospital that offers emergency cardiac care. If you are trained in cardiopulmonary resuscitation (CPR) and the patient is not breathing or does not have a pulse, call 911 or the emergency medical service in your area, and then start CPR immediately. In any cardiac emergency, rapid action is essential.

---

every three people suffers from hypertension—that is, more than 73 million people (1). Unfortunately, the symptoms of hypertension, such as severe headaches or dizziness, don't show up in everyone, so many people are unaware that they are hypertensive. In fact, without annual medical checkups or blood pressure screenings, hypertension may go undiagnosed for years. For this reason, hypertension is often called the "silent killer."

FIGURE 9.5
One in three Americans will develop hypertension.

Source: Heart disease and stroke statistics—2009 update. *Circulation* 119:e21–e181, 2009.

Make sure you know...

> Cardiovascular disease is the number-one cause of death in the United States.

> The term *cardiovascular disease* refers to any disease that affects the heart or blood vessels.

> The four major cardiovascular diseases are arteriosclerosis, coronary heart disease, stroke, and hypertension.

What Are the Risk Factors Associated with Coronary Heart Disease?

Because CHD is the leading contributor to heart attacks, researchers are focused on reducing its occurrence and understanding its causes. They have identified a number of major and contributory risk factors that increase the chance of developing both CHD and stroke. Major risk factors (also called *primary risk factors*) are directly related to the development of CHD and stroke. In contrast, contributory risk factors (or *secondary risk factors*) are those that increase the risk of CHD but whose direct contribution to the disease process has not been precisely determined.

hypertension High blood pressure.

Major Risk Factors

Each year the American Heart Association publishes new information concerning the major risk factors associated with the development of CHD and stroke. The most recent list includes tobacco smoking, hypertension, high blood cholesterol levels, physical inactivity, obesity and overweight, diabetes mellitus, heredity, gender, and increasing age (1). The greater the number of CHD risk factors an individual has, the greater the likelihood that he or she will develop CHD (Figure 9.6).

Smoking A smoker's risk of developing CHD is more than twice that of a nonsmoker (1). Smoking is also considered the biggest risk factor for sudden death due to cardiac arrest, a heart attack, or irregular heartbeats **(arrhythmias).** In addition, smoking promotes the development of atherosclerosis in peripheral blood vessels (such as in the arms or legs), which can lead to hypertension and increased risk of stroke. Finally, smokers who have a heart attack are more likely to die suddenly (within an hour after the attack) than are nonsmokers. Numerous studies have also concluded that passive inhalation of cigarette smoke can increase the risk for both cardiovascular and lung disease (4).

Cigarette smoking can influence your risk of CHD in at least four ways. First, the nicotine in cigarette

CONSIDER THIS!

Within 10 years of quitting smoking, a person's risk of death from CHD is reduced to a level equal to that of someone who has never smoked.

smoke increases both heart rate and blood pressure. Second, smoking increases the stickiness of the platelets in your blood, increasing the likelihood of clotting and raising the risk of heart attack. Third, nicotine also influences the way your heart functions, leading to arrhythmias, which can in turn lead to sudden cardiac death. Finally, cigarette smoking increases your chance of developing atherosclerosis by elevating the amount of cholesterol in the blood and encouraging fat deposits in arterial walls (4). Women who smoke and take birth control pills are at an even higher risk. Furthermore, studies show that they have a much greater risk of heart attack and are much more likely to have a stroke than women who don't smoke (1).

Hypertension Hypertension is unique because it is both a disease in its own right and a risk factor for stroke and CHD. It contributes to CHD by accelerating the rate of atherosclerosis development (3, 5).

A diet high in sodium (such as from processed foods and/or table salt) increases the risk of developing hypertension. High plasma levels of sodium expand the blood volume and therefore increase blood pressure. Although sodium is a required micronutrient, the daily requirement for most people is small (less than one-fourth teaspoon, or 400 mg). Some individuals are more sodium sensitive than others, and sodium-sensitive individuals with hypertension can often lower

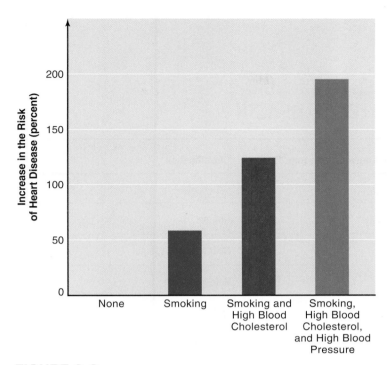

FIGURE 9.6
Your risk of developing CHD increases as the number of risk factors increases.

more than 1 teaspoon of per day are at risk for developing hypertension.

Even athletes or laborers who lose large amounts of water and electrolytes via sweat rarely require more than 1.5 teaspoons (3000 mg) of salt per day. Currently, many U.S. citizens consume more than 6 teaspoons (12,000 mg) of salt per day; clearly, this level of sodium intake is beyond the amount needed for normal body function.

The key to lowering your sodium intake is avoiding foods that are high in salt. Table 9.1 lists some common foods that are high in sodium. Take the time to learn which foods contain a lot of sodium, and limit your intake of sodium to less than 1 teaspoon per day (6). Because of the link between hypertension and salt intake, the National Institutes of Health has developed a Dietary Approach to Stop Hypertension (called DASH). This DASH eating plan is recognized as an excellent approach to prevent and lower hypertension. For more details on the DASH eating plan, see www.nhlbi.nih.gov/health/public/heart/hbp/dash/new_dash.pdf.

their blood pressure by reducing their salt intake. For example, people who ingest less than 1/2 teaspoon of sodium each day typically do not develop hypertension. In contrast, sodium-sensitive people who consume

High Blood Cholesterol Levels   As discussed in Chapter 7, cholesterol is a type of lipid that can either be consumed in foods or be synthesized in the body, and it is a primary risk factor for CHD. The risk of CHD increases as the blood cholesterol increases.

Because cholesterol is not soluble in blood, it is combined with proteins in the liver so it can be transported in the bloodstream. This combination of cholesterol and protein results in two major forms of cholesterol: **low-density lipoproteins (LDL)** and **high-density lipoproteins (HDL).** The association between elevated blood cholesterol and CHD is due primarily to LDL. Individuals with high blood LDL levels have an increased risk of CHD, whereas those with high levels of HDL have a decreased risk of CHD (1, 3, 7, 8). Because of these relationships, LDL has been called "bad cholesterol," whereas HDL has been called "good cholesterol."

TABLE 9.1
Sodium Content of Selected Foods

Food	Serving Size	Sodium Content (mg)
Bologna	2 oz	700
Cheese		
American	1 oz	305
Cheddar	1 oz	165
Parmesan	1 oz	525
Frankfurter	1	495
Hamburger patty	1 small	550
Pickle (dill)	1 medium	900
Pizza (cheese)	1 slice (14-inch diameter)	600
Potato chips	20	300
Pretzels	1 oz	890
Canned soup		
Chicken noodle	1 cup	1010
Vegetable beef	1 cup	1046
Soy sauce	1 tablespoon	1320

arrhythmia An irregular heartbeat.

low-density lipoproteins (LDL) A combination of protein, fat, and cholesterol in the blood, composed of relatively large amounts of cholesterol. LDLs promote the fatty plaque accumulation in the coronary arteries that leads to heart disease; also called "bad" cholesterol.

high-density lipoproteins (HDL) A combination of protein, fat, and cholesterol in the blood, composed of relatively large amounts of protein. Protects against the fatty plaque accumulation in the coronary arteries that leads to heart disease; also called "good" cholesterol.

A CLOSER LOOK BLOOD CHOLESTEROL GUIDELINES FROM THE NATIONAL INSTITUTES OF HEALTH

In response to studies conclusively showing that lowering blood LDL ("bad cholesterol") levels can reduce the risk of heart disease by 40% (7), the National Institutes of Health (NIH) has released guidelines for optimal blood levels of LDL and HDL. Even though the major focus of the guidelines is recommendations for managing blood LDL levels, NIH included recommendations for blood levels of HDL ("good cholesterol") because HDL can carry cholesterol away from arteries and back to the liver. The guidelines are summarized in the table.

In short, the guidelines consider LDL levels of 100 mg/dl or lower to be optimal for reducing the risk of developing CHD, whereas LDL levels above 190 mg/dl are considered indicative of a high risk for CHD. Because the presence of HDL can lower LDL levels, low blood levels of HDL can indicate an increased risk of developing CHD. Accordingly, the guidelines consider blood HDL levels below 40 mg/dl to be low and undesirable in terms of CHD risk.

Cholesterol Concentration (mg/dl)	Classification
LDL	
<100	Optimal
100–129	Near or above optimal
130–159	Borderline high
160–189	High
>190	Very high
HDL	
<40	Low (undesirable)
>60	High (very desirable)

Even though the risk of developing CHD is best predicted from LDL and HDL levels in the blood, measurement of total blood cholesterol (the sum of all types of cholesterol) also provides a good indication of CHD risk (1, 3, 8). A total blood cholesterol concentration that is less than 200 mg/dl (milligrams per deciliter) indicates a low risk of developing CHD, whereas a concentration that is greater than 240 mg/dl indicates a high CHD risk (3, 8). Unfortunately, because of high-fat diets and lack of exercise, more than 34 million people in the United States have total blood cholesterol levels above 240 mg/dl (1).

The National Institutes of Health released new guidelines for assessing CHD risks using blood levels of LDL and HDL. For a brief overview of these guidelines, see the Closer Look box above.

Physical Inactivity The first evidence that physical activity reduces the risk of heart disease emerged more than 50 years ago (9). An interesting study compared the rates of CHD between bus conductors and bus drivers in London, England. Whereas the conductors spent their days walking up and down the stairs of "double-decker" London buses collecting tickets, the bus drivers remained seated and sedentary throughout the workday. This study found that the rate of CHD was much higher in the sedentary bus drivers than in the more physically active conductors. Since this initial study, numerous investigations have consistently reported that regular physical activity reduces the risk of developing CHD (8, 10–14).

Although it is well known that exercise reduces the risk of CHD, the mechanism by which this works is unclear. Possible explanations include improvements in

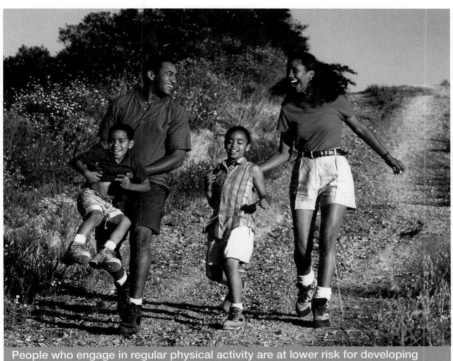
People who engage in regular physical activity are at lower risk for developing heart disease.

ment of CHD. The physiological reason for the link between CHD and regional fat distribution may be that people with high waist-to-hip circumference ratios often eat high-fat diets, which elevate blood cholesterol levels.

Possible causes of hypertension in obese individuals include high sodium intake, which elevates blood pressure, and increased vascular resistance, which results in the need for higher pressure to pump blood to the tissues (3).

Heredity Children of parents with CHD are more likely to develop CHD than are children of parents who do not have CHD (1, 3). Evidence suggests that the familial risk for CHD may be linked to factors such as high blood cholesterol, hypertension, diabetes, and obesity. People with a family history of CHD are not doomed to develop this disease, but to reduce their risk, they will have to work harder to develop a healthy lifestyle.

Gender Up to age 55, men have a greater risk of developing CHD and stroke than do women. Much of the protection against CHD in women is linked to the female sex hormone estrogen, which may elevate HDL cholesterol. Although the risk of CHD increases markedly in women after menopause, it never becomes as great as for men (3).

Increasing Age As you get older, your risk for developing CHD will increase. This is partly due to the fact that the buildup of arterial plaque is an ongoing process; the longer one lives, the greater the buildup. In fact, more than 83% of people who die of CHD are age 65 or older (11). Increasing age also increases your risk of stroke. The risk of stroke increases by 200% in both men and women over the age of 55 (1).

Contributory Risk Factors

Contributory risk factors are risk factors that increase your risk of developing a major risk factor. The American Heart Association recognizes stress and alcohol as contributory risk factors for CHD.

body weight, blood pressure, and lipid profile and the reduced risk of diabetes (6, 14–17), all of which are associated with exercise. Collectively, these changes can greatly reduce the overall risk of developing CHD.

Diabetes Mellitus As we saw in Chapter 1, diabetes is a disease that results in elevated blood sugar levels due to the body's inability to use blood sugar properly. Diabetes occurs most often in middle age and is common in people who are overweight. The link between diabetes and CHD is well established; about 75% of all individuals with diabetes die from some form of cardiovascular disease. The role that diabetes plays in increasing risk of CHD may be tied to the fact that people with diabetes often have elevated blood cholesterol levels, have hypertension and are inactive (11).

Obesity and Overweight Compared with individuals who maintain their ideal body weight, overweight and obese individuals are more likely to develop CHD, even if they have no other major risk factors. Furthermore, obesity is often associated with elevated blood cholesterol levels and may contribute to hypertension (11).

Of particular interest is the fact that a person's fat distribution pattern affects the risk of CHD. Waist-to-hip circumference ratios greater than 1.0 for men and 0.8 for women indicate a significant risk for develop-

Stress Stress contributes to the development of several major CHD risk factors. For example, stress may be linked to smoking habits. People under stress may start smoking in an effort to relax, or stress could influence smokers to smoke more than they normally would. Further, stress increases the risk of developing both hypertension and elevated blood cholesterol. The physiological connection between stress and hypertension appears to be the stress-induced release of hormones that elevate blood pressure.

Alcohol Consumption Although there is some evidence that moderate alcohol consumption (one drink per day for women and two drinks per day for men) may lower risk for heart disease, drinking too much alcohol raises risk. People who drink too much alcohol are more likely to suffer high blood pressure, heart failure, and stroke. Excessive alcohol consumption can also contribute to high triglycerides, cancer, and other diseases. The American Heart Association recommends that nondrinkers continue to abstain from alcohol and that moderate drinkers not increase their intake (11).

Make sure you know...

> Researchers have identified several major and contributory risk factors that increase the chance of developing both coronary heart disease (CHD) and stroke.

> Major risk factors for CHD and stroke include smoking, hypertension, high blood cholesterol levels, physical inactivity, diabetes mellitus, obesity and overweight, heredity, gender, and increasing age.

> Contributory risk factors for CHD and stroke include stress and alcohol.

How Can You Reduce Your Risk of Heart Disease?

Although cardiovascular disease remains the number-one killer in the United States, incidence of the disease has declined over the past 30 years (1). This drop has occurred primarily because people have reduced their risk factors for CHD. Table 9.2 lists the major and contributory CHD risk factors discussed earlier in the chapter. Note that six of the nine major risk factors, and both of the contributory factors, can be modified by behavior. Therefore, you can modify 70% of CHD risk factors to reduce your risk of developing cardiovascular disease.

The more risk factors you avoid or eliminate, the less your risk for developing CHD. Let's discuss the actions you can take today to eliminate these risk factors.

Don't Smoke

As soon as a smoker quits smoking, CHD risk drops. If you don't currently smoke, the best advice is not to start. If you do smoke, you need to stop. Unfortunately, for most people, smoking is a difficult habit to break.

TABLE 9.2
Major and Contributory Risk Factors for Developing Coronary Heart Disease

Risk Factor	Classification	Is Behavior Modification Possible?	Behavior Modification to Reduce Risk
Tobacco smoke	Major	Yes	Smoking cessation, avoiding secondhand smoke
Hypertension	Major	Yes	Exercise, proper diet, and stress reduction
High blood cholesterol	Major	Yes	Exercise, proper diet, and medication
Diabetes mellitus	Major	Yes	Proper nutrition, exercise
Obesity and overweight	Major	Yes	Weight loss, proper nutrition, exercise
Physical inactivity	Major	Yes	Exercise
Heredity (including ethnicity)	Major	No	
Gender (male)	Major	No	
Increasing age	Major	No	
Stress	Contributory	Yes	Stress management, exercise
Alcohol	Contributory	Yes	Moderate consumption

Source: Data from American Heart Association. *Risk factors and coronary heart disease.* www.americanheart.org, 2009.

Smoking cessation requires major behavior modification to stop smoking and remain smoke-free for the rest of your life.

Lower Your Blood Pressure

Hypertension can be combated in several ways. In some instances, medication may be required to control high blood pressure. However, in many cases of hypertension, exercise and a healthy diet low in sodium can assist in lowering blood pressure. Because stress can also contribute to hypertension, maintaining low levels of daily stress is also important. Chapter 10 discusses approaches to stress management in detail.

Eat a Healthy Diet

High blood cholesterol levels are a key factor in risk of CHD, and the best way to reduce blood levels of cholesterol is through diet and exercise. Decreasing your intake of saturated fats and cholesterol may significantly reduce your blood cholesterol levels. Saturated fats stimulate cholesterol synthesis in the liver and therefore contribute to elevated blood cholesterol. Saturated fats are found mostly in meats and dairy products, so avoiding high intake of these foods can reduce your blood cholesterol levels. Table 9.3 lists the cholesterol content of selected foods. If diet and exercise are not effective in lowering blood lipid levels to a desirable range, cholesterol-lowering drugs are available.

Eating a healthy diet, particularly one that's low in sodium, saturated fat, and cholesterol, can reduce your risk for heart disease.

Be Physically Active

Regular exercise has been shown to improve blood lipid profiles in most people. Even modest levels of exercise (e.g., 30 minutes of walking performed 3 to 5 times per week) have been shown to reduce the risk of CHD development due to physical inactivity (1, 3, 10–12). In addition, regular aerobic exercise has been shown to modify other CHD risk factors by positively influencing blood pressure, body composition, insulin resistance, and blood cholesterol levels.

Although even small amounts of exercise can provide some protection against CHD, studies reveal that the risk of death from CHD decreases as the total physical activity energy expenditure increases from 500 to 3500 kilocalories per week (14). Further, whereas total energy expenditure from exercise is important in preventing CHD, the intensity of exercise is also important. A study of Harvard alumni reported that individuals engaged in regular vigorous exercise (50% $\dot{V}O_2$max or higher) were better protected against CHD than people exercising at much lower levels

(18). Other studies have also reported a strong link between exercise intensity and reduction in death from CHD (14).

Remember, "regular" exercise (3 or more days per week) is the key. Sporadic bouts of exercise (3–4 days per month) will not reduce the risk of CHD. Moreover, cessation of exercise will result in a loss of exercise-induced protection from heart disease (19–21). So, make a commitment to a consistent and lifelong exercise program today. You heart will love you for it!

Reduce Your Stress Level

Relaxation techniques (discussed in Chapter 10) can help counteract the effects of a stressful lifestyle and therefore reduce the risk for developing CHD. Every lifestyle contains stressful elements. For example, college students are often posed with "school stress" related to such factors as studying for exams and completing course assign-

A CLOSER LOOK

FREQUENTLY ASKED QUESTIONS ABOUT EXERCISE, DIET, AND HEART DISAESE

CAN DIETARY MODIFICATIONS OR REGULAR EXERCISE SLOW THE PROGRESSION OF ATHEROSCLEROSIS?

Several studies have concluded that a diet low in saturated fat will retard the development of atherosclerotic plaque in blood vessels. Further, regular endurance exercise also slows the progression of atherosclerosis (3). It follows that a lifestyle that includes both regular exercise and a low-fat diet would be a good strategy to slow the collection of atherosclerotic plaque in blood vessels.

WHAT IF DIET AND EXERCISE AREN'T ENOUGH TO LOWER MY CHOLESTEROL TO DESIRABLE LEVELS?

When diet and exercise alone are not successful in lowering blood cholesterol, drug therapy may help. The most effective and widely tested cholesterol drugs are a class of drugs called *statins*. These drugs work by preventing the formation of cholesterol in the liver and also help remove cholesterol from the blood. Statins can reduce the "bad cholesterol" (i.e.,

LDL) level by 20–45% depending on the drug used and the dosage (22, 25). Although statins have been shown to reduce the risk of atherosclerosis in many people, statins can produce some potentially serious side effects (22). Therefore, if diet and exercise alone cannot successfully lower your cholesterol, you and your physician can decide together whether a statin drug is right for you. For more information on the treatment for high cholesterol, consult the National Cholesterol Education Program online at www.nhlbi.nih .gov/about/ncep/index.htm.

SOME DOCTORS RECOMMEND ASPIRIN TO REDUCE THE RISK OF HEART ATTACK. HOW DOES ASPIRIN REDUCE THE RISK OF HEART ATTACK?

Extensive research indicates that taking aspirin daily (80–325 mg/day) can help prevent heart attacks by preventing blood platelets from sticking together, thereby reducing the likelihood of blood clots.

However, taking aspirin daily is not risk free. For example, people with bleeding disorders, liver disease, kidney

disease, or peptic ulcers and individuals who are allergic to aspirin should not take it.

ARE SOME PEOPLE AT RISK FOR SUDDEN CARDIAC DEATH DURING EXERCISE?

Yes, although regular physical activity reduces the risk of developing coronary heart disease, vigorous exercise can acutely increase the risk of both sudden cardiac death and heart attacks in susceptible persons (23). For example, people with advanced heart disease might have an increased risk for sudden death during exercise because of blockage in a major coronary artery. Further, individuals with hereditary cardiac abnormalities may also be at risk during exercise (23). A medical exam can usually identify whether the person is at risk for sudden cardiac death during exercise. Specifically, a medical history and a physical exam from a qualified physician can detect hidden heart disease that could pose a risk for participating in regular exercise.

TABLE 9.3
Cholesterol and Saturated Fat Content of Selected Foods

Food	Serving Size	Cholesterol (mg)	Saturated Fat (g)
Bacon	2 slices	30	0.7
Beef (lean)	8 oz	150	12
Butter	1 Tablespoon	32	0.4
Cheese (American)	1 oz	27	5.4
Cheese (cheddar)	1 oz	30	5.9
Egg	1 (boiled)	113	2.8
Frankfurter	1	30	5.2
Hamburger	1 small patty	68	5.9
Milk (whole)	1 cup	33	5
Milkshake	10 oz	54	8.2
Pizza (meat)	1 slice (14″ diameter)	31	8
Sausage	3 oz	42	8.6

STEPS FOR
BEHAVIOR CHANGE

What's your risk for cardiovascular disease?

Although you are probably young and healthy and can't imagine the day when you'll have high blood pressure or diabetes, you do have a chance of developing one or more of these conditions during your lifetime. Take this quiz to determine whether your current habits put you at higher risk for developing CVD.

Y N

☐ ☐ Do you get up and move around often enough to accumulate 30 minutes of physical activity per day?

☐ ☐ Do you usually avoid eating high-fat foods?

☐ ☐ Do you watch your sodium intake and refrain from using too much salt during cooking and at the table?

☐ ☐ Do you monitor your stress level and practice stress management when necessary?

☐ ☐ Do you avoid smoking cigarettes and using other tobacco products?

If you answered yes to three or more of these questions, congratulations! You are on your way to developing a lifetime of healthy habits. If you answered no to most of these questions, you may already be at increased risk for CVD.

TIPS TO LOWER YOUR CVD RISK

☑ Start an exercise program. Even a half hour per day a few days a week will go a long way in improving heart health. And you'll look and feel better, too.

☑ Watch your diet. Although the occasional fast-food meal isn't the end of the world, in general, you should eat whole foods, such as fruits, vegetables, and whole grains, and avoid deep-fried or other high-fat foods.

☑ Eat less salt. Sodium is an essential nutrient for several body processes, but you actually need very little of it to be healthy, and too much sodium has been linked to high blood pressure. To lower your sodium intake, use pepper at the table instead of salt, and use spices to flavor foods during cooking.

☑ De-stress. Too much stress is linked not only to increased risk of CVD, but also to high blood pressure. Try some of the techniques in Chapter 10 to manage your stress level.

☑ Quit smoking. Tobacco use leads to numerous health problems. For the sake of your heart, your lungs, your breath, and those around you, you should avoid smoking. If you don't smoke, don't start; and if you do, stop.

---

ments. If you are stressed about school-related issues, try exercising (e.g., going for a run) at the end of the day to reduce tension. If you find yourself getting angry or hostile easily, consider scheduling counseling sessions with a school counselor trained in anger management.

Make sure you know...

> Although heart disease remains the number one killer in the United States, the incidence of heart disease has declined during the past 30 years. This reduction in CHD has occurred because people have modified their behavior to reduce their risk factors for CHD.

> You can reduce your risk of developing CHD by not smoking, by controlling your blood pressure, by eating a healthy diet, by being physically active, and by reducing your stress level.

Summary

1. Heart disease is the number-one cause of death in the United States, where almost one of every two deaths is due to heart disease.

2. Cardiovascular disease refers to any disease that affects the heart and blood vessels. Common cardiovascular diseases include atherosclerosis, coronary heart disease, stroke, and hypertension.

3. CHD risk factors are classified as either major or contributory. Major risk factors are those that directly increase the risk of coronary heart disease. Contributory risk factors may increase your chance of developing coronary heart disease by promoting the development of a major risk factor.

4. Major risk factors for developing coronary heart disease include smoking, hypertension, high blood cholesterol, physical inactivity, diabetes mellitus, obesity and overweight, heredity, gender, and increasing age.

5. Contributory risk factors for the development of coronary heart disease include stress and alcohol.

6. You can reduce your risk of developing coronary heart disease by not smoking, by eating a healthy diet (particularly avoiding saturated fat and dietary cholesterol in foods), by being physically active, by maintaining a healthy body weight, and by reducing stress.

Study Questions

1. Which of the following CHD risk factors is NOT a major risk factor?
   a. smoking
   b. hypertension
   c. high blood cholesterol
   d. resting pulse rate

2. Which of the following blood pressure measurements would be considered hypertension?
   a. 100/80
   b. 110/80
   c. 130/80
   d. 140/90

3. Cholesterol exists in several forms in your blood. The form of blood cholesterol that is classified as "good cholesterol" is called
   a. total cholesterol.
   b. HDL cholesterol.
   c. LDL cholesterol.
   d. EDL cholesterol

4. The leading cause of death in the United States is
   a. AIDS.
   b. cancer.
   c. cardiovascular disease.
   d. accidents.

5. Which of the following risk factors for CHD cannot be modified by a change in behavior?
   a. obesity
   b. heredity
   c. hypertension
   d. stress

6. Define the following terms:
   cardiovascular disease
   coronary heart disease
   coronary artery disease
   hypertension

7. What are the major and contributory risk factors for developing CHD?

8. Discuss the difference between major and contributory risk factors for developing coronary heart disease.

9. Why are high-density lipoproteins known as "good" cholesterol? Conversely, why are low-density lipoproteins labeled "bad" cholesterol?

10. Which major coronary heart disease risk factors can be modified?

11. Which contributory coronary heart disease risk factors can be modified?

12. How does a high-sodium diet contribute to hypertension?

13. What is the link between diet and blood cholesterol?

14. How does smoking increase your risk of developing cardiovascular disease?

15. How are arteriosclerosis and atherosclerosis related?

Suggested Reading

Bybee, K., J. Lee, and J. O'Keefe. Cumulative clinical trial data on atorvastatin for reducing cardiovascular events: The clinical impact of atorvastatin. *Current Medical Research Opinion* 24:1217–1229, 2008.

Franklin, B., J. Trivax, and T. Vanhecke. New insights in preventive cardiology and cardiac rehabilitation. *Current Opinion in Cardiology* 23:477–486, 2008.

Gotto, A. Statins: Powerful drugs for lowering cholesterol. *Circulation* 105:1514–1516, 2002.

Heart and Stroke Facts. Dallas: American Heart Association, 2003.

Heart Disease and Stroke Statistics—2009 update. At-A-Glance. Dallas: American Heart Association, 2009.

Heart Facts 2007: Latino/Hispanic Americans. Dallas: American Heart Association, 2006.

Know the Facts, Get the Stats. Dallas: American Heart Association, 2007.

Löllgen, H., A. Böckenhoff, and G. Knapp. Physical activity and all-cause mortality: An updated meta-analysis with different intensity categories. *International Journal of Sports Medicine* 30:213–224, 2009.

Peterson, J. A. Take ten: 10 ways to protect your heart. *ACSM's Health and Fitness Journal* 4 (2):48, 2000.

Powers, S., and E. Howley. *Exercise Physiology: Theory and Application to Fitness and Performance*, 7th ed. New York: McGraw-Hill, 2009.

Powers, S., Z. Murlasits, M. Wu, and A. Kavazis. Ischemia-reperfusion-induced cardiac injury: A brief review. *Medicine and Science in Sports and Exercise* 39:1529–1536, 2007 .

Waisted: Abdominal obesity and your health. *Harvard Men's Health Watch* 13:1–6, 2009.

For links to the organizations and websites listed below, visit The Total Fitness and Wellness Website at www.pearsonhighered.com/powers.

Mayo Clinic Health

Contains wide-ranging information about diet, fitness, and health.

American Medical Association

Contains many sources of information about a wide variety of medical problems, including heart disease.

WebMD

Presents information about a wide variety of diseases and medical problems, including heart disease.

American Heart Association

Contains information about a variety of topics related to both heart disease and stroke.

References

1. American Heart Association. Heart Disease and Stroke Statistics—2009 update. *Circulation* 119:e21–e181, 2009.

2. Centers for Disease Control and Prevention. *Heart disease and stroke prevention: Addressing the nation's leading killers, At-A-Glance 2009*, www.cdc.gov/NCCDPHP/publications/aag/dhdsp.htm, 2009.

3. Powers, S., and E. Howley. *Exercise Physiology: Theory and Application to Fitness and Performance*, 7th ed. New York: McGraw-Hill, 2009.

4. American Cancer Society. *Fifty Most Often Asked Questions about Smoking and Health and the Answers*. New York: American Cancer Society, 1990.

5. Pollack, M., and D. Schmidt. *Heart Disease and Rehabilitation*. Champaign, IL: Human Kinetics, 1995.

6. Durstine, J. L., and R. Thompson. Exercise modulates blood lipids and exercise plan. *ACSM's Health and Fitness Journal* 4(4):44–46, 2000.

7. Third report of the National Cholesterol Education Program Expert Panel on Detection, Evaluation, and Treatment of High Blood Cholesterol in Adults. *Journal of the American Medical Association* 285(19):1–19, 2001.

8. Thomas, T., and T. LaFontaine. Exercise, nutritional strategies, and lipoproteins. In *ACSM's Resource Manual for Guidelines for Exercise Testing and Prescription*, 4th ed., ed. J. Roitman. Philadelphia: Lippincott Williams & Wilkins, 2001.

9. Morris, J., J. Heady, P. Raffle, C. Roberts, and J. Parks. Coronary heart disease and physical activity of work. *Lancet* Ii:1053–1057, 1953.

10. Blair, S. N., H. W. Kohl, R. S. Paffenbarger, D. G. Clark, K. H. Cooper, and L. W. Gibbons. Physical fitness and all-cause mortality: A prospective study of healthy men and women. *Journal of the American Medical Association* 262:2395–2401, 1989.

11. American Heart Association. *Risk factors and coronary heart disease*. www.americanheart.org, 2009.

12. Paffenbarger, R. S., R. T. Hyde, A. L. Wing, and C. C. Hsieh. Physical activity, all-cause mortality of college alumni. *New England Journal of Medicine* 314:605–613, 1986.

13. Kohl, H. Physical activity and cardiovascular disease: Evidence for a dose-response. *Medicine and Science in Sports and Exercise* 33(Suppl.): S472–S483, 2001.

14. Powers, S., S. Lennon, J. Quindry, and J. L. Mehta. Exercise and cardioprotection. *Current Opinion in Cardiology* 17:495–502, 2002.

15. Wood, P. Physical activity, diet, and health: Independent and interactive effects. *Medicine and Science in Sports and Exercise* 26:838–843, 1994.

16. Durstine, J., and W. Haskell. Effects of training on plasma lipids and lipoproteins. *Exercise and Sport Science Reviews* 22:477–521, 1994.

17. Batty, G., and I-Min Lee. Physical activity and coronary heart disease. *British Medical Journal* 328:1089–1090, 2004.

18. Lee, I., C. Hsieh, and R. Paffenbarger. Exercise intensity and longevity in men: The Harvard Alumni Health Study. *Journal of American Medical Association* 273:1179–1184, 1995.

19. French, J., K. Hamilton, J. Quindry, Y. Lee, P. Upchurch, and S. Powers. Exercise-induced protection against myocardial apoptosis and necrosis: MnSOD, calcium-handling proteins, and calpain. *The FASEB Journal* 22:2862–2871, 2008.

20. Quindry, J., K. Hamilton, J. French, Y. Lee, Z. Murlasits, N. Tumer, and S. Powers. Exercise-induced HSP-72 elevation and cardioprotection against infarct and apoptosis. *Journal of Applied Physiology* 103:1056–1062, 2007.

21. Powers, S., J. Quindry, and A. Kavazis. Exercise-induced cardioprotection against myocardial ischemia-reperfusion injury. *Free Radical Biology and Medicine* 44:193–201, 2008.

22. Gotto, A. Statins: Powerful drugs for lowering cholesterol. *Circulation* 105:1514–1516, 2002.

23. Thompson, P.D., et al. Exercise and acute cardiovascular events placing the risks into perspective: A scientific statement from the American Heart Association Council on Nutrition, Physical Activity, and Metabolism and Council on Clinical Cardiology. *Circulation* 115:2358–2368. 2007.

24. Powers, S., Z. Murlasits, M. Wu, and A. Kavazis. Ischemia-reperfusion-induced cardiac injury: A brief review. *Medicine and Science in Sports and Exercise* 39:1529–1536, 2007.

25. Bybee, K., J. Lee, and J. O'Keefe. Cumulative clinical trial data on atorvastatin for reducing cardiovascular events: The clinical impact of atorvastatin. *Current Medical Research Opinion* 24:1217–1229, 2008.

Videos

Log on to www.pearsonhighered.com/powers to view these chapter-related videos.

Cardiovascular Disease

Heart Disease in America

NAME _____ DATE _____

Finding Your Cholesterol Plan

The following two-step program will guide you through the National Cholesterol Education Program's treatment guidelines. The first step helps you establish your overall coronary risk; the second uses that information to determine your LDL treatment goals and how to reach them. You'll need to know your blood pressure, your total LDL and HDL cholesterol levels, and your triglyceride and fasting glucose levels. If you're not sure of those numbers, ask your doctor and, if necessary, schedule an exam to get them. (Everyone should have a complete lipid profile every 5 years, starting at age 20.)

Step 1: Take the Heart-Attack Risk Test

This test will identify your chance of having a heart attack or dying of coronary disease in the next 10 years. (People with previously diagnosed coronary disease, diabetes, aortic aneurysm, or symptomatic carotid artery disease or peripheral artery disease already face more than a 20 percent risk; they can skip the test and go straight to step 2.) The test uses data from the Framingham Heart Study, the world's longest-running study of cardiovascular risk factors. The test is limited to established, major factors that are easily measured. Circle the point value for each of the risk factors shown.

Age

Years	Women	Men
20–34	−7	−9
35–39	−3	−4
40–44	0	0
45–49	3	3
50–54	6	6
55–59	8	8
60–64	10	10
65–69	12	11
70–74	14	12
75–79	16	13

Total Cholesterol

mg/dL	Age 20–39 Women	Age 20–39 Men	Age 40–49 Women	Age 40–49 Men	Age 50–59 Women	Age 50–59 Men	Age 60–69 Women	Age 60–69 Men	Age 70–79 Women	Age 70–79 Men
<160	0	0	0	0	0	0	0	0	0	0
160–199	4	4	3	3	2	2	1	1	1	0
200–239	8	7	6	5	4	3	2	1	1	0
240–279	11	9	8	6	5	4	3	2	2	1
280+	13	11	10	8	7	5	4	3	2	1

High-Density Lipoprotein (HDL) Cholesterol

mg/dL	Women and Men
60+	−1
50–59	0
40–49	1
<40	2

Systolic Blood Pressure (the Higher Number)

Mm/Hg	Treated		Untreated	
	Women	Men	Women	Men
<120	0	0	0	0
120–129	1	0	3	1
130–139	2	1	4	2
140–159	3	1	5	2
>159	4	2	6	3

Smoking

Age 20–39		Age 40–49		Age 50–59		Age 60–69		Age 70–79	
Women	Men	Women	Men	Women	Men	Women	Men	Women	Men
9	8	7	5	4	3	2	1	1	1

Total Your Points _____

Now find your total point score in the men's or women's column to locate your 10-year risk (the far-right column).

Ten-Year Risk for Heart Disease

Women's Score	Men's Score	Your 10-Year Risk
<20	<12	<10%
20–22	12–15	10–20%
>22	>15	>20%

Step 2: Find Your Low-Density Lipoprotein (LDL) Treatment Plan

Consult the table on the next page to learn whether your overall CHD risk indicates that you need to lower your LDL cholesterol level and, if you do, by how much. First, locate your CHD risk in the left column. (That's based on the 10-year heart-attack risk that you just calculated, as well as your CHD risk factors and any heart-threatening diseases you may have.) Then look across that row to see whether you should make lifestyle changes and take cholesterol-lowering medication, based on your current LDL level.

LDL Treatment Plan

CHD Risk Group	Start lifestyle changes if your LDL level is . . .*	Add drugs if your LDL level is . . .
Very High 1. Ten-year heart-attack risk of 20% or more *or* 2. History of coronary heart disease, diabetes, peripheral-artery disease, carotid-artery disease, or aortic aneurysm.	100 mg/dl or higher. (Aim for an LDL under 100.) Get retested after 3 months.	130 or higher. (Drugs are optional if your LDL is between 100 and 130.)
High 1. Ten-year heart-attack risk of 10% to 20% *and* 2. Two or more major coronary risk factors.†	130 or higher. (Aim for an LDL under 130.) Get retested after 3 months.	130 or higher and lifestyle changes don't achieve your LDL goal in 3 months.
Moderately High 1. Ten-year heart-attack risk under 10% *and* 2. Two or more major coronary risk factors.†	Same as above.	160 or higher, and lifestyle changes don't achieve your LDL goal in 3 months.‡
Low to Moderate 1. One or no major coronary risk factors.†§	160 or higher. (Aim for an LDL under 160.) Get retested after 3 months.	190 or higher, and lifestyle changes don't achieve your LDL goal in 3 months. (Drugs are optional if your LDL is between 160 and 189.)

*People who have the metabolic syndrome should make lifestyle changes even if their LDL level alone doesn't warrant it. You have the metabolic syndrome if you have three or more of these risk factors: HDL under 40 in men, 50 in women; systolic blood pressure of 130 or more or diastolic pressure of 85 or more; fasting glucose level of 110 to 125; triglycerides level of 150 or more; and waist circumference over 40 inches in men, 35 inches in women. People with the syndrome should limit their carbohydrate intake, get up to 30 to 35 percent of their calories from total fat (more than usually recommended), and make the other lifestyle changes, including restriction of saturated fat.

†The major coronary risk factors are cigarette smoking; coronary disease in a father or brother before age 55 or a mother or sister before age 65; systolic blood pressure of 140 or more, a diastolic pressure of 90 or more, or being on drugs for hypertension; and an HDL level under 40. If your HDL is 60 or more, subtract one risk factor. (High LDL is a major factor, of course, but it's already figured into the table.)

‡Although the goal is to get LDL under 130, the use of drugs in these people usually isn't worthwhile, even if lifestyle steps fail to achieve that goal.

§People in this group usually have a 10-year risk of less than 10%. Those who have higher risk should ask their doctor whether they need more aggressive treatment than shown here.

Source: From Rebecca Donatelle, *Access to Health,* 8th ed. Copyright © 2004. Reprinted by permission of Pearson Education, Inc.

NAME _____ DATE _____

Understanding Your Risk for Cardiovascular Disease

Each of us has a unique level of risk for various diseases. Some of these risks you can take action to change; others are risks that you need to consider as you plan a lifelong strategy for overall risk reduction. Complete each of the following questions, and total your points in each section. If you score between 1 and 5 in any section, consider your risk. The higher the number, the greater your risk. If you answered "Don't know" for any question, talk to your parents or other family members as soon as possible to find out whether you have any unknown risks.

Part I: Assess Your Family Risk for CVD

1. Do any of your primary relatives (mother, father, grandparents, siblings) have a history of heart disease or stroke?

   Yes _____ (1 point)   No _____ (0 points)   Don't know _____

2. Do any of your primary relatives (mother, father, grandparents, siblings) have diabetes?

   Yes _____ (1 point)   No _____ (0 points)   Don't know _____

3. Do any of your primary relatives (mother, father, grandparents, siblings) have high blood pressure?

   Yes _____ (1 point)   No _____ (0 points)   Don't know _____

4. Do any of your primary relatives (mother, father, grandparents, siblings) have a history of high cholesterol?

   Yes _____ (1 point)   No _____ (0 points)   Don't know _____

5. Would you say that your family consumed a high-fat diet (lots of red meat, dairy products, butter or margarine) during your time spent at home?

   Yes _____ (1 point)   No _____ (0 points)   Don't know _____

Total points _____

Part II: Assess Your Lifestyle Risk for CVD

1. Is your total cholesterol level higher than it should be?

   Yes _____ (1 point)   No _____ (0 points)   Don't know _____

2. Do you have high blood pressure?

   Yes _____ (1 point)   No _____ (0 points)   Don't know _____

3. Have you been diagnosed as prediabetic or diabetic?

   Yes _____ (1 point)   No _____ (0 points)   Don't know _____

4. Do you smoke?

   Yes _____ (1 point)   No _____ (0 points)   Don't know _____

5. Would you describe your life as being highly stressful?

   Yes _____ (1 point)   No _____ (0 points)   Don't know _____

Total points _____

Part III: Assess Your Additional Risks for CVD

1. How would you best describe your current weight?

   a. Lower than what it should be for my height and weight. (0 points)

   b. About what it should be for my height and weight. (0 points)

   c. Higher than it should be for my height and weight. (1 point)

2. How would you describe the level of exercise that you get each day?

   a. Less than what I should be exercising each day. (1 point)

   b. About what I should be exercising each day. (0 points)

   c. More than what I should be each day. (0 points)

3. How would you describe your dietary behaviors?

   a. Eating only the recommended number of calories per day. (0 points)

   b. Eating less than the recommended number of calories each day. (0 points)

   c. Eating more than the recommended number of calories each day. (1 point)

4. Which of the following best describes your typical dietary behavior?

   a. I eat from the major food groups, trying hard to get the recommended fruits and vegetables. (0 points)

   b. I eat too much red meat and consume too much saturated fat from meats and dairy products each day. (1 point)

   c. Whenever possible, I try to substitute olive oil or canola oil for other forms of dietary fat. (0 points)

5. Do you have a history of *Chlamydia* infection?

   a. Yes. (1 point)

   b. No. (0 points)

Total points _____

NAME _____   DATE _____

Assessing Your Genetic Predisposition for Cardiovascular Disease

The following is a family tree that allows you to fill in risk factors and conditions for heart disease in your family members. Remember that heart disease has a genetic component, so examining your relatives' health and lifestyles will provide insight into your future susceptibility to heart disease. Write in risk factors directly related to heart disease. Examples include hypertension, high blood cholesterol, diabetes, stroke, obesity, and heart attack.

Your Family History of Heart Disease

Grandparents
_____
_____
_____

Grandparents
_____
_____
_____

Aunts/Uncles
_____
_____
_____

Mother

Father

Aunts/Uncles
_____
_____
_____

_____
_____
_____

_____
_____
_____

Sisters
_____
_____
_____

You
_____
_____
_____

Brothers
_____
_____
_____

Note: This family tree can be copied and used for other diseases with an inheritable component, such as cancer.

In the space below, list any diet, behavior, or lifestyle risks in your life that may contribute to heart disease. Examples include high stress level, high-fat diet, physical inactivity, high sodium intake.

_____

_____

_____

_____

Interpretation

Inherited traits can increase your risk of cardiovascular disease. The good news is that you are not destined to develop heart disease or any of the conditions present in your relatives. Lifestyle changes that include moderate exercise and proper diet can reduce your risk of developing cardiovascular diseases. Being aware of health concerns and problems within your family that may be passed on genetically will make you a more informed, health-conscious individual.

LABORATORY

Stress Management

true or false?

1. All stress is bad for your health and should be eliminated.
2. Chronic stress increases your risk for heart disease.
3. Many everyday situations can cause you to feel stressed.
4. Good time management can help you manage stress.
5. Your personality has no effect on your level of stress.

Answers appear on the next page.

Do you tend to get sick during finals, or do you have difficulty sleeping when a big term paper is due? Does a fight with your boyfriend or girlfriend leave you unfocused? Do you feel muscle tension while sitting frustrated in rush-hour traffic? These familiar, everyday situations often lead to stress and the negative physical symptoms associated with stress. On the other hand, you may have noticed that if you do not feel some stress before a test, competition or performance, you do not do your best. A certain amount of stress is good. The goal is not to eliminate all stress, but to manage it well so it does not have a negative impact on your health and performance.

Have you thought about the specific physical responses your body undergoes during a period of stress? Are you aware of the potential long-term effects stress can have on your health? We will discuss these topics and more in this chapter as we analyze the complex topics of stress and stress management.

What Are Stress and the Stress Response?

Most people are familiar with the term *stress*, but few are aware of its precise definition. Let's find out how scientists define the term.

CONSIDER THIS!

In one survey, 33% of students experienced stress to the point that their academic performance was negatively affected.

Defining Stress

During **stress**, the body is in a state of mental and physical tension, and the balance (homeostasis) of the body's systems is disrupted. Stress is caused by one or more **stressors**, which can be physical (such as an injury) or mental (such as emotional distress resulting from a personal relationship). Regardless of the nature of the stressor, the body's physiological and mental responses usually include feelings of strain, tension, and anxiety. Our bodies' reactions to stress, called the **stress response,** prepare us to deal with stressors so balance can be restored. People are stressed by numerous stressors during daily life, and different people are stressed by different things. For example, you might find a long commute to work stressful, but someone else might enjoy the alone time.

There are different classifications of stressors, and each can affect our behaviors, health, and life. Stressors can be acute (such as the death of a loved one), cumulative (such as a series of events that lead to a breakup with a boyfriend or girlfriend), or chronic (such as daily job- or school-related pressures). Although it is clear that chronic or extreme stress is unhealthy, some degree of stress is required to maximize performance. For any type of "performance" activity there is an optimal level of stress that pushes us to perform and excel. This level is specific to the individual,

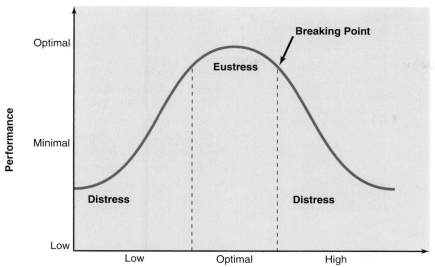

FIGURE 10.1
Eustress is positive stress that helps you achieve optimal performance. Distress (negative stress) hurts performance. Too much or too little stress also hurts performance.

and it is motivating and energizing. Stress that is positive and that is associated with improved performance is called **eustress.**

Although some level of stress is desirable and beneficial, too much stress or poorly managed stress can have a negative impact on health and lead to poor performance and decisions. This idea is illustrated in Figure 10.1. When we are out of the range that leads to optimal performance, stress can have a negative impact. This negative stress is called **distress.** For example, regular exercise can be described as a positive stressor. However, regular exercise at very high frequency or intensity increases the risk for injury and emotional tension, and it can be considered a negative stressor because performance often suffers.

Physiological Changes of the Stress Response

You are driving home, and another driver runs a stop sign and just barely misses hitting your car. Your body will have a set of predictable reactions to this acute stressor: Your heart rate increases, your senses heighten, and **endorphins** are released, to name a few of the changes that take place. These reactions are part of the stress response. The body's responses to stress are mediated by an area in the brain called the *hypothalamus* and are initiated when the hormones **epinephrine, norepinephrine**, and **cortisol** are released into the bloodstream. The hormones cause a number of physiological changes, some of which are illustrated in Figure 10.2. Hence the two body systems

primarily responsible for the changes that occur during the stress response are the *nervous system* and the **endocrine system.**

Your nervous system controls both your voluntary movements (such as your raising your hand in class) and your involuntary bodily processes (such as your heartbeating and digestion). The involuntary actions are controlled by the **autonomic nervous system.** There are two branches of the autonomic nervous system, the **parasympathetic** branch and the **sympathetic** branch. The parasympathetic branch is in control of body processes and functions when you are relaxed or resting. Maintaining your resting heart rate and blood pressure, growth, digestion, and storing energy are examples of processes under control of the parasympathetic nervous system. The sympathetic branch is the excitatory division of the autonomic nervous system. This branch is activated when you need to react and

stress A state of physical and mental tension in response to a situation that is perceived as a threat or challenge.

stressor A factor that produces stress.

stress response The physiological and behavioral changes that take place when a person is presented with a stressor.

eustress A stress level that results in improved performance; also called *positive stress.*

distress Negative stress that is harmful to performance.

endorphins A group of hormones (endogenous opioids, or "painkillers") released during the stress response.

epinephrine A hormone secreted by the inner core (medulla) of the adrenal gland; also called *adrenaline.*

norepinephrine A hormone secreted by the inner core (medulla) of the adrenal gland.

cortisol A hormone secreted by the outer layer (cortex) of the adrenal gland.

endocrine system Series of glands and tissues in the body that secrete hormones to regulate bodily processes.

autonomic nervous system The branch of the nervous system that controls basic bodily functions that do not require conscious thought; includes the parasympathetic and sympathetic branches.

parasympathetic branch The division of the autonomic nervous system that is dominant at rest and controls the energy conservation and restoration processes.

sympathetic branch The division of the autonomic nervous system that is in control when we need to react or respond to challenges; the excitatory branch.

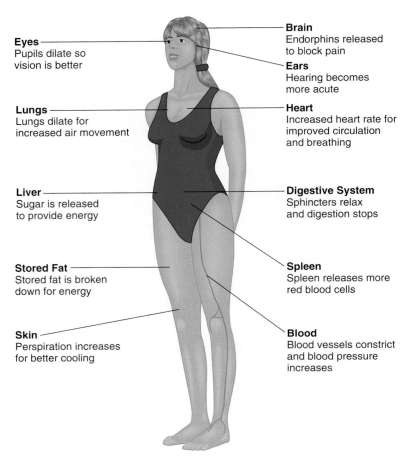

Eyes
Pupils dilate so
vision is better

Lungs
Lungs dilate for
increased air movement

Liver
Sugar is released
to provide energy

Stored Fat
Stored fat is broken
down for energy

Skin
Perspiration increases
for better cooling

Brain
Endorphins released
to block pain

Ears
Hearing becomes
more acute

Heart
Increased heart rate for
improved circulation
and breathing

Digestive System
Sphincters relax
and digestion stops

Spleen
Spleen releases more
red blood cells

Blood
Blood vessels constrict
and blood pressure
increases

FIGURE 10.2
The body's physiological responses to stress.

produce energy. The increase in heart rate, faster breathing, perspiration, and initial release of epinephrine are some of the changes produced by the activation of the sympathetic division.

As part of the stress response, the sympathetic nervous system activates the endocrine system, which in turn releases hormones. The main stress hormone released by the system is cortisol. This hormone is more predominant during distress and prolonged stress situations. Cortisol helps make glucose and break down fat for energy, increase the production of epinephrine and norepinephrine, and suppress an immune response.

The Fight-or-Flight Response

Together the responses of the autonomic nervous system and the endocrine system make up the **fight-or-flight response.** This initial response to stress was first discovered by Harvard physiologist Walter Canon (1) and later elaborated on by the biologist Hans Selye (2). Canon described the stress response as an inborn, automatic, and primitive response designed to prepare individuals to face (fight) or run away (flight) from any

type of perceived threat or challenge to survival. According to Canon, once a person perceives a threat, the brain initiates a sequence of physiological and physical changes that ready the body for action. However, the challenge does not have to be a matter of life or death. The stressors we are presented with in everyday life can also evoke the fight-or-flight response.

Imagine you are at home asleep and the telephone rings. You answer the phone and hear your professor's voice asking why you did not take the final exam. You look at your clock and realize you overslept and missed class! Suddenly your heart is racing, you are sweating profusely, your blood pressure rises, and your hands become cold and clammy. These responses prepare you to deal with the threatening or stressful situation. Do you try to explain the situation to your professor (fight) or quickly hang up and never return to school again (flight)?

Your body has "activation" responses to enable you to fight or flee (Figure 10.2). In addition to the changes already mentioned, blood is directed away from the digestive tract and redirected into the muscles to provide extra energy for fighting or fleeing. You will have an increased awareness of your surroundings, quickened impulses, and diminished pain perception. Your body physically and mentally prepares to "battle" the stressor. After you successfully cope with your stressor or no longer perceive it as threatening, the body returns to homeostasis. However, if the situation is not resolved, you will stay in this aroused state.

During the fight-or-flight response, people are in an "attack mode" and are focused on short-term "survival." Primitive people were required to exert physical activity while fighting or fleeing from wild animals, and physical exertion related to the act of fighting or fleeing would rid the body of excess levels of stress hormones, allowing it to return to homeostasis. However, today's modern stressors, such as congested roads, too few parking spaces, missing an exam, bouncing a check, or having an argument with your significant other, do not typically require physical exertion. People living highly stressful lives can experience chronic stress in which they have some level of arousal from stress almost constantly. There is often no release from these stressors in the form of physical exertion, and over time the stress hormones accumulate in the body, causing illness and chronic disease. We'll discuss the relationship between chronic stress and disease later in the chapter.

TABLE 10.1
Personality Behavior Patterns and Their Risks for Heart Disease

Personality Behavior Pattern	Qualities	Risk for Heart Disease
A	Impatient, competitive, aggressive, highly motivated, and sometimes hostile	High
B	Patient, with low aggression, and easygoing	Low
C	Competitive, highly motivated, high level of confidence, and constant level of emotional control	Low
D	Negative, anxious, worried, and socially inhibited	High

Make sure you know...

> Stress is a mental and physical response to situations we perceive as pressures or challenges.

> Stressors can come from many sources, and they can be positive (eustress) or negative (distress). Some degree of stress is required to maximize performance.

> The autonomic nervous system and the endocrine system are responsible for the changes that occur during the stress response. The parasympathetic branch of the autonomic nervous system is in control at rest, and the sympathetic branch is activated when you need to react. Cortisol is the main stress hormone produced by the endocrine system.

> The changes in the body that occur during the stress response prepare our bodies to fight or flee the stressful situation. These responses are collectively referred to as the fight-or-flight response.

What Factors Affect Your Stress Level?

Although everyone feels stress, life events and situations do not affect everyone the same way. Our personalities, past experiences, and gender are three influences on the way we perceive situations and cope with stress. For example, your grandmother who recently recovered from a hip fracture might experience stress when she enters a setting with a lot of stairs and uneven terrain. However, as a young healthy adult, you do not find that environment threatening. You might have the tendency to freak out during finals, whereas your roommate remains calm. We will discuss some of the factors that impact your ability to handle stressful situations next.

Personality Behavior Patterns

People's different reactions to the same stressful situation can be due to personality differences and how they have learned to respond.

There are many different ways to describe personalities and behavior patterns. Note that although there is no one specific (or completely reliable) way of identifying stress-prone personality patterns, one of the most common, and easily interpreted, classification groupings describes individuals as having characteristics that fit into one of four behavior pattern categories: Type A, Type B, Type C, and Type D (Table 10.1). This classification system describes the four most common behavior patterns.

People who exhibit Type A behavior pattern (TABP) are highly motivated, time-conscious, hard-driving, impatient, and sometimes hostile, cynical, and angry. They have a heightened response to stress, and their hostility and anger, especially if repressed, place them at a greater risk for heart disease (3, 4). Individuals with Type B behavior pattern are easygoing, nonaggressive, and patient, and they are not prone to hostile episodes like their TABP counterparts. People with Type B behavior pattern are less likely to perceive everyday annoyances as significant stressors and are at low risk for heart disease from stress.

Most people have heard of TABP and Type B behavior pattern, but you might not be familiar with the other behavior patterns. People with Type C behavior pattern have many of the positive qualities of TABP. They are confident, highly motivated, and competitive. However, individuals with Type C behavior pattern typically do not express the hostility and anger seen with TABP, and they use their personality characteristics to maintain a constant level of emotional control and to

fight-or-flight response A series of physiological reactions by the body to prepare to combat a real or perceived threat.

channel their ambition into creative directions. People with Type C behavior pattern have the positive characteristics of TABP but do not express their negative emotions and feelings in the same manner. As a result, individuals with Type C behavior pattern experience the same low risk for stress-related heart disease as do those with Type B behavior pattern. However, a person with Type C behavior pattern who keeps emotions in and does not express them can face a higher risk for heart disease.

Individuals with Type D behavior pattern also are considered to be at greater risk for stress-related disease. These individuals are prone to worry and anxiety and also tend to be socially inhibited and uneasy when interacting with others. Their social clumsiness results in a chronic state of anxiety, which places them at greater risk for heart disease (5, 6). You can see a summary of the different personality behavior patterns, and their corresponding risks for heart disease, in Table 10.1.

Past Experiences

Discovering aspects of one's personality can be interesting and entertaining, but we must keep in mind that ultimately it is our perception of a stressor and the way we react to it that will determine any resulting health effects. We learn from our experiences, and what we learn can help us respond more positively in future situations. For example, finals time is a common stressor. You would expect a person with TABP to be extremely stressed during the time leading up to finals. However, a person with TABP who has learned that too much stress leads to unfocused study time and poor grades might plan to manage and structure study time weeks in advance to avoid the last-minute stress. Likewise, a student with type B behavior who performed poorly in the past because she was too relaxed during finals and did not prepare well might learn to prepare more diligently for future finals to improve her performance.

Gender

Gender is another factor that impacts the way we react to stressors. There are no sex differences in the physiological responses to stress, but gender might affect the way we perceive situations and how we react to

CONSIDER THIS!

About 15% of college students say their academic performance has been impaired because of Internet use or computer games.

stressors. For example, our society has traditionally deemed it more acceptable for women to express their emotions openly. Therefore, a woman might feel more comfortable discussing stressors and be better able to cope with them than a man who has been socialized to "keep his feelings in." Conversely, a woman might have been taught that certain responses, such as explosive anger, are not "ladylike" and therefore refrain from expressing her anger, leading to greater stress. Participating in activities outside traditional gender roles also might produce stress. A man who decides to be a stay-at-home dad or work from home so his wife can pursue her career, for example, might experience higher levels of stress because his choice does not fit with societal norms. Gender-related reactions to stress also might vary in different cultures.

Regardless of your personality characteristics, past experiences, and gender, you can learn ways to deal with the stress in your life, and the first step is to examine your stress level. A convenient way to do this is to complete a questionnaire designed to evaluate your stress level, such as Laboratory 10.1 at the end of this chapter. If the results suggest that you are under unhealthy levels of stress, you should implement stress management and stress reduction techniques.

Common Causes of Stress

Recognizing the everyday life situations that contribute to your stress level is important in managing stress. The pressure of performing well in your classes, along with competing deadlines for papers, projects, and tests, can be a source of stress, especially if you do not have strong time management skills. Choosing a major and planning for your future after graduation are also stressful processes. Making use of career services and talking with your professors and faculty advisors can help you find the best options for your strengths and interests.

Interpersonal relationships often change when you enter college. If you move to go to college, getting connected within the college community and developing new relationships can be a source of stress. Leaving family and friends also can be a challenge. If you did not have to move, your existing relationships still might be affected as you balance your time with schoolwork, new friends, and other responsibilities of college life.

Financial responsibilities can be a source of stress in many stages of life. Costs associated with college tuition, fees, and books are high, and you may have to rely on student loans to assist with college expenses.

with the demands of school. Nontraditional students—for example, people who have returned to school after several years—may feel out of place and experience additional stress related to those feelings. In addition to balancing the demands of school, work, and relationships, some students engage in leisure activities, such as spending time on the Internet, which affect productivity and, in turn, may lead to stress. Students with disabilities are likely to face stressors in learning to navigate a college campus that might not adequately accommodate their specific disabilities.

Make sure you know...

> Personality can impact the way we perceive situations and respond to stress. Type A and Type D behavior patterns are associated with higher risk for heart disease.

> Past experiences and gender also influence our reactions to situations we perceive as stressful.

> College life can present many stressors. Some of the most common include academic responsibilities, poor time management, the demands of relationships, and finances.

Stress and Health

Chronic (persistent) stress is related to some of the most significant health problems in the United States. Heart disease, depression, and migraines are all associated with stress and have significant direct and indirect health care costs. Stress is a risk factor for depression and anxiety, and up to 25% of the U.S. adult population suffers from these and other mental health problems every year (7). Approximately 75–90% of all physician visits are for stress-related complaints, and millions of people take medication for stress-related illnesses (8). From a medical standpoint, stress can affect both emotional and physical health. Chronic stress has been linked to elevated blood pressure, heart disease, hormonal imbalances, reduced resistance to disease, and emotional disorders (9–11) (Figure 10.3).

Stress-related problems cost both businesses and government billions of dollars every year in the form of employee absenteeism and health care costs. Stress can suppress the immune system, making a person more susceptible to illness. Acute stress also can impact productivity. Headaches and tension might cause a person to miss work or class or be less focused. Therefore, stress is a major health problem that affects individual lives and the economy as a whole.

Hans Selye developed one of the earliest scientific theories to explain the relationship between stress and disease. Selye proposed that humans adapt to stress in

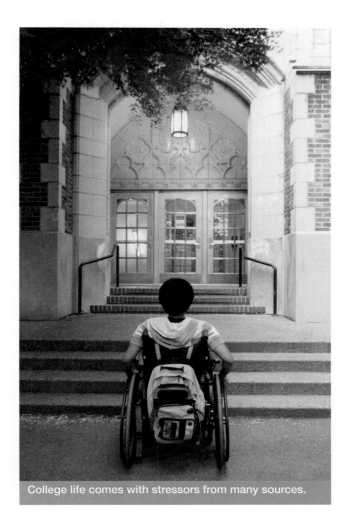
College life comes with stressors from many sources.

Work-study and other college programs can relieve some of the financial burden but place additional demands on your already limited time. Maybe you are among the many students who have to work during the school year and summers to make money for school. These work demands can be a significant source of stress, because they affect relationships, time, and schoolwork. Also, when selecting your major, you have to consider job opportunities and earning potential of the career paths that interest you. The need to attend graduate school or take low-paying or nonpaying internships can further add to financial strain and stress. Budgeting and planning for expenses are important skills to develop. Avoiding credit card debt also reduces stress of the financial burden of college.

Other common college stressors include traffic, parking on campus, and adjusting to college life. (See the Closer Look box on page 300 for a discussion of road rage, one common source of traffic stress). Students who are married with families have the combined stresses of managing home and family responsibilities

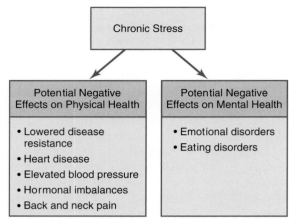

FIGURE 10.3
Chronic stress can have negative effects on both physical and mental health.

a response he termed the **general adaptation syndrome,** which involves three stages: an alarm stage, a resistance stage, and an exhaustion stage (2).

During the alarm stage, the fight-or-flight response, discussed earlier, occurs. There is a release of the stress hormones, and their effects on the body can cause anxiety, headaches, and disrupted patterns of sleeping and eating (2). During this phase, the body is more susceptible to disease and more prone to injury.

With continued exposure to stress, the individual reaches the resistance stage. During this stage, the body's resistance to stress is higher than normal, and mechanisms are activated that allow the body to resist disease effectively. In short, the resistance stage represents an improved ability to cope with stress (2).

However, if the stress persists, the individual reaches the exhaustion stage. Note that "exhaustion" in this sense refers to the depletion of the physical and psychological resources to cope with stress that occurs with chronic exposure to stress. Selye suggests that the body is vulnerable to disease during this stage because the resources for responding to stress are depleted. During this phase, physical symptoms that appeared in the alarm stage can reappear, but they now are more serious and can sometimes compromise health.

Although Selye's model of adaptation to stress is still viewed as an important contribution to our understanding of the stress response, newer research findings have improved our understanding of the relation-

A CLOSER LOOK
ROAD RAGE

WHAT IS ROAD RAGE?

Road rage refers to extreme acts of aggression resulting from disagreements between drivers. Typical road rage behaviors include tailgating, headlight flashing, obscene gestures, deliberately blocking other vehicles, verbal abuse, and its most extreme form—physical assault. According to estimates, aggressive driving injures or kills at least 1500 people each year. Road rage is a serious problem and a criminal offense.

WHAT CAUSES ROAD RAGE?

For many of us, driving is our most stressful daily activity. Roadways are crowded, and we must deal with all levels of drivers—good and bad. Everyone makes traffic mistakes at times, whether intentionally or unintentionally. Often, road rage starts as a simple misunderstanding between drivers and then escalates into a more serious situation. Usually, the driving incident is not the immediate cause of anger. For some, mounting professional or personal troubles, plus frustration over another driver's "stupid" mistakes, is enough to cause them to erupt in anger. Drivers in a "bad mood" before they get behind the wheel are more likely to have strong reactions to the actions of other drivers. Researchers believe that some personality characteristics are more prone to aggressive driving.

If you drive aggressively, the following tips can help you reduce your traffic stress:

- Avoid driving during times of heaviest congestion.

- Allow yourself plenty of time so you do not have to speed, run traffic lights, or roll through stop signs.

- Drive in comfort. Use your air conditioner, get a comfortable seat cover, and listen to classical music during your drive. Do not listen to emotionally stimulating radio talk shows. Enjoy audio books.

- Do not drive when you are angry or upset.

- When in traffic, concentrate on being relaxed. Practice breathing for relaxation.

STEPS FOR
BEHAVIOR CHANGE

How well do you manage your time?

Take the quiz below to find out whether you are a good time manager.

Y N

☐ ☐ Do you procrastinate?

☐ ☐ Do you take on more responsibilities than you can handle?

☐ ☐ Are you consistently late for class, appointments, or work?

☐ ☐ Do you need more hours in the day to accomplish all of your daily tasks?

☐ ☐ Do you have little time for fun with friends or family?

If you answered yes to most or all of these questions, you can probably use some tips for better time management.

TIPS TO IMPROVE YOUR TIME MANAGEMENT SKILLS, REDUCE STRESS, AND INCREASE PRODUCTIVITY

☑ Plan ahead. Plan your day by using a PDA or daily planner to organize tasks. Make a schedule you are able to implement, and allow time for unscheduled events and delays.

☑ Delegate responsibility. If you are involved with clubs or group projects, share and delegate responsibility to lower stress. Also, learn to say no to activities that prevent you from achieving your goals. Before accepting a new responsibility, complete your current task or eliminate an unnecessary project.

☑ Establish goals. Establish a list of goals you plan to accomplish. Include short- and long-term goals.

☑ Prioritize. List your tasks in order of their importance (high priority to low priority), and then follow that list. Establish a daily goal of accomplishing the three most important tasks on your priority list.

☑ Schedule time for you. Find time each day to relax and do something you enjoy. Regularly evaluate your ratio of work time to home and leisure time, and make sure you maintain balance.

---

ship between stress and disease. We now know that the underlying cause of many stress-related diseases is the body's inability to respond to stress the normal way, not because of depletion of resources. The repeated and/or prolonged response to stress results in the continual activation of the the nervous, endocrine, and immune systems. This long-term activation includes the continual release of stress hormones, including cortisol.

The ideas of **allostasis** and **allostatic load** are better explanations of the relationship between stress and disease. Allostasis refers to the body's ability to change and adapt in stressful situations. With long-term stress, we do not adapt as well. The allostatic load is the point at which there is too much stress, which taxes the system's stress response (12). The constant

level of activation or the repeated activation causes stress response to become inefficient.

One's risk of developing a stress-related illness increases because high levels of cortisol in the blood impair the immune system's ability to fight infections over time (12–15). As you have realized by now, prolonged stress places an individual at greater risk for illness and

general adaptation syndrome A pattern of responses to stress that consists of an alarm stage, a resistance stage, and an exhaustion stage.

allostasis The ability to maintain homeostasis through change.

allostatic load The inability to respond appropriately to stress; leads to compromised health.

STEPS FOR
BEHAVIOR CHANGE

Are you getting enough sleep?

Making sure that you get enough sleep will help you effectively deal with your daily stressors and may also help improve your grades. Answer these questions to find out whether you are getting enough sleep.

Y   N

☐ ☐ Do you fall asleep as soon as your head hits the pillow?

☐ ☐ Do you find yourself dozing in class or at other inappropriate times of the day?

☐ ☐ Do you frequently take naps during the day?

☐ ☐ Do you have an irregular bedtime?

☐ ☐ Do you "binge" sleep on the weekend?

☐ ☐ Do you have difficulty waking in the morning?

If you answered yes to more than two of the above questions, you may not be getting enough sleep at night.

TIPS TO HELP YOU GET CONSISTENT, RESTFUL SLEEP

☑ Avoid drinking caffeinated beverages after 4:00 PM.

☑ Avoid stimulating reading or television/movies in the evening. Instead, try meditating or listening to soothing music to help you unwind and relax.

☑ Keep a regular bedtime.

☑ Avoid disrupting your regular sleep pattern. Long naps during the day and using the weekend to play "catch up" on sleep missed during the week can disrupt sleep patterns.

☑ Use bright light in the morning to help you wake up.

☑ Sleep in a comfortable environment. A cool, dark room with little noise is recommended for a good night of sleep.

other associated problems. As a result, understanding and implementing stress management skills are important for maintaining a high level of wellness.

Make sure you know...

> Depression and anxiety have a significant impact on the U.S. adult population, and stress is a risk factor for both conditions.

> General adaptation syndrome, which includes alarm, resistance, and exhaustion stages, was one of the first theories proposed about the relationship between stress and disease.

> The concept of the allostatic load is that long-term and repeated exposure to stress and the continual activation of the stress response compromise health.

How Can You Manage Stress?

Once you know your stress level, you can cope with stress by using stress management techniques. There are two general steps to managing stress: Reduce the

FIGURE 10.4
Rest, exercise, and meditation are all techniques you can use to reduce your stress level.

amount of stress in your life, and cope with stress by improving your ability to relax (16). Let's discuss each of these steps individually.

Manage Stressors

The first significant way to lower the impact of stress on your life is to reduce the number of stressors you encounter (see the Closer Look box, page 304). Although you will not be able to avoid all sources of stress, you can eliminate many "unnecessary" forms of stress. The first step is to recognize those factors that produce daily stress. Use Laboratory 10.1 to assess your stressors and to help determine which ones you can most readily work to eliminate, avoid, or better manage. Getting adequate amounts of rest and sleep and exercising regularly, are also important factors in managing your stress levels.

One example of a stressor that you can eliminate is overcommitment, a frequent cause of stress in college students. If you plan your time carefully and prioritize your activities, you can avoid feeling overwhelmed by having too much to do and not enough time to do it. You can plan a daily schedule that allows you to accomplish the things you need to without being distracted by less important activities. The Steps for Behavior Change box on page 301 can help you determine how well you manage your time.

Another common stressor that you may be able to better manage is financial pressure. You cannot eliminate the high costs associated with paying tuition, rent (or room and board), or buying textbooks and materials, but you can strive to minimize the amount of debt you accrue as a student, particularly credit card debt. Avoiding overuse of credit cards and developing a budget are two very important strategies for preventing

excessive debt. Look for ways to reduce your everyday costs, and do not buy the expensive clothes or gadgets if you do not have the money to pay for them, no matter how popular they may be.

Rest and Sleep

One of the most effective means of reducing stress and tension is to get an adequate amount of rest and sleep. How much sleep do you need? Although individual needs vary greatly, adults typically need 7 to 9 hours of restful sleep per night. Because of the body's natural hormonal rhythms, you should also try to go to bed at approximately the same time every night. See the Steps for Behavior Change box on page 302 to help determine whether you're getting enough sleep.

In addition to a good night's sleep, 15 to 30 minutes of rest during the day can help reduce stress. You can do this by simply putting your feet up on a desk or table and closing your eyes. A well-rested body is the best protection against stress and fatigue.

Exercise

Light to moderate exercise can reduce many types of stress and anxiety. Even if you are not an experienced exerciser, you can benefit from the calm feeling that comes after an exercise session. The recommended types of exercise for optimal stress reduction are low-to-moderate-intensity aerobic exercises, such as brisk walking, swimming, and cycling. The guidelines for this type of exercise prescription are presented in Chapter 3. Yoga, tai-chi, and Pilates are other popular types of exercise that help you reduce stress and relax. Many gyms and health clubs offer classes in these forms of exercise.

Studies have shown that exercise is a very effective for stress reduction (17–19). Figure 10.4 compares the effects of a 30-minute session of exercise (running) to other common forms of stress reduction: rest, reading, and meditation. In this study, meditation provided the greatest stress reduction, with exercise finishing a close second (17). Other studies have shown that exercise reduces stress about as much as other types of relaxation techniques (20). Also, the relaxing effects of exercise can last for hours after an exercise session (21).

Although we consistently see that people feel more relaxed after exercise, we do not know exactly how exercise reduces stress. Several ideas have been proposed. One theory is that exercise causes the brain to release several natural tranquilizers (endorphins), which can produce a calming effect (22). Another theory is that exercise may be a diversion or break from your stressors and worries of life. The improved physical fitness and self-image that you enjoy as a result of regular exercise also increases your resistance to stress. A final possibility is that all of these factors may contribute to the beneficial effects of exercise on stress management. The next time you feel stressed, try exercising; you will feel and look better as a result.

Use Relaxation Techniques to Cope with Stress

Stress management techniques can help reduce the potentially harmful effects of stress. Most of these techniques are designed to relax you and thereby reduce your stress level. When trying to relax, ask yourself two questions: (a) What prevents me from relaxing? And (b) What am I not doing that could help me relax? (9). Your answers can help you determine how and where to focus your efforts to manage your stress. Lowering your levels of stress and practicing effective stress management techniques will increase your overall level of wellness (14). The following are some of the more common approaches used in stress management.

Progressive Relaxation   Progressive relaxation is a stress reduction technique that uses exercises to reduce muscle tension. (Muscle tension is a common symptom of stress.) You practice the technique while sitting quietly or lying down. First you contract muscle groups, and then you relax them one at a time, beginning with your feet and then moving up your body to your hands and neck, until you achieve a complete state of muscle relaxation. You can find specific directions for one progressive relaxation exercise in the Closer Look box on the following page.

The proponents of progressive relaxation techniques argue that relaxing the muscles in this manner will also relax the mind and therefore relieve stress.

A CLOSER LOOK

HOW MUCH STRESS IS TOO MUCH?

The number of stressors that each of us can deal with, as well as our reaction to the stressors, is very individual. Even so, there are some common signs of being overstressed. People who experience chronic stress or very high levels of stress and its associated feelings of anxiety can experience **burnout** (21). If you recognize any of the following warning signals of burnout in your own life, begin practicing the stress management techniques offered in this chapter.

1. **Changes in sleeping patterns.** You might sleep too much or too little. Also, you might have trouble falling asleep and/or staying asleep. Waking up during the night with difficulty returning to sleep is especially a concern. During these periods of waking, you typically find yourself thinking about events or activities that are causing you stress.

2. **Changes in eating habits.** You either overeat or undereat. During stressful times some people gain weight, especially in the abdominal area. However, others lose weight. Once again, this response is highly individual.

3. **Greater susceptibility to illness.** You begin to notice more frequent headaches (migraines), stomachaches, muscle tension, and other aches or pains. Over time you may be more susceptible to colds or other viral and bacterial infections. In addition, you do not recover as quickly as you once did.

4. **Intense cravings.** Specific cravings depend on your preferences and habits. Common cravings include coffee (caffeine), cigarettes, alcohol, and special "comfort" foods, such as chocolate, ice cream, and other high-fat, high-calorie foods. You might find that to relieve your anxiety, it takes larger quantities of these substances than you would normally use or consume. Sometimes the behavior or food does not relieve the negative feelings caused by stress.

5. **Increased feelings of hopelessness and exhaustion.** Over time, the lack of sleep, coupled with the ever-increasing unhealthy lifestyle and its negative consequences, can make you to want to "give up." If you get to this point, you may find yourself thinking about dropping a class, quitting your job or school, leaving your mate, moving, or doing anything that may relieve some of the stress in your life.

PROGRESSIVE RELAXATION TRAINING

There are many types of progressive relaxation training methods, and over 200 different exercises have been described. The basic technique involves contracting and relaxing muscle groups, starting in your lower body and moving toward your upper body. The following technique is one of the many forms that you can use.

1. Find a quiet, comfortable, and private place. Remove your shoes. Wear loose, comfortable clothing, or loosen any tight clothing. The first few times you can expect emerging thoughts and emotions to distract your attempts to relax. After some practice, you will be able block distractions. Listening to soothing music during your relaxation sessions is one way to help you relax and filter distractions; there are many commercial relaxation music CDs available. You may also read the instructions into a tape recorder and use them to guide you through your relaxation session. Using this strategy you will avoid having to remember the steps involved.

2. Assume a relaxed position (either sitting or lying down). Close your eyes, and begin by focusing on your breathing. Become aware of how it feels to breathe in and breathe out. Breathe deeply and slowly through your nose, and imagine that you are breathing in good, healing air and breathing out stress and muscle tension. While developing your breathing you may find it useful to inhale to a count of 7, 1-2-3-4-5-6-7, and exhale to the same count. Breathe this way several minutes before starting your progressive relaxation exercise.

3. Without speaking, focus on relaxing each part of your body. You are consciously "telling" each part of your body to relax. Contracting the muscles in each body part first and then relaxing them can help you to feel the difference, because sometimes we are not aware of tension we carry in our muscles. Do not move on to the next area until you have relaxed the part you are focusing on.

   Proceed by relaxing your body in the following order:
   a. Toes of left foot
   b. Toes of right foot
   c. Left foot
   d. Right foot
   e. Left ankle
   f. Right ankle
   g. Lower left leg
   h. Lower right leg
   i. Left thigh
   j. Right thigh
   k. Buttocks
   l. Abdomen
   m. Chest
   n. Left shoulder
   o. Right shoulder
   p. Left arm
   q. Left hand
   r. Left fingers
   s. Right arm
   t. Right hand
   u. Right fingers
   v. Neck
   w. Face

4. Now you should be completely relaxed. Continue breathing for the next few minutes. Try not to let your mind wander—remain in this relaxed state.

5. At the end of your session, take a deep breath. Slowly bring yourself out of your relaxed state. Stand up and stretch. You should feel renewed and refreshed.

The theory behind this concept is that an anxious (stressed) mind cannot exist in a relaxed body.

Breathing Exercises Breathing exercises can also help you relax. The following is a sample step-by-step breathing exercise for reducing stress:

1. Assume a comfortable position, sitting or lying down, with your eyes closed.

2. Begin to slowly inhale and exhale. Count from 1 to 3 during each inhalation and each exhalation to maintain a slow and regular breathing pattern.

3. Next, combine stretching and breathing to provide greater relaxation and stress reduction. For example, stretch your arms toward the ceiling as you inhale, then lower your arms as you exhale.

Try this exercise for 5 to 15 minutes in a quiet room.

burnout The loss of physical, emotional, and mental energy, which, if ignored, can lead to emotional exhaustion and withdrawal.

Assuming a relaxed position in a quiet setting is central to several relaxation techniques.

Meditation   **Meditation** has been practiced for ages to help people relax and achieve inner peace. There are many types of meditation, and there is no scientific evidence that one form is superior to another. Most types of meditation have the same common elements: sitting quietly for 15 to 20 minutes twice a day, concentrating on a single word or image, and breathing slowly and regularly. The goal is to achieve a complete state of physical and mental relaxation.

Although beginning a successful program may require the help of an experienced instructor, the following is a brief overview of how to practice meditation:

1. First, choose a word or sound, called a *mantra*, to repeat during the meditation. The idea of using a mantra is that this word or sound should become your symbol of complete relaxation. Choose a mantra that has little emotional significance for you, such as the word *red*.

2. Next, find a quiet area and sit comfortably with your eyes closed. Take several deep breaths, and concentrate on relaxing; let your body go limp.

3. Concentrate on your mantra. This means that you should not hear or think about anything else. Repeat

your mantra over and over again in your mind, and relax. Avoid distracting thoughts, and focus only on the mantra.

4. After 15 to 20 minutes of concentration on the mantra, open your eyes, and begin to move your thoughts away from the mantra. End the session by making a fist with both hands and saying to yourself that you are alert and refreshed.

Visualization   **Visualization** (sometimes called *imagery*) uses mental pictures to reduce stress. The idea is to create an appealing mental image (such as a quiet mountain setting) that promotes relaxation and reduces stress. To practice visualization, follow the instructions presented for meditation, but substitute a relaxing mental scene for the mantra. If you fail to reach a complete state of relaxation after your first several sessions, do not be discouraged. Achieving complete relaxation with this technique may require numerous practice sessions.

Develop Spiritual Wellness

As we discussed in Chapter 1, spiritual wellness is associated with better recovery from illness and improved mental health. Spiritual wellness can provide a sense of peace. People who report high levels of spiritual wellness often practice behaviors such as prayer, meditation, or enjoying the beauty of nature to reduce stress and anxiety.

Develop a Support Network

Having a network of friends and family to help you cope with stressors can help to reduce or eliminate stress. Sometimes just talking through your stressful situation can help you think more clearly about the situation and develop an effective plan to address your stressors. Others who have your best interest as a concern will likely help you with a plan for stress management. When you are dealing with stressors that cannot be eliminated, your network will be there for support while you work through your period of stress.

Avoid Counterproductive Behaviors

Some people choose poor health behaviors, such as smoking cigarettes or drinking alcohol, in an attempt to manage stress. However, these behaviors are counterproductive and can lead to more cumulative stress in the long term.

Using Tobacco   Many people say that they smoke cigarettes "to relax," but the nicotine in cigarettes and other tobacco products is actually a stimulant that produces responses similar to the fight-or-flight response. Additionally, nicotine is an addictive substance that has serious long-term effects. As discussed earlier, smoking is the leading cause of preventable death, increasing the risk for lung and other types of cancer and the risk for heart disease. Smoking and tobacco also are very costly habits.

Using Alcohol or Other Drugs   Using alcohol or other substances might make you briefly forget about problems or stressors, but these behaviors do not eliminate or reduce the stressor. In some cases they might add to your level of stress. Alcohol (especially binge drinking) or drug use can affect your sleep patterns and productivity. Using alcohol or other substances to solve or cope with your problems can lead to abuse. Even legal substances, such as caffeine, also can cause problems instead of solving them.

Disordered Eating Patterns   *Disordered eating patterns* are eating patterns that are not healthy, but that do not meet the clinical definitions for eating disorders. These patterns can lead to the development of an eating disorder. Undereating or overeating can be disordered eating. Skipping meals will result in lack of nutrients and energy, which can affect how well you can focus and cope with stressors. Overeating, binge eating, or using "comfort foods" to cope with stress can lead to weight gain and health problems. Also, blood glucose levels can be affected, resulting in fluctuations in your energy levels and decreased ability to focus on managing your stress.

Make sure you know...

> The two general steps involved in stress management are reducing the sources of stress and using relaxation techniques to help you cope with stress.

> The ideal way to lessen the effects of stress on your life is to reduce the sources of stress.

> Getting more rest and sleep; engaging in exercise; and practicing progressive muscle relaxation, breathing exercises, meditation, and visualization are some of the many relaxation techniques that can help you cope with stress.

> Developing your spiritual and social wellness can be very important in managing stress.

> Adopting unhealthy behaviors, such as smoking or drinking alcohol, to relax will lead to higher levels of stress in the long term.

CONSUMER CORNER

CAN NUTRITIONAL SUPPLEMENTS REDUCE EMOTIONAL STRESS?

Currently, there is no scientific evidence that any specific nutritional supplement, including megadoses of vitamins, will reduce emotional stress. According to researchers at the University of Texas Southwestern Medical Center at Dallas, most "stress formulas" contain B vitamins, such as niacin and riboflavin, which are meant to aid in recovery from physical stress (e.g., injuries), not emotional stress. The B vitamins are sometimes used to supplement the diets of people recovering from surgery. However, emotional stress does not increase the body's energy or nutrient needs, so taking vitamins will not calm us down.

Getting plenty of rest and exercising regularly, combined with a healthy diet, are the best ways to deal with emotional stress. Combining healthy lifestyle practices with stress management techniques such as those offered in this chapter can help you deal with life's stressors.

Although numerous nutritional products are marketed as stress relievers, none have been proven effective for stress reduction.

meditation A method of relaxation that involves sitting quietly, focusing on a word or image, and breathing slowly.

visualization A relaxation technique that uses appealing mental images to promote relaxation and reduce stress; also called *imagery*.

Summary

1. Stress is defined as a physiological and mental response to things in our environment that we perceive as threatening. Any factor that produces stress is called a stressor.

2. Excessive stress or poorly managed stress can lead to headaches, digestive problems, heart disease, and mental health problems.

3. The autonomic nervous system consists of the parasympathetic and sympathetic branches and works with the endocrine system to produce the stress response. The combined physiological responses of these systems result in the fight-or-flight response, which prepares the body to fight or flee.

4. Common stressors include academic and financial responsibilities, managing interpersonal relationships, and everyday life hassles.

5. Personality factors, past experiences, and gender can affect the way we perceive situations and behave in response to stressors.

6. Two steps in managing stress are to reduce stressors in your life and to learn to cope with stress by improving your ability to relax.

7. Common relaxation techniques to reduce stress include rest and sleep, exercise, progressive relaxation, breathing exercises, meditation, visualization. Developing spiritual wellness and a social network can also help you better manage stress. Avoiding unhealthy habits for reducing stress is key to maintaining manageable stress levels.

Study Questions

1. Which of the following is a physical symptom of stress?
   a. muscle tension
   b. headaches
   c. anxiety
   d. all of the above

2. Positive stress that is associated with optimal performance is called _____.
   a. distress
   b. visualization
   c. eustress
   d. productive stress

3. Which of the following is not a hormone that is part of the stress response?
   a. dopamine
   b. cortisol
   c. epinephrine
   d. norepinephrine

4. Common stressors include _____.
   a. financial responsibilities
   b. interpersonal relationship problems
   c. academic pressures
   d. all of the above

5. Which of the following is not a healthy way to cope with stress?
   a. exercise
   b. alcohol
   c. meditation
   d. progressive muscle relaxation

6. Define *stress*. Define *stressor*, and name common stressors.

7. Why is stress management important to health?

8. List the steps in stress management. Identify some common stress management (relaxation) techniques.

9. Discuss the concept of eustress.

10. Explain potential ways exercise is useful in reducing stress.

11. List the key guidelines for the development of a time management program.

Suggested Reading

Atkinson, D. *Live Right! Beating Stress in College and Beyond.* San Francisco: Benjamin Cummings, 2008.

Barrett, S., W. Jarvis, M. Kroeger, and W. London. *Consumer Health: A Guide to Intelligent Decisions*, 7th ed. New York: McGraw-Hill, 2002.

Benson, H. *The Relaxation Response.* New York: Avon, Wholecare, 2000.

Daniel, E. (Ed.). *Annual Editions: Health*, 25th ed. Guilford, CT: McGraw-Hill, 2004.

Donatelle, R. *Health: The Basics*, 8th ed. San Francisco: Benjamin Cummings, 2009.

Greenberg, J. *Comprehensive Stress Management*, 10th ed. Dubuque, IA: McGraw-Hill, 2006.

For links to the organizations and websites listed below, visit The Total Fitness and Wellness Website at www.pearsonhighered.com/powers.

American College Counseling Association

Offers information related to counseling and college students.

American College Health Association (ACHA)

Offers health-related information for college students.

National Institute of Mental Health

Working to improve mental health through biomedical research on mind, brain, and behavior.

Weil Lifestyle

Provides a wide range of wellness information.

Mayo Clinic Health

Contains wide-ranging information about stress, diet, fitness, and mental health.

American Medical Association

Includes many sources of information about a wide variety of medical problems, including stress-related disorders.

WebMD

Contains information about a wide variety of diseases and medical problems, including stress-related disorders.

American Psychological Association

Provides information on stress management and psychological disorders.

References

1. Canon, W. *The Wisdom of the Body.* New York: Norton Publishing, 1932.

2. Selye, H. *The Stress of Life*, revised edition. New York: McGraw-Hill, 1978.

3. Friedman, M., and R. H. Rosenman. Type A behavior pattern: Its association with coronary heart disease. *Annals of Clinical Research* 3(6):300–312, 1971.

4. Knox, S. S., G. Wiedner, A. Adelman, S. M. Stoney, and R. C. Ellison. Hostility and physiological risk in the National Heart, Lung, and Blood Institute Family Heart Study. *Archives of Internal Medicine* 164(22): 2442–2448, 2004.

5. DeFruyt, F., and J. Denollet. Type D personality: A five factor model perspective. *Psychology and Health* 17(5): 671–683, 2002.

6. Albus, C., J. Jordan, and C. Herrmann-Lingen. Screening for psychosocial risk factors in patients with coronary heart disease—Recommendations for clinical practice. *European Journal of Cardiovascular Rehabilitation* 11(1):75–79, 2004.

7. Kessler, R. C., W. T Chui, O. Demler, K. R. Merikangas, and E. E. Walters. Prevalence, severity, and comorbidity of 12-month DSM-IV disorders in the National Comorbidity Survey Replication Study. *Archives of General Psychiatry* 62:590–592, 2005.

8. American Psychological Association HelpCenter. How does stress affect us? www.apahelpcenter.org, accessed May 2007.

9. Weil, A. Stress and relaxation: An introduction. www.drweil.com/drw/u/id/ART00534, accessed June 2007.

10. Margen, S., et al. (Eds.). *The Wellness Encyclopedia.* Boston: Houghton Mifflin, 1992.

11. Lovallo, W. R. *Stress and Health: Biological and Psychological Interactions.* Thousand Oaks, CA: Sage Publications, 1997.

12. McEwen, B. S. Allostasis and allostatic load: Implications for neuropsychopharmacology. *Neuropsychopharmacology* 22:108–124, 2000.

13. Abercrombie, H., et. al. Flattened cortisol rhythms in metastatic breast cancer patients. *Psychoneuroendocrinology* 29(8):1082–1092, 2004.

14. Holroyd, K. A., et al. Management of chronic tension-type headache with tricyclic antidepressant medication, stress management therapy, and their combination: A randomized trial. *Journal of the American Medical Association* 285(17):2208–2215, 2001.

15. Sewitch, M., et al. Psychological distress, social support, and disease activity in patients with inflammatory bowel disease. *American Journal of Gastroenterology* 96(5): 1470–1479, 2001.

16. Howley, E., and B. D. Franks. *The Fitness Professional's Handbook,* 5th ed. Champaign, IL: Human Kinetics, 2007.

17. Tsai, J. C., et al. The beneficial effects of tai chi chuan on blood pressure and lipid profile and anxiety status in a randomized controlled trial. *Journal of Alternative Complementary Medicine* 9(5):747–754, 2003.

18. Berger, B., and D. Owen. Stress reduction and mood enhancement in four exercise modes: Swimming, body conditioning, hatha yoga, and fencing. *Research Quarterly for Exercise and Sport* 59:148–159, 1988.

19. Oliver, S., and D. Alfermann. Effects of physical exercise on resources evaluation, body self-concept and well-being among older adults. *Anxiety, Stress, and Coping* 15(3):311–320, 2002.

20. Breus, M. J., and P. J. O'Connor. Exercise-induced anxiolysis: A test of the "time out" hypothesis in high anxious females. *Medicine and Science in Sports and Exercise* 30(7):1107–1112, 1998.

21. Petruzzello, S. J., D. M. Landers, B. D. Hatfield, K. A. Kubitz, and W. Salazar. Meta-analysis on the anxiety-reducing effects of acute and chronic exercise: Outcomes and mechanisms. *Sports Medicine* 11:143–182, 1991.

22. Farrell, P. Enkephalins, catecholamines, and psychological mood alterations: Effects of prolonged exercise. *Medicine and Science in Sports and Exercise* 19:347–353, 1987.

Videos

Log on to www.pearsonhighered.com/powers to view these chapter-related videos.

Stress Management
The Multi-tasking Myth
Stress at Work and Home

NAME _____ DATE _____

Stress Index Questionnaire

The purpose of this stress index questionnaire is to increase your awareness of stress in your life. Circle either yes or no to answer each of the following questions.

Yes   No   1. I have frequent arguments.

Yes   No   2. I often get upset at work.

Yes   No   3. I often have neck and/or shoulder pains due to anxiety/stress.

Yes   No   4. I often get upset when I stand in long lines.

Yes   No   5. I often get angry when I listen to the local, national, or world news or read the newspaper.

Yes   No   6. I do not have a sufficient amount of money for my needs.

Yes   No   7. I often get upset when driving.

Yes   No   8. At the end of a workday I often feel stress-related fatigue.

Yes   No   9. I have at least one constant source of stress/anxiety in my life (e.g., conflict with boss, neighbor, mother-in-law).

Yes   No   10. I often have stress-related headaches.

Yes   No   11. I do not practice stress management techniques.

Yes   No   12. I rarely take time for myself.

Yes   No   13. I have difficulty in keeping my feelings of anger and hostility under control.

Yes   No   14. I have difficulty in managing time wisely.

Yes   No   15. I often have difficulty sleeping.

Yes   No   16. I am generally in a hurry.

Yes   No   17. I usually feel that there is not enough time in the day to accomplish what I need to do.

Yes   No   18. I often feel that I am being mistreated by friends or associates.

Yes   No   19. I do not regularly perform physical activity.

Yes   No   20. I rarely get 7 to 9 hours of sleep per night.

Scoring and Interpretation

Answering yes to any of the questions means that you need to use some form of stress management techniques (see the text for details). Total your yes answers, and use the following scale to evaluate the level of stress in your life.

Number of Yes Answers	Stress Category
6–20	High stress
3–5	Average stress
0–2	Low stress

1. Are you satisfied with your score? If not, name the areas you could target to reduce your level of stress.

_____

_____

_____

2. If you named areas you want to target in the previous question or you are in the high-stress category, what techniques will you employ to help lower your stress level? Write out a specific plan for how you will attempt to use at least of one of the stress management strategies for a specific stressor that you face.

_____

_____

_____

_____

_____

_____

LABORATORY

NAME _____ DATE _____

Keeping a Stress Diary

For this exercise, you will need seven copies of this worksheet. Keep a daily stress diary for one week. Indicate the time of day the stressor occurred, your perceived level of stress (10 is the worst stress you have ever felt), any symptoms you experienced, and your response to the symptoms. A response can include, for example, practicing a relaxation technique, getting angry, or doing nothing. At the end of 7 days, analyze your stress diary to determine the greatest sources of stress and the times that they occur. Once you have done this, you will be ready to practice effective stress management techniques.

Date: _____

Time	Level of Perceived Stress (0 to 10)	Cause of Stress	Symptoms of Stress	Your Response
7:00 AM				
8:00				
9:00				
10:00				
11:00				
12:00 PM				
1:00				
2:00				
3:00				
4:00				
5:00				
6:00				
7:00				
8:00				

1. What are the greatest sources of stress in your life, and when do they occur?

_____

_____

2. What are some specific steps you can take to eliminate or minimize these stressors?

_____

_____

NAME _____ DATE _____

Managing Time and Establishing Priorities

Often people feel that that there are not enough hours in the day. They feel that at some future point, such as "when I graduate," they will have more time to focus on priorities. Delaying things until the future results in lack of completion. Use the following time management tool to help you budget your time and organize your priorities.

Step 1: Establish Priorities

Rank each priority that applies to you in the list below. Use 1 for the highest priority, 2 for the second highest, and so on. You may add priorities as necessary.

Priority	Rank	Priority	Rank
More time with family	_____	More time for exercise and physical activity	_____
More time with friends	_____	More time to relax	_____
More time for work and professional pursuits	_____	More time to study	_____
More time for leisure and recreation	_____	More time for myself	_____
More time with boyfriend/girlfriend/spouse	_____	Other: _____	_____

Step 2: Monitor Your Current Time Use

Pick one day of the week, and track what you do each hour of the day.

Time	Activity
5:00 AM	
6:00	
7:00	
8:00	
9:00	
10:00	
11:00	
12:00 PM	
1:00	
2:00	

LABORATORY

Time	Activity
3:00	
4:00	
5:00	
6:00	
7:00	
8:00	
9:00	
10:00	
11:00	
12:00 AM	

Step 3: Analyze Your Current Time Use

1. In what activity can you spend less time? For example, did you watch TV for 3 hours?

   _____

   _____

2. What can you do to spend less time in these activities? How can you replace those activities with ones on your prioritized list?

   _____

   _____

3. During which hours can you spend time doing activities that are important to you?

   _____

   _____

Step 4: Make a Schedule

Write in your planned activities for the next day, and try to stick closely to this schedule.

Time	Activity
5:00 AM	
6:00	
7:00	
8:00	
9:00	
10:00	
11:00	
12:00 PM	
1:00	
2:00	
3:00	
4:00	
5:00	
6:00	
7:00	
8:00	
9:00	
10:00	
11:00	
12:00 AM	

Were you able to modify your schedule to find time for your priorities? If not, state how you will modify your plan to accommodate your priority activities.

_____

_____

NAME _____ DATE _____

Assessing Your Personality Behavior Pattern

Circle the position that you feel best reflects your typical behavior in the situations described. Behaviors exhibited by extreme Type A behavior pattern fall to the left, and those exhibited by extreme Type B behavior pattern fall to the right.

Extreme Type A Behavior Pattern						Extreme Type B Behavior Pattern
Fast at doing things	1	2	3	4	5	Slow at doing things (eating, talking, walking)
Unable to wait patiently	1	2	3	4	5	Able to wait patiently
Never late	1	2	3	4	5	Unconcerned about being on time
Very competitive	1	2	3	4	5	Not competitive
Poor listener (I finish other people's sentences for them)	1	2	3	4	5	Good listener
Always in a hurry	1	2	3	4	5	Never in a hurry
Always do two or more things at once	1	2	3	4	5	Take one thing at a time
Speak quickly and forcefully	1	2	3	4	5	Speak slowly and deliberately
Need recognition from others	1	2	3	4	5	Don't worry about what others think
Push myself (and others) hard	1	2	3	4	5	Easygoing
Don't express feelings	1	2	3	4	5	Good at expressing feelings
Few interests outside school or work	1	2	3	4	5	Many hobbies and interests
Very ambitious	1	2	3	4	5	Not ambitious
Eager to get things done	1	2	3	4	5	Deadlines don't bother me

Interpretation

- If the majority of your responses are 1s, then you fall in the **Extreme Type A Behavior Pattern.** This personality behavior pattern is described as extremely competitive, highly committed to work, with an extreme sense of time urgency. Such individuals are extremely goal oriented, and can become hostile if someone gets between them and a goal they have established.

- If the majority of your responses are 2s with a few 1s, then you fall in the **Type A Behavior Pattern.** Type A behavior pattern is characterized by the traits listed for Extreme Type A behavior pattern, but they are moderated somewhat. People who exhibit this behavior pattern are ambitious, competitive, and goal oriented, with a sense of time urgency.

- If your responses are a mixture of the behavior patterns, you are described as a **Balanced Personality.** People with this type of personality get things done, but not at all costs. They can compete but do not feel they have to. They are more laid-back and inclined to give people the benefit of the doubt. They balance leisure time and work time.

- If the majority of your responses are 4s with some 5s, then you fall in the **Type B Behavior Pattern.** People with Type B behavior pattern are easygoing and lack a strong sense of time urgency. They don't like to compete and won't let deadlines interfere with vacation or leisure time. It is not that they are less ambitious than those with Type A behavior pattern; they are just more relaxed.

- If the majority of your responses are 5s, then you fall in the **Extreme Type B Behavior Pattern.** This personality behavior pattern is very relaxed, with no sense of time urgency. In fact, Extreme Type Bs typically don't wear a watch. They try to avoid competition at all costs and never mix leisure time and work time.

Remember: This inventory is only one aspect of your personality. If your responses indicate Type A tendencies, you may want to assess your lifestyle and address some of the more stressful areas.

NAME _____ DATE _____

Assessing Your Risk for Stress-Related Illness

In 1967, Drs. Holmes and Rahe developed a scale of life change events to study the relationship between stress and illness. These events have been updated through the years to better reflect the amount of stress that life changes can bring about. To identify the level of stress in your life, circle each of the following life change events that you have experienced during the past 12 months. Add the assigned life change unit (LCU) values to determine your total LCU score. Refer to the scoring chart below the table to determine your risk of developing a stress-related illness.

Life Event	Life Change Units (LCUs)
Death of spouse, parent, boyfriend/girlfriend	100
Divorce (yourself or your parents)	65
Pregnancy (or causing pregnancy)	65
Marital separation or breakup with boyfriend/girlfriend	60
Jail term or probation	60
Death of other family member (other than spouse, parent, boyfriend/girlfriend)	60
Broken engagement	55
Engagement	50
Serious personal injury or illness	45
Marriage	45
Entering college or beginning next level of school	45
Change in independence or responsibility	45
Any drug or alcohol use	45
Fired at work or expelled from school	45
Change in alcohol or drug use	45
Reconciliation with spouse or significant other	40
Trouble at school	40
Serious health problem of a family member	40
Working while attending school	35
Working more than 40 hours per week	35
Changing course of study	35
Change in frequency of dating	35
Sexual adjustment problems (confusion of sexual identity)	35

Life Event	Life Change Units (LCUs)
Gain new family member (new baby born or parent remarries)	35
Change in work responsibilties	35
Change in financial state	30
Death of a close friend (not family member)	30
Change to a different kind of work	30
Change in number of arguments with spouse, significant other, family, or friends	30
Sleeping fewer than 8 hours per night	25
Trouble with in-laws or family of significant other	25
Outstanding personal achievement (e.g., awards, grades, promotion)	25
Significant other or parents start or stop working	20
Begin or end school	20
Change in living conditions (e.g., visitors in home, change in roommates)	20
Change in personal habits (start or stop a habit, such as smoking or dieting)	20
Chronic allergies	20
Trouble with boss	20
Change in work hours	15
Change in residence	15
Change in religious activity	15
Change to a new school (other than graduation)	10
Going into debt (you or your family)	10
Change in frequency of family gatherings	10
Vacation	10
Currently in winter holiday season	10
Minor violation of the law	5
Total Life Change Events	

Scoring

- Fewer than 150 LCUs   37% chance of developing a stress-related illness
- 150–299 LCUs   51% chance of developing a stress-related illness
- Over 300 LCUs   80% chance of developing a stress-related illness

Remember: This score indicates your probability or risk of developing a stress-related illness. It does not guarantee that you will develop a stress-related illness. Persons with a low stress tolerance may develop a stress-related illness with fewer than 150 LCUs, and others may remain healthy in spite of high numbers of LCUs. It is your perception of the stressors, as well as your ability to effectively manage them, that influences your chance of developing a stress-related illness. Developing a realistic perception of the stressor(s), plus employing effective coping strategies such as those presented in this chapter, will lessen your chances of becoming ill. If after evaluating the level of stress in your life you would like to learn more about stress management or contact a professional for help in this area, refer to the websites listed at the end of this chapter.

Source: Reprinted from T. H. Holmes and R. H. Rahe, "The Social Readjustment Rating Scale," Journal of Psychosomatic Research, Vol. 11, Issue 2, Aug 1967, pp. 213–218, © 1967, with permission from Elsevier Limited.

Exercise and the Environment

true or false?

1. Someone suffering from heat exhaustion might have pale, clammy skin.

2. Heat stroke can be a life-threatening emergency.

3. Exercise in hot or humid conditions can be more dangerous than exercise in cooler, drier environments.

4. Exercising in extreme cold can damage your lungs.

5. You breathe faster and deeper during exercise at altitudes above 5000 feet.

Answers appear on the next page.

Have you ever had a hard time catching your breath after a run on a hot day? Or have you ever felt woozy after just a few minutes of hiking in the mountains? You probably know that your environment can affect your exercise performance and that exercising in hot weather, at a high altitude, or in the midst of air pollution can elevate your heart rate, promote labored breathing, and impair your tolerance. But do you know why? In this chapter, we discuss common environmental hazards that you should consider when planning workouts or strenuous outdoor activities, and we'll outline ways to cope with environmental stress. In particular, we focus on heat and humidity, cold, altitude, and air pollution. Let's start with how your environment affects your workout.

Why Does the Environment Matter during Exercise?

Air temperature matters during exercise because humans are **homeotherms;** that is, our body temperature is regulated to remain close to a set point—98.6°F, or 37°C. If body temperature falls too far below or rises too far above this "normal" temperature, serious bodily injury can result (Figure 11.1). The body must maintain precise control over its temperature to avoid a life-threatening situation.

Other environmental factors that can affect exercise performance are altitude and air pollution. The further you rise above sea level, the less oxygen gets into the blood. Your body has to work harder to pull in adequate amounts of oxygen, and breathing and heart rate can be affected. For anyone who exercises in high-population areas, air pollution can be a problem during outdoor exercise. We will discuss each of these environmental factors in more depth next.

Make sure you know...

> Environmental factors matter during exercise. Air temperature has a significant impact on the body's ability to regulate its core temperature, and altitude can affect the body's ability to circulate oxygen in the bloodstream.

Exercising in a Hot Environment

During exercise, your muscles produce heat as a by-product of muscular contractions. High-intensity exercise using large muscle groups produces more body heat than low-intensity exercise involving small muscle groups. Thus, when large muscle groups are vigorously exercised under hot conditions, the body produces excess heat that it must release in order to prevent a dangerous rise in body temperature. If the body cannot eliminate enough heat to keep body temperature from exceeding 105°F (41°C), then heat injury can ensue (1). There are several types of heat injury, and their various symptoms can include cramps; dizzyness; nausea; clammy skin; rapid heartbeat; lack of sweating; seizures; and hot, dry skin.

Answers

1. TRUE Because blood volume and circulatory control are compromised during heat exhaustion, blood flow to the skin is reduced, which can cause a pale, clammy appearance.

2. TRUE Heat stroke can be an extremely serious condition, because the body stops sweating and therefore cannot release heat. A rising core body temperature can lead to brain damage or even death.

3. TRUE Increased sweating during exercise in hot, humid conditions causes rapid decreases in blood volume. This decrease can lead to heat exhaustion or heat stroke.

4. FALSE The air you breathe is warmed before it gets to the gas exchange areas of the lung, so its being cold when you first breathe it in will have no effect on your body.

5. TRUE The lower atmospheric pressure at altitudes above 5000 feet significantly reduces the forcing of oxygen into the blood. You will breathe faster and more deeply to provide more oxygen to exercising muscles.

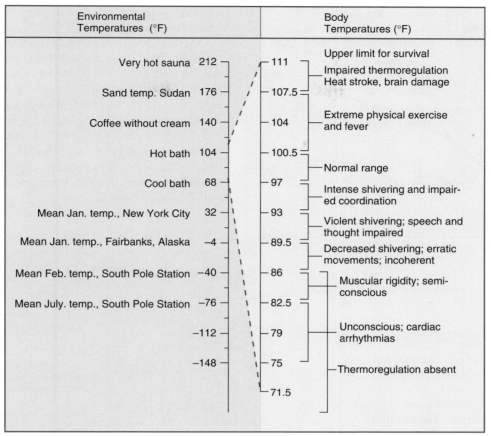

FIGURE 11.1

A comparison of temperature extremes: the environment (at left) and the body (at right). Note that even the relatively small changes in body temperature can have serious consequences.

Source: Adapted from Brooks, G., T. Fahey, K. Baldwin, and T. White. *Exercise Physiology: Human Bioenergetics and Its Applications.* Mountain View, CA: Mayfield, 1996.

Heat Loss during Exercise

There are two primary means of heat loss during exercise: convection and evaporation. The body loses heat by **convection** when air or water moves around the body. Convective heat loss occurs only when the air or water molecules moving over the surface of the body are cooler than skin temperature; the faster the flow of cool air or water around the body, the greater the heat loss. Minimal convective cooling occurs during exercise in a hot environment where there is limited air movement (riding a stationary exercise bicycle, for example). In contrast, bicycling outdoors on a cold day or swimming in cool water results in a large amount of convective cooling.

During **evaporation,** the body releases heat when sweat on the skin is converted to a gas (water vapor). On a warm day with limited air movement around the body, evaporation is the most important means of body heat loss (1). The evaporation of sweat on the skin's surface removes heat from the body, even

if the air temperature is higher than body temperature, as long as the air is dry. However, if the air temperature is high and the **humidity** is also high (i.e., the air is relatively saturated with water), then evaporation is limited and the body cannot release as much heat. Under these conditions, the body retains the heat produced by the contracting muscles and body temperature increases gradually throughout the exercise session. Prolonged exercise in a hot and humid environment can result in a dangerously high increase

homeotherms Animals that regulate their body temperature to remain close to a set point. Humans regulate their body temperature around the set point of 98.6°F or 37°C.

convection Heat loss by the movement of air or water over the surface of the body.

evaporation The conversion of water (sweat) to a gas (water vapor); the most important means of releasing heat from the body during exercise.

humidity The amount of water vapor in the air.

FIGURE 11.2
Body temperature responses to prolonged exercise under three different environmental conditions.

in body temperature. Figure 11.2 illustrates the differences in body temperature rise during exercise in a high-temperature/ high-humidity environment, a high-temperature/low-humidity environment, and a low-temperature/low-humidity environment.

Short-term exposure (30–60 min) to an extremely hot environment is sufficient to cause heat injury in some people (2), especially those at high risk. (Older adults and people with low cardiovascular fitness levels are most susceptible.) Even individuals who are physically fit and accustomed to the heat are at risk if they exercise in a hot environment.

In addition to air temperature, humidity can also be a significant factor during heat stress (Figure 11.3). The higher the humidity, the higher the "effective" temperature— that is, the temperature that the body senses. At high levels of humidity, sweat on the skin cannot evaporate into the air, impairing the body's ability to release heat. This causes body temperature to increase above what it would be on a less humid day at the same air temperature.

Although it is obviously dangerous to exercise at high air temperatures (130°F, 55°C), it may not be obvious that the body undergoes the same heat stress at only 90°F (29°C) when the relative humidity approaches 100%. In other words, the effective temperature remains at 130°F. Thus, high humidity

causes the body to sense a moderately high air temperature as extremely hot.

The best way to determine whether environmental conditions are imposing a heat load on your body is to monitor your heart rate. An increase in body temperature during exercise in a hot environment will result in larger increases in heart rate than during exercise in a cooler environment. This point is illustrated in Figure 11.4, which shows the large differences in how exercise heart rates respond to three different conditions. A temperature-induced increase in exercise heart rate is significant because it makes staying within your target heart rate zone more difficult.

Category	Heat Index	General Effect of Heat Index on People in Higher Risk Groups
1	130° or higher	Heat/sunstroke highly likely with continued exposure
2	105°–130°	Sunstroke, heat cramps, or heat exhaustion likely and heatstroke possible with prolonged exposure and/or physical activity
3	90°–105°	Sunstroke, heat cramps, and heat exhaustion possible with prolonged exposure and/or physical activity
4	80°–90°	Fatigue possible with prolonged exposure and/or physical activity

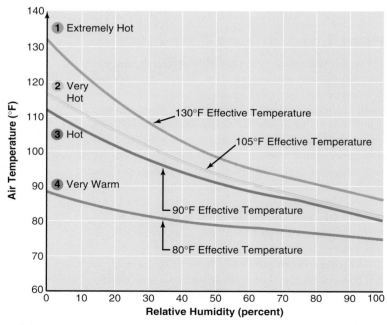

FIGURE 11.3
The concept of "heat index" or "effective" temperature.

What to Wear: Exercise Clothing for Hot Environments

You can reduce your risk of heat injury during exercise in a hot environment by wearing the proper clothing (3). The first rule is to minimize the amount of clothing you wear so that you maximize the exposed body surface area for evaporation. Clothing should be lightweight and made from materials that readily absorb moisture and allow air to move through them freely, features that promote both evaporative and convective cooling. Cottons and linens are best for these purposes.

You also don't necessarily want to switch to dry clothing when your initial clothing becomes saturated with sweat, because wet clothing promotes heat exchange better than dry clothing. Thus, switching to dry clothing delays the resumption of evaporative cooling. Heavy clothing and clothing made of rubber or plastic trap humid air next to the skin and also impair evaporative heat loss. Finally, wearing light-colored clothing when exercising outdoors will lessen the amount of radiant heat you absorb from the sun.

Be aware of the signs of heat injury. Distance runners and athletes who wear heavy equipment in hot conditions are especially prone to the serious effects of heat injury.

Heat Acclimatization

Exercise in a hot, or even a moderately hot, environment will cause the body to adapt, or **acclimatize,** to this condition, thereby decreasing the likelihood of heat injury. When the body is in a hot environment and needs to dissipate more heat, sweating begins earlier, more sweat is produced (to facilitate more evaporative cooling), and blood volume increases (3). Within 10 to 12 days of heat exposure, the physiological responses to exercise in the heat are drastically altered (3). The result is that heat acclimatization promotes a decrease in exercise heart rate and in body temperature.

Heat injury can occur when the exercise heat load exceeds the body's ability to regulate body temperature. It is a serious condition and can result in damage to the nervous system and, in extreme cases, death. The following are the most common types of heat injury.

- *Heat cramps* are characterized by muscle spasms or twitching of limbs. They usually occur in people who are unacclimatized to the heat. Anyone with these symptoms should be moved to a cool place, laid down, and given 1 to 2 glasses of water with 1/2 teaspoon of salt added to each glass.

FIGURE 11.4
Changes in heart rate during prolonged exercise.

acclimatize To undergo the physiological adaptations that help the body adjust to environmental extremes.

heat injury Bodily injury that can occur when the heat load exceeds the body's ability to regulate body temperature. Also called *heat illness*.

A CLOSER LOOK

GUIDELINES FOR FLUID INTAKE DURING EXERCISE IN A HOT ENVIRONMENT

Because the sweat you lose during exercise is replaced with water from the blood, the ultimate danger during prolonged exercise in the heat is **dehydration** and decreased blood volume. The best strategy for preventing a decrease in blood volume is maintaining a regular schedule of fluid intake during exercise. You cannot rely on thirst as an indicator for when additional fluid is necessary, because the thirst mechanism lags behind fluid loss. Your body does not recognize a need for fluid until the composition of the blood has changed. Therefore, you should begin to drink within 10 to 20 minutes after beginning exercise, before a fluid deficit accumulates (4). The following fluid replacement schedule will help you meet your body's need for water during exercise:

CONTENTS OF FLUID

The drink should:

- Be low in sugar (generally less than 8 grams per 100 ml of water).

- Contain only a small amount of electrolytes (sodium and potassium).

- Be free of alcohol.

In general, water is the optimal fluid to drink during short duration exercise. For longer or more intense exercise sessions, an electrolyte-containing sport drink may be beneficial. Alcoholic beverages can impair performance and should be avoided for 24 hours before exercise.

FLUID INTAKE BEFORE WORKOUT

Drink approximately 16 ounces (2 cups) of fluid about 2 hours prior to the workout.

FLUID INTAKE DURING WORKOUT

Drink approximately 4 to 8 ounces (1/2 to 1 cup) every 10 to 20 minutes during exercise, regardless of whether you feel thirsty.

FLUID REPLACEMENT AFTER WORKOUT

In general, you should consume 30 ml (about 1 ounce) of fluid for every minute of exercise performed. Another means to estimate how much fluid you need is to weigh yourself before exercising and immediately after your cool-down period. The difference in body weight is a measure of how much fluid you lost via sweating, and you should replace more than that amount. In fact, each ounce of body weight lost due to sweating is equivalent to 1 fluid ounce. For example, a body weight difference of 1 pound indicates that your body lost 16 ounces of sweat during exercise. Therefore, you would need to consume more than 16 fluid ounces (2 cups) of fluid to replenish body fluid stores (4).

- *Heat exhaustion* results in general weakness, fatigue, a possible drop in blood pressure, blurred vision, occasionally a loss of consciousness, and profuse sweating from pale, clammy skin. Heat exhaustion can occur in an acclimatized individual. First aid should consist of moving the victim to a cool place, removing the clothing, applying cold water or ice, and giving 1 cup of water containing 1/2 teaspoon of salt every 15 minutes for 1 hour.

- *Heat stroke* is a life-threatening emergency. A person experiencing heat stroke stops sweating, and the skin is hot and red. Muscles are limp. Signs include involuntary limb movement, seizures, diarrhea, vomiting, and a rapid, strong heartbeat. The individual may hallucinate and eventually lapse into a coma. Any of these signs should be taken very seriously. Seek emergency medical assistance immediately, and administer first aid by moving the victim to a cool place,

removing clothing, and lowering body temperature as rapidly as possible (by giving liquids, immersing in water or ice, and/or fanning).

Each of these conditions is initiated by heat exposure and involves significant loss of water and electrolytes. The body also stores additional heat, as indicated by a high core temperature. Note that you can minimize loss of water by drinking plenty of fluids whenever it's hot. Inattention to any of the signs of heat injury can lead to heat stroke and finally to death. Do not take these symptoms lightly!

You can exercise in hot and/or humid conditions, but be sure to keep the following in mind:

- Start exercising slowly, and keep your exercise session relatively short (15 to 20 minutes).

- Monitor your exercise heart rate often, and keep your exercise intensity low so that you stay within your target heart rate zone.

EFFECTS OF DEHYDRATION

Exercise in the heat can be extremely dangerous, depending on exercise intensity, ambient temperature, relative humidity, clothing, and state of hydration. The table in this box shows how weight loss during exercise can be a predictor of some of the dangers associated with exercise in the heat. The loss of body weight during exercise in the heat is due to water loss through sweating. Thus, prolonged, profuse sweating is the first warning signal of impending dehydration.

% Body Weight Loss	Symptoms
0.5	Thirst
2	Stronger thirst, vague discomfort, loss of appetite
3	Concentrated blood, dry mouth, reduced urine output
4	Increased effort required during exercise, flushed skin, apathy
5	Difficulty in concentrating
6	Impaired temperature regulation, increased heart rate
8	Dizziness, labored breathing during exercise, confusion
10	Spastic muscles, loss of balance, delirium
11	Circulatory insufficiency, decreased blood volume, kidney failure

- Wear appropriate clothing.
- To avoid dehydration, drink plenty of fluids before, during, and after the exercise session (see the Closer Look boxes for guidelines for fluid intake and the effects of dehydration).
- Exercise in the morning or evening, when outside air temperatures are cooler because of less radiant heat from the sun. If you must exercise during the heat of the day, try to find a shaded area. This might mean exercising indoors or hiking/jogging in a wooded area.

Make sure you know...

> Evaporation is the most important means of heat loss during exercise in a hot environment.

> Heat acclimatization occurs after several days of exposure to a hot environment. It increases the body's ability to cool itself and thus reduces the likelihood of heat injury.

> Heat cramps, heat exhaustion, and heat stroke can all result from the body's failure to release enough heat during exercise; each of these conditions is potentially serious and needs to be treated immediately.

> You can exercise safely in a hot environment as long as you follow safety guidelines, such as wearing loose, light-colored clothing and drinking plenty of fluids.

Exercising in a Cold Environment

Just as exercising in too hot an environment can potentially lead to heat injury, exercising in too cold an environment can also cause problems. Below an air temperature of about 60°F, you need to wear warm clothing and retain muscle heat to prevent too much loss of body heat.

Maintaining Body Temperature in a Cold Environment

If you do not retain enough body heat in extremely cold temperatures, you are more likely to experience **hypothermia,** which can be life-threatening (1). Exercise in the cold for long periods (e.g., 1–4 hours) or swimming in cold water may overwhelm the body's ability to prevent heat loss, resulting in hypothermia. Severe hypothermia can result in a loss of judgment, which increases the risk of further cold injury.

dehydration Loss of too much body water, resulting in impaired function.

hypothermia A significant decline in body temperature due to exposure to cold.

A CLOSER LOOK

EXERCISE IN THE COLD—BUT DON'T GET WET!

Exercise in a cool or cold environment can be safe as well as pleasurable if the proper clothing is worn. If the intensity of the exercise causes a person to sweat or if a person gets wet in the rain, hypothermia could occur. One study examined the effects of cold, rain, and wind on exercise tolerance and hypothermia. Subjects were asked to attempt a 5-hour walk at 41°F (5°C) at a brisk pace. At the end of 1 hour, the subjects were exposed to constant rain and wind in addition to the cold. These conditions were severe enough that only 5 of 16 subjects could complete the 5-hour walk.

During the first hour of walking, body temperature actually rose 1 degree. However, with the onset of wind and rain, body temperature started to decrease, even when some subjects began shivering. The shivering produced weakness and loss of manual dexterity. Over the last 2 hours, body temperature was variable in subjects completing the walk. Of the five subjects who completed the walk, two experienced a severe decrease in body temperature as they were not able to maintain the walking pace because of fatigue from shivering.

This study illustrates the importance of the interaction between air temperature, wind, and water. If clothing gets wet, it conducts heat from the body so fast that the heat produced during exercise may not be sufficient to maintain body temperature. The subjects in this study were not wearing protective rainwear. Any type of waterproof clothing would have given them significant additional time to exercise in the wind and rain.

Source: Thompson, R. L., and J. S. Hayward. Wet-cold exposure and hypothermia: Thermal and metabolic responses to prolonged exercise in the rain. *Journal of Applied Physiology* 81(3):1128–1137, 1996.

Hypothermia can be avoided by limiting the duration of exercise in a cold environment, dressing appropriately, and staying out of cold water (if you're in water that makes you shiver, then it's too cold). See the Closer Look box on this page for details of one study on the effects of cold and rain on exercise performance.

Contrary to popular belief, exercising in the cold will not damage your lungs. Research suggests that exercise when the temperature is between 15°F and 32°F does not present a major risk to lung tissues (5). Inhaled cold air is rapidly warmed by the nasal passages and airways, so that by the time it reaches the lungs, it is close to normal body temperature.

What to Wear: Exercise Clothing for Cold Environments

The key to exercising in the cold is to wear the proper clothing—that is, clothing that

CONSIDER THIS!

You lose 30–40% of your body heat through the head, so wearing a hat is often important.

traps just enough of the heat produced during exercise to maintain normal body temperature, but not enough to overheat the body. The ideal clothing permits sweat to be transferred from the skin to the outer surface of the clothing, so that it does not evaporate from your skin and cause too much heat loss.

The best way to trap heat is to layer—to wear multiple layers of clothing so that air, an excellent insulator, is trapped between the layers. The thicker the zone of trapped air between the body and the outside of the clothing, the more effective the insulation; thus, several layers of lightweight clothing provide much greater insulation than a single bulky coat.

Dressing the upper body in layers is critical to maintaining the body's core temperature. Each layer has a purpose (Figure 11.5). The base layer (underwear) should remove moisture from your skin and move it to the next layer (a process called "wicking"). This is critical because wet clothing can lose its insulating properties (see Consumer Corner on page 334). Be sure to avoid cotton clothing for the base layer, because cotton will get wet and stay wet when you perspire, chilling you to the bone.

BASE LAYER: Undershirt
Purpose: Wicks moisture away from the body
Made From: Lightweight non-cotton, e.g., polypropylene, silk, polyester, Thermax, Thinsulate, wool

MID LAYER: Looser shirt
Purpose: Provides insulation
Made From: Heavier material, e.g., down, polyester, fleece, wool, Polartec, Thermax

OUTER LAYER: Jacket
Purpose: Protects from wind and water
Made From: Lightweight, breathable, windproof, water-resistant microfiber e.g., Gore-Tex

FIGURE 11.5
Layering is the key to maintaining body temperature during exercise in a cold environment.

The primary purpose of the middle layer is to further insulate the body while still wicking moisture outward. Middle layers are often a bit heavier than the base layer. They should be used only in very cold conditions and should fit loosely over the base layer. The middle layer should be easy to remove for changing environmental conditions. Suggested fabrics include Polartec, Thermax, and fleece.

The outer layer should protect you from wind and water. The wind makes the "effective" temperature colder than the actual air temperature (called the wind-chill effect; Figure 11.6). Water causes virtually the same effect by conducting heat away from the body more rapidly than air. Thus, the outer layer should be a lightweight, microfiber, well-ventilated, windproof jacket. This type of material will protect you against cold, wind, rain, or snow while still allowing perspiration to evaporate. The final layer of clothing should be the hats, scarves, and gloves that protect your extremities from frostbite and keep heat from escaping through your head and neck.

The proper amount of clothing to provide comfort during exercise varies with the temperature, the wind speed, and the intensity and duration of exercise. If you wear too little clothing, your body will lose too much heat. Too much clothing, in contrast, can limit your freedom of movement and, even more important, can trap so much heat that you sweat. If you sweat during extreme cold, the loss of body heat can lead to hypothermia, which can be fatal (3).

Make sure you know...

> Exercise in the cold can be safe and enjoyable, provided that exercisers take the necessary precautions to maintain heat balance and avoid hypothermia: limit the duration of exercise, avoid cold water, and dress in layers of the appropriate amounts and types of clothing.

	Ambient Temperature, °F*														
	40	35	30	25	20	15	10	5	0	−5	−10	−15	−20	−25	−30
Wind Speed, mph	Effective Temperature, °F*														
Calm	40	35	30	25	20	15	10	5	0	−5	−10	−15	−20	−25	−30
5	37	33	27	21	16	12	6	1	−5	−11	−15	−20	−26	−31	−35
10	28	21	16	9	4	−2	−9	−15	−21	−27	−33	−38	−46	−52	−58
15	22	16	11	1	−5	−11	−18	−25	−36	−40	−45	−51	−58	−65	−70
20	18	12	3	−4	−10	−17	−25	−32	−39	−46	−53	−60	−67	−76	−81
25	16	7	0	−7	−15	−22	−29	−37	−44	−52	−59	−67	−74	−83	−89
30	13	5	−2	−11	−18	−26	−33	−41	−48	−56	−63	−70	−79	−87	−94
35	11	3	−4	−13	−20	−27	−35	−43	−49	−60	−67	−72	−82	−90	−98
40	10	1	−6	−15	−21	−29	−37	−45	−53	−62	−69	−76	−85	−94	−101
	Little Danger					**Danger**					**Great Danger**				

*°C = 0.556 (°F − 32)
Convective heat loss at wind speeds above 40 mph have little additional effect on body cooling.

FIGURE 11.6
The "wind-chill" index.

Source: McArdle, W. D., F. I. Katch, and V. L. Katch. *Exercise Physiology: Essentials of Exercise Physiology,* 3rd ed. Philadelphia: Lippincott Williams and Wilkins, 2005.

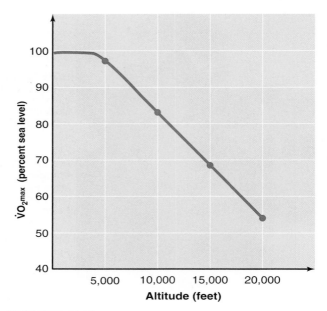

FIGURE 11.7
The effects of altitude on maximal exercise capacity.

CONSUMER CORNER

ADVANCES IN COLD-WEATHER CLOTHING

Even though wearing several layers of clothing is beneficial while exercising in the cold (because the air trapped between layers provides great insulation), exercising in the cold can be extremely dangerous if the clothing gets wet from perspiration. Thus materials that help remove moisture from the skin are better when worn next to the skin than are materials that absorb moisture, such as cotton.

New high-tech fabrics combine several layers to provide insulation, breathability, and water resistance. One example is the ComforMax™ fabric. The polyester fiberfill in the center of the fabric traps pockets of warm air, providing insulation, while the nonwoven membrane retains and reflects the body's own radiant heat. The open-pore structure of the membrane allows perspiration to pass out of the fabric and evaporate easily. An outer shell provides additional protection from both wind and water. Materials like ComforMax™ are used in many types of active wear that require warmth, insulation, and weather-resistance without excessive bulk.

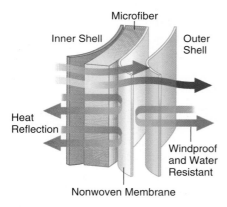

Source: DuPont™ ComforMax™ Premium is a trademark of DuPont. Illustration used by permission of DuPont.

Exercising at High Altitudes

The number of people going to high altitudes for hiking, skiing, camping, mountain climbing, and other activities is growing yearly. In fact, according to the National Ski Area Association, over 57 million visits are made to ski slopes alone each year. How does the body respond to exercise at high altitudes, and how can you adjust your exercise prescription?

The primary concern with exercise at high altitude is that the lower barometric pressure limits the amount of oxygen transported in blood (1). As a result, less oxygen reaches the exercising muscles, and therefore both exercise tolerance and $\dot{V}O_2$max are reduced. As shown in Figure 11.7, at altitudes above about 5000 feet (which is the approximate elevation of Denver, Colorado), the reduction increases as a function of increasing altitude: The higher the altitude, the more $\dot{V}O_2$max and exercise tolerance decline.

FIGURE 11.8
The effect of elevation on heart rate and ventilation during moderate exercise.

To cope with this decrease in oxygen delivery to the exercising muscles, the body makes several physiological adjustments (Figure 11.8). Breathing becomes deeper and faster in an attempt to maximize oxygen transfer from the lungs to the blood. Exercise heart rate rises to increase blood flow and oxygen delivery to the exercising muscles. To stay within your target heart rate zone during exercise at high altitude, it is necessary to lower your exercise intensity to a level below your normal intensity. In general, there is little need to alter your duration or frequency of training during a brief stay at high altitude. However, the air is very dry at high altitudes, so your body loses more water during breathing (1). In addition, the body decreases its water content as a way of coping with the stress of altitude exposure. Be sure to drink plenty of fluids during and after exercise.

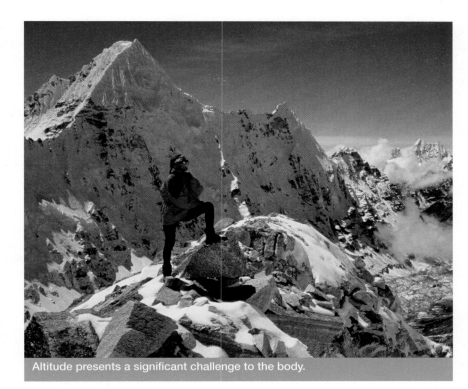

Altitude presents a significant challenge to the body.

A problem associated with recreation at very high altitude (above approximately 8000 ft) is *acute mountain sickness (AMS)*. This occurs in about 20% of people going above this altitude and may occur in as many as 80% of those who fly into areas with elevations of 12,000 feet. AMS is characterized by severe headaches, nausea, weakness, and dizziness, which, if not corrected, can cause fluid to collect in the brain or lungs, a life-threatening condition. The major cause of AMS is going too high too fast, with the result that your body doesn't have time to adjust the rate and depth of breathing.

If you know you get AMS, or if you want to reduce your chance on your first trip, try these strategies before your next trip to the mountains:

- Ascend slowly. (Hiking is best; if you drive, try to spread the trip over several days; if you fly, remain at that altitude for at least 24 hours.)
- If you go above 10,000 feet, increase your altitude by no more than 1000 feet per day.
- Sleep at the lowest elevation possible.
- If you feel the onset of AMS, don't go higher—if symptoms get worse, get off of the mountain.
- Drink plenty of water. Mountain air is typically dry, and you can dehydrate without sweating (make sure urine output is normal and clear).
- Avoid tobacco, alcohol, and other depressants, because they decrease your rate of breathing.

- Eat a high-carbohydrate diet.
- If you know you get AMS, see your doctor. There are medications that can help with acclimatization.

Make sure you know...

> Exercise at high altitude reduces the amount of oxygen in the blood, which in turn reduces oxygen transport to the working muscles and lowers both $\dot{V}O_2$max and exercise tolerance.

> At high altitudes, it is necessary to reduce the intensity of exercise to stay within your target heart rate range. However, there is little need to reduce your duration or frequency of exercise training during brief stays.

> If possible, make your ascent to high altitudes gradually, so your body can acclimatize to the lower air pressure.

Exercise and Air Pollution

Air pollution is a growing problem in many parts of the world. Particulate matter in the air can lead to respiratory problems. The increase in rate and depth of breathing during exercise increases the exposure of your lungs to the polluted air. If you exercise outdoors in a polluted environment, you should take measures to minimize pollution's effects.

11 A.M. – 3 P.M.
Ozone Levels
Are High

7 A.M. – 8 A.M.
Carbon Monoxide
Levels Are High
in Traffic Areas

5 P.M. – 6 P.M.
Carbon Monoxide
Levels Are High
in Traffic Areas

FIGURE 11.9
Times of day to avoid exercise because of high levels of
ozone and carbon monoxide.

Major Forms of Air Pollution

Two major pollutants that affect exercise performance
are ozone and carbon monoxide (6). **Ozone** is a gas
produced primarily by a chemical reaction between
sunlight and the hydrocarbons emitted from car exhaust. This form of pollution is extremely irritating to
the lungs and airways, causing tightness in the chest,
coughing, headaches, nausea, throat and eye irritation,
and, worst of all, bronchoconstriction (6). In fact,
exposure to ozone can trigger an asthma attack.

To protect citizens from air pollution, many cities
monitor air quality and issue health alerts when it is
poor. Stage 1 health alerts are issued when ozone
reaches 0.2 ppm (parts per million), and stage 2 alerts
are issued at 0.35 ppm. These alerts suggest that anyone with lung problems, such as asthma, should not exercise outdoors. Many large metropolitan areas now
have stage 1 alerts on more than 100 days out of the
year. Although the long-term effects of ozone exposure
are not clear, research suggests that chronic exposure
to ozone diminishes lung function.

Carbon monoxide is a gas produced during the
burning of fossil fuels, such as gasoline and coal, and it
is also present in cigarette smoke. This pollutant binds
to hemoglobin in the blood and reduces the blood's
oxygen-carrying capacity. High levels of carbon monoxide can impair exercise performance by reducing oxygen delivery to the exercising muscles (6). In cities
where traffic is heavy and congested, carbon monoxide
can be a serious deterrent to exercise. For example, re-

search suggests that runners in large metropolitan
areas exhibit carbon monoxide levels in the blood
that are twice the level necessary to negatively affect
exercise performance (6).

Coping with Air Pollution

The best way to minimize the effects of air pollution
during exercise is to avoid exercising when ozone or
carbon monoxide levels are highest (Figure 11.9). On
hot summer days, ozone levels are highest during midday (11:00 AM to 3:00 PM), when the sun's ultraviolet
rays are strongest. Avoid exercising during this time
and also when automobile traffic is heavy. Carbon
monoxide levels reach approximately 35 ppm in moving
traffic and can exceed 100 ppm in slow and congested
conditions (6). Because these levels can extend 20 to 30
yards away from traffic, exercisers should avoid heavily
traveled roads and stay at least 30 yards away from the
road if possible. Exposure to carbon monoxide (from
sitting in traffic with the windows down or being in a
smoke-filled room) can be detrimental before exercise,
too, because carbon monoxide leaves the blood slowly.
In fact, the body may need more than 6 hours to remove significant amounts of carbon monoxide from the
blood (6). See the Steps for Behavior Change box to
help determine whether you can lessen your exposure
to air pollution during exercise.

Air pollution is not always visible. Therefore, you
must be aware of the times of day at which various
pollutants are in highest concentrations and avoid
exercising then. Pollutants not only affect exercise
performance, but also, with chronic exposure, are
hazardous to your health. So, don't simply try to avoid
pollution; do what you can to reduce pollution so that
you have a cleaner environment in which to exercise.
Walk or take public transportation rather than driving
whenever possible. Recycle waste, and don't burn
leaves or garbage.

Make sure you know...

> Ozone is produced by a chemical reaction between
sunlight and automobile exhaust. Carbon monoxide
is produced by the burning of fossil fuels. Both
forms of air pollution can impair exercise tolerance.

> Avoid exercising during the times of day when ozone
or carbon monoxide levels are highest. Ozone levels
are highest during midday on hot summer days.
Carbon monoxide levels are highest when
automobile traffic is heavy.

STEPS FOR
BEHAVIOR CHANGE

How exposed are you to air pollution during exercise?

Are you minimizing your exposure to air pollution during exercise? Answer the following questions to find out.

Y N

☐ ☐ Do you work out late in the afternoon?

☐ ☐ Do you exercise outdoors when air pollution is high?

☐ ☐ Do you jog near congested roadways?

If you answered yes to any of the above questions, you may be able to avoid exposing yourself to excess air pollution by making a few changes.

TIPS TO REDUCE YOUR EXPOSURE TO AIR POLLUTION

☑ Work out during the early morning hours. Ozone levels are highest during the heat of the day. Also, pollution levels tend to be lower in the morning because overnight there is less traffic and industrial emissions are lower, and air movement may move polluted air out of the area.

☑ Exercise indoors. A good indoor health facility will have air filters and conditioned air.

☑ Avoid exercising near congested traffic. Automobile emissions contain pollutants that can both harm your lungs and decrease your exercise capacity.

ozone A gas produced by a chemical reaction between sunlight and the hydrocarbons emitted from car exhausts.

carbon monoxide A gas produced during the burning of fossil fuels such as gasoline and coal; also present in cigarette smoke.

Summary

1. Evaporation is the most important means of heat loss during exercise in a hot environment. Maximizing the body surface area exposed to the air, such as by wearing appropriate clothing, will help ensure adequate release of body heat through evaporation.

2. The body becomes acclimatized to heat after several days of exposure to a hot environment. Acclimatization increases the body's ability to lose heat and reduces the likelihood of heat injury. During exercise in hot environments, it is important to drink plenty of fluids to avoid dehydration.

3. Although long-term exercise in a cold environment can result in hypothermia, short-term exercise in a cold environment does not generally pose a serious threat to heat balance. The key to avoiding hypothermia when exercising in a cold environment is to dress in layers of clothing.

4. Exercise at high altitude reduces the amount of oxygen in the blood, which reduces oxygen transport to the working muscles and lowers both $\dot{V}O_2$max and exercise tolerance.

5. At high altitudes, it is necessary to reduce the intensity of exercise so that you stay within your target heart rate range. However, there is little need to reduce your duration or frequency of exercise training during brief stays at high altitudes.

6. Ozone is produced by a chemical reaction between sunlight and automobile exhaust. Carbon monoxide is produced by the burning of fossil fuels. Both forms of air pollution can impair exercise tolerance. The best way to minimize the effects of air pollution during exercise is to avoid exercising when ozone or carbon monoxide levels are highest.

Study Questions

1. Which of the following is a major mechanism of heat loss during exercise?
   a. conduction
   b. radiation
   c. evaporation
   d. diffusion

2. During exercise, body temperature would rise to the highest level in which of the following environmental conditions?
   a. high temperature and low humidity
   b. high temperature and high humidity
   c. low temperature and high humidity
   d. low temperature and low humidity

3. The best strategy for dressing to exercise in the cold is to
   a. wear the thickest garment available.
   b. wear light-colored clothes.
   c. wear clothing that prevents moisture penetration.
   d. wear layers of clothing.

4. The greatest danger of exercising in the cold is
   a. reduced oxygen intake.
   b. increased likelihood of hypothermia.
   c. sweating too little.
   d. none of these.

5. Which of the following occur to help the body cope with the stress of altitude?
   a. decrease in heart rate
   b. increase in breathing
   c. both of these
   d. none of these

6. Define the term *homeotherm.*

7. How is body heat lost during swimming?

8. What is the most important means to dissipate heat during exercise in a hot environment?

9. List key guidelines for exercising in the heat.

10. List guidelines for fluid intake during and after exercise in hot environments.

11. Describe the appropriate clothing for exercising in hot and cold environments.

12. Outline the major types of heat injury, and list the symptoms of each.

13. Why does exercise at high altitude increase heart rate and breathing rate more than the same exercise performed at sea level?

14. Discuss the effects of air pollution on exercise tolerance.

15. What guidelines should you follow to minimize your exposure to air pollution?

16. Define the term *acclimatize.*

Suggested Reading

American College of Sports Medicine. Position stand: Exercise and fluid replacement. *Medicine and Science in Sports and Exercise* 28:1, 1996.

American College of Sports Medicine. Position stand: Exertional heat illness during training and competition. *Medicine and Science in Sports and Exercise* 39(3): 556–572, 2007.

American College of Sports Medicine. Position stand: Prevention of cold injuries during exercise. *Medicine and Science in Sports and Exercise* 38(11):2012–2029, 2006.

Bärtsch P, and B. Saltin. General introduction to altitude adaptation and mountain sickness. *Scandinavian Journal of Medicine and Science in Sports* 18(Suppl 1):1–10, 2008.

Hargreaves, M. Physiological limits to exercise performance in the heat. *Journal of Science and Medicine in Sport* 11(1):66–71, 2008.

Mäkinen, T. Human cold exposure, adaptation, and performance in high latitude environments. *American Journal of Human Biology* 19(2):155–164, 2007.

Maughan, R., S. Shirreffs, and P. Watson. Exercise, heat, hydration and the brain. *Journal of the American College of Nutrition* 26(5):604S–612S, 2007.

Mazzeo, R. Physiological responses to exercise at altitude: An update. *Sports Medicine* 38(1):1–8, 2008.

Murray, B. Hydration and physical performance. *Journal of the American College of Nutrition* 26(5 Suppl): 542S–548S, 2007.

Sharman, J., J. Cockcroft, and J. Coombes. Cardiovascular implications of exposure to traffic air pollution during exercise. *QJM: An International Journal of Medicine* 97(10):637–643, 2004.

For links to the organizations and websites listed below, visit The Total Fitness and Wellness Website at www.pearsonhighered.com/powers.

Northern Outfitters

Contains links to the sites for several cold-weather clothing outfitters.

Sportsmedicine.About.com

Information about various aspects of training and nutrition with special topics on proper hydration for exercise in the heat.

American Lung Association

Information on air pollution and exercise, including who is vulnerable, how it affects your body, and ways to minimize your risk.

References

1. Brooks, G., T. Fahey, and K. Baldwin. *Exercise Physiology: Human Bioenergetics and Its Applications*, 4th ed. Dubuque, IA: McGraw-Hill, 2005.

2. American College of Sports Medicine. Position stand: Exertional heat illness during training and competition. *Medicine and Science in Sports and Exercise* 39(3):556–572, 2007.

3. McArdle, W. D., F. I. Katch, and V. L. Katch. *Exercise Physiology: Nutrition, Energy, and Human Performance*, 7th ed. Philadelphia: Lippincott Williams and Wilkins, 2009.

4. American College of Sports Medicine. Position stand: Exercise and fluid replacement. *Medicine and Science in Sports and Exercise* 39(2):377–390, 2007.

5. American College of Sports Medicine. Position stand: Prevention of cold injuries during exercise. *Medicine and Science in Sports and Exercise* 38(11):2012–2029, 2006.

6. Carlisle, A. J., and N. C. Sharp. Exercise and outdoor ambient air pollution. *British Journal of Sports Medicine* 35(4):214–222, 2001.

Videos

Log on to www.pearsonhighered.com/powers to view this chapter-related video.

Environmental Health

NAME _____ DATE _____

Exercising in Harsh Environments

Answer the following true-or-false questions related to exercise and the environment. If a statement is false, change it to make it true. You can check your answers against those provided on the next page.

TRUE or FALSE

1. Evaporation is the primary means of heat loss during exercise in a hot environment.

   T F _____

2. When exercising in a hot, humid environment, you should wear loose, dark-colored clothing.

   T F _____

3. Exercise at high altitude increases the amount of oxygen in the blood.

   T F _____

4. At high altitude, it is necessary to reduce the intensity of exercise to stay within your target heart rate range.

   T F _____

5. Ozone levels are highest during cool winter days.

   T F _____

6. Humans regulate their body temperature around the set point of 98.6°F.

   T F _____

7. Low-intensity exercise using small muscle groups produces more body heat than high-intensity exercise incorporating large muscle groups.

   T F _____

8. An increase in body temperature during exercise in a hot environment will result in larger increases in heart rate than will exercise in a cool environment.

   T F _____

9. The strategy for exercising in the cold is to wear enough clothing necessary to trap just enough heat to maintain body temperature, but not to overheat.

   T F _____

10. Heat injuries are nonfatal conditions that result in cramps and fatigue.

   T F _____

ANSWERS

1. True

2. False: When exercising in a hot, humid environment, you should wear loose, light-colored clothing.

3. False: Exercise at high altitude reduces the amount of oxygen in the blood.

4. True

5. False: Ozone levels are highest during hot summer days.

6. True

7. False: High-intensity exercise using large muscle groups produces more body heat than low-intensity exercise incorporating small muscle groups.

8. True

9. True

10. False: Heat injuries are serious and can result in damage to the nervous system and, in extreme cases, death.

Answer the three questions below to help you increase your awareness of safety issues in harsh environments.

1. If your friend planned to exercise in a warm, high humidity environment, what safety advice would you give to him or her?

   _____

   _____

2. What advice would you give to a friend exercising in a cold climate?

   _____

   _____

3. What can you do to minimize the amount of air pollution in your immediate environment?

   _____

   _____

Preventing Exercise-Related and Unintentional Injuries

true or false?

1. Sprains **involve damage to bone.**

2. **Tendonitis refers to** inflammation **of the cartilage in joints.**

3. **Runners often get** shin splints.

4. **Falls are the number one cause of unintentional** injuries **for young adults.**

5. **The first step in** treating **an injury is always CPR.**

Answers appear on the next page.

Many of the physical recreational activities that Americans most enjoy, from bungee jumping and snowboarding to contact sports and rollerblading, involve some risk of injury. As Americans have increased their participation in these activities, their risk of injury has also increased. Each year about 20 million weekend athletes and another 10 million school children experience sports injuries (1). For runners, the incidence of injuries ranges from 25% to 75%.

In addition to exercise-related injuries, Americans are also at risk of unintentional injuries involving their cars, motorcycles, firearms, and even the stairs in their homes. In 2004, unintentional injuries accounted for approximately 7% of deaths (2) and, as with exercise-related injuries, most can easily be prevented. In this chapter we discuss the cause, prevention, and treatment of exercise-related and unintentional injuries.

The Risk and Causes of Injury from Increased Physical Activity

Unfortunately, the more you exercise, the more likely you are to suffer from an exercise-related injury. Although many factors have been blamed for the injuries that recreational and competitive athletes experience, there is convincing evidence that only a few actually do cause injuries: improper training techniques, inadequate shoes, and alignment abnormalities in the legs and feet (3). Of these, improper training techniques account for two-thirds of all injuries (4).

One result of improper training techniques can be **overtraining syndrome,** a major cause of exercise-related injuries. Overtraining is associated with too much exercise and not enough recovery time between workouts. The signs and symptoms may include increased resting heart rate, reduced appetite, weight loss, irritability, disturbed sleep, elevated blood pressure, frequent injuries, increased incidence of colds and flu, and chronic fatigue.

To prevent overtraining, a good rule of thumb is to increase your exercise intensity or duration by no more than 10% over a 2-week period. In addition, listen to your body. If you notice any of the overtraining signs or symptoms, reduce your training intensity and/or duration, and increase your rest intervals. By avoiding overtraining, you can greatly reduce your chance of injury and help maintain a positive attitude about fitness.

Two other common causes of exercise-related injuries are alignment problems in the legs or feet and inappropriate footwear. Although little can be done about alignment abnormalities, a change in shoes can help prevent injury in many cases. Approximately one-third of runners experience a decrease in injuries after changing to proper shoes (3) because of the increased cushioning and support for the arch of the foot. Using shoes specially designed for such activities as tennis or aerobic dance can also reduce injuries.

Several aerobic programs such as water aerobics, low-impact aerobics, step aerobics, and specific dance aerobics, carry a fairly high risk for injury. Approximately one-half of all participants in traditional aerobic dance classes report injuries (5), which occur at a rate of approximately one injury per 100 hours of dancing. One study found that more than three sessions per week, improper shoes, and nonresilient surfaces were the primary causes of injury (5).

Answers

1. FALSE Sprains are defined as damage to soft tissue of the joint, typically the ligaments.

2. FALSE Like it sounds, tendonitis is an inflammation of the tendons that attach muscle to bone, not the cartilage in joints.

3. TRUE A repetitive movement such as running can often result in stress to the connective tissue surrounding the utilized muscle. Shin splints are caused by irritation and inflammation of the connective tissue of the front of the lower leg.

4. FALSE Although falls do result in numerous injuries every year, the number-one cause of unintentional injuries for young adults between the ages of 15 and 34 is motor vehicle accidents.

5. FALSE The treatment for any injury should be determined by the cause. CPR is beneficial only if the heart has stopped.

Risk Factors for Sports Injuries

Intrinsic Risk Factors

Age. Risk increases with age. As you age, soft tissues become less elastic, and injuries are more likely.

Body size and composition (weight, body fat). More weight puts more stress on joints, bones, and connective tissue, thereby increasing risk of injury.

Physical fitness. Risk is greater in unfit individuals. As you become more fit, bones and muscles get stronger and more resistant to damage.

Bone density and structure. Less dense or weaker bones are more prone to fracture and break.

Gender (sex hormones, menarche). Women are at greater risk of injury than men. Hormonal differences may cause women to be at higher risk of lower leg injuries during exercise.

Muscle flexibility and strength. Less flexibility and strength predispose you to risk.

Extrinsic Risk Factors

Environmental factors (terrain, surface, weather). Rough terrain or poor weather conditions increase risk for injury.

Equipment (footwear, clothing). Improper shoes can lead to joint injuries in the leg, and inadequate or inappropriate clothing can lead to overheating in the summer or hypothermia in the winter.

Type of activity. Competitive activities are more likely to result in injury than are leisure activities.

Intensity and amount of activity. Intense activity and fatigue cause more injuries.

Warm-up. Some evidence suggests that a warm-up before exercise decreases risk.

Source: Adapted from Murphy, D. F., D. A. Connolly, and B. D. Beynnon. Risk factors for lower extremity injury: A review of the literature. *British Journal of Sports Medicine* 37(1):13–29, 2003.

As you can see, improper exercise techniques (e.g., excessive distance or duration, drastic changes in the exercise routine) are the major causes of injuries. Excessive distance or duration may cause wear to tissues, such as connective tissue in joints. Drastic changes in training routines may put greater stress on and tear tissues. See the box above for additional extrinsic and intrinsic risk factors for injury during physical activity.

Make sure you know...

> The factors most closely associated with exercise-related injuries are improper training techniques, inadequate shoes, and alignment problems in the legs and feet.
> The one factor most likely to cause exercise-related injury is overtraining.
> Factors associated with injuries in aerobic dance are participating in more than three sessions per week, improper shoes, and nonresilient surfaces.

Common Conditions and Injuries

Although many injuries can result from overtraining, some are more common than others. This section discusses the cause and prevention of many general types of injuries and conditions associated with exercise training.

Back Pain

One of the most common complaints among athletes and nonathletes alike is back pain, especially in the lower back. Back pain can range from a vague ache to a searing, sharp pain that shoots up the spine. As with other injuries, there are mild and severe forms, and the degree to which back pain interferes with your physical activity can vary accordingly.

overtraining syndrome A phenomenon in which too much exercise and not enough recovery time between workouts results in exercise-related injuries.

Cause Recall from Chapter 5 that one important cause of back pain is inadequate muscle strength in the abdomen and lower back. For someone experiencing back pain, exercise may be extremely helpful or extremely harmful. For example, exercise has been effectively used in pain clinics for treating back pain (6) and can sometimes prevent or correct back problems by strengthening weak muscles and stretching the stronger ones (see Chapter 5). However, if you have any type of back pain, you should attempt to find the cause before starting an exercise program. Certain types of exercise may compound the problem and thus should be avoided.

Prevention Exercises to increase flexibility and strength, reduce body fat, improve muscle balance between the abdominal and back muscles, and prevent osteoporosis can decrease your risk of developing back problems (6). In addition, these exercises can help alleviate back pain that you may already be experiencing.

Use the following guidelines to help prevent back problems from getting worse or to prevent the onset of back pains:

- Maintain a healthy body weight and body composition. Obesity puts great strain on the lower back.
- Warm up before engaging in any physical activity.
- Do exercises to strengthen the abdominal muscles.
- Do exercises to stretch the lower back and hamstring muscles.
- When lying down, lie on your side with your knees and hips bent. Try to avoid lying on your back, but if you do, place a pillow under your knees.
- During prolonged standing, try to take the strain off of the lower back by propping one foot on an object such as a rail or box, which bends the leg at the hip and knee.
- Avoid quick, jerking movements of the spine.
- Do not overextend the neck or lower back or overflex the neck.
- Avoid stretching the long or weak muscles, especially the abdominal muscles.
- Be especially careful when being passively stretched by another person. Avoid passive back or neck stretches or any ballistic passive stretches (Chapter 5).
- Avoid movements that place forces on spinal disks, such as extending and rotating the spine simultaneously, trunk and neck circling, and double leg lifts.
- Avoid forceful hyperextension and flexion of the spine.
- Avoid improper lifting. Squat to lift any object, and never bend at the waist.

Acute Muscle Soreness

Acute muscle soreness is not an injury but a form of fatigue, and it is a common condition among athletes who are training vigorously. Once exercise ceases, the athlete is left with a temporary feeling of weakness and stiffness.

Cause Acute muscle soreness may develop during or immediately following an exercise session that has been too long or too intense. As someone who is exercising to improve your fitness, you should not train hard enough to cause acute soreness. If you do feel local muscle weakness or stiffness after a workout, this may be a sign that your workout was a bit more strenuous than anticipated.

Despite popular belief, lactic acid is not the cause of this type of soreness (7). Instead, it is more likely caused by other alterations in the chemical balance within muscle, increased fluid accumulation in muscle, or injury to muscle tissue.

Prevention Abnormally strenuous or prolonged exercise is likely to cause acute muscle soreness. Novice exercisers should be particularly cautious in this regard when beginning an exercise training program. These changes can be further prevented by gradually beginning and ending each exercise session. All exercise sessions should begin with a warm-up period of 5 to 15 minutes to allow muscles to increase their internal temperature slowly to avoid damage during the more stressful exercise training session. Finally, a post-exercise cool-down is important to allow the muscles to return to their normal, pre-exercise condition.

Delayed-Onset Muscle Soreness

Delayed-onset muscle soreness (DOMS), as the name implies, does not occur immediately after exercise, but rather, 1–2 days after the exercise session. Acute muscle soreness is likely to be present as well, but the cause of each is different.

Cause DOMS develops after a bout of exercise that is excessive in duration or intensity (8). It is also common following new or unique physical activities that use muscle groups unaccustomed to exercise. For example, it is not unusual for a runner to experience soreness in the upper body after beginning a weight-training program.

DOMS is likely caused by microscopic tears in the muscle (8), which lead to swelling and pain. Many investigators believe that this type of injury occurs primarily during the lengthening phase (the eccentric portion) of muscular contraction. The damage apparently is due to the greater force placed on the muscle during this phase of the contraction. For example, an individual who runs downhill (which emphasizes such contractions) without being accustomed to this type of exercise will generally experience soreness in the leg muscles after the exercise session. Similarly, DOMS is likely to occur in people unaccustomed to walking up and down steps if they begin a program that involves this form of exercise.

Prevention   As with acute muscle soreness, DOMS can be prevented by refraining from exercise that is more strenuous or more prolonged than normal. Start with a warm-up, and limit both the intensity and duration of the first several workouts. Remember that eccentric contractions are more likely to result in muscle damage than are concentric (shortening) contractions. Therefore, in the beginning stages of an exercise program, try to avoid heavy weights for exercises that involve large amounts of eccentric contractions (e.g., walking down steps, running downhill, and performing certain movements during weight lifting).

Muscle Strains

Commonly referred to as a "pulled muscle," a muscle **strain** can occur with any type of unaccustomed movement involving a load that is abnormally high. Strains occur fairly frequently among weight lifters and other people engaged in activities that involve lifting heavy loads. Depending on the severity of the damage, recovery can take from a few days to many weeks.

Cause   If a muscle is overstretched or forced to shorten against an extremely heavy weight (as when lifting a heavy box), muscle fibers may be damaged. The resulting strain can range from minor to major damage to the muscle (9). The following are the degrees of muscle strain:

> **First-degree strain.** Only a few muscle fibers are stretched or torn. Movement is painful, but a full range of motion is still possible.
>
> **Second-degree strain.** Many muscle fibers are torn, and movement is extremely painful and limited. The torn area may be apparent as a soft, sunken area in the muscle. Swelling may occur around the tear as a result of hemorrhage (bleeding).
>
> **Third-degree strain.** The muscle is torn completely (Figure 12.1). The tear can be in the belly of the muscle, in the tendon, or at the point where the tendon attaches to the bone. Movement is generally impossible. Initial pain is intense but quickly subsides because nerve fibers are also damaged. Surgery is usually necessary for repair.

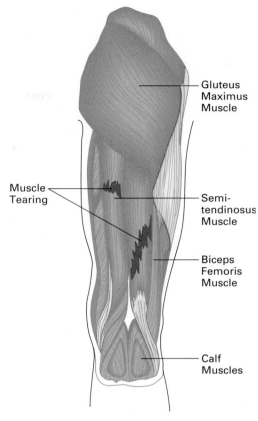

FIGURE 12.1
A third-degree muscle strain involves a complete tear of the muscle and loss of function. Surgery may be necessary to repair this degree of muscle strain.

Source: Adapted from Karren, K. J., B. Q. Haffen, D. Limmer, and J. J. Mistovich. *First Aid for Colleges and Universities,* 9th ed., p. 212. Benjamin Cummings. Copyright © 2008. Reprinted by permission of Pearson Education, Inc.

Prevention   Because strains occur when muscles must generate excessive force, it follows logically that strains can be prevented by limiting the amount of stress placed on muscles. But note that it is not possible to predict just how much force is needed to cause muscle damage; moreover, warm muscles are more pliable (that is, more easily stretched and less likely to tear) than cold muscles. Therefore, before lifting a heavy object or engaging in any activity that requires

acute muscle soreness A condition that may develop during or immediately following an exercise session that has been too long or too intense.

delayed-onset muscle soreness (DOMS) A condition that develops within 24 to 48 hours after an exercise session that is excessive in duration or intensity.

strain Damage to a muscle that can range from a minor separation of fibers to a complete tearing of the muscle.

(a) 1st Degree

(b) 2nd Degree

(c) 3rd Degree

FIGURE 12.2
The extent of damage in the three categories of sprains, which involve damage to the ligaments that support the joint. (a) First-degree sprain at the shoulder, with minimal disruption of ligament. (b) Second-degree sprain with severe tearing and loss of joint stability. (c) Complete separation.

quick, jerking movements, warm up thoroughly for 5 to 15 minutes. Even though a good warm-up should prevent muscle strains, remember that muscle contractions that are more strenuous than normal may result in DOMS.

Tendonitis

Tendonitis, which is the inflammation or swelling of a tendon, is one of the most common exercise-related injuries (9). Because tendons are located around joints, activities that stress the joints, such as tennis or jogging, are often the culprit behind these injuries.

Cause   As muscles shorten and pull on tendons, the tendons move across other tendons, muscles, and soft tissue. This movement, if unfamiliar, can cause irritation and swelling in the tendon. Once tendonitis develops, pain associated with movement is the first symptom. Swelling, redness, and warmth generally follow. Tendonitis can occur in a number of areas, such as the elbow and shoulder. It is a common injury in weight lifters as well as in runners and tennis players.

Prevention   Tendonitis is generally caused by strenuous, prolonged muscle contractions to which an individual is unaccustomed. Therefore, the best prevention of tendonitis is to avoid overuse. If you feel tendon pain or discomfort during a workout, stop exercising. This will prevent further irritation and reduce the severity of tendon damage. If you cannot stop using the muscle and tendon causing the pain, follow the measures for managing injuries, discussed at the end of this chapter.

Ligament Sprains

A **sprain** is caused by damage to a ligament (9). Recall that ligaments connect the bones, provide joint support, and determine the direction and range of motion of joints.

Cause   Ligament damage can occur if excessive force is applied to a joint. One of the most common sites of ligament damage is the ankle. When walking or running on an uneven surface, it is easy to "turn" the ankle, which means that the ankle joint is rotated such that much of the body weight is placed on the side of the foot. Because the ankle joint is not designed to rotate to that degree, the stress on the joint damages the ligaments. As with muscle strains, the degrees of ligament damage are classified as follows:

First degree: Stretching and separation of a limited number of ligament fibers, resulting in minor instability of the joint (Figure 12.2a). Minor pain and swelling are the likely result.

Second degree: Tearing and separation of a significant number of ligament fibers (Figure 12.2b). Moderate instability of the joint, with definite pain, swelling, and stiffness, occurs.

Third degree: Total tearing or separation of the ligament, causing major instability of the joint (Figure 12.2c). Nerves may be damaged, and pain may subside quickly. Considerable swelling generally occurs.

Prevention   Lightweight metal braces can provide added support to joints and therefore some protection

A CLOSER LOOK

ARTHROSCOPIC SURGERY: A HIGH-TECH APPROACH TO JOINT REPAIR

As many professional basketball, football, and soccer players can tell you, severe damage to a ligament or cartilage in a joint, such as the knee, can be extremely painful. In addition to the pain, such injuries used to cost players much time off the field because of the required surgery and recuperation involved with repairing the injury. However, thanks to advanced surgical techniques, this is no longer necessarily the case.

Traditional surgical techniques required the surgeon to cut the joint open to repair it, causing additional trauma to the joint and resulting in prolonged recuperation and rehabilitation. Today, a commonly used surgical technique called **arthroscopic surgery** allows surgeons to repair joint injuries with significantly less trauma to the joint.

In arthroscopic surgery, surgeons insert micro-optic devices through two or three small incisions. These devices allow them to see inside the joint and insert a microsurgery tube that enables them to cut and remove damaged tissue and sew the remaining tissue together. The small incisions cause less surgical damage, which translates into less pain and a shorter recovery and rehabilitation period than with conventional surgical techniques.

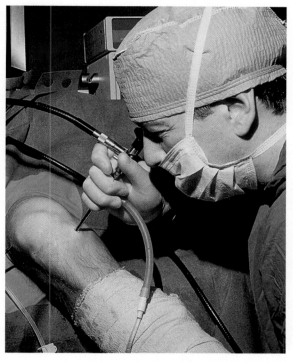

Arthroscopic surgery is relatively painless and requires much less recovery time than conventional surgery.

from ligament damage. These braces are commonly used in football, a sport recognized for inducing knee damage. Without these expensive, high-tech devices, the best protection against torn ligaments is to refrain from activities that may subject a joint to high stress, including tennis, soccer, racquetball, and basketball. In addition, if you have a particular joint that has been injured previously or is weak, work to maintain maximum strength in the muscles surrounding the joint, because strong muscles provide additional support.

Torn Cartilage

Cartilage on the end of bones in certain joints, such as the elbow, knee, and ankle, acts as a shock absorber to cushion the weight of one bone on another and to protect the bones from the friction due to joint movement. Torn cartilage does not commonly result from a fitness program, but swelling and pain can indicate that damage has been done.

Cause   Unusually high forces or unusual movements can tear cartilage, resulting in joint pain. This is usually seen in athletes who undergo high-force activities while a joint is stretched. Damaged cartilage can also result from abnormal wear with misaligned bones or from excess wear due to weak musculature around a joint. This type of injury, and severe ligament damage as well, normally requires surgical correction.

To learn about a high-tech procedure that makes surgical repair of joints less invasive, see the Closer Look box above.

tendonitis Inflammation or swelling of a tendon.

sprain Damage to a ligament that occurs if excessive force is applied to a joint.

arthroscopic surgery A common surgical procedure that can repair joint injuries without causing undue trauma to the joint.

The Patella Glides Along Its Track

The Patella Moves Off Its Track

FIGURE 12.3
When the thigh muscles pull correctly (left), the kneecap stays in place and glides easily in its track. With patellofemoral pain syndrome, or PFPS (right), the thigh muscles pull unevenly, and the kneecap gets "off track." This results in uneven pressure on the back of the kneecap, which causes excessive wear and pain.

Prevention The good news is that you don't need to incorporate into a general fitness program activities that put you at high risk for torn cartilage. Walking, swimming, and biking are examples of activities that don't put much strain on the joint and therefore do not usually result in torn cartilage. So to avoid cartilage injury, limit activities that produce excess stress on the joint or forceful movements that take the joint outside its normal range of motion.

Make sure you know...

> Exercise can play an important role in preventing back pain and rehabilitating back problems. Exercises to increase flexibility and strength, reduce body fat, improve muscle balance between the abdominal and back muscles, and prevent osteoporosis can decrease your risk of developing back problems.

> Acute muscle soreness, which occurs during or immediately after exercise, may be due to muscle damage, accumulation of fluid within the muscle, and/or chemical imbalances within the muscle itself.

> Delayed-onset muscle soreness (DOMS) usually occurs 24 to 48 hours after an exercise session. Eccentric exercise is a common cause of DOMS.

> When muscle is forced to contract against excessive resistance, the resulting damage to muscle fibers is called a strain. Such damage can range from a minor separation of fibers to a complete tear in the muscle. A sprain is caused by damage to a ligament.

> Tendonitis is one of the most common of all overuse problems associated with physical activity; torn cartilage is not that common but can be extremely painful when it does occur.

Common Injuries to the Lower Extremities

We have discussed the cause and prevention of several general exercise-related injuries. Because many fitness programs involve weight-bearing activities that involve the legs, such as running, walking, and aerobic dance, let's take a closer look at some specific injuries of the lower body.

In general, walking does not result in a large number of injuries. However, running can lead to a myriad of injuries. More than one-third of runners develop orthopedic injuries serious enough to reduce weekly running mileage (3). Approximately 60% of those injuries involve the foot and knee. One of the major factors responsible for this type and number of injuries is the severity of stress on the legs and feet. In fact, the impact of the foot on the running surface is approximately 2.5 times the body weight of the runner (3). In the case of a 150-pound runner, the amount of force generated when the foot strikes the pavement is 375 pounds! In addition, the incidence of injury increases with running mileage (3). If you run 15 miles a week, you can expect one injury every 2 years.

You can probably imagine how injuries might occur with this level of stress. In the following paragraphs we discuss the cause and prevention of the most common lower extremity injuries.

Patellofemoral Pain Syndrome

Patellofemoral pain syndrome (PFPS) is a common exercise-induced injury that manifests as pain behind the patella, or kneecap (9). Also known as "runner's knee," PFPS may account for almost 10% of all visits to sports injury clinics and 20–40% of all knee problems (10).

Cause PFPS results when the patella gets "off track" (Figure 12.3), which causes excessive wear of the patella and pain. Among the several factors that predispose an individual to PFPS are misalignments of the thigh muscles that extend the knee, overuse or prolonged immobilization of the muscles, acute trauma, obesity, and genetics.

When these factors are present, the increased forces and repetitive movements of exercise result in pain and possibly also in cracking and popping sounds during movement. Over time and with increased use, the articular (joint) cartilage may begin to degenerate, which eventually may lead to osteoarthritis.

Prevention   You can prevent PFPS by avoiding stress on the knee due to excessive amounts of running, jumping, aerobic dancing, and stair climbing. Further, you can reduce your chances of developing PFPS by strengthening the front thigh muscles (quadriceps); this improves the tracking of the patella and reduces wear on the patellar surface.

The two best exercises seem to be knee extension exercises over the last 20 degrees of extension and/or isometric contractions of the quadriceps muscles with the leg fully extended (try to press the back of the knee to the floor while lying on your back) (9). Remember, avoid unnecessary stresses on the knee, such as squatting.

Finally, PFPS is one injury that may be prevented by using the proper athletic footwear. If you develop any of the symptoms of PFPS, see your physician or a podiatrist (foot specialist) to determine whether footwear may be contributing to the problem.

Treatment   An aggressive rehabilitation program that includes quadriceps exercises, rest, and anti-inflammatory drugs has proved beneficial for most PFPS patients. Although ice neither prevents PFPS nor rehabilitates the joint, it (like anti-inflammatory agents) may provide some relief from the pain and inflammation.

Shin Splints

Shin splints is a generic term referring to pain associated with injuries to the front of the lower leg (9). The condition is common among runners, particularly distance runners, and can be quite painful.

Cause   Three of the most common injuries that cause shin splints are strain and irritation of one or several muscles and tendons located in the lower leg (Figure 12.4); inflammation of tissue connecting the two bones of the lower leg, the tibia and the fibula; and microscopic breaks (called stress fractures; discussed next) in either the tibia or the fibula.

Prevention   Shin splints can be avoided by running on soft surfaces; by wearing well-padded, shock-absorbing shoes; and by slowly advancing exercise in-

FIGURE 12.4
Locations of the muscles and tendons that are often irritated in shin splints.

Peroneus Longus

Tibia

Tibialis Anterior

Extensor Digitorum Longus

Tendons of Lower Leg

Gastrocnemius

tensity from walking to running. If shin pain develops, it could be due to a fracture or break of bones and therefore should not be regarded lightly. High-impact activities such as running should be stopped and replaced with low-impact activities such as cycling or swimming. Stretching muscles located in the front and back of the lower leg may help prevent the problem.

Stress Fractures

Stress fractures are tiny cracks or breaks in bone. Although stress fractures can occur in any leg bone, the long bones of the foot extending from the bones in the heel to the toes (the metatarsal bones) are especially

patellofemoral pain syndrome (PFPS) A common exercise-induced injury, sometimes called "runner's knee," that manifests as pain behind the kneecap (patella).

shin splints Generic term referring to pain associated with injuries to the front of the lower leg.

stress fractures Tiny cracks or breaks in the bone.

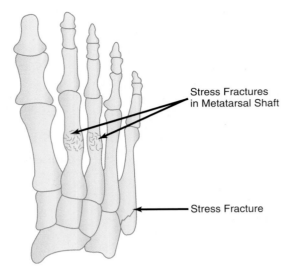

Stress Fractures
in Metatarsal Shaft

Stress Fracture

FIGURE 12.5
Metatarsal stress fractures can result in pain during any
weight-bearing movement.

susceptible (Figure 12.5). In fact, these are the most
common sites of stress fractures in the body.

Cause Stress fractures result from excessive force
applied to the leg and foot during running or other
types of weight-bearing activities (11). The most likely
candidates for this injury are individuals who have high
arches or poor flexibility of the lower body and who increase training intensity or duration too rapidly.

Prevention People with high arches should seek
exercise advice from their physician or a podiatrist,
who might prescribe arch supports to help prevent a
stress-related problem. Again, a key factor in preventing stress fractures is to avoid overtraining by increasing your training load gradually (by no more than
5–10% per week). Often, lack of flexibility in the hips
and the back of the legs causes the body's weight to
shift such that some bones become chronically over-
loaded and fracture. Thus, maintaining flexibility in the
back of the legs and hips will reduce your chances of
developing a stress fracture. If pain in the foot or leg
makes you suspect a stress fracture, stop activities that
involve the injured area. See your physician to get an
X-ray examination of the area. If a stress fracture is
present, only rest can assist the healing process.

Although recognizing and understanding all of the
injuries we've discussed so far is important, the best
strategy to address exercise-related injuries is to reduce
your risk of sustaining them. See the Closer Look box
on page 354 to learn ways to reduce your overall risk.
Finally, to assess your exercise program with respect to
the risks of injury it may pose, see Laboratory 12.1 on
page 363.

Make sure you know...

> Common injuries to the lower extremities include
  PFPS, in which the articular cartilage on the
  back of the kneecap (patella) may be damaged
  by chronic use during exercise; shin splints, a
  condition that encompasses several different injuries
  to the front of the lower leg; and stress fractures,
  which are microscopic breaks in the bone.

> To reduce your risk of developing an exercise-
  related injury, engage in a program of muscle-
  strengthening exercises to maintain balance in
  strength around joints; warm up before and
  cool down after each workout; use the proper
  equipment (especially proper footwear); increase
  exercise intensity and duration slowly throughout
  your exercise training program; maintain the proper
  rest-to-exercise ratio; and do not overtrain.

Managing Injuries

As mentioned earlier, almost everyone who engages in
regular physical activity will experience some type of
injury. In the following sections we discuss injury treatment and provide an overview of the rehabilitation
process.

Any injury that results in extreme pain or the possibility of a broken bone should be examined by a
physician, who will likely order X-ray exams to determine whether there are any broken bones. The following treatment regimen should be followed for less
severe injuries (first-degree strains and sprains,
tendonitis, and so on).

Initial Treatment of Exercise-Related Injuries

The objectives of the initial treatment of exercise-
related injuries are to decrease pain, limit swelling,
and prevent further injury (9). These objectives can be
met by a combination of **r**est, **i**ce, **c**ompression, and
elevation **(RICE).** Rest will help prevent further injury. Moving injured tissues will aggravate the injury
and result in further damage. Any movement that
causes pain should be avoided.

Applying ice to an injury reduces swelling by
reducing blood flow to the cooled area. Minimizing
swelling will reduce the pain and lead to more rapid
healing. Place ice (or an ice pack) in a cloth wrap to
guard against skin damage due to frostbite, and apply it
for 30-minute periods, three to four times a day, for 2
days after the injury.

Compressing the injured area also reduces
swelling. The amount of compression should be

FIGURE 12.6
The steps of the cryokinetics procedure for rehabilitating injuries.

enough to reduce fluid collection around the damaged area, but not severe enough to inhibit blood flow. Snugly wrapping the injured area with an elastic bandage is sufficient to control swelling. Placing a bag of ice in the last two or three wraps of the elastic bandage incorporates pressure and cools at the same time.

Finally, elevating the injured area, above the level of the heart if possible, reduces blood pressure and may therefore reduce swelling. Approximately 3 days following the injury, start an exercise rehabilitation program, as outlined in the next section. If you have any doubts about whether the injury is ready for rehabilitation, delay another 24 to 48 hours.

Rehabilitation

The rehabilitation of minor injuries occurs naturally. That is, after an injury has healed and swelling has subsided, most people will begin to move the injured area at a rate according to how much pain is involved. As the pain subsides, more movement can occur, until a normal range of motion is restored. However, this rehabilitation regimen has several drawbacks. First, it is very slow. Depending on the injury, the natural rehabilitation process may take five to ten times as long as an aggressive rehabilitation program. Second, the damaged area may be reinjured because many people attempt to return to full use of the injured area too quickly. This secondary injury results in much greater damage than the first injury and can even weaken the tissue and lead to recurring injuries throughout life. Third, for many types of injury, the lack of an aggressive rehabilitation program can prevent the return of full function because the scar tissue that develops limits the normal range of motion. Fortunately, these problems may be overcome by an active rehabilitation process.

A relatively new rehabilitation technique that is implemented after the RICE procedures have been followed is called **cryokinetics** (12). Ice is applied for approximately 12 minutes, followed by 3 minutes of light exercise, followed by another 3 minutes of cold. The 3 minutes of exercise and 3 minutes of ice should be repeated for five cycles. Exercise of the injured limb during this treatment must be guided by the pain associated with its use. Start with an exercise intensity that provides little or no pain, increasing intensity gradually as long as no increase in pain occurs. If pain increases during the cryokinetic therapy, stop the treatment and resume the RICE procedures until the pain subsides (Figure 12.6).

The initial management of an injury is critical and determines how much time is required to complete the rehabilitation process. For example, a regimen of cryokinetics initiated after a third-degree ankle sprain (2–3 days post injury) results in complete recovery within 2 weeks. In contrast, if the cryokinetic treatment starts late (5–7 days post injury), the recovery may take 4 to 5 weeks.

As pain subsides and the range of motion returns, you may accelerate full recovery by adding a program of weight-training and flexibility exercises. This is especially true for muscle injuries, because the healing process may cause the muscle to shorten and thereby limit flexibility. An injury that does not heal properly may cause recurring pain during activity and may persist for years. Therefore, for stubborn injuries, you should seek the treatment advice of a trained professional (athletic trainer, physical therapist, or physician).

RICE An acronym representing a treatment protocol for exercise-related injuries. It stands for a combination of **r**est, **i**ce, **c**ompression, and **e**levation.

cryokinetics A rehabilitation technique that incorporates alternating periods of treatment using ice, exercise, and rest.

A CLOSER LOOK

REDUCING YOUR RISK OF EXERCISE-RELATED INJURY

Here are five key ways to reduce your risk of injury due to exercise training.

1. Engage in a program of muscle-strengthening exercises using all major muscle groups. Maintaining a balance of muscular strength around joints will prevent muscular imbalance and reduce the incidence of injury.

2. Warm up before and cool down after all workouts. Stretching during the warm-up may help prevent injuries, and stretching during the cool-down will help maintain flexibility.

3. Use the proper footwear. Good shoes are important for activities such as running and aerobic dance and can reduce your chance of injury.

4. Do not overtrain! Improper training techniques, which include overtraining, are the main culprits in exercise-related injuries. Gradual progression of exercise intensity and duration is essential in preventing injuries.

5. Incorporate the proper amount of recovery time into your training routine. Rest is an important part of any successful training program.

Make sure you know...

> For treating injuries, remember the RICE protocol: rest, ice, compression, and elevation.

> Cryokinetics is a rehabilitation technique that involves alternating periods of applying ice to and exercising the injured area.

Preventing Unintentional Injuries

In addition to the exercise-related injuries that result from overstressing bones, muscles, ligaments, and tendons during physical activity, many Americans suffer from other **unintentional injuries** every year.

Unintentional injuries are the number-one killer of people aged 15 to 34 in the United States (Table 12.1). Each year, unintentional injuries claim the lives of more than 5100 children, or about 14 per day (13). In addition, for children under age 14, unintentional injuries result in about 6.2 million emergency room visits each year (13).

Although most unintentional injuries may seem to result from chance or "accidents," this is not the case. In fact, public health officials prefer using the term *unintentional injury* instead of **accident,** because the latter implies random events, bad luck, and an inability to change the outcome through modifying events or behavior (14). Keep in mind that *accident* refers to the sequence of events that lead up to the injury, whereas the injury is the health consequence of the accident. You can modify your behavior to control many risk fac-

tors and reduce your risk of unintentional injury. Let's examine some of the most common risk factors.

Risk Factors for Unintentional Injury

One of the most important injury risk factors is an unsafe attitude, which promotes risk-taking behaviors. For example, people who are overly confident in their driving skills may speed on a winding or wet road and increase their risk of being in a motor vehicle crash.

TABLE 12.1

Five Leading Causes of Death among Young Adults

Rank	Ages 15–24	Ages 25–34
1	Unintentional injury: Motor vehicle crash: 69.6% Poisoning: 14.6% Drowning: 3.7% Other: 12.1%	Unintentional Injury: Motor vehicle crash: 52.4% Poisoning: 27.9% Drowning: 3.0% Other: 16.7%
2	Homicide	Malignant neoplasms
3	Suicide	Heart disease
4	Malignant neoplasms	Suicide
5	Heart disease	Homicide

Source: National Center for Injury Prevention and Control. *CDC Injury Fact Book.* Atlanta: Centers for Disease Control and Prevention, 2006; and National Center for Health Statistics. *Health, United States, 2008 with Chartbook.* Hyattsville, MD: National Center for Health Statistics, 2009.

Similarly, people who are overconfident in their job skills may take unnecessary risks at work.

Some people crave excitement or the sensation of danger. This type of thrill-seeking attitude increases the risk of accidents. Such people often engage in high-risk physical activities, such as skydiving, auto racing, or rock climbing, which increase their risk of injury due to accidents.

Stress also increases your risk of accidents. During periods of emotional or physical stress, people tend to be less careful. If you find yourself having a series of small mishaps or "near misses" when performing routine activities such as yardwork, house cleaning, or sports activities, this may be an indication that you should reduce your stress level by resting and using stress management techniques.

Alcohol and other drugs also increase your risk of accidents. Drug use alters your judgment and decreases both reaction speed and motor coordination. Alcohol use is also involved in about 25–50% of deaths among adolescents and adults due to water recreation accidents, and among adolescent men, alcohol is a contributing factor in 50% of drowning deaths (15). Sun exposure and heat increase the effects of alcohol on balance, coordination, and judgment. Similarly, cocaine and marijuana use are associated with a wide range of accidents, including falls, drownings, fires, and automobile accidents.

A number of environmental factors can increase your risk of accident. For example, storing combustible materials close to a heater and failing to have properly operating smoke detectors both increase your risk of injury due to fire. Other factors, such as failing to properly maintain ladders or steps around your home or workplace, may increase your risk of falls or other accidental injury.

Reducing Your Risk of Accidents

You can take a number of steps to reduce your risk of injury. The key is to increase your awareness of the risk factors. See the Steps for Behavior Change box on page 356 to find out whether your behaviors put you at increased risk of unintentional injuries. Use the tips

there and in the box on page 358 to reduce your risk of injury from vehicular accidents, fire, falls, drowning, and poisoning.

Make sure you know...

> Behavior and attitude can have a large impact on your likelihood of sustaining an unintentional injury. Motor vehicle accidents, falls, drowning, and poisoning are the most common types of unintentional injuries.

> Avoiding or minimizing alcohol intake can reduce your risk of unintentional injury.

CONSIDER THIS!

Every 33 minutes, someone in the United States dies in an alcohol-related motor vehicle crash, and every 2 minutes someone is nonfatally injured.

Treating Unintentional Injuries

If you find yourself in a situation where you or someone else has sustained an unintentional injury, prompt attention and treatment can be essential. The best training is usually through a first aid or CPR course, such as those given through the Red Cross, community colleges, or local hospitals. Even if you can't take such a course, you should know the basics of how to assist someone who is choking, is drowning, or has stopped breathing. The following paragraphs describe the basics of first aid. However, note that all treatments can do more harm than good if not done correctly. You should therefore consult a trained professional for guidance on how to perform the following (and possibly earn your certification).

Choking

Choking occurs when something in the mouth becomes lodged in the trachea (windpipe), thereby blocking air passage from the nose and mouth to the lungs. In

unintentional injury Injury resulting from unplanned actions; preferred term for accidental injury.

accident Sequence of events producing unintended injury, death, or property damage; refers to the event and not the consequences of the event.

STEPS FOR
BEHAVIOR
CHANGE

Does your behavior increase your likelihood of an unintentional injury?

Are you taking unnecessary risks that put you in danger of injury? Take this quiz to find out.

Y **N**

☐ ☐ I often engage in thrill-seeking activities, such as bungee jumping, sky diving, and downhill skiing.

☐ ☐ I am a very confident driver and sometimes speed, or drive fast under subprime conditions, because I know I can handle it.

☐ ☐ I have driven a car after consuming alcohol.

☐ ☐ I quicken my pace when going up or down stairs or navigating a hill or other uncertain terrain.

☐ ☐ I don't read package labels or directions when using a new cleaning product, gadget, or appliance.

If you answered yes to more than one of the above, you're probably on the road to some sort of unintentional injury.

TIPS TO REDUCE YOUR RISK

☑ Adopt a realistic attitude toward sports and extracurricular activities. If you engage in a high-risk activity, such as sky diving, make sure you thoroughly understand the risks and proper precautions necessary to avoid injury. Also, be sure to undergo adequate training by a qualified individual prior to trying a new activity.

☑ Obey the rules of the road, and drive defensively. Always wear your seat belt; always drive within the legal speed limit. Do not drive when emotionally upset, and do not respond to aggressive drivers.

☑ Never drive while or after using drugs or alcohol.

☑ Use handrails when going up and down stairs, and never run up or down stairs. Additionally, do not attempt to climb ladders or stairs when you are ill or physically impaired because of alcohol or drug use.

☑ When using a new medication, always read the label carefully to find out whether you need to avoid certain foods or substances. Don't use multiple medications without the express advice of your health care provider.

☑ Always read the directions. When using a new gadget or appliance (particularly electrical ones) for the first time, don't assume you know how it works.

short, the victim cannot breathe. To assist a choking victim, you have to dislodge the trapped object, usually by performing abdominal thrusts.

Abdominal thrusts (also known as the "Heimlich maneuver") are a series of under-the-diaphragm thrusts, usually given from behind. To perform the maneuver, the rescuer stands behind the victim and circles his arms around the victim's waist. The rescuer clasps his hands together and administers quick thrusts to the victim's abdomen (Figure 12.7).

These thrusts are recommended for rescuers to use on conscious adults and children over the age of 1. They are not recommended for choking in infants under age 1 (alternative measures are recommended for choking infants; see the Mayo Clinic website at www.mayoclinic.com for guidance on treating choking infants). Abdominal thrusts lift the diaphragm and force enough air from the lungs to create an artificial cough. The cough is intended to expel the obstructing foreign body from the airway.

Poisoning

Poisoning often occurs when children accidentally ingest medications, cleaning products, or other household items during a moment of lax adult supervision. However, adults can also inadvertently be exposed to toxic or corrosive chemicals.

For poisoning accidents, always check the label for first aid information, and contact your poison control center. You may also need to contact 911 or a medical professional. For some nonemergency situations, or before you call for medical attention, the following strategies may be useful:

- *Poisons in the eye.* Flood the eye with lukewarm (never hot) water poured from a large glass 2 or 3 inches from the eye. Continue for 15 minutes. Blink the eye as much as possible during the flooding. Do not force the eyelid open, and do not allow the eyes to be rubbed. If lukewarm water is not available, rinse the eye quickly using a gentle stream from a hose for at least 15 minutes.

- *Poisons on the skin.* Any poisons that come in contact with the skin must be removed as quickly as possible. Remove contaminated clothing, and flood the skin area with water for 10 minutes. Then gently wash the skin area with soap and water and rinse. Later, destroy contaminated clothing. For a chemical burn, rinse the area with lots of water, remove the clothes, and cover with a soft, clean cloth. Do not apply grease or ointments.

- *Inhaled poisons.* Inhaled poisons are very serious because of the damage they can cause to the lungs and other tissues of the body. Minimize your risk of exposure, and immediately get the person to fresh air. Loosen the victim's clothing. Send someone for help as quickly as possible. If the victim is not breathing, start CPR, and continue it until the victim is breathing or help arrives. Open the doors and windows so that no one else will be poisoned by the fumes.

- *Swallowed poisons.* If you suspect that someone has swallowed a poisonous substance, first look into the victim's mouth and remove all tablets, powder, or any material that may be present. Examine the mouth for cuts, burns, swelling, unusual coloring, or odor. Rinse and wipe out the mouth with a cloth. If the person is awake and able to swallow, give one-half glassful of water.

Keep in mind that antidotes recommended on many product labels may be outdated or incorrect, so you should not rely on them. In addition, salt water, mustard water, and many other home remedies are ineffective and may be dangerous. Do not use them. Although in the past ipecac syrup was sometimes used as

FIGURE 12.7
The Heimlich maneuver is performed by administering quick abdominal thrusts on someone who is choking.

a home remedy to induce vomiting, currently experts disagree as to whether this is a safe and effective strategy. As of 2003, the American Academy of Pediatrics advises parents against keeping ipecac syrup in the home (16).

Bleeding

Although everyone experiences minor cuts and scrapes, and the accompanying bleeding, from time to time, massive blood loss is an extremely serious condition that can quickly lead to unconsciousness and even death. If you or someone near you experiences a wound that bleeds heavily, immediate attention will be necessary. For cuts, punctures, and abrasions, follow these steps until medical help is available (17):

1. **Have the injured person lie down.** If possible, position the person's head slightly lower than the trunk, or elevate the legs. This position reduces the risk of fainting by increasing blood flow to the brain. If possible, elevate the site of bleeding.

2. **While wearing gloves, remove any obvious dirt or debris from the wound.** Don't remove any large or more deeply embedded objects. Don't probe the wound or attempt to clean it at this point. Your principal concern is to stop the bleeding.

3. **Apply pressure directly on the wound.** Use a sterile bandage, clean cloth, or even a piece of clothing. If nothing else is available, use your hand.

Reducing Your Risk of Unintentional Injury

Bicycle or Motorcycle Accidents

- Always wear a helmet and use reflectors and protective clothing when riding.
- Ride with the traffic, or use bike paths when available.

Motor Vehicle Crashes

- Do not drive when you are overly tired or sleepy.
- Maintain your motor vehicle in good mechanical condition.
- If you need assistance, stay in your car and wait for help.

Falls

- Maintain ladders and steps in good working condition.
- Use skidproof backing on rugs that are not attached to the floor.
- Use handrails or nonslip mats in the bathtub and shower.

Poisoning

- Properly label all drugs.
- Never take more of any drug than is recommended.
- Keep all drugs out of the reach of children.
- Use only nontoxic cleaning materials.
- Discard old or expired prescriptions.
- Do not combine drugs.
- Keep the poison control center's telephone number near your phone.
- Store all drugs and chemicals in their proper containers.

Fire

- Store combustible materials in a safe place.
- Maintain smoke detectors, fire extinguishers, and sprinkler systems in proper working condition.
- Know how to use a fire extinguisher properly.
- Practice safe evacuation procedures from your home and workplace.
- Never leave portable heaters unattended.
- Do not overload electrical outlets.

Drowning

- Never allow children to swim unsupervised.
- Learn to swim, and learn proper water safety procedures.
- Do not swim alone or in the dark.
- Dive only in designated areas.
- Do not swim immediately after eating or when tired.
- Do not swim when using drugs of any kind.
- Avoid swimming in dangerous waters, such as rivers with strong currents.
- Learn cardiopulmonary resuscitation.
- Make sure residential pools are fenced.

4. **Maintain pressure until the bleeding stops.** Hold continuous pressure for at least 20 minutes without looking to see whether the bleeding stopped. You can maintain pressure by binding the wound tightly with a bandage (or a piece of clean clothing) and adhesive tape.

5. **Don't remove the gauze or bandage.** If the bleeding continues and seeps through the gauze or other material you are holding on the wound, don't remove it. Instead, add more absorbent material on top of it.

6. **Immobilize the injured body part once the bleeding has stopped.** Leave the bandages in place, and get the injured person to the emergency room as soon as possible.

Stopped Breathing or Heartbeat

Cardiopulmonary resuscitation (CPR) may be necessary when an accident victim has stopped breathing or the heart has stopped. You need to take a course in CPR to be fully qualified to treat these victims. In short, here is what the rescuer should do:

1. First, check the victim for responsiveness. If there is no response, Call 911 and return to the victim. In most locations, the emergency dispatcher can assist you with CPR instructions.

2. The following is what you will likely be instructed to do. Tilt the head back, and listen for breathing. If the victim is not breathing normally, pinch the nose, cover the mouth with yours, and blow until you see

the chest rise. Give two breaths. Each breath should take 1 second.

3. If the victim is still not breathing normally, coughing, or moving, begin chest compressions. Push down on the chest 1 1/2 to 2 inches 30 times between the nipples. Pump at the rate of 100 compressions per minute, faster than once per second.

4. Continue with two breaths and 30 pumps until help arrives.

Make sure you know...

> In the event of an unintentional injury, there are a few key first-aid procedures that you should know, including the Heimlich maneuver and what to do in the case of poisoning or severe bleeding. You should take a course in first aid and CPR to be sufficiently qualified to administer these procedures.

Summary

1. Overtraining poses the greatest risk of developing an exercise-related injury. Injuries associated with running occur primarily in the foot and knee because of the excessive stress placed on the legs and feet. The factors most closely associated with running injuries are improper training techniques, inadequate shoes, and alignment problems in the legs and feet.

2. Exercise can play an important role in preventing back pain and rehabilitating some back problems. Exercises to increase flexibility and strength, reduce body fat, improve muscle balance between the abdominal and back muscles, and prevent osteoporosis can decrease your risk of developing back problems.

3. Acute muscle soreness may occur during or immediately after an exercise session. This type of injury may be due to muscle damage, accumulation of fluid within the muscle, and/or chemical imbalances within the muscle.

4. Delayed-onset muscle soreness (DOMS) sometimes occurs 24 to 48 hours after an exercise session. Eccentric exercise is a common cause of DOMS.

5. When a muscle is forced to contract against excessive resistance, fibers are damaged. This damage is referred to as a strain and can range from a minor separation of fibers to a complete tear.

6. Tendonitis, or inflammation of a tendon, is one of the most common of all overuse problems associated with physical activity.

7. A sprain is caused by damage to a ligament, a type of connective tissue that provides support for joints. In contrast, torn cartilage refers to damage to the tough, connective tissue that serves as a cushioning pad between the ends of bones.

8. Common injuries to the lower extremities include patellofemoral pain syndrome (PFPS), in which the articular cartilage on the back of the kneecap (patella) may be damaged by chronic use during exercise; shin splints, a condition that encompasses several different injuries to the front of the lower leg; and stress fractures, which are microscopic breaks in the bone.

9. For treating injuries, remember the RICE protocol: rest, ice, compression, and elevation. Cryokinetics treatment calls for alternating periods of cold applications and exercise.

10. The five most common types of unintentional injuries are motor vehicle crashes, fires, drownings, poisonings, and falls. Risk factors for accidents and injuries include unsafe attitudes, stress, drug use, and an unsafe environment.

11. Basic first aid involves knowing how to do the Heimlich maneuver and treat bleeding and poisonings. You should not perform CPR unless you have been trained and certified through the American Red Cross or other accredited program.

Study Questions

1. Which of the following factors are associated with running injuries?
   a. improper shoes
   b. improper training techniques
   c. alignment abnormalities
   d. all of the above

2. Which of the following plays a major role in preventing back pain?
   a. exercise
   b. increasing body fat
   c. reducing hip flexibility
   d. all of the above

3. Pain developing immediately after exercise that has been too long or intense is referred to as
   a. delay-onset muscle soreness.
   b. acute muscle soreness.
   c. overtraining syndrome.
   d. none of the above.

4. Which of the following can help prevent shin splints?
   a. run on a soft surface
   b. wear well-padded shoes
   c. slowly advance exercise intensity
   d. all of the above

5. The primary means of preventing ligament sprains is to
   a. wear a joint brace.
   b. consume large amounts of protein.
   c. avoid intense exercise.
   d. refrain from activities that place a strain on joints.

6. What are considered the primary causes of running injuries?

7. Compare and contrast a strain and a sprain.

8. Define *tendonitis*, and describe the best method of preventing or treating it.

9. What is the cause of PFPS, and how should it be treated?

10. Define the RICE protocol, and discuss its use.

11. Define the following terms:
    arthroscopic surgery
    cartilage
    ligament
    stress fracture
    overtraining syndrome

12. Describe the proper first-aid response for the following:
    choking
    puncture wound with profuse bleeding
    swallowing of poison
    drowning victim who has stopped breathing

Suggested Reading

Chou, L. H., V. Akuthota, D. F. Drake, S. D. Toledo, and S. F. Nadler. Sports and performing arts medicine: Lower-limb injuries in endurance sports. *Archives of Physical Medicine and Rehabilitation* 85(3 Suppl 1): S59–66, 2004.

da Costa, B. R., and E. R. Viera. Stretching to reduce work-related musculoskeletal disorders: A systematic review. *Journal of Rehabilitation Medicine* 40(5):321–328, 2008.

Garrick, J., J. T. Bell, and P. Radetsky. *Anybody's Sports Medicine Book: The Complete Guide to Quick Recovery from Injuries*, 2nd ed. Tampa, FL: IFPA, 2009.

Herbert, R. D., and M. Gabriel. Effects of stretching before and after exercising on muscle soreness and risk of injury: Systematic review. *British Medical Journal* 325(7362):468, 2002.

Houglum, P. *Therapeutic Exercise for Athletic Injuries*, 2nd ed. Champaign, IL: Human Kinetics, 2005.

Howatson, G., and K. A. van Someren. The prevention and treatment of exercise-induced muscle damage. *Sports Medicine* 38(6):483–503, 2008.

Hreljac, A. Impact and overuse injuries in runners. *Medicine and Science in Sports and Exercise* 36(5):845–849, 2004.

Thacker, S. B., J. Gilchrist, D. F. Stroup, and C. D. Kimsey. The prevention of shin splints in sports: A systematic review of literature. *Medicine and Science in Sports and Exercise* 34(1):32–40, 2002.

For links to the organizations and websites listed below, visit The Total Fitness and Wellness Website at www.pearsonhighered.com/powers.

WebMD
Provides information about preventing and treating exercise-related injuries.

FamilyDoctor.org
Provides information on basic exercise injuries and sports safety.

Fitness Files
Contains information concerning fitness fundamentals, flexibility and contraindicated exercises, exercise nutrition, and the treatment of exercise injuries.

The Running Page
Contains information about racing, running clubs, places to run,

running-related products, running magazines, and treating running-related injuries.

Meriter Fitness
Presents information concerning injury prevention and treatment, weight training, flexibility, exercise prescriptions, and more.

Sportsmedicine.About.com
Provides information on basic exercises for rehabilitating common exercise- or sports-related injuries.

References

1. Radomski, M. Sports injuries. *Wellness Options* 6:52, 2003.

2. Bergen G., L. H. Chen, M. Warner, and L. A. Fingerhut. *Injury in the United States: 2007 Chartbook.* Hyattsville, MD: National Center for Health Statistics, 2008.

3. Murphy, D. F., D. A., Connolly, and B. D. Beynnon. Risk factors for lower extremity injury: A review of the literature. *British Journal of Sports Medicine* 37(1): 13–29, 2003.

4. Dugan, S. A., and K. P. Bhat. Biomechanics and analysis of running gait. *Physical Medicine and Rehabilitation Clinics of North America* 16(3):603–621, 2005.

5. Macintyre, J., and E. Joy. Foot and ankle injuries in dance. *Clinics in Sports Medicine* 19(2):351–368, 2000.

6. Maher, C. G. Effective physical treatment for chronic low back pain. *Orthopedic Clinics of North America* 35(1):57–64, 2004.

7. Powers, S., and E. Howley. *Exercise Physiology: Theory and Application to Fitness and Performance*, 7th ed. New York: McGraw-Hill, 2009.

8. Connolly, D. A., S. P. Sayers, and M. P. McHugh. Treatment and prevention of delayed onset muscle soreness. *Journal of Strength and Conditioning Research* 17(1): 197–208, 2003.

9. Prentice, W. E. *Therapeutic Modalities: For Sports Medicine and Athletic Training.* New York: McGraw-Hill, 2009.

10. Adirim, T. A., and T. L. Cheng. Overview of injuries in the young athlete. *Sports Medicine* 33(1):75–81, 2003.

11. Dugan, S. A., and K. M. Weber. Stress fractures and rehabilitation. *Physical Medicine and Rehabilitation Clinics of North America* 18(3):401–416, 2007.

12. Bleakley, C., S. McDonough, and D. MacAuley. The use of ice in the treatment of acute soft-tissue injury: A systematic review of randomized controlled trials. *American Journal of Sports Medicine* 32(1):251–261, 2004.

13. Safe Kids USA. *Report to the Nation: Trends in Unintentional Childhood Injury Mortality and Parental Views on Child Safety.* Washington, DC: Safe Kids Worldwide, 2008.

14. Institute of Medicine. *Reducing the Burden of Injury: Advancing Prevention and Treatment.* Washington, DC: National Academies Press, 1999.

15. National Center for Injury Prevention and Control. *CDC Injury Fact Book.* Atlanta, GA: Centers for Disease Control and Prevention, 2006.

16. Kennedy, K. Parents should dispose of ipecac syrup: New AAP policy. *AAP News* 23:145–154, 2003.

17. Mayo Clinic. First aid guide. www.mayoclinic.com/health/first-aid-severe-bleeding/FA00038.

Videos

Log on to www.pearsonhighered.com/powers to view these chapter-related videos.

Injury Prevention and Emergency Care

Hip Flexor Stretch

Abdominal Curl

Abdominal Curl (stability ball)

Hamstrings Stretch (seated)

Modified Hurdler Stretch

Low Back Knee-to-Chest Stretch

Torso Twist and Hip Stretch

Back Bridge

Cat Stretch

NAME _____ DATE _____

Preventing Injuries during Exercise

This lab will help you identify and eliminate ways in which your exercise program may cause injuries. The following measures are associated with preventing exercise-related injury. Check those you have incorporated into your exercise program (and, in some cases, into your life in general). For any measure you do not check, write in the space provided exactly what changes you plan to implement to reduce or eliminate the risks associated with that measure.

I always wear the proper shoes for the activity.   Yes ___   No ___

Changes to implement: _____

I always perform a proper warm-up before the exercise activity.   Yes ___   No ___

Changes to implement: _____

I always stretch the muscles that will be involved in the activity.   Yes ___   No ___

Changes to implement: _____

All muscle groups involved in the activity are strengthened and balanced.   Yes ___   No ___

Changes to implement: _____

I avoid overstretching my neck and back.   Yes ___   No ___

Changes to implement: _____

I avoid extending and rotating my spine.   Yes ___   No ___

Changes to implement: _____

I avoid lifting heavy objects.   Yes ___   No ___

Changes to implement: _____

I avoid quick, jerking movements.   Yes ___   No ___

Changes to implement: _____

My training program has been properly designed.   Yes ___   No ___

Changes to implement: _____

I use the appropriate frequency of exercise.   Yes ___   No ___

Changes to implement: _____

I use the appropriate intensity of exercise.   Yes ___   No ___

Changes to implement: _____

I use the appropriate duration of exercise.   Yes ___   No ___

Changes to implement: _____

I use proper exercise techniques.   Yes ___   No ___

Changes to implement: _____

I run only on a firm, level surface.   Yes ___   No ___

Changes to implement: _____

I include a proper cool-down after exercising.   Yes ___   No ___

Changes to implement: _____

NAME _____ DATE _____

Assessing Flexibility and Back Pain Risk

Back pain is a multifactoral problem that is preventable in most cases. There are many sources of back pain, including improper lifting techniques, weak muscles, poor posture, inflexibility, and bone disorders. The following tests will assess the flexibility in your lower back, hamstrings, and hip flexors. Choose a partner, and use extreme caution in applying force.

Stretches and exercises to alleviate back pain or prevent future back injury are suggested in the Interpretation sections below. Log on to **www.pearsonhighered.com/powers** to view demonstration videos of these exercises. ▷

Test 1: Back to Wall

Stand with your back against a wall so that your head, shoulders, calves, and heels are all touching the wall. Try to flatten your neck and the hollow of your back by pressing your buttocks down. Your partner should be able to place just a hand between the wall and the small of your back.

Pass _____   Fail _____

Interpretation

If this space is greater than the thickness of a flattened hand, you may have lumbar lordosis (increased curvature in the lower back with a forward pelvic tilt) with shortened lumbar and hip flexor muscles. To correct or prevent lumbar lordosis, flexibility exercises to lengthen the hip flexor muscles, as well as strength and endurance exercises for the abdominal muscles, are generally recommended. See the descriptions and videos for Hip Flexor Stretch, Abdominal Curl, and Abdominal Curl (stability ball). ▷

Test 2: Straight Leg Lift

Lie on your back with your hands behind your neck. Your partner will kneel on your left side and stabilize your right leg by placing his or her right hand on your knee. With the left hand, your partner should grasp your left ankle and raise your left leg as near to a right angle (90 degrees) as possible. In this position, your lower back should be in contact with the floor, and your right leg should remain straight and on the floor. Repeat this test on the opposite side.

Left side: Pass _____   Fail _____
Right side: Pass _____   Fail _____

Interpretation

If your left leg bends at the knee, your hamstring muscles are short. If your back arches and/or your right leg does not remain on the floor, short lumbar muscles, short hip flexors, or both are implicated. To correct this condition, perform exercises to stretch your hamstrings; lower back stretches can be used to lengthen the lumbar muscles. See the descriptions and videos for Hamstrings Stretch (seated), Modified Hurdler Stretch, Low Back Knee-to-Chest Stretch, Torso Twist and Hip Stretch, Back Bridge, and Cat Stretch. ▷

→

Test 3: Knee to Chest

(No partner is needed.) Lie on your back on a table or bench, with your right leg extended beyond the edge of the table (about one-third of your thigh is off the table). Bring your left knee to your chest, and grasp the back of your thigh, pulling down tightly toward your chest. Your right thigh should remain in contact with the table. Repeat this test on the opposite leg.

Left side: Pass _____   Fail _____
Right side: Pass _____   Fail _____

Interpretation

If your right thigh lifts off the table while you hug your knee to your chest, you have a tight right hip flexor muscle; if your left thigh lifts, then you have a tight left hip flexor. To stretch the right hip flexor, place the left knee directly above the left ankle, and stretch the right leg backward so that the right knee touches the floor. Press your pelvis forward and downward. Do not bend your front knee more than 90 degrees. Repeat on the opposite side to stretch the left hip flexor. See the description and video for Hip Flexor Stretch (thigh stretch). ⊳

Summary

Awareness of flexibility problems may help you alleviate back pain or prevent future back discomfort. Remember that exercises designed to increase flexibility and strength, reduce body fat, improve muscle balance between the trunk flexors and extensors, and prevent osteoporosis can decrease your risk of developing back problems.

Cancer

13

true or false?

1. Your diet can influence your risk for cancer.

2. Breast cancer is the leading cause of cancer deaths in women.

3. Black Americans have the highest rates of cancer deaths of U.S. adults.

4. Cancer can be caused by a virus.

5. Using a tanning bed is a safe way to tan without increasing your risk for skin cancer.

Answers appear on the next page.

Do you eat a low-fat, high-fiber diet? Do you use sunscreen and avoid sun exposure between 10.00 AM and 4.00 PM? Do you limit alcohol consumption and avoid cigarette smoking and tobacco products? If you answered yes to these questions, then you are making some healthy behavior choices that can reduce your risk for some of the most common types of cancers. Determining your risk for cancer and participating in cancer screenings are important wellness behaviors. In this chapter, we will define and discuss the most common types of cancers. You will also learn about the significant risk factors, signs and symptoms, and procedures for screening and early detection of cancer.

What Is Cancer?

Cancer is the second leading cause of death in the United States, accounting for almost 25% of all deaths (1). Since 2002 the rate of cancer deaths has been on the decline, the first time that's happened since 1930. Cancer rates have stabilized for men and have slightly increased for women since the mid-1990s. An estimated one in two men and one in three women will develop cancer at some point in their lifetime (1). Cancer can strike at any age, but it occurs more frequently in older people. The most common cancer among young people is leukemia.

As awareness of risk factors for cancer has increased, and as early detection, prevention, and treat-

ment methods have improved, the survival rates for cancer have also risen. In the mid-1970s cancer survival rates were around 50%, but they increased to approximately 66% by 2002 (1). According to the American Cancer Society, more than 11.1 million Americans have survived cancer. The key is early detection. If more cancers were diagnosed earlier, over one-half of cancer patients could be saved!

In addition to unhealthy behaviors such as smoking, drinking alcohol, and eating a less than optimal diet, environmental factors, such as cancer-causing chemicals in water and food supplies, are linked to increased cancer risk (1–3).

Cancer is not a single disease but a collection of over 100 related diseases that are characterized by rapid, uncontrolled cell growth. Cancer can occur in almost every tissue and organ in the body (4, 5). Groups of abnormal cells can form **tumors** that can be **benign tumors** or **malignant tumors.** Generally, benign tumors are not serious health threats because the cells in them grow and divide less quickly and do not spread throughout the body. However, depending on the location, they might interfere with normal body functions and still require medical treatment. Cells of malignant tumors are cancer cells, though not all cancers form tumors (e.g., leukemia). Once a tumor is detected, a **biopsy** is used to determine whether the cells are cancerous.

Cancer cells increase in size and often spread, invading neighboring tissues or other locations in the body after being transported in blood or lymph. The growing cancer cells damage healthy tissue and interfere with normal organ functioning, which may eventually result in organ failure and death. The spread of

Answers

1. **TRUE** What you eat (or don't eat) can have a significant impact on your risk for cancer. Excess consumption of dietary fat and processed foods and inadequate consumption of fiber, fruits, and vegetables can increase your risk for cancer.

2. **FALSE** In both women and men, lung cancer kills more people than any other cancer. Although more women are diagnosed with breast cancer per year than lung cancer, breast cancer is typically detected earlier and is more treatable than lung cancer.

3. **TRUE** Black adults have higher rates of cancer deaths than other racial or ethnic groups. In some cases, the rates are over two times higher. Asian and Pacific Islander men and women have the lowest rates of cancer deaths.

4. **TRUE** Viruses can damage DNA, leading to cancer. Types of leukemia, lymphomas, and cervical cancer are examples of cancers linked to viruses.

5. **FALSE** Like natural sunlight, tanning beds expose you to harmful ultraviolet rays. To minimize your risk for skin cancer, you need to avoid tanning beds and use sunscreen when outdoors.

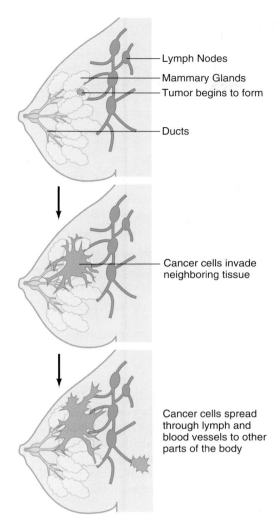

Lymph Nodes
Mammary Glands
Tumor begins to form

Ducts

Cancer cells invade
neighboring tissue

Cancer cells spread
through lymph and
blood vessels to other
parts of the body

FIGURE 13.1
Growth and metastasis of a malignant breast tumor.

cancer cells throughout the body is a process called
metastasis.

Although cancer cells spread and form new tumors
throughout the body, a cancer diagnosis is always
named after the site of origin, or primary site. For example, cancer cells that develop into a tumor in the
breast are called breast cancer. If the cells metastasize
to another organ, such as the lungs, the cancer is breast
cancer that has metastasized to the lungs, and the lungs
are the secondary site (Figure 13.1). Metastasis
significantly reduces a cancer patient's chances of
survival because it is more difficult to treat cancer in
more than one location.

Make sure you know...

> Cancer is not a single disease but a collection of
diseases that can affect almost every body tissue.

> Cancer is the uncontrolled growth and spread of
abnormal cells; a group of these abnormal cells is
called a tumor.

> Cancer cells can spread through the bloodstream
and lymphatic system in a process called metastasis.

How Do Normal Cells Become Cancerous?

Cell growth and division is controlled by DNA within
the cells. Normal functioning DNA carefully regulates
cell growth and division in a slow and steady manner. If
DNA is damaged by **carcinogens,** it can result in cell
division that escalates out of control. A number of environmental agents, such as radiation, chemicals, and
drugs, can lead to the DNA damage that causes a normal cell to become an abnormal cancer cell (Figure
13.2). Although cancer cells grow rapidly, tumors take
time to develop. A tumor the size of a pea contains
approximately a billion cells, so it may take years for a
tumor to become large enough to be detected.

Tumors in superficial tissues such as the breasts or
testes can be felt as a lump during self-exams or clinical
exams. However, tumors of deeper tissues or organs
are not as easily detected and can develop into much
larger masses before symptoms are present. This is why
knowing the seven warning signs (see the box on page
370) and seeking medical treatment is important for
early detection of cancer. Additionally, getting regular
screenings at the recommended ages and time intervals
is a key factor for early detection. As we discuss
specific types of cancer in the next sections, we will
discuss specific risk factors and the recommended early
detection screenings.

Make sure you know...

> Cell growth and division are regulated by DNA, and
the uncontrolled growth of cancer cells is caused by
damaged DNA.

cancer A collection of over 100 different diseases that can
affect almost every body tissue. Cancer is the uncontrolled
growth and spread of abnormal cells.

tumor A group of abnormal cells.

benign tumor A tumor of cells that are not cancerous.

malignant tumor A tumor of cells that are cancerous.

biopsy The surgical removal of a small sample of a tumor for
laboratory analysis.

metastasis The spreading of cancer cells throughout the
body.

carcinogens Cancer-causing agents, which include
radiation, chemicals, drugs, and other toxic substances.

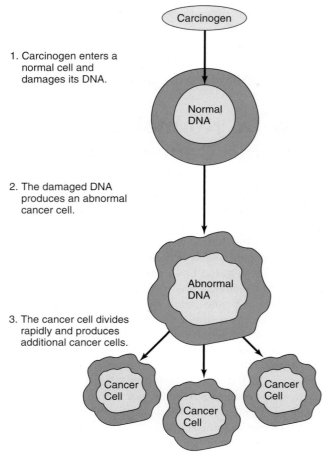

1. Carcinogen enters a normal cell and damages its DNA.

2. The damaged DNA produces an abnormal cancer cell.

3. The cancer cell divides rapidly and produces additional cancer cells.

FIGURE 13.2
The transformation of a normal cell into a cancer cell.

> DNA can be damaged by various cancer-causing substances called carcinogens.

> Tumors in superficial tissue can be detected with self-exams and clinical exams, whereas tumors in deeper tissues can only be detected with X-ray exams or other screening procedures.

Types of Cancer

Cancer can develop in almost any organ (4). The most common cancers are skin cancers, followed by prostate cancer in men and breast cancer in women. However, skin cancers are very

CONSIDER THIS!

Over 80% of lung cancers are linked to smoking, but risk is reduced 65% after 10 years of being smoke-free.

Seven Warning Signs of Cancer

Early detection is key to surviving cancer, and early detection can be easier if you are familiar with the warning signs. One way to remember seven of the most common warning signs is to use the following mnemonic device:

CAUTION

*C*hange in bowel or bladder habits

*A*rea or sore that does not heal or that heals slowly

*U*nusual bleeding or discharge from the bowel, nipples, or vagina, or unexplained blood in the urine

*T*hickening or lump in the breast or elsewhere

*I*ndigestion, difficulty swallowing, or loss of appetite that persists

*O*bvious change in size or color of a wart or mole

*N*agging or persistent cough or hoarseness

You should see your health care provider if you have any of these symptoms.

treatable and curable, so they do not contribute to as many cancer deaths as other types of cancers (1). Other common cancer sites include the lungs, colon and rectum, uterus, kidneys, and liver (Figure 13.3). Let's examine some specific types of cancer in depth, beginning with the most common killer, lung cancer.

Lung Cancer

The number of new cases of lung cancer has decreased for men and has leveled off for women in the recent past. However, lung cancer is still the leading cause of cancer deaths for men and women. As you can see in Figure 13.4 on page 372, lung cancer has been the leading cause of cancer deaths in men since 1960, but it is only since the mid-1980s that lung cancer surpassed breast cancer as the leading cause of cancer deaths for women. The rise in lung cancer in women is likely due to the rise in the number of female smokers over this time period. Estimates indicate close to 160,000 men and women died from lung cancer in 2009 and there were more than 200,000 new cases diagnosed (1). More cases of skin, prostate, and breast cancer are diagnosed each year compared to lung cancer, but there are more deaths due to lung cancer than prostate, breast, and colon cancers combined (6).

Estimated New Cases*		Estimated Deaths*	
Male	**Female**	**Male**	**Female**
Prostate 192,280 (25%)	Breast 192,370 (27%)	Lung & bronchus 88,900 (30%)	Lung & bronchus 70,490 (26%)
Lung & bronchus 116,090 (15%)	Lung & bronchus 103,350 (14%)	Prostate 27,360 (9%)	Breast 40,170 (15%)
Colon & rectum 75,590 (10%)	Colon & rectum 71,380 (10%)	Colon & rectum 25,240 (9%)	Colon & rectum 24,680 (9%)
Urinary bladder 52,810 (7%)	Uterine corpus 42,160 (6%)	Pancreas 18,030 (6%)	Pancreas 17,210 (6%)
Melanoma of the skin 39,080 (5%)	Non-Hodgkin lymphoma 29,990 (4%)	Leukemia 12,590 (4%)	Ovary 14,600 (5%)
Non-Hodgkin lymphoma 35,990 (5%)	Melanoma of the skin 29,640 (4%)	Liver & intrahepatic bile duct 12,090 (4%)	Non-Hodgkin lymphoma 9,670 (4%)
Kidney & renal pelvis 35,430 (5%)	Thyroid 27,200 (4%)	Esophagus 11,490 (4%)	Leukemia 9,280 (3%)
Leukemia 25,630 (3%)	Kidney & renal pelvis 22,330 (3%)	Urinary bladder 10,180 (3%)	Uterine corpus 7,780 (3%)
Oral cavity & pharynx 25,240 (3%)	Ovary 21,550 (3%)	Non-Hodgkin lymphoma 9,830 (3%)	Liver & intrahepatic bile duct 6,070 (2%)
Pancreas 21,050 (3%)	Pancreas 21,420 (3%)	Kidney & renal pelvis 8,160 (3%)	Brain & other nervous system 5,590 (2%)
All Sites 766,130 (100%)	**All Sites 713,220 (100%)**	**All Sites 292,540 (100%)**	**All Sites 269,800 (100%)**

*Excludes basal and squamous cell skin cancers and in situ carcinoma, except urinary bladder.

FIGURE 13.3
Leading sites of new cancer cases and deaths—2009 estimates.

Source: American Cancer Society. *Cancer Facts and Figures 2009.* Atlanta: American Cancer Society, 2009, p. 10 Reprinted by permission of the American Cancer Society, Inc. Modification is prohibited.

Why does lung cancer contribute to so many more deaths than other cancers? One factor is lack of methods for early detection. Lung cancer symptoms are often not present until the cancer has become more advanced and has spread. Although new screening procedures are being studied, no good screening methods have been developed to catch lung cancer in early stages. Therefore, it is more difficult to treat lung cancer than other types of cancer, and mortality rates are higher. The American Cancer Society reports that 6 out of 10 people diagnosed with lung cancer will die within 1 year of being diagnosed, and 7 to 8 will die within 2 years of diagnosis.

Because early detection of lung cancer is difficult, knowing how to limit your risk factors, and to spot the early signs and symptoms, is extremely important. The most significant thing you can do to reduce your risk of lung cancer is to not smoke. Smoking has long been linked to lung cancer, and the more and longer a person smokes, the greater the risk. However, the good news is that stopping smoking will lower risk if cancer has not already developed. It is not just cigarette smoking that increases the risk for lung cancer; smoking pipes, cigars, or marijuana also increases risk, as does exposure to secondhand smoke. Other risk factors include exposure to asbestos, radon, air pollution, and workplace carcinogens such as gasoline, diesel exhaust, and coal products. Some research suggests that a diet rich in fruits and vegetables may help reduce the risk for lung cancer (7). See the box on page 373 for several specific signs and symptoms that may be indicators of lung cancer.

Colon and Rectal Cancer

Colon and rectal cancer, or colorectal cancer, is the third leading cause of cancer deaths for both men and women, contributing to approximately 9% of cancer

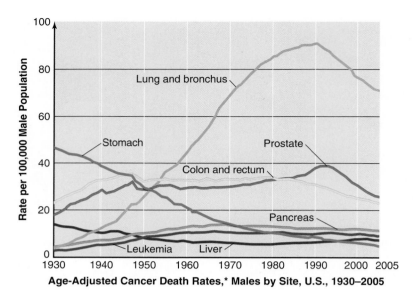

Age-Adjusted Cancer Death Rates,* Males by Site, U.S., 1930–2005

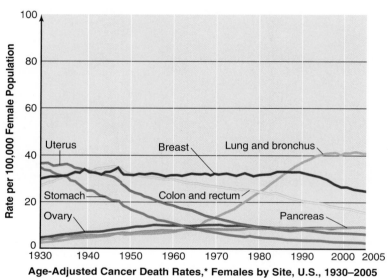

Age-Adjusted Cancer Death Rates,* Females by Site, U.S., 1930–2005

FIGURE 13.4

Death rates for some cancers have leveled off, and even declined, in the last decades as people have become more aware of their risk and screening measures have improved chances of early detection.

*Per 100,000, age-adjusted to the 2000 U.S. standard population.

Note: Because of changes in ICD coding, numerator information has changed over time. Rates for cancer of the liver, lung and bronchus, colon and rectum, and ovary are affected by these coding changes.

Source: National Center for Health Statistics, Centers for Disease Control and Prevention. *U.S. Mortality Public Use Data Tapes 1960 to 2005, U.S. Mortality Volumes 1930 to 1959.* 2008.

deaths among men and 9% among women. The number of deaths is on the decline because of better screening procedures that can detect **polyps** and early stages of cancer, thereby making early treatment possible. Because risk increases with age, adults should begin getting regular screenings at age 50. However, indi-

viduals at high risk might need to start screenings at younger ages as recommended by their health care providers.

There are several screening procedures that can be performed. The American Cancer Society recommends a fecal stool blood test or a fecal immunochemical test annually and a flexible sigmoidoscopy every 5 years. The fecal tests assess blood in the stool, which is an indicator of polyps or cancer. The flexible sigmoidoscopy involves the insertion of a thin tube into the rectum and colon to visually check for the presence of polyps and tumors. A colonoscopy is another commonly used procedure that is similar to the flexible sigmoidoscopy, but a longer tube is used that can examine a larger portion of the colon. This procedure is recommended every 10 years.

Although early detection for colon and rectal cancer is easier than for lung cancer, prevention is still the key. Regular exercise and a high-fiber, low-fat diet are two behavioral factors that can reduce your risk for developing these two types of cancer. Engaging in the recommended 30 minutes of moderate activity at least 5 days of the week is associated with a lower risk of colon cancer. Diets that are rich in a variety of fruits and vegetables and whole grains will provide the fiber associated with lowering the risk for colon and rectal cancers. Other factors that might reduce your risk include consuming adequate calcium, vitamin D, and possibly a multivitamin that includes folic acid.

Risk factors for colon and rectal cancer include nonmodifiable factors, such as heredity, and modifiable factors, such as the diet and exercise behaviors mentioned above. Ashkenazi Jews of Eastern European descent have the highest rates in the world, and blacks have the highest death rates from colon cancer in the United States (8). A family or personal history of colon and rectal cancer and a personal history of polyps are also associated with increased risk, and people with diabetes are at greater risk. In addition to exercise and diet, modifiable risk factors include heavy alcohol consumption, being overweight, and smoking.

Breast Cancer

Breast cancer is the most common type of cancer in women (after skin cancers) and is the second leading cause of cancer deaths for women. The American Can-

Signs and Symptoms of Specific Cancers

Lung Cancer

- A cough that does not go away
- Chest pain, often aggravated by deep breathing, coughing, and even laughing
- Hoarseness
- Weight loss and loss of appetite
- Bloody or rust-colored sputum (spit or phlegm)
- Shortness of breath
- Recurring infections such as bronchitis and pneumonia
- New onset of wheezing

Colon and Rectal Cancer

- Change in bowel habits, such as diarrhea, constipation, or narrowing of the stool, that lasts for more than a few days
- A feeling that you need to have a bowel movement that doesn't go away even after you do have a bowel movement
- Bleeding from the rectum or blood in the stool
- Cramping or gnawing stomach pain
- Decreased appetite
- Weakness and fatigue
- Jaundice (yellow-green color of the skin and the white part of the eye)

Breast Cancer

- A new lump or mass
- Generalized swelling of part of a breast (even if no distinct lump is felt)
- Skin irritation or dimpling
- Nipple pain or retraction (turning inward)
- Redness or scaliness of the nipple or breast skin
- A discharge other than breast milk

Prostate Cancer

- Blood in the urine (hematuria)
- Difficulty getting an erection (impotence)
- Pain in the hips, spine, ribs, or other areas if it spreads to the bones
- Weakness or numbness in the legs or feet, or even loss of bladder or bowel control if it spreads to the spine and affects spinal nerves

Testicular Cancer

- A slight enlargement of one of the testicles
- A change in the consistency of a testicle
- A dull ache in the lower abdomen or groin (may not occur in all cases of testicular cancer)
- The sensation of dragging and heaviness in a testicle

cer Society estimates that 1 in 8 women will develop breast cancer in her lifetime, and 1 in 33 will die from breast cancer. Fortunately, death rates from breast cancer are decreasing. Women today are more aware of the importance of regular screenings and of minimizing their risk. Hence this type of cancer is increasingly detected in its earlier, more treatable stages. Although breast cancer occurs primarily in women, men too can develop breast cancer.

As with most cancers, breast cancer risk increases with age. Approximately 80% of the cases are in women 50 years and older. However, younger women can also develop breast cancer. Women should get to know their breasts well and perform regular self-exams so they can readily detect a lump or growth if one develops. Over 95% of all breast cancers are discovered by women themselves during routine self-exams. (See the Closer Look box on page 374 for more on breast self-exams.)

Women in their 20s and 30s should get regular clinical exams at least every 3 years. Typically your health care provider will perform a clinical breast exam

when you have your annual Pap test. Beginning at age 40, women should have annual **mammograms.** Women at higher risk might need to start mammograms earlier as recommended by their health care providers.

Knowing the signs and symptoms of breast cancer is very important for early detection. If you notice changes in your breasts or detect any of the signs during a self-exam, you should see your health care provider. Many of the lumps detected are not cancerous, but you cannot tell without a biopsy. If a lump is determined to be cancerous, there are multiple courses of treatment. The removal of the lump, and potentially

polyps Growths from mucous membranes; commonly found in the colon and rectum, where they can be indicators of colon cancer.

mammograms Low-radiation X-ray films of the breast used to check for tumors that cannot be detected by self-exams or clinical exams.

A CLOSER LOOK

BREAST SELF-EXAMINATION

The best time for a woman to examine her breasts is just after her menstrual period, when the breasts are not tender or swollen. Sticking to the same time every month will also help you remember to do the exam. Women who are pregnant, breast-feeding, or have breast implants should still examine their breasts regularly.

Take the following steps to perform your self-exam:

1. Lie down, and place your right arm behind your head. Lying down allows the breast tissue to spread evenly over the chest wall so it is as thin as possible. This will make it easier to thoroughly examine the entire breast.

2. Use the pads (fingertips) of the three middle fingers on your left hand to feel for lumps in the right breast. Use overlapping dime-sized circular motions to feel all of the breast tissue.

3. Use three different levels of pressure at each spot so you're sure to examine all tissue. Light pressure is needed to feel the tissue closest to the skin; medium pressure to feel a little deeper; and firm pressure to feel the tissue closest to the chest and ribs. A firm ridge in the lower curve of each breast is normal. Your health care provider can help you determine the pressure if you are not sure.

4. Move around the breast in an up-and-down pattern, starting at an imaginary line drawn straight down your side from the underarm and moving across the breast to the middle of the chest bone. Be sure to check the entire breast area, going down until you feel only ribs, and going up to the neck or collar bone (clavicle). There is some evidence that the up-and-down pattern (sometimes called the vertical pattern) is the most effective pattern for covering the entire breast without missing any breast tissue.

5. Repeat the exam on your left breast, using the finger pads of the right hand.

6. While standing in front of a mirror with your hands pressing firmly down on your hips, look at your breasts for any changes of size, shape, contour, or dimpling. (Pressing down on the hips contracts the chest wall muscles and enhances any breast changes.) Continue to look for changes with your arms down at your sides and then with your arms raised up over your head with your palms pressed together.

7. Examine each underarm while sitting up or standing and with your arm only slightly raised so you can easily feel in this area. (Raising your arm straight up tightens the tissue in this area and makes it difficult to examine.)

Use pads of the fingers, and move in an up-and-down pattern when performing a breast self-exam.

Source: American Cancer Society. How to perform a breast self-exam. 2007. www.cancer.org/docroot/CRI/content/ CRI_2_6x_How_to_perform_a_breast_self_exam_ 5.asp?sitearea=.

the surrounding tissues and lymph nodes, is a typical first step. The specific surgical procedure will be determined by the stage and spread of the cancer and the woman's level of risk. Surgical procedures are typically followed by radiation and/or chemotherapy to kill any remaining cancer cells.

Many of the risk factors for breast cancer are non-modifiable. Being a woman over 50 years and having a family or personal history are risk factors. There are also genetic risk factors in that women with certain specific genes have significantly higher risk for breast cancer than those without those genes. Race has differential associations with breast cancer. White women are more likely to develop breast cancer than other racial or ethnic groups. Asian, Hispanic, and Native American women have lower rates than other groups. Black women, however, are more likely to die from breast cancer than other racial groups. Starting menstruation before age 12 and going through menopause after age 55 have been linked to increased breast cancer risk as well.

Lifestyle and behavioral factors can also influence breast cancer risk. Having no children, or having a first child after age 30 is associated with slightly elevated risk. By contrast, more than one pregnancy and pregnancy at a young age are associated with lower breast cancer risk. Breast-feeding also is linked to lower risk. The use of hormones, especially over a long term, such as taking oral contraceptives or hormone replacement therapy, has been linked to increased risk. There is evidence that regular exercise reduces the risk for breast cancer, so meeting the general exercise recommendations for health is suggested. Women who consume 2 to 5 alcoholic drinks per day have a risk one and a half times greater than that of women who do not consume alcohol (9). As with many types of cancer, obesity and a high-fat diet increase the risk for developing breast cancer.

Prostate Cancer

The prostate gland is a small gland, about the size of a walnut, that produces seminal fluid in men. Cancer of the prostate is second only to skin cancer in the number of cases diagnosed per year in men, accounting for approximately 25% of cancers. After an increase in the early 1990s, rates have leveled off in the recent past, thanks to better early detection methods. Death rates of prostate cancer are second to lung cancer in men.

Prostate cancer is typically a slowly developing cancer, and there are two tests available for screenings: the digital rectal exam (DRE) and the prostate-specific antigen (PSA) blood test. During a DRE, a health care provider inserts a gloved, lubricated finger into the rectum to feel for tumors. If a tumor is detected, then a biopsy will be performed to determine whether the mass is cancerous. The PSA test is a blood test in which levels of PSA are assessed. Higher levels are associated with prostate cancer.

The American Cancer Society recommends that health care providers offer the tests annually to healthy men beginning at age 50. It is not necessarily recommended that all men get the screening but that men and their health care providers discuss the benefits and the risks associated with the tests and decide whether to have them done. Men at higher risk should begin testing at younger ages as recommended by their health care providers.

Risk for prostate cancer increases with age, and most cases occur in men over 65 years. Race is a significant risk factor, with rates higher among black men in the United States compared to other racial or ethnic groups. Asian men tend to have lower rates than white men. Rates for prostate cancer are higher in North America and northwestern Europe than in Asia, Africa, and South and Central America. Family history is another nonmodifiable risk factor for prostate cancer. Diet is a behavioral risk factor. Diets high in red meat and high-fat dairy products are associated with increased risk for prostate cancer.

There are several signs and symptoms for advanced prostate cancer, but there are typically no symptoms with early stages (refer back to the box on page 373). If you experience any of the symptoms, you should see your health care provider.

Testicular Cancer

Although testicular cancer is not a common type of cancer overall, it is one of the most common cancers in men 15 to 34 years of age (1), and it accounts for 12% of all deaths in this group. Testicular cancer is treatable and curable. Again, early detection is key to being a cancer survivor.

Lumps in the testes can be detected though routine self exams (see the Closer Look box on page 376). Men should also have a clinical examination of the testes performed during their regular physical exam. Risk factors for testicular cancer are primarily nonmodifiable. An undescended testicle, which is present at birth, is the most common risk factor. Other risk factors include race, previous testicular cancer, and family history. In regard to race, white men have higher rates than black, Asian, and Hispanic men. Because the risk factors are not behavioral, there is little that can be done to prevent testicular cancer. Knowing your risk factors and participating in the recommended screenings are important for early detection and prompt treatment.

Skin Cancer

Skin cancers are the most common types of cancer, but they are very treatable and curable. There are two types of skin cancers, **melanoma** and **nonmelanoma.** Melanoma is the more serious type of skin cancer because it spreads quickly. Although melanoma only makes up about 3% of skin cancers, it is one of the

melanoma Less common, more serious type of skin cancer, which spreads.

nonmelanoma More common, less serious type of skin cancer, which typically doesn't spread.

A CLOSER LOOK

TESTICULAR SELF-EXAMINATION

Young men should perform a monthly testicular self-examination. The exam is best performed shortly after a warm shower or bath, when the skin of the scrotum (the sac surrounding the testicles) is most relaxed. The examination is performed by rolling each testicle between the thumb and fingers (see the figure). Lumps are generally found on the side or front of the testicle.

The presence of a lump does not necessarily indicate cancer, but you should call your health care provider immediately to schedule a medical exam if you feel a lump.

A testicular self-exam.

Source: From Michael Johnson, *Human Biology: Concepts and Current Issues,* 3rd ed. Copyright © 2006. Reprinted by permission of Pearson Education, Inc.

most common cancers in young people under 30 years. Melanoma develops in the melanocytes (located in the epidermis of the skin) as brown or black tumors on the skin's surface.

Nonmelanoma is more common and develops on the basal (deep in the epidermis) or squamous (main cells of the epidermis) cells. However, these cancer cells rarely spread and are considerably less serious than melanoma.

The most reliable way to catch skin cancer early is to perform routine self-exams (see the Closer Look box on the next page). In addition to examining existing moles, you should examine blemishes and birthmarks for changes or new growths. Treatment for skin cancer varies depending on the type and severity. Possible treatments might include surgery, topical medications, chemotherapy, radiation, and other procedures to remove the cancerous cells.

The keys to preventing both types of skin cancer are to avoid excessive exposure to ultraviolet (UV) light and, when you are exposed, to adequately protect your skin with sunscreen. In addition to wearing an

CONSIDER THIS!

Melanoma skin cancer is the leading cause of cancer deaths in women aged 25–30.

adequate sunscreen (**SPF** 15 or higher), you should also avoid sunlight between 10.00 AM and 4.00 PM, wear protective clothing, and wear sunglasses when outdoors.

Although sunlight is the most common source of UV light, tanning beds also produce harmful UV rays that can damage your skin and increase your risk for skin cancer. Because there is no health benefit from tanning, you should avoid using these beds. Exposure to radiation and certain chemicals that might be present in the workplace also is associated with increased risk for skin cancer.

There are also nonmodifiable risk factors for both types of skin cancer. Men have higher rates than women. People with fair skin, especially those who freckle or sunburn easily, have higher rates than people with darker skin. However, individuals with darker skin can develop skin cancer, so it is important for all people to use protective measures when exposed to UV light. Family history, personal history, and a weakened or suppressed immune system are risk factors for both types of skin cancer. Moles are an additional risk factor for melanoma. Risk for nonmelanoma is increased with smoking and certain types of skin conditions.

A CLOSER LOOK

EARLY DETECTION OF SKIN CANCER

The key to early detection of skin cancer is self-examination. This exam should be performed monthly and should include the entire body, particularly those areas exposed to the sun. When examining your skin, begin by examining moles. Although moles are quite common and typically harmless, a change in a mole's appearance is a sign that you should see your health care provider.

When examining moles, use the simple ABCD rule to remember the important signs of melanoma and other skin cancers:

A is for Asymmetry: Does one-half of a mole not match the other half?

B is for Border: Is the border of the mole irregular, ragged, or notched?

C is for Color: Is the color of the mole not the same all over? That is, does the mole have differing shades of black, brown, and sometimes patches of red or white?

D is for Diameter: Is the diameter of the mole larger than 6 millimeters (about the size of a pencil eraser)? And does the mole appear to be growing in size?

Note that some skin cancers may not fit the ABCD rule, so it is particularly important for you to notice any changes in skin lesions or the appearance of a new skin lesion. Other warning signs of skin cancer include the following:

- A sore that does not heal
- A new growth of any kind
- Spread of pigment from the border of a spot to the surrounding skin
- Redness or a new swelling beyond the border of a mole
- Change in sensation on the skin, such as itchiness, tenderness, or pain

- Change in the surface of a mole, such as scaliness, oozing, bleeding, or the appearance of a bump or nodule

Schedule an appointment with your health care provider as soon as possible if you observe any of these changes in your skin. Remember that many skin cancers can be successfully treated, but early detection is the key in treatment of any cancer.

These four moles are examples of abnormalities that fit the ABCD rule for melanoma.

Uterine, Ovarian, and Cervical Cancer

Cancers of the female reproductive organs include uterine, ovarian, and cervical cancers. The most common type of uterine cancer is endometrial cancer, a cancer of the lining of the uterus. Many risk factors for endometrial cancer are similar to those for breast cancer, but certain hormone therapies are associated with lower risk. Uterine cancer also includes cancer of the muscles and tissues of the uterus. They are less common than endometrial cancer, and risk factors are similar to those of endometrial cancer.

Ovarian cancer is the fifth leading cause of cancer deaths in women. Age, obesity, a longer menstrual his-

SPF Abbreviation for "sun protection factor." A sunscreen with an SPF of 15 provides you with 15 times more protection than unprotected skin.

tory, family history, infertility, and breast cancer are risk factors for ovarian cancer. The use of birth control pills, breast-feeding, one or more pregnancies, and a diet high in vegetables are associated with lower risk. During a routine pelvic exam, a health care provider will check for lumps on the ovaries. Health care providers may have women at higher risk get other clinical tests, such as an ultrasound, to screen for ovarian cancer.

Cervical cancer is most strongly linked to **human papillomavirus (HPV),** a sexually transmitted virus that can cause genital warts. Smoking, long-term use of birth control pills, HIV infection, chlamydia, having many full-term pregnancies, a diet low in fruits and vegetables, low socioeconomic status, and family history are additional factors associated with increased risk for cervical cancer. In general, women should begin having Pap tests 3 years after they start having intercourse or at age 21, whichever is earlier, to screen for cervical cancer (10).

Other Cancers

The previously discussed cancers tend to be the ones you most frequently hear about, but numerous other cancers are routinely diagnosed, and some carry high rates of fatality. As with all cancers, early detection and treatment are the keys for survival.

Oral cancers include cancers of the lips, mouth, throat, and tongue. These cancers are strongly associated with tobacco use and alcohol consumption. Men are more likely to develop oral cancers than women. Exposure to UV light and HPV also increases risk. Early detection typically occurs through routine dental appointments and physical exams. Symptoms such as sores or a toothache may indicate oral cancer. Treatment options depend on the location and stage of the cancer and can include surgery, radiation, chemotherapy, and other medications.

Leukemia is cancer of the blood. A tumor does not develop, but leukemia is still characterized by rapid abnormal cell growth. There are several types of leukemia that can develop in children and in adults. Because leukemia affects the blood and the production of blood cells, anemia and fatigue can be symptoms. Easy bruising, bleeding from the gums, and nosebleeds might be other indicators. White blood cells that fight infection can also be affected, so leukemia also impairs the body's ability to fight infection. The treatment will vary depending on the type of leukemia but can include bone marrow transplants, radiation, and chemotherapy.

Cancer of the pancreas is the fourth leading cause of cancer deaths for men and women. Increased risk is associated with age, family history, and race (blacks have higher rates compared to whites). Behavioral risk factors include smoking, obesity, physical inactivity, work exposure to pesticides and dyes, and diets high in fat, red meat, and pork. Early detection is difficult for pancreatic cancer, but signs and symptoms include digestive problems, pain, jaundice, and weight loss. Treatment for pancreatic cancer may include surgery, radiation, and/or chemotherapy.

Make sure you know...

> Common sites for cancers include the skin, colon, rectum, lungs, prostate, and breasts.

> Prevention and early detection are important for the most effective treatment of cancer. Screening procedures vary according to the site of the cancer and level of individual risk.

What Are the Risk Factors for Cancer, and How Can You Reduce Your Risk?

The cause of specific cancers is often unknown, but studies have revealed that a variety of carcinogens can damage normal cells and start the cancer process. Several factors have been linked to an increased risk of cancer (1, 3, 11). We have already mentioned risks for specific cancers, but in this section we will discuss in more depth some of the factors commonly associated with several types of cancers. These factors include heredity, race, diet, radiation exposure, viruses, tobacco use, alcohol use, occupational carcinogens, and ultraviolet light.

Factors You Cannot Control

You cannot eliminate all of your risk for cancer. For instance, you cannot control your heredity or race, both of which are risk factors for many types of cancer. However, knowing your family history and whether you have nonmodifiable risk factors is important so you can discuss the best screening procedure with your health care provider. Often screenings are recommended at earlier ages for individuals at high risk. You may not be able to prevent cancer by modifying your behaviors, but early detection will increase your likelihood for successful treatment if cancer is detected.

Heredity   If a close relative, such as your father or mother, has had cancer, your chances of developing cancer are three times greater than average (11). Although the exact link between heredity and cancer remains unclear, cancers of the breast, stomach, colon, prostate, uterus, ovaries, and lungs appear to run in families. Whether these patterns of increased cancer risk are due to genetics or to the fact that people in the same family experience similar environmental risks remains unclear. It is important that you learn as much about your family's cancer history as you can. For many types of cancer, there are different screening recommendations for individuals with a family history, and your health care provider will help you determine the best plan for early detection.

Race   Race is another factor which may affect your risk for developing cancer and over which you have no control. The overall incidence and death rates of cancer are higher among blacks than whites (1, 12). However, there are differences according to specific sites (e.g., skin cancer and breast cancer). The reason why death rates in blacks are higher is unclear, but it may be linked to the fact that cancers in whites are often detected at an earlier, more treatable stage. Fortunately, there has been a decline in death rates among black adults. The decline is especially noted in men. One of the goals for the *Healthy People* objectives is to address health disparities, so increasing the awareness of cancer risk, preventive measures, and early detection procedures among blacks is important in addressing the disproportionately high rates of cancer. The Appreciating Diversity box on page 380 provides more information about the role that race plays in various cancer risks.

Factors You Can Control

Approximately 80% of all cancers are related to lifestyle and environmental factors, that is, factors you can control (1, 13). According to the National Cancer Institute, people who lead a healthy lifestyle have one-third to one-half the rate of cancer deaths compared with the general population. The first step in reducing your risk of cancer is identifying the risk factors that apply to you (see Laboratory 13.1). The next step is to modify those aspects of your environment and lifestyle that increase your chances of developing cancer. You can refer to Chapter 1 for behavior change strategies.

Diet   Your diet is probably the most important behavioral factor in controlling your risk of cancer (13). According to the National Academy of Sciences, diet is implicated in 60% of the cancers in women and 40% of the cancers in men (13). A high-fat diet has been

A diet rich in fruits and vegetables can provide antioxidants and other nutrients that help protect against cancer.

linked to breast, colon, and prostate cancer. A high-fat diet contributes to obesity, which is a risk factor for colon, breast, and uterine cancer. Additionally, salt-cured, smoked, and nitrite-cured foods have been linked to cancers of the esophagus and stomach.

Just as there are foods that increase cancer risk, there are foods and nutrients that seem to have a protective effect against cancer. For example, the antioxidant vitamins A, E, and C appear to protect cells against damage by free radicals (14). Free radicals, when produced in large quantities, promote the development of cancer by binding to DNA and altering cell structure and function (refer back to Figure 13.2). Antioxidants remove free radical cells, preventing DNA damage. Therefore, many cancer experts recommend a diet that is high in antioxidants.

Consumption of a high-fiber diet lowers your risk of colon and rectal cancers. A high-fiber diet increases the frequency of bowel movements, which decreases the time the colon and rectum are exposed to dietary carcinogens, reducing the risk of cancer.

A high-fat diet has been hypothesized to be a risk factor for colon and rectal cancer, but recent studies suggest that fat itself is not a major risk factor in most cancers (15–18). These studies indicate that consuming more than 4 oz of red meat or more than 1 oz of processed meat per day increases your risk of colon and rectal cancers by 12–49%. The biological link between cancer and the ingestion of red meat remains

human papillomavirus (HPV) A sexually transmitted virus that can cause cervical cancer.

APPRECIATING DIVERSITY RACE AND THE RISK OF CANCER IN THE UNITED STATES

More than 1.4 million Americans will be diagnosed with cancer this year, and more than 550,000 Americans are expected to die from it. Blacks in the United States are more likely to die from cancer than individuals of any other racial or ethnic group (see figure). Data indicate that blacks are 33% more likely to die of cancer than Asians and Pacific Islanders, Native Americans, and Hispanics. Additionally, the incidence of many cancer types is higher in blacks compared to other racial and ethnic groups.

Blacks have the highest incidence of colon, rectum, and lung cancers in the United States, and black men are 50% more likely to develop prostate cancer than men of any other racial or ethnic group.

In most cases we do not have an explanation for the racial differences in the incidence and death rates. However, we do know that some risk factors for several types of cancers are higher in blacks than in other groups. Rates of physical inactivity and obesity are higher in blacks compared to whites and the general population, especially in black women.

Also, disproportionate numbers of blacks live in low socioeconomic status (SES) environments. Typically, people who have a low SES also have less access to quality health care and are more likely to be uninsured. These conditions potentially decrease the likelihood of routine screening procedures that would detect cancer early and increase survival rates. Additionally, behaviors such as eating a diet high in fat and low in fresh fruits and vegetables and smoking are more common among individuals living in a low SES environment. Increasing awareness about cancer risk, prevention, and screening are key in addressing the high rates of cancer among black Americans.

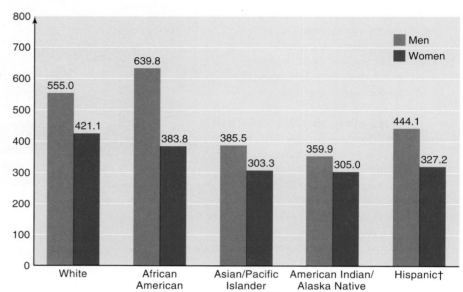

Cancer Incidence Rates* by Race and Ethnicity, U.S., 1999–2003

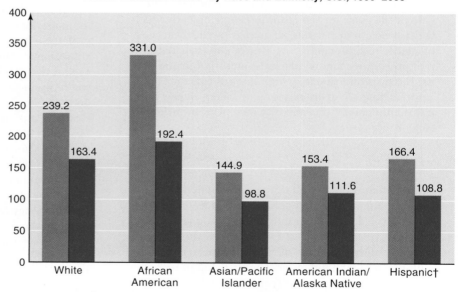

Cancer Death Rates* by Race and Ethnicity, U.S., 1999–2003

* Per 100,000, age-adjusted to the 2000 U.S. standard population.

† Persons of Hispanic origin may be of any race.

Source: From the Division of Cancer Control and Population Sciences, National Cancer Institute, 2006. www.cancer.gov.

A CLOSER LOOK

DIETARY AND PHYSICAL ACTIVITY GUIDELINES FOR LOWERING CANCER RISK

The American Cancer Society has issued nutritional guidelines for lowering your risk of cancer. The following guidelines were developed by the American Cancer Society 2006 Nutrition and Physical Activity Guidelines Advisory Committee:

- *Maintain a healthy weight throughout life.*
  Balance caloric intake with physical activity.
  Avoid excessive weight gain throughout life.
  Achieve and maintain a healthy weight if you are currently overweight or obese.

- *Adopt a physically active lifestyle.*
  Adults: Engage in at least 30 minutes of moderate to vigorous physical activity, above usual activities, on 5 or more days of the week; 45 to 60 minutes of intentional physical activity are preferable.
  Children and adolescents: Engage in at least 60 minutes of moderate to vigorous physical activity at least 5 days per week.

- *Eat a healthy diet, with an emphasis on plant sources.*
  Choose food or beverages in amounts that help achieve and maintain a healthy weight.

Eat 5 or more servings of a variety of vegetables and fruits every day.
Choose whole grains in preference to processed (refined) grains.
Limit consumption of processed and red meats.

- *If you drink alcoholic beverages, limit consumption.*
  Drink no more than 1 drink per day if you are a woman or 2 per day if you are a man.

Source: American Cancer Society. At a Glance—Nutrition and Physical Activities: ACS Guidelines for Nutrition and Physical Activity for Cancer Prevention. www.cancer.org/docroot/PED/ped_3_1x_ACS_Guidelines.asp?sitearea=PED.

---

unclear and is the focus of intensive research. Dietary recommendations for lowering your risk of cancer are presented in the Closer Look box above.

Alcohol Use Heavy use of alcohol increases the risk for oral, esophagus, liver, and breast cancer (19, 20). Even moderate drinking is linked to a slightly increased risk of breast cancer in women.

Because moderate alcohol consumption may increase your risk for some cancers, it is best to abstain from alcohol. If you choose to drink alcohol, it is important to limit not just the quantity, but also the frequency of consumption. Having a drink one or two days a week is better than consuming alcohol on a daily basis. Also, consider other high-risk behaviors often associated with drinking. Many people combine drinking and smoking, creating an even greater risk for developing cancer. Even if you do not smoke, parties and bars are environments where you are likely to be exposed to secondhand smoke. Enjoying a drink at home with friends or at a smoke-free restaurant is an alternative to a smoke-filled bar.

Tobacco Use Tobacco use is the single largest cause of cancer deaths (approximately 25%) (1). Heavy smokers are 15 to 25 times more likely to die of cancer than are nonsmokers (1). Smoking also puts you at an increased risk for oral cancers (e.g., cancers of the

mouth, pharynx, larynx, and esophagus), as well as cancers of the pancreas, bladder, and colon (1). The average life expectancy for a chronic smoker is 7 years shorter than for a nonsmoker (21).

Cigarette smoking is responsible for 87% of all lung cancer cases (1). The risk of developing lung cancer and other smoking-related cancers is related to the total lifetime exposure to cigarette smoke (22–24). Lifetime exposure is measured by factors such as the number of cigarettes smoked each day and the number of years a person has smoked. Risk of developing smoking-related cancer is greatest in heavy smokers with a long history of smoking. However, remember that stopping smoking at any time decreases your risk. Secondhand tobacco smoke is also carcinogenic. So, living with a smoker or working in an environment where people smoke increases your risk for cancer, too.

Cigarettes do not pose the only risk from tobacco. Pipes, cigars, and smokeless tobacco also increase the risk for lung and oral cancers, and the use of chewing tobacco increases your risk of cancer of the mouth, larynx, throat, and esophagus (1). You can greatly reduce cancer risk by abstaining from all tobacco products. If you have never used any tobacco products, don't start. If you use tobacco products, stopping can reverse your risk. Your risk of cancer decreases with each additional year you do not smoke. Even long-term smokers who quit after age 50 substantially reduce their risk of dying

Cancer Deaths in Men and Women

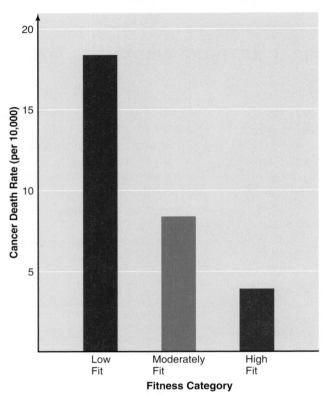

FIGURE 13.5
The declining risks of dying from cancer associated with increased exercise-related fitness.

Source: Data are adapted from Thune, I., and A. Furberg. Physical activity and cancer risk: Dose-response and cancer, all sites and site specific. *Medicine and Science in Sports and Exercise* 33:S530–S550, 2001. Also, Bauman, A. Updating the evidence that physical activity is good for health: An epidemiological review 2000–2003. *Journal of Science and Medicine in Sports* 7:6–19, 2004.

early from cancer (23, 24). Therefore, it is never too late to quit.

Physical Inactivity Some studies show that regular exercise may provide some protection against dying from cancer (Figure 13.5) (2, 25–29). The strongest evidence comes from studies that have shown that regular exercise lowers the risk for colon cancer (27). Other studies show a relationship between exercise and the reduced risk for developing breast and uterine cancer in women (26).

So how does exercise reduce the risk of cancer? One potential mechanism is an effect of exercise on the immune system. Tumors are normally formed in everyone from time to time, but the immune system typically destroys the abnormal cells before they increase in number. Therefore, a strong immune system acts to reduce the risk of cancer, whereas a weak immune system may increase your risk of cancer. Numerous studies suggest that physically active individuals have an increased resistance to infection and a decreased

incidence of certain forms of cancer (2, 25, 26, 30). However, scientific evidence that exercise positively alters the immune system is limited (31, 32). Therefore, it may be that factors other than adaptation of the immune system are responsible for the observed association between exercise and a reduced risk of cancer.

There are other potential explanations for the relationship between regular exercise and the reduced risk for cancer. Regular exercise also helps you maintain a healthy body weight, and obesity is a risk factor for several types of cancer. Effects on hormones or menstrual status might play a role in breast cancer. Exercise is associated with increased bowel motility. Exercise has an effect like that of a high-fiber diet, in that it can help you have more regular bowel movements, thereby reducing your exposure to the carcinogens in the waste. Although we do not completely understand the relationship between exercise and all types of cancer, we do see a relationship between exercise and cancer risk reduction. Therefore, maintaining an activity program at the recommended levels is an important health behavior in lowering your cancer risk.

Exposure to Ultraviolet Light Prolonged exposure to ultraviolet light from any source can damage your skin and increase your risk of cancer (33). Ultraviolet radiation from the sun and artificial tanning is responsible for over 700,000 new cases of skin cancer each year (1). Tanning machines and sunlamps produce ultraviolet rays and present as much risk as does the sun. Some tanning salons claim their equipment is less dangerous, but that is not true! If a sunlamp causes you to tan or burn, it is just as dangerous as the sun.

Limiting your sun exposure and avoiding tanning salons are the obvious ways to avoid the carcinogenic effect of ultraviolet light. However, most people cannot completely avoid being in the sun. When you are exposed to the sun for work or recreation, wear protective clothing and use a sunscreen on exposed skin to block the effects of ultraviolet light.

There is no such thing as a safe tan. All ultraviolet exposure to your skin can be damaging, whether you tan quickly or accumulate it slowly over time. Although most people recognize the need to protect skin from the sun, they often associate skin protection with only the occasional extreme exposure (e.g., a day at the beach). However, long-term day-to-day sun exposure also increases your risk for skin cancer. Studies show that over the course of a lifetime, a person will receive tens of thousands of doses of damaging ultraviolet radiation (33). This cumulative exposure greatly increases your risk of developing skin cancer (34). Therefore, you need to protect yourself with everyday basic sunscreen protection. Research shows that daily use of even low-level sunscreen (i.e., SPF 4–10) can reduce your lifetime ultraviolet exposure by 50% or more (35). See the

STEPS FOR
BEHAVIOR CHANGE

Do you protect your skin from ultraviolet light?

Taking the necessary precautions is very important to protect yourself against skin cancer. Answer the following questions to see how well you are doing in shielding your skin from ultraviolet light:

Y   N

☐ ☐   Do you wear sunscreen every time you know you will be exposed to the sun?

☐ ☐   Do you avoid the use of tanning beds?

☐ ☐   Do you avoid being in the sun between 10:00 AM and 4:00 PM?

☐ ☐   Do you wear protective clothing when exposed to the sun?

If you answered yes to all of these questions, you are doing a good job of protecting your skin.

TIPS TO PROTECT YOUR SKIN FROM UV LIGHT

☑   Use a sunscreen of at least SPF 15 on skin exposed to the sun. Reapply sunscreen during prolonged sun exposure. Make sure you use sunscreen on your face and lips.

☑   Use sunscreen when exercising outside in the sun.

☑   Avoid sun exposure from 10:00 AM to 4:00 PM, when the UV rays are the strongest.

☑   Use a sunless tanner instead of tanning in the sun or on a tanning bed.

☑   Keep your skin covered, and wear a hat with a brim and sunglasses to protect your skin from exposure to the sun.

Steps for Behavior Change box to determine whether you are taking the necessary steps to protect your skin.

Viruses   Viruses can cause cancer by invading cells and damaging DNA. Research demonstrates that viruses play a role in several blood cancers (leukemias) as well as cancers of the lymphatic system (lymphomas). Evidence also suggests that viruses can cause liver, cervical, nose, and pharynx cancer. (1). How can viruses be a factor you can control? In regard to the virus associated with cervical cancer, you do have some control. Cervical cancer is largely associated with HPV, a sexually transmitted virus. Abstaining from sex, using condoms during intercourse, and limiting the number of sexual partners can reduce your risk for cervical cancer. Recently, an HPV vaccine for women has become available that may prevent certain types of cervical cancer.

Radiation Exposure   Up to 5% of all cancers may be caused by radiation exposure due to medical X-rays, occupational exposure through computer moni-

tors, and environmental radiation (34). Further, many modern conveniences that emit electromagnetic fields may increase cancer risk. For example, electric blankets and low-frequency radio waves, such as those associated with cellular telephones, have been implicated in causing cancer. You can reduce your cancer risk by taking the recommended safety precautions if you work in an environment where you are exposed to radiation. Avoiding use or excessive use of items that expose you to radiation can lower your risk (e.g., electric blankets, computer games, cell phones).

Occupational Carcinogens   Factory workers and people living near factories may have an increased risk of cancer due to specific types of chemicals used or produced in the factory. Industrial chemicals known to be carcinogenic include benzene, nickel, chromate, asbestos, and vinyl chloride (34). One of the most common occupational carcinogens is asbestos, a substance formerly used in the building and automobile industries. Additionally, working with coal tars in mining or working near airborne carcinogens, such as in auto painting, is also dangerous. Many chemicals used to kill weeds (herbicides) and insects (pesticides) contain potential carcinogens and are found in excessive amounts in some water supplies.

Some professions require people to work around industrial pollutants, but being aware of your risk and following safety procedures can help lower your risk. In particular, avoid exposure to industrial agents such as radon, dioxins, nickel, chromate, asbestos, and vinyl chloride. If you have questions concerning the carcinogenic risks of chemical exposure in your workplace, contact the Environmental Protection Agency (EPA; see www.epa.gov). The EPA can provide you with a complete list of cancer-causing chemicals and identify those used in your workplace.

Make sure you know...

> Even though the cause of specific cancers is often unknown, many cancer risk factors have been identified.

> Some cancer risk factors, such as heredity and race, cannot be controlled.

> Consuming a healthy diet, limiting alcohol intake, avoiding tobacco products and secondhand tobacco smoke, exercising regularly, and avoiding radiation (e.g., UV radiation) and occupational carcinogens will all reduce your risk for developing multiple types of cancers.

Summary

1. Currently, cancer is the number-two cause of death in the United States. Skin cancer is the most frequently diagnosed cancer per year, and lung cancer is the leading cause of cancer deaths.

2. Cancer is the uncontrolled growth and spread of abnormal cells. Groups of abnormal cells can form a tumor, which can be classified as benign or malignant. Benign tumors are abnormal growths that are generally not life-threatening, whereas malignant tumors consist of cancerous cells that can spread to other tissues and disrupt organ function.

3. Carcinogens are cancer-causing agents. Normal cells become cancerous when DNA becomes damaged by carcinogens, resulting in uncontrolled cell division.

4. Common sites of cancer include the breasts, lungs, colon, prostate gland, cervix, testes, pancreas, and mouth.

5. Heredity and race are nonmodifiable risk factors for cancer. Modifiable behavioral risk factors for cancer include exposure to carcinogens such as radiation, viruses, tobacco, alcohol, occupational carcinogens, and ultraviolet light. Other behaviors that increase cancer risk include a low-fiber diet and lack of physical activity.

6. Approximately 80% of all cancers are related to lifestyle and environmental factors.

7. Diet is probably the most important factor in controlling your risk of cancer. Among the primary nutrients in foods that offer protection from cancer are the antioxidant vitamins A, E, and C, which reduce the risk of cancer by removing free radicals.

8. Exercise has been shown to reduce the risk of colon, uterine, and breast cancer.

9. Participating in cancer screenings is important for early detection of cancer. Recommendations for cancer screenings are based on age, sex, and the presence of risk factors.

Study Questions

1. What cancer causes the most deaths for women in the United States?
   a. breast
   b. lung
   c. skin
   d. cervical

2. _____ is the spread of cancerous cells throughout the body
   a. Benign tumor
   b. Malignant tumor
   c. Carcinogen
   d. Metastasis

3. Which of the following is not a behavioral risk factor for developing cancer?

    a. poor diet

    b. physical inactivity

    c. doing breast self-exams

    d. excessive alcohol consumption

4. What is the most common type of cancer?

    a. skin

    b. leukemia

    c. lung

    d. colon

5. Which of the following is not one of the seven warning signs of cancer?

    a. nagging cough or hoarseness

    b. a sore that does not heal

    c. unusual bleeding or discharge

    d. all are warning signs of cancer

6. How do normal cells become cancerous?

7. How do antioxidants reduce the risk of cancer?

8. Discuss the signs of skin cancer.

9. Outline the dietary guidelines for reducing your risk of cancer.

Suggested Reading

American Cancer Society. *Cancer Facts and Figures 2009*. Atlanta: American Cancer Society, 2009, www.cancer.org.

Bauman, A. Updating the evidence that physical activity is good for health: An epidemiological review 2000–2003. *Journal of Science and Medicine in Sports* 7:6–19, 2004.

Bostwick, D. G. *The American Cancer Society: Prostate Cancer*. Atlanta: American Cancer Society, 1999.

Eyre, H, et al. Preventing cancer, cardiovascular disease, and diabetes. *Stroke* 35:1–12, 2004.

Nole, G., and A. Johnson. An analysis of cumulative lifetime solar ultraviolet radiation exposure and the benefits of daily sun protection. *Dermatology Therapy* 17:57–62, 2004.

Tannock, I., R. P. Hill, R. G. Bristow, and L. Harrington. *The Basic Science of Oncology*. St. Louis: McGraw-Hill, 1998.

Thune, I., and A. Furberg. Physical activity and cancer risk: Dose-response and cancer, all sites and site specific. *Medicine and Science in Sports and Exercise* 33: S530–S550, 2001.

Stix, G. Overcoming self: A company tries to turn the immune system against cancer. *Scientific American* 291:40–41, 2004.

Willett, W. Diet and cancer: One view at the start of the millennium. *Cancer, Epidemiology, Biomarkers and Prevention* 10:3–8, 2001.

For links to the organizations and websites listed below, visit The Total Fitness and Wellness Website at www.pearsonhighered.com/powers.

Mayo Clinic Health
Provides wide-ranging information about cancer and many other health-related issues.

American Medical Association
Presents many sources of information about a wealth of medical problems, including cancer.

WebMD
Contains information on a wide variety of diseases and medical problems, including cancer.

American Cancer Society
Includes up-to-date information, including cancer statistics, risk factors, and current treatments.

References

1. American Cancer Society. *Cancer Facts and Figures 2009*. Atlanta: American Cancer Society, 2009.

2. Gerhardsson, M., S. E. Norell, H. Kiviranta, N. L. Pedersen, and A. Ahlbom. Sedentary jobs and colon cancer. *American Journal of Epidemiology* 123:775–780, 1986.

3. American Institute for Cancer Research. *Diet and Cancer*. www.aicr.org/site/PageServer?pagename=dc_home.

4. Robbins, S., and V. Kumar. *Basic Pathology*. Philadelphia: W. B. Saunders, 1997.

5. Tannock, I., R. P. Hill, R. G. Bristow, and L. Harrington. *The Basic Science of Oncology*, 4th ed. St. Louis: McGraw-Hill, 2005.

6. American Cancer Society. What are the key statistics about lung cancer? October 2008; www.cancer.org.

7. American Cancer Society. Can non-small cell lung cancer be prevented? October 2008. www.cancer.org.

8. American Cancer Society. What causes colorectal cancer? May 2009. www.cancer.org.

9. American Cancer Society. What causes breast cancer? May 2009. www.cancer.org.

10. American Cancer Society. Can cancer of the cervix be prevented? May 2009. available at www.cancer.org.

11. American Cancer Society. What are the risk factors for cancer? February 2009. www.cancer.org.

12. American Cancer Society. Cancer facts and figures for African Americans, 2009–2010. 2009. www.cancer.org.

13. *Surgeon General's Report on Nutrition and Health*. Washington, DC: Diane Publishing Co., 1994.

14. Kanter, M. Free radicals and exercise: Effects of nutritional antioxidant supplementation. *Exercise and Sport Science Reviews* 23:375–397, 1995.

15. Willett, W. C. Diet and cancer. *Oncologist* 5:393–404, 2000.

16. Sandu, M., I. White, and K. McPherson. Systematic review of prospective cohort studies on meat consumption and colorectal cancer risk: A meta-analytical approach. *Cancer, Epidemiology, Biomarkers and Prevention* 10:439–496, 2001.

17. Norat, T., and E. Roboli. Meat consumption and colorectal cancer: A review of epidemiological evidence. *Nutritional Reviews* 59:37–47, 2001.

18. Willett, W. Diet and cancer: One view at the start of the millennium. *Cancer, Epidemiology, Biomarkers and Prevention* 10:3–8, 2001.

19. Brown, L. M. Epidemiology of alcohol-associated cancers. *Alcohol* 35:161–168, 2005.

20. McPherson, K. Moderate alcohol consumption and cancer. *Annals of Epidemiology* 17:S46–S48, 2007.

21. Bernhard, D., C. Moser, A. Backovic, and G. Wick. Cigarette smoke—an aging accelerator? *Experimental Gerontology* 42:160–165, 2007.

22. Edwards, R. The problem of tobacco smoking. *British Medical Journal* 328:217–219, 2004.

23. Westmaas, J., and T. Brandon. Reducing risk in smokers. *Current Opinion in Pulmonary Medicine* 10:284–288, 2004.

24. Stein, C., and G. Colditz. Modifiable risk factors for cancer. *British Journal of Cancer* 90:299–303, 2004.

25. Paffenbarger, R. S., R. T. Hyde, A. L. Wing, and C. C. Hsieh. Physical activity, all-cause mortality of college alumni. *New England Journal of Medicine* 314:605–613, 1986.

26. Frisch, R. E., G. Wyshak, N. L. Albright, et al. Lower prevalence of breast cancer and cancers of the reproductive system among former college athletes compared to non-athletes. *British Journal of Cancer* 52:885–891, 1985.

27. Blair, S., H. Kohl, R. Paffenbarger, D. Clark, K. Cooper, and L. Gibbons. Physical fitness and all-cause mortality: A prospective study of healthy men and women. *Journal of the American Medical Association* 262:2395–2401, 1989.

28. Thune, I., and A. Furberg. Physical activity and cancer risk: Dose-response and cancer, all sites and site specific. *Medicine and Science in Sports and Exercise* 33:S530–S550, 2001.

29. Bauman, A. Updating the evidence that physical activity is good for health: An epidemiological review 2000–2003. *Journal of Science and Medicine in Sports* 7:6–19, 2004.

30. Nash, M. Exercise and immunology. *Medicine and Science in Sports and Exercise* 26:125–127, 1994.

31. Woods, J., and M. Davis. Exercise, monocyte/macrophage function, and cancer. *Medicine and Science in Sports and Exercise* 26:147–157, 1994.

32. Shepard, R., S. Rhind, and P. Shek. The impact of exercise on the immune system: NK cells, interleukins 1 and 2, and related responses. *Exercise and Sport Sciences Reviews* 23:215–241, 1995.

33. Nole, G., and A. Johnson. An analysis of cumulative lifetime solar ultraviolet radiation exposure and the benefits of daily sun protection. *Dermatology Therapy* 17:57–62, 2004.

34. American Cancer Society. Radiation. 2009. www.cancer.org.

35. Eyre, H, et al. Preventing cancer, cardiovascular disease, and diabetes. *Stroke* 35:1–12, 2004.

Videos

Log on to www.pearsonhighered.com/powers to view these chapter-related videos.

Cancer

Treating Cancer with Bone Drugs

Possible Melanoma Treatment

Human Papillomavirus Vaccine Mandatory

NAME _____ DATE _____

Determining Your Cancer Risk

The purpose of this laboratory is to increase your awareness of your risk of developing all forms of cancer. Complete the following questions by putting a check under either "Yes" or "No."

The more times you check "yes," the more risk factors you have for developing cancer. If you check "yes" even once, you should take steps to modify your lifestyle and reduce your risk for cancer. For some specific information about lowering your cancer risks, see the text of this chapter.

	Yes	No
Do you have a family history of cancer?	____	____
Do you have a fair complexion?	____	____
Are you regularly exposed to occupational carcinogens or various types of radiation?	____	____
Is your skin regularly exposed to excessive sunlight?	____	____
Do you consume more than 4 oz of red meat or 1 oz of processed meat per day?	____	____
Do you regularly eat smoked foods?	____	____
Is your diet low in fiber?	____	____
Are you obese?	____	____
Do you consume an excessive amount of alcohol?	____	____
Do you use tobacco products or breathe secondhand tobacco smoke?	____	____

1. How many "yes" responses do you have?

_____

2. Name any behaviors you can modify or change to reduce your risk for cancer.

_____

_____

3. Select one of your modifiable risk factors, and write out steps to change your behavior to reduce your risk. Use the strategies for behavior change you learned in Chapter 1 to address your risk factor, if applicable.

_____

_____

_____

_____

LABORATORY

NAME _____ DATE _____

Early Detection

Early detection of cancer is very important in getting prompt and effective treatment. Several screening procedures outlined in this chapter are recommended for early detection of cancer. The purpose of this lab is to assess your behaviors related to early detection of cancer. Check the appropriate box to indicate your current level of participation for each screening.

	Never	Sometimes	As Recommended	N/A
Breast self-exam	____	____	____	____
Clinical breast exam	____	____	____	____
Mammogram	____	____	____	____
Testicular self-exam	____	____	____	____
Clinical testicular exam	____	____	____	____
Colon cancer screening	____	____	____	____
PSA test	____	____	____	____
Pap test	____	____	____	____
Skin exam	____	____	____	____

1. Do you meet the recommendations for cancers screenings based on your age, sex, and risk level?

   _____

2. If not, what screenings do you need to start? Make a plan to begin the appropriate screenings recommended for early detection of cancer.

   _____

   _____

   _____

   _____

Sexually Transmitted Infections

true or false?

1. The most common sexually transmitted infection (STI) in the United States is HIV.

2. If you're not sexually promiscuous, you will not contract an STI.

3. All STIs are easily treated with antibiotics.

4. Using condoms prevents all STIs.

5. Among sexual behaviors, anal intercourse carries the highest risk of transmitting HIV between partners.

Answers appear on the next page.

Have you ever asked a potential sexual partner about his or her sexual history? If you have, were you nervous about the conversation or worried about offending the other person? Were you surprised by his or her responses, and did you learn anything that caused you to reconsider entering into a sexual relationship?

Such conversations may seem uncomfortable for some people, but they are an essential component of practicing responsible sexual behavior. Asking questions, taking precautions, and educating yourself about the risks associated with sexual activities are the keys to protecting yourself from sexually transmitted infections. In this chapter, we will discuss the symptoms and transmission routes of some of the most common **sexually transmitted infections** (STIs). We will also address strategies you can employ to ensure that any sexual activity you choose to engage in will not result in the unpleasant, and sometimes deadly, sexually transmitted infections.

What Are Sexually Transmitted Infections?

STIs are infections that you can get and pass to others through vaginal, oral, or anal sex. STIs can be caused by viruses, bacteria, or parasites. Many STIs, such as those caused by bacteria or parasites, can be treated with antibiotics or other drugs, but STIs caused by viruses remain with the host for life.

STIs are more than just an embarrassing problem. In many cases, they can be life-altering and life-threatening. STIs can lead to infertility, complications during pregnancy, and cervical and other cancers. They can be passed on even when there are no symptoms present. These silent but sometimes deadly infections affect both men and women of all ages, races, and socioeconomic backgrounds.

STIs are often "silent" diseases, because early symptoms can be ignored and go untreated. Further, although STIs can be diagnosed through medical testing, routine screening programs are not widespread, and social stigmas about STIs often prevent infected individuals from visiting health care professionals for testing (1). Therefore, many cases of STIs go unreported, resulting in an underestimation of the total number of people infected with STIs.

STIs are a major public health challenge in the United States. The Centers for Disease Control and Prevention (CDC) estimates that 19 million new infections occur each year, almost half of them among young people aged 15–24 (2). Because young people are among the groups most affected by STIs, one of the national health objectives for *Healthy People 2010* was to promote responsible sexual behavior among adolescents. Compared with other countries, the rate of STIs in the United States far exceeds those of every other industrialized nation. Lack of education and lack of public awareness of the dangers of STIs play a role in the high incidence of STIs in the United States. Statistics indicate that one in four Americans will contract at least one STI in their lifetime. STIs also pose a major health problem in many other countries (see the Appreciating Diversity box on page 397).

Answers

1. **FALSE** Although HIV rates are increasing rapidly worldwide, human papillomavirus (HPV) is still the most common sexually transmitted infection in the United States.

2. **FALSE** Although monogamy greatly reduces your chance of infection, your risk is not eliminated unless both you and your partner have had no previous sexual partners. When you engage in sexual intercourse with someone, you are effectively being exposed to every sexual partner she or he has had (and vice versa).

3. **FALSE** Some STIs, specifically those caused by bacterial infections, can be treated and cured with antibiotics. However, STIs that are caused by viral infections, such as HIV and genital herpes, cannot be cured by antibiotics.

4. **FALSE** Although condoms greatly reduce the risk of STI transmittal, they do not eliminate it completely. Condoms sometimes fail and are more likely to break during anal intercourse than during any other type of sex.

5. **TRUE** Anal intercourse can result in small tears and bleeding in the anal membrane. Infectious agents can enter the body through these tears.

In addition to the health threat they pose, STIs pose an economic burden as well. Current estimates are that STIs add an estimated $14.7 billion dollars to health care costs in the United States each year (2). Some of the most common STIs include human immunodeficiency virus (HIV), trichomoniasis, chlamydia, hepatitis B, gonorrhea, genital warts, genital herpes, and syphilis (3) (Figure 14.1). Because of its important worldwide health ramifications, we begin our discussion of STIs with a detailed look at HIV.

Make sure you know...

> Every year millions of people in the United States are infected by one or more sexually transmitted infections (STIs).

> STIs can go undiagnosed for some time because of lack of symptoms and/or lack of screening, and they can be passed along even when no symptoms are present.

> The most common STIs in the United States include HIV, trichomoniasis, chlamydia, hepatitis B, gonorrhea, genital warts, genital herpes, and syphilis.

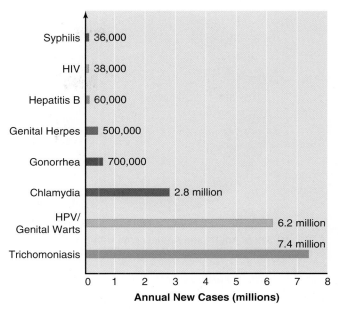

FIGURE 14.1
The most common STIs in the United States, as estimated by annual new cases of the infection.

Source: Data are from the Centers for Disease Control and Prevention, 2007. www.cdc.gov/std/healthcomm/fact_sheets.htm.

HIV/AIDS

In 1981, physicians in San Francisco, Los Angeles, and New York began noticing repeated occurrences of rare diseases among previously healthy young men. It was quickly determined that these problems were the result of a severely impaired immune system. Even before the virus responsible for the breakdown in the immune system was discovered, this disease was given the name **acquired immunodeficiency syndrome,** or **AIDS.**

AIDS is caused by a **virus,** called *human immunodeficiency virus (HIV)*. When HIV enters the bloodstream, immune cells rush to the virus in an attempt to destroy this invading agent. However, HIV enters the circulating immune cells and uses them as a host to replicate itself. The entry of HIV into immune cells eventually disarms the immune cells and impairs the body's ability to fight infections. Over time, the level of HIV in the blood increases, and the immune system becomes weaker and weaker, resulting in immunodeficiency and the development of AIDS.

Incidence of HIV/AIDS

At the end of 2003, the CDC estimated that 1 to 1.1 million people in the United States were living with HIV/AIDS. In addition, an estimated 56,300 Americans became infected with HIV in 2006 (4). In 2005, the total number of deaths from AIDS had decreased

because of improved drug treatment; however, the number of AIDS diagnoses increased (4). This increase in AIDS diagnoses may be due to an increased emphasis on testing.

In the beginning of the AIDS epidemic in the United States, the disease was predominant among homosexual men; however, the incidence of AIDS among heterosexual Americans is on the rise. AIDS is the leading cause of death for black women aged 25–34, the third leading cause of death among Hispanic men aged 35–44, and the fourth leading cause of death among Hispanic women in the same age group (5). See Figure 14.2 for a look at the race and gender distributions of new HIV infections in the United States.

sexually transmitted infections (STIs) A group of more than 25 infections that are generally spread through sexual contact.

acquired immunodeficiency syndrome (AIDS) A fatal disease that develops from infection by the human immunodeficiency virus, or HIV.

virus An infectious microorganism that cannot live independently and must invade a host cell to survive. Viruses cannot be killed with antibiotics.

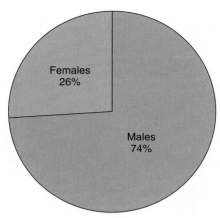

No. = 42,495

(a) Sex of Adults and Adolescents with HIV/AIDS Diagnosed During 2007

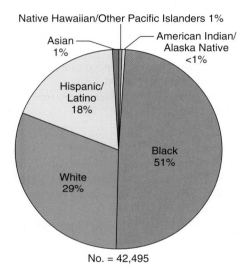

No. = 42,495

(b) Race/Ethnicity of Persons (Including Children) with HIV/AIDS Diagnosed During 2007

FIGURE 14.2

Each year, over 40,000 Americans become infected with HIV. The pie charts above indicate that certain groups of Americans are becoming infected with HIV disproportionately compared to other groups. For example, even though men make up about half of the population, three-fourths of new HIV infections each year occur in men **(a)**. Moreover, although African Americans account for only 13% of the U.S. population, almost half of all new HIV infections occur in that group **(b)**.

Note: Based on data from 33 states with long-term, confidential, name-based HIV reporting.

Source: From Centers for Disease Control and Prevention, "HIV/AIDS in the United States," 2009. www.cdc.gov/hiv/resources/factsheets/PDF/us.pdf.

HIV/AIDS is a major health problem not just in the United States; the number of people infected with HIV is increasing all over the world. Current estimates are that over 33 million people worldwide are infected with HIV, more than 22 million in Africa alone. New

HIV infections in eastern Europe and central Asia have risen by more than 50% since 2004 (5). Africa remains the global epicenter of the AIDS **pandemic.** In many African countries, HIV prevention programs are not reaching the people most at risk of infection because levels of knowledge about HIV transmission and safe sex remain low. The World Health Organization (WHO) reports that two-thirds or more of young women (aged 15–24) lack comprehensive knowledge of HIV transmission (5). Access to HIV treatment varies significantly throughout Africa, and treatment still lags in the countries with the highest levels of poverty. According to a 2008 UNAIDS/WHO report on the AIDS epidemic, there were 2.7 million new HIV infections in 2007, 1.9 million (70%) of which occurred in sub-Saharan Africa (6). (See the figure in the Appreciating Diversity box on page 397.)

Stages of HIV Infection

Many people infected with HIV are unaware that they carry the virus because symptoms may not appear for months or even years after infection. Evidence suggests that in many cases, the virus remains dormant in the body for 5 to 10 years before creating health problems (7, 8). After this incubation period, the virus begins to multiply and eventually damages specific cells within the immune system. Because an impaired immune system is incapable of preventing infections, the body becomes vulnerable to a variety of diseases, from the common cold to cancer. When serious disease symptoms appear as a result of HIV infection, the individual has developed AIDS.

Once an individual is infected with HIV, the infection progresses into AIDS in three stages (Figure 14.3). The first stage after HIV enters the body is the silent stage. During this stage, there are no physical symptoms, and the only evidence of HIV is the development of HIV antibodies in the blood. Typically, HIV antibodies are formed within 2 weeks after infection, but it can take up to 6 to 8 weeks before antibody levels are high enough to be detected by a blood test.

The second phase of HIV infection is called the symptomatic infection stage. This stage consists of several symptoms that may include constant fatigue, fever, weight loss, swollen lymph nodes, and sore throat. Symptoms that develop later in the second stage include night sweats, chronic infections, skin disorders, and ulcers of the membranes lining the nose, mouth, and other body cavities.

Unless medical research can develop a cure for HIV, all HIV-infected individuals will eventually progress to the third and final stage of HIV infection, AIDS. AIDS is characterized by all of the general symptoms associated with the second phase of HIV in-

Stages in the Development of AIDS

Stage 1: Silent Stage
HIV infection with no physical symptoms
HIV antibodies form in the blood

↓

Stage 2: Symptomatic Infection Stage
Symptoms may include constant fatigue, fever,
weight loss, swollen lymph nodes, sore throats,
night sweats, and chronic infections

↓

Stage 3: AIDS
Final stage of HIV infection: AIDS

FIGURE 14.3
Stages in the development of AIDS.

fection, plus one or more opportunistic diseases such as pneumonia or selected types of cancer such as Kaposi's sarcoma (Table 14.1). Moreover, in this final stage of HIV infection, it is common for HIV to cross the blood–brain barrier and cause personality changes, deterioration of memory and judgment, and brain tumors.

Although AIDS is a fatal disease, people now live with it for many years. This is possible because of improved medications, coupled with superior clinical management of the disease. In recent years, the National Institutes of Health has devoted millions of research dollars toward developing a cure for AIDS. Because of this investment in AIDS research and the scientific progress that has been achieved, some researchers have concluded that eventually AIDS will be considered a chronic disease (like hypertension or diabetes) that can be controlled by appropriate medical treatment. For more about AIDS research, see A Closer Look: The Search for a Cure for AIDS on page 398.

CONSIDER THIS!

The only diseases that cause more deaths in women than HIV/AIDS are cancer and heart disease.

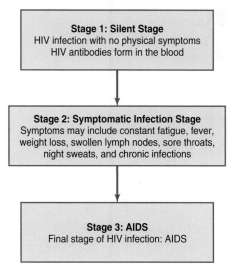

How HIV Is Transmitted

For HIV to replicate in the body, the virus must enter the bloodstream. Therefore, any exchange of body fluids such as blood, semen, or vaginal secretions is a possible mode for transmission of HIV (Figure 14.4). The three most common modes of HIV transmission are the following:

1. Vaginal or anal intercourse without using a condom.
2. Sharing needles contaminated with HIV-infected blood during injected drug use, tattooing, or body piercing.
3. Passage of the virus from mother to fetus in the uterus (20–50% chance) or in blood during delivery.

In addition to these common routes of transmission, the virus can also be spread from an HIV-infected mother to a baby by breast-feeding. Moreover, it is also possible to transmit the virus by sharing sex toys if they are not properly disinfected and cleaned. Finally, HIV can be transmitted through accidental contamination when infected blood enters the body through the mucous membranes of the eyes or mouth or through breaks in the skin (i.e., cuts, abrasions, or punctures). Although there were formerly cases in which individuals contracted the virus through a blood transfusion, today's screening methods of all donated blood have minimized this risk.

Myths about HIV Transmission

Several myths about how HIV is transmitted create unnecessary fears in many people. This fear has caused some individuals to avoid any type of contact with infected individuals. It is critically important to understand both how HIV *can* be transmitted and how HIV *cannot* be transmitted. You cannot get HIV from any of the following:

- *Casual contact with HIV-infected individuals.* Normal household or social contact does not transmit HIV. Shaking hands, hugging, and providing personal care such as bathing, feeding, or dressing someone with HIV are unlikely to transmit the virus.

pandemic An illness or infection that occurs over a wide geographic area and affects an exceptionally high proportion of the population.

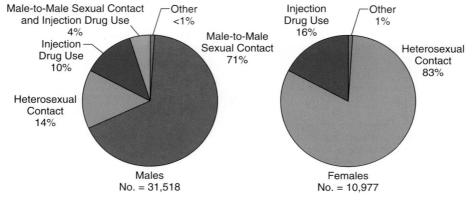

Transmission Categories of Adults and Adolescents with HIV/AIDS Diagnosed During 2007

FIGURE 14.4

Sexual contact is the most common mode of transmitting HIV/AIDs in both men and women.

Note: Based on data from 33 states with long-term, confidential, name-based HIV reporting.

Source: From Centers for Disease Control and Prevention, "HIV/AIDS in the United States," 2009. www.cdc.gov/hiv/resources/factsheets/PDF/us.pdf.

- *Contact with inanimate objects.* HIV cannot live outside the body. Therefore, HIV cannot survive on toilet seats, drinking fountains, countertops, doorknobs, or other areas. Alcohol, bleach, Lysol, or hydrogen peroxide can be used to disinfect a surface if it becomes contaminated with blood or semen containing HIV.

- *Sports participation.* To date, there are no documented cases of HIV transmission through sports. Further, HIV is not found in sweat of HIV-positive individuals, and HIV exists in only limited quantities in tears. According to the CDC, there is limited risk of contracting HIV during contact sports, even when bleeding occurs.

- *Saliva.* Although small amounts of HIV have been found in saliva and tears, there is no evidence that HIV has ever been transmitted from one person to another by kissing or by drinking from water fountains or beverage containers used by HIV-infected individuals.

- *Swimming pools, hot tubs, or whirlpool baths.* HIV cannot live or replicate in water. Therefore, HIV cannot be transmitted by contact with water contained in hot tubs, whirlpools, or swimming pools.

- *Contact with animals.* Household pets and farm animals cannot contract the HIV virus. Therefore, these animals cannot spread HIV to humans.

TABLE 14.1

Common Opportunistic Diseases Associated with the Development of AIDS

Disease	Symptoms of Disease
Kaposi's sarcoma (type of cancer)	Brown or purple lesions on the skin that resemble bruises but do not heal.
Primary lymphoma of the brain (type of cancer)	Headache, loss of memory, personality changes, impaired vision
Tuberculosis (bacterial infection)	Fever, night sweats, fatigue, cough, weight loss
Pneumocystis pneumonia (rare form of pneumonia)	Chest pain, dry cough, difficulty breathing
Cytomegalovirus (viral infection)	Viral infection that can occur in the lung, gastrointestinal tract, or central nervous system; symptoms vary depending on the location of the infection
Atypical mycobacterium (bacterial infection)	High fever, night sweats, fatigue, weakness

APPRECIATING
DIVERSITY SEXUALLY TRANSMITTED INFECTIONS ARE A WORLDWIDE PROBLEM

STIs are a major health problem in countries around the world. Nonetheless, the incidence of STIs varies widely: Some countries report a relatively low incidence, whereas other countries report a high prevalence of STIs (19–22). For example, the incidence tends to be relatively low in many highly industrialized countries, whereas STIs constitute a large health risk for most developing countries. Each year there are an estimated 340 million new cases of curable STIs around the world, and more than 75% (255 million) of these cases occur in developing countries (19).

The reasons for the differences in the incidence of STIs between industrialized and developing countries are numerous and complex. Behavior changes in young people, such as not having sex before age 15, increasing use of condoms, and having fewer sexual partners provide possible explanations of why STI incidence is lower in industrialized coun-

tries (5). Social and cultural norms surrounding a woman's role in the family in some developing nations can contribute to her increased risk, because she has less control over her own sexual activity and no control over her partner's promiscuity. Some people may also be at increased risk if they do not have access to condoms or decline to use them because it conflicts with their religious beliefs regarding birth control.

Lack of knowledge of safe sex and HIV remains low in many countries, and large proportions of the population do not believe they are at risk of becoming infected. However, lack of education does not always explain the high rates of STI transmission. A study by the World Health Organization reported that sub-Saharan Africa had the highest incidence of HIV infection in the world (see the figure). However, the majority of HIV infections occurred in the most literate men and women of this region.

One reason may be that in some regions of the world, more education is associated with economic and cultural changes that result in behaviors that increase the risk of developing STIs. For example, increased education may result in a better job with higher income to support high-risk behaviors such as paying for prostitutes, paying for and using injectable illicit drugs, or maintaining a number of different sexual partners.

The good news is that government support for expanded access to HIV treatment and new drug therapy programs are having a positive impact on reducing the number of new HIV cases globally. Programs that are focused and adapted to reach people most at risk are demonstrating the most progress in preventing HIV. For example, in China special programs for sex workers have led to increases in condom use and decreases in rates of STIs (5).

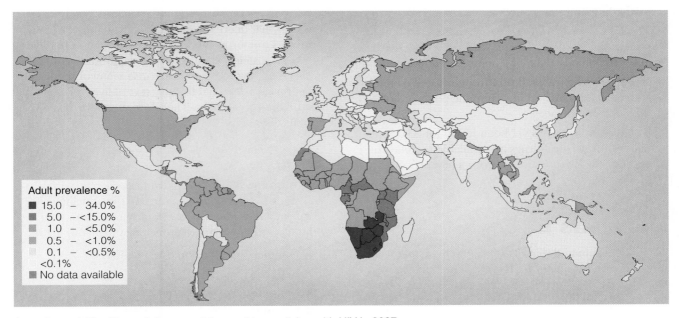

Adult prevalence %
- 15.0 – 34.0%
- 5.0 – <15.0%
- 1.0 – <5.0%
- 0.5 – <1.0%
- 0.1 – <0.5%
- <0.1%
- No data available

An estimated 33 million adults around the world were living with HIV in 2007.

Source: UNAIDS. UNAIDS 2008 Report on the Global AIDS Epidemic: Executive Summary. Geneva, Switzerland: UNAIDS, 2008.

THE SEARCH FOR A CURE FOR AIDS

Current estimates are that 39.5 million people worldwide are infected with HIV. In 2006, 2.9 million people died of AIDS-related illnesses (23). Without a cure for this disease, even more people will die, typically within 7–12 years after acquiring the virus.

A major problem confronting scientists in the treatment for HIV is that the virus is capable of mutating into many different strains. That is, the virus can change its characteristics, which makes developing a drug to kill all strains of the virus extremely difficult. Although no cure has yet been developed, advances in AIDS treatment (such as the use of anti-retroviral drugs) have diminished the mortality and morbidity of the disease. Many scientists remain optimistic that a cure for the AIDS virus will be found (24, 25).

The best way to address the spread of HIV infection is to prevent it, but prevention works best when efforts are focused and sustained. In countries where a concerted effort has been made to address behavioral issues to stop the spread of HIV, such as promoting the use of condoms and encouraging monoga-mous relationships, rates of new HIV infections have decreased. In addition, worldwide funding to fight the spread of HIV had increased to $10 billion in 2007, more than six times the amount spent in 2001 (6). This has allowed for greater access to antiretroviral treatments, from 240,000 people in 2001 to 3 million people in low- and middle-income countries in 2007 (6). However, an estimated $20 billion will be needed annually to achieve the 2010 United Nations goal of halting and beginning to reverse the HIV epidemic (27).

- *Insect bites.* Studies have found that biting insects such as mosquitoes, biting flies, and bedbugs cannot transmit the HIV virus.

Make sure you know...

> AIDS is a fatal disease that develops from infection by the human immunodeficiency virus (HIV).

> The HIV virus is transmitted when infected body fluids, such as blood, semen, and vaginal secretions, enter the bloodstream of a noninfected individual.

> HIV cannot be transmitted through casual contact, kissing, water (such as in swimming pools or hot tubs), or dry surfaces.

> Although no cure has yet been found for AIDS, many antiretroviral drugs are available to delay the onset of the disease and improve a patient's quality of life.

Hepatitis B

The CDC estimated that in 2007, 43,000 people were infected with **hepatitis B (HBV),** a virus that causes liver disease (3). Hepatitis B virus can be transmitted by contact with infected blood, blood products, semen, vaginal secretions, and saliva. Consequently, people at risk for contracting hepatitis B include individuals having sex with a partner who is infected with HBV, shar-ing personal items such as razors or toothbrushes, shooting drugs, or working in a job that involves handling human blood or other body fluids. The risk of contracting hepatitis B is higher for people who engage in sexual relations with more than one partner. Individuals who are at risk for contracting hepatitis B are often advised to be vaccinated against the disease.

Hepatitis promotes an inflammatory response in the liver that decreases normal liver function. The liver performs numerous bodily functions, such as regulating blood glucose levels between meals, producing bile, and detoxifying the blood. Because many of the liver's functions are essential for life, severe liver dysfunction can be life-threatening. Therefore, hepatitis B is a very serious disease.

Symptoms

Approximately 30% of the individuals infected with hepatitis B do not develop symptoms. In the remaining 70% of infected individuals, a variety of symptoms may be present. Common symptoms include the following (9):

- Jaundice (eyes or skin turn yellow)
- Reduced appetite
- Nausea
- Vomiting
- Stomach and/or joint pain
- Chronic fatigue

Although the mortality rate for hepatitis B is typically lower than for some other forms of hepatitis, it is estimated that over 5000 people die each year in the United States from this disease.

Diagnosis and Treatment

Hepatitis B is diagnosed by a blood test for antibodies that indicate an infection with the hepatitis B virus. Unfortunately, there is currently no cure for hepatitis B. Therefore, prevention of this disease is critical. Once hepatitis B is diagnosed, the treatment consists of rest and consuming sufficient amounts of fluid to ensure adequate hydration. For some people with the hepatitis B virus, the liver can become severely compromised; for those who do develop severe liver disease from hepatitis B infection, two drugs (alpha interferon and lamivudine) have been shown to be effective in reducing symptoms.

Human Papillomavirus (Genital Warts)

Genital *human papillomavirus (HPV)* refers to a group of over 30 strains of sexually transmitted virus that can infect the genitals. Most infected individuals do not realize they are infected because the virus lives in the skin or mucous membranes and usually causes no symptoms (1). However, some people may get visible **genital warts.** Genital warts appear as soft pink or flesh-colored swellings that can be raised or flat. Infection generally occurs through sexual contact with an infected individual; after exposure, the virus penetrates the skin or mucous membranes of the genitals or anus, and warts may appear within 3–9 weeks (7, 10).

HPV is one of the most common causes of STIs in the world and the most common cause of STIs in the United States. Current estimates are that more than 20 million people in the United States are infected with HPV (11). Moreover, approximately 6.2 million Americans get a new genital HPV infection each year (3). The incidence of HPV varies across the population, with the highest rates in people aged 19–30. In particular, studies suggest that the incidence of HPV in college students is extremely high.

Symptoms

Many people infected with HPV are asymptomatic. In others, HPV can cause genital warts or precancerous changes in the cells of the cervix, vulva, anus, or penis. On dry areas of the external genitals (such as the penis and vulva), warts may develop as a series of small itchy bumps on the skin and may range in size from that of a

pinhead to that of a pencil eraser. Men and women can detect these warts by routinely examining their genitals for suspicious growths. In women, a physician can often detect HPV infection during a routine Pap smear.

Treatment

Genital warts can be treated with several different types of medication, which cause the warts to dry up within a few days, or they can be removed by cryosurgery (freezing them), laser surgery, or excision surgery. Removing the wart does not remove the virus from the individual's system. In fact, because the virus can remain dormant in cells, in some cases warts can reappear within months or even years after treatment. Unfortunately, the extent to which an individual can spread the virus after the visible warts have been removed is currently unknown.

Many HPV infections will disappear without medical treatment. The greatest risk from them is that in women, HPV infection increases the risk of uterine and cervical cancer. Exactly how HPV results in cancer is unclear. Nonetheless, what is known is that within 5 years after infection, about 30% of all untreated HPV results in precancerous growth. Among precancerous growths that remain untreated, 70% will lead to cancer (7, 10).

In 2006, the U.S. Food and Drug Administration (FDA) approved the first vaccine to help prevent cervical cancer caused by some types of HPV (3). The HPV vaccine is recommended for girls before the onset of sexual activity. The vaccine can also be administered to women who have not been infected with HPV.

Genital Herpes

Genital **herpes** infections are caused by the herpes simplex virus, a family of more than 70 herpesviruses (7). In the 1960s, it was discovered that two specific forms of herpes simplex virus generally cause genital herpes; these viruses are labeled as type I herpes simplex virus (HSV-1) and type II herpes simplex virus (HSV-2). In general, type I infections are more common above the waist (e.g., sores on the lips or

hepatitis B (HBV) A viral infection that attacks the liver.

genital warts Warts caused by a small group of viruses called human papillomavirus; after exposure, the virus penetrates the skin or mucous membranes of the genitals or anus, and warts appear within 6–8 weeks; also known as *venereal warts*.

herpes A general term for a family of highly contagious diseases caused by herpes simplex viral infections.

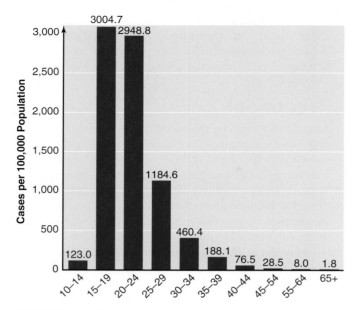

FIGURE 14.5
Women between the ages of 15 and 24 show the highest rates of chlamydia.

Source: Centers for Disease Control and Prevention. Trends in Reportable Sexually Transmitted Diseases in the United States, 2007. 2009. www.cdc.gov/STD/stats07/trends.htm.

mouth, known as fever blisters or cold sores) whereas type II infections are more common below the waist (e.g., genital lesions).

Genital herpes is highly contagious and can be transmitted through any form of sexual contact (such as hand-to-genital contact, oral sex, or intercourse). The incidence of genital herpes in the United States is greatest among white teens and young adults. Over 1 million new cases of herpes are reported in the United States each year, and it is estimated that genital herpes affects approximately 45 million Americans, or about 17% of the population (3). Healthy People 2010 has set a goal to reduce the incidence of herpes infection from 17% to fewer than 14% of the population (12).

Symptoms

For most people infected with the herpes simplex virus, the initial infection is the most severe. The first symptoms of herpes infection generally appear within 3–20 days after exposure (3). Symptoms of herpes vary from sores (blisters) on the mouth, rectum, and genitals, to fever and swollen glands. Symptoms may disappear and then reappear without warning. Although symptoms may come and go, the virus remains in the body for life.

Treatment

At present, there is no cure for herpes, but newly developed drugs show promise. Although treatment with cold-sore medication reduces the pain and irritation of the sore, rubbing anything on the herpes blister increases the chance of spreading herpes-laden fluids to other body parts or to other people.

Make sure you know...

> In addition to AIDS, several other STIs are caused by viruses, including hepatitis B, genital warts, and genital herpes. Some viral STIs are treatable, but none are curable.

> Hepatitis B is a liver disease that can be transmitted by sexual activity. Symptoms of Hepatitis B include jaundice, reduced appetite, nausea, and vomiting.

> Genital warts are caused by the human papillomavirus (HPV), which is typically spread by sexual contact with an infected individual; the warts can be treated with medication and/or surgery. Untreated HPV in women will increase their risk of uterine and cervical cancer. A vaccine against some types of HPV is available.

> Herpes is a viral STI that can be transmitted through any form of sexual contact; symptoms generally include sores on the mouth, rectum, and genitals.

Chlamydia

Among the STIs caused by **bacteria, chlamydia** is one of the most common STIs among heterosexual people worldwide (3). The disease is caused by infection within the reproductive organs and is spread through vaginal, anal, and oral sex. The incidence of chlamydia infection in the United States experienced a rapid growth between 1980 and 2000. A report from the Centers for Disease Control and Prevention reveals that chlamydia is the most common bacterial STI in the United States, with 2.8 million new cases occurring each year (2). Equally alarming is the estimate that about 20% of all college students may have chlamydia; college-aged women are the most susceptible. Figure 14.5 shows the rates of chlamydia for women of all ages; note that high school and college-aged women make up the bulk of the cases (3). The good news is that the infection rates of chlamydia in the United States may be on the decline (3). The Healthy People 2010 objective for chlamydia is to reduce the incidence of this infection to fewer than four cases of chlamydia per 100,000 people.

Symptoms

Symptoms of chlamydia often go unnoticed and may vary among individuals. In fact, over 75% of the women and 50% of the men infected do not develop symptoms and are unaware that they carry the bacteria. For both men and women, early symptoms occur within 7–21 days after infection. Early symptoms of infection in women may include the following:

- Unusual vaginal discharge
- A burning sensation when urinating
- Unexplained vaginal bleeding between menstrual periods

Later symptoms, typically occurring several months after infection, include the following:

- Lower back pain
- Lower abdominal pain
- Pain during intercourse
- Low-grade fever

Up to 50% of all men infected with chlamydia do not develop symptoms when first infected. However, several months after infection, the following symptoms may occur:

- Unusual discharge from the penis
- Burning sensation when urinating
- Low-grade fever
- Pain and swelling of the testicles

Diagnosis and Treatment

Chlamydia can be diagnosed by a blood test or a Pap test, in which the bacteria responsible for the infection are grown in a tissue culture. Fortunately, chlamydia can be cured with antibiotics. If untreated, chlamydia can result in infertility in both men and women. Further, untreated chlamydia in women can lead to **pelvic inflammatory disease (PID),** an inflammatory infection of the lining of the abdominal and pelvic cavity. Common symptoms of pelvic inflammatory disease include pain in the lower abdominal cavity, fever, and menstrual irregularities. PID can lead to internal abscesses and long-lasting, chronic pain, and it can damage the fallopian tubes enough to cause infertility or increase the risk of ectopic pregnancy (3).

All sexually active women should be screened yearly, and all pregnant women should have a screening

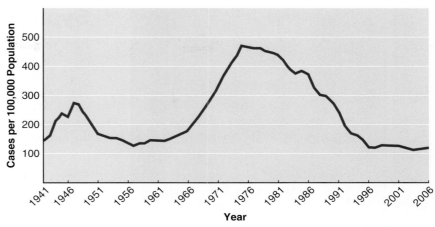

FIGURE 14.6

Reported rates of gonorrhea in the United States from 1941 to 2007. Notice the rise in gonorrhea infections in the 1970s and the subsequent decline during the period from 1976 to 1996.

Source: Centers for Disease Control and Prevention. Trends in Reportable Sexually Transmitted Diseases in the United States, 2006. 2007. CDC, 2009. www.cdc.gov/STD/stats07/trends.htm.

test for chlamydia. Early treatment of chlamydia is important to prevent potentially serious long-term health consequences.

Gonorrhea

Gonorrhea (also known as "the clap") is another common STI, and it is estimated that over 700,000 cases of gonorrhea will be reported in the United States each year (3). In comparison to other STIs, the incidence of gonorrhea ranks it as the second most common communicable bacterial infection. Only chlamydia is more prevalent. Fortunately, the rate of gonorrhea infection in the United States has declined over the past 25 years (Figure 14.6). The decline in gonorrhea may be due to improved testing and more frequent condom use. The Healthy People 2010 goal for gonorrhea is to reduce the incidence of this infection from the current annual rate of approximately 120 infections per 100,000 people to fewer than 20 infections per 100,000 individuals.

bacteria Microorganisms that can cause infectious diseases. STIs caused by bacteria can be cured with antibiotics.

chlamydia The most common sexually transmitted disease among heterosexuals in the United States; is caused by a bacterial infection within the reproductive organs.

pelvic inflammatory disease (PID) An inflammatory infection of the lining of the abdominal and pelvic cavities in women.

gonorrhea A common sexually transmitted disease caused by the *Neisseria gonorrhoeae* bacterium; curable with antibiotics.

A chancre on the site of the initial infection is a symptom of primary syphilis.

The bacterium that causes gonorrhea is called *Neisseria gonorrhoeae* and grows well within mucous membranes in the body. This bacterium cannot grow outside the body because it requires a warm and moist environment. Therefore, gonorrhea cannot be spread by contact with toilet seats, doorknobs, or other inanimate objects. However, gonorrhea can be transmitted through vaginal, anal, or oral sex.

Symptoms

Over 80% of men develop symptoms within 2–10 days after sexual contact with an infected person. Typical symptoms include a milky discharge from the penis and painful urination (10). Moreover, in some men, lymph glands in the groin become inflamed and swollen. In contrast, only 20% of infected women develop symptoms. When symptoms are present, they include painful urination and an occasional fever (10). The lack of symptoms in women poses a serious problem because the woman is unaware that she has been infected and may continue to spread the disease to her sexual partners.

Diagnosis and Treatment

Gonorrhea can be diagnosed by a tissue culture of the discharge from the penis or vagina and is curable with antibiotics. When diagnosed early and treated with appropriate medication, gonorrhea can be easily cured. However, untreated gonorrhea may spread to the prostate, testicles, kidney, and bladder and can result in sterility in both men and women (3, 10). Like chlamydia, gonorrhea is a common cause of PID in women. As with all other STIs, early detection and treatment of gonorrhea are essential to prevent serious negative health consequences.

Syphilis

Each year thousands of new cases of **syphilis** are reported in the United States (3). Like chlamydia and gonorrhea, syphilis is caused by a bacterial infection. The spiral-shaped bacterium responsible for syphilis is called *Treponema pallidum*. This bacterium requires a warm and moist environment, such as the genitals or the mucous membranes of the mouth, to survive.

Symptoms

The symptoms of untreated syphilis vary because the disease generally progresses through four stages: primary syphilis; secondary syphilis; latent syphilis; and tertiary syphilis. The early symptoms of primary syphilis generally include a dime-sized, painless sore, called a **chancre,** located at the initial site of infection, such as the penis, vaginal walls, or mouth. In both men and women, this chancre will completely disappear in 3–6 weeks.

Within 6 weeks after the disappearance of the chancre, symptoms associated with secondary syphilis appear. These include a skin rash or white patches on the mucous membranes of the mouth, throat, or genitals. Hair loss may also occur, lymph glands may become swollen, and infectious sores may develop around the mouth or genitals.

If syphilis is not treated, stage 2 symptoms typically disappear, and stage 3—latent syphilis—begins. During this phase, the infected person may not experience symptoms or may experience symptoms that are vague and difficult to diagnose without a blood test to screen for the bacteria.

Stage 4, or tertiary syphilis, is rarely seen in the United States because medical treatment usually prevents the disease from progressing to this stage. Nonetheless, if untreated, the infected individual may spend several years in the latent stage of syphilis while the infection slowly spreads to organs throughout the body, leading to stage 4. This last stage of untreated syphilis may result in heart damage, blindness, deafness, paralysis, and mental disorders.

Diagnosis and Treatment

Syphilis can be diagnosed with a blood test and can be cured by antibiotics. However, because of the progressive nature of this infection, early treatment of syphilis is important to prevent serious and long-term health problems.

Make sure you know...

> Commons STIs caused by bacterial infections include chlamydia, gonorrhea, and syphilis.

Bacterial STIs can be treated and cured with antiobiotics.

> Chlamydia is the most common STI among heterosexuals and is caused by a bacterial infection within the reproductive organs. Symptoms of chlamydia vary among individuals; more than 75% of infected women and 50% of infected men do not develop symptoms and are unaware that they carry the bacteria.

> More than 80% of men infected with gonorrhea develop symptoms within 2–10 days after sexual contact with an infected person; typical symptoms include a milky discharge from the penis and painful urination. Only 20% of women infected with gonorrhea develop symptoms. When symptoms are present, they include painful urination and occasional fever.

> Syphilis infections progress through four stages. Symptoms of untreated syphilis vary depending on the stage of the infection; early symptoms in stages 1 and 2 may include a painless sore, called a chancre, followed by hair loss, swollen lymph glands, and infectious sores around the mouth or genitals. The third stage of syphilis is a latent stage in which no symptoms may be present, but the infection spreads throughout the body. Stage 4 symptoms include heart and nervous system damage.

Other Sexually Transmitted Infections

In addition to the previously discussed STIs, numerous other sexually transmitted infections also exist. In this section, we present a brief discussion of four other common STIs caused by organisms other than viruses or bacteria.

Trichomoniasis

Trichomonas vaginalis is a one-celled organism (protozoan) that infects the vaginal or urinary mucosa to cause a vaginal infection called **trichomoniasis (trich).** Trichomoniasis is a very common infection that affects approximately 7 million people each year (3). The most common mode of transmission is by vaginal intercourse or sexual contact with an infected person. Women can acquire the disease from infected men or women, whereas men usually acquire the disease from infected women (3).

Trichomoniasis can also be contracted by prolonged exposure to moisture (e.g., exposure to wet bathing suits or other clothing infected with the protozoan). *Trichomonas vaginalis* is a very hardy organism that can live for several hours on wet towels or toilet

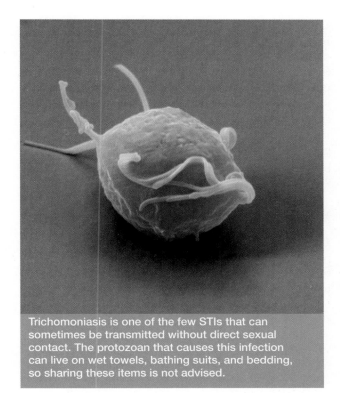

Trichomoniasis is one of the few STIs that can sometimes be transmitted without direct sexual contact. The protozoan that causes this infection can live on wet towels, bathing suits, and bedding, so sharing these items is not advised.

seats. Because trichomoniasis can be contracted by means other than sexual intercourse, this infection is often referred to as a sexually related infection.

Symptoms Most men and women experience symptoms of infection within days after contact with *Trichomonas vaginalis*. For women, common symptoms include the following:

• Yellow-green (often foamy) vaginal discharge with a strong odor

• Irritation and itching of the genital area

• Pain or irritation during intercourse

Men may experience the following symptoms:

• Irritation inside the penis

• Discharge from the penis

• Burning sensation during urination or after ejaculation

syphilis A sexually transmitted disease caused by the *Treponema pallidum* bacterium; curable with antiobiotics.

chancre A sore that appears at the site of infection in stage 1 syphilis.

trichomoniasis (trich) A sexually transmitted disease that is caused by a single-celled protozoan parasite.

Diagnosis and Treatment Trichomoniasis can be diagnosed by a simple medical test. When trichomoniasis is detected, all sexual partners should also be treated for this infection, because the infection can be passed back and forth between partners (called the *ping-pong effect*). Infection with trichomoniasis can be treated with an oral dose of the prescription drug metronidazole (3). Although trichomoniasis is not generally considered a life-threatening infection, prolonged and untreated trichomoniasis is associated with an increased risk of cancer.

Pubic Lice

Pubic lice, or "crabs," are usually transmitted from person to person by sexual contact but can also be transmitted from infected bed linen, clothes, or even toilet seats. These organisms grip pubic hair and feed on blood from tiny blood vessels in the surrounding skin. Once an infection occurs, pubic lice reproduce, and the numbers of lice in the infected area grows. When large numbers of lice are present, they can be seen as brown spots on pubic hairs and the surrounding skin.

As the pubic lice feed on blood vessels in the pubic area, they irritate the skin, causing itching and sometimes swelling. Fortunately, both over-the-counter and prescription skin medications are available to eliminate pubic lice. In addition to applying a topical lotion to kill the lice, an infected individual also needs to wash all clothing and bed linen to avoid reinfection.

Scabies

Scabies is caused by a tiny mite that infects the skin between the fingers, on the wrist, under the breasts, and the pubic area. Once an infection occurs, the female mite burrows under the skin, causing irritation and itching. Skin-to-skin contact (including sexual contact) with an infected individual can spread these parasites. Unlike pubic lice, scabies is rarely contracted from clothing, bedding, or toilet seats.

A physician can diagnose scabies by scraping the infected area and performing a microscopic test to determine whether mites are present. Once diagnosed, scabies can be treated with several topical medications (2). Typically, one or more treatments eliminate the invading mites.

Candidiasis

Candidiasis is a common form of vaginitis (inflammation of the vagina) caused by a fungus called *Candida albicans*. Although this fungus is normally found in small quantities in the vagina, its rapid growth can result in a "yeast infection" that is characterized by itching, discomfort, and a thick vaginal discharge. This fungus can be spread from person to person by sexual contact and can also manifest itself in the mouth and throat. Candidiasis requires different treatments depending on the location of the infection, but it is curable regardless of location with the appropriate antifungal medication.

See the Closer Look box on page 406 for answers to additional questions about STIs.

Make sure you know...

> Trichomoniasis ("trich") is a common STI caused by infection with a protozoan called *Trichomonas vaginalis.*

> Symptoms of *trichomoniasis* include a yellow-green vaginal discharge for women and a discharge from the penis for men. Trichomoniasis is treatable with medication.

> Pubic lice, or "crabs," are parasites that infect the pubic area.

> Scabies is caused by a tiny mite that can infect skin between fingers, under the breasts, and in the pubic area.

> Candidiasis (yeast infection) is a common form of vaginitis that can also manifest in the mouth and throat.

Reducing Your Risk for Sexually Transmitted Infections

There is no cure for viral infections such as HIV, HPV, or genital herpes, and although many STIs can be treated, prevention is the best approach. The keys to preventing STIs are education and responsible action. You can assess your risk for contracting STIs with the Steps for Behavior Change box on page 407 and Laboratory 14.1 at the end of the chapter. These questionnaires will help make you aware of the attitudes and behaviors that increase the risk of infection via sexual activity.

In the following sections, we discuss several steps that you can take to avoid infection with an STI.

Abstinence

Because all forms of sexual activity, including anal and oral sex, carry some risk of transmitting STIs, the only 100% effective means of preventing STIs is abstinence.

If abstinence is not an option, there are several strategies that can help minimize the risk of infection.

Limiting the Number of Sexual Partners

Maintaining a monogamous relationship with a sexual partner that is not infected with an STI is one way to avoid STIs. The keys to success with this strategy are that both partners be free of STIs and that the relationship remain monogamous. Failure of one member of the relationship to maintain monogamy will increase the risk of contracting an STI for *both* partners.

Limiting your number of sexual partners will also decrease your risk of contracting an STI. The rationale behind this statement is simple: The more sexual partners you have, the greater your odds of being exposed to an STI. Therefore, limiting your number of sexual partners will help reduce your risk.

Using Male Latex Condoms

The pores of latex condoms are too small for most microorganisms to pass through; they therefore limit the transmission of many STIs. Consistent and proper use of a latex condom during all sexual activity (including oral sex, anal sex, or vaginal intercourse) will reduce the risk of contracting and spreading an STI.

How effective are latex condoms in preventing the transmission of STIs? A study by the American Public Health Association revealed that use of latex condoms during sexual activities is effective against the transmission of HIV and gonorrhea in both men and women (13). Further, although definitive evidence is not available, it appears likely that the use of male condoms will also reduce the risk of other STIs, including syphilis and chlamydia (14). However, latex condoms will not prevent the transmission of parasites such as scabies and pubic lice. Also, chancres, HPV, and genital herpes infections can occur in areas not covered by condoms. Therefore, although using condoms will reduce your risk for many STIs, it will not provide absolute protection against all STIs (13, 14).

Using Female Condoms

A laboratory study conducted by the CDC has indicated that female condoms are effective mechanical barriers against viruses, including HIV (14). From these studies, the CDC has concluded that when used consistently and correctly, female condoms may reduce the risk of STIs including HIV (14). However, clinical studies proving that female condoms prevent the spread of STIs are not currently available. Nonetheless,

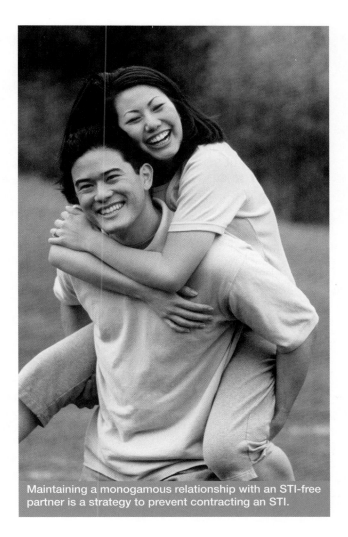

Maintaining a monogamous relationship with an STI-free partner is a strategy to prevent contracting an STI.

the CDC recommends that when male condoms cannot be used, sexual partners should consider the use of female condoms to reduce the risk of STIs (14).

Discussing Sexually Transmitted Infections with Sexual Partners

Prior to engaging in sexual activity with a new partner, you should talk about your concerns regarding STIs. Ask whether the person has been recently medically screened for an STI or has engaged in high-risk

pubic lice   STI caused by a parasitic insect that grips the hair in the pubic area; also called "crabs."

scabies   Infection caused by a parasitic mite that can burrow under the skin between the fingers, on the wrist, under the breasts, and the pubic area.

A CLOSER LOOK

ANSWERS TO FREQUENTLY ASKED QUESTIONS ABOUT SEXUALLY TRANSMITTED INFECTIONS

ARE STIS BECOMING MORE COMMON OR LESS COMMON IN THE UNITED STATES?

It depends on the STI. Many cases of STIs go undiagnosed, and some highly prevalent viral infections, such as human papillomavirus and genital herpes, are not reported at all. Although the estimated incidence of HIV/AIDS is holding constant at about 40,000 new cases per year, the numbers of new cases of syphilis and chlamydia are increasing. Fortunately, the rates of new cases of gonorrhea have plateaued in recent years.

WHICH STIS ARE THE MOST SERIOUS FOR WOMEN?

Although HIV/AIDS is a serious problem in women, they bear a larger burden than do men with respect to gonorrhea, chlamydia, and genital warts because women suffer more frequent and more serious complications from those infections. For example, 10–20% of women with gonorrhea or chlamydia will develop

pelvic inflammatory disease, which can lead to chronic pelvic pain and infertility. Women infected with human papillomavirus also have an increased risk of cervical cancer. Finally, women infected with an STI during pregnancy can experience early onset of labor and premature birth, which is the leading cause of infant death and disability in the United States.

WHO SHOULD GET TESTED FOR HIV?

Anyone who is at risk for HIV infection should get tested. You are at risk if (a) you have had unprotected sex with anyone who has not been involved in a long-term, mutually monogamous relationship with you; (b) either you or your partner has had unprotected sex with other people during the past several years; (c) you have shared needles or syringes with anyone for injecting drugs; or (d) you received a blood transfusion before 1985.

Getting tested for HIV if you are at risk is important because many people carrying HIV don't know they are infected, and because early treatment for HIV can improve the outcome of the infection. Testing is available from several sources, including any physician, your student health clinic, Planned Parenthood, and your local public health department. Taking the test itself is simple: It involves taking a small blood sample that is sent to a laboratory for analysis. Costs of these tests are generally between $50 and $100. Another option—home testing kits—is available from several manufacturers. Home testing kits provide a sterile lancet (needle) to prick the finger to obtain a few drops of blood and a sterile storage container for sending the blood sample to a lab for analysis. Whenever choosing a home testing kit, select only those clearly marked as approved by the federal Food and Drug Administration (FDA).

---

behaviors (such as having multiple sexual partners) that would increase the risk of being infected. This kind of conversation can lead to a mutual concern for preventing STIs and in some cases, result in the decision to refrain from sexual activity until medical screening for STIs has been completed.

Avoiding Drugs and Alcohol

The use of psychoactive drugs and alcohol prior to engaging in sexual activity can impair your reasoning and increase your risk of engaging in risky sexual activity and/or failing to use condoms during sex. Because drugs and alcohol weaken your ability to reason, you should refrain from abusing these substances to reduce your risk of contracting STIs.

Other Protective Measures

In addition to the previously discussed actions, there are several other steps that you can take to reduce your risk of contracting an STI:

- Inspect yourself and your partner for signs of STIs.
- Do not share needles, scissors, or razors.
- Wash your genitals before and after sex.
- Do not handle towels, wet bedding, or underclothing that has been in contact with an individual who may be infected with an STI.

Note that vaginal spermicides containing nonoxynol 9 are not effective against preventing most STIs, including gonorrhea, HIV, or chlamydia. In fact, evidence indicates that nonoxynol 9 can increase the risk of contracting STIs by irritating the vaginal or anal lining and increasing the ease of entry of infectious

STEPS FOR
BEHAVIOR CHANGE

Are you at increased risk for a sexually transmitted infection?

Answer the following questions to assess whether some of your behaviors put you at increased risk for an STI.

Y N

☐ ☐ I sometimes end up having sex with someone without intending to, on the spur of the moment.

☐ ☐ I am an intravenous drug user, and I have shared used needles with other drug users.

☐ ☐ I am too uncomfortable to discuss STIs and sexual history with new sexual partners, so I do not address the topic.

☐ ☐ I don't worry about using condoms during sexual intercourse.

☐ ☐ I haven't been tested for STIs, because I know there's no chance I have one, even though I am or have been sexually active.

If you answered yes to any of the above, then you could do more to protect yourself from an STI.

TIPS TO LESSEN YOUR RISK OF CONTRACTING STIS

☑ Before entering a situation where spontaneous sex may occur, ask yourself whether or not you are willing to engage in sex and under what circumstances this would be acceptable. If you do decide to have sex, make sure you are protected.

☑ Never share needles when using drugs or anabolic steroids.

☑ Always use a condom.

☑ Get tested if there's even a slight chance of your having an STI. If you are sexually active, have periodic medical examinations that include blood, urine, and/or pelvic exams.

☑ Always discuss your sexual histories with a new sexual partner. Remember that you're having sex not just with them; you're having sex with everyone they've had sex with.

---

agents into the body. The CDC recommends avoiding condoms containing nonoxynol 9 (15).

If you suspect that you have been exposed to an STI, you should contact your physician immediately for medical screening. Never try to diagnose an STI yourself, and do not delay seeking medical attention if you develop symptoms of any STI. Early diagnosis and treatment are essential to ensure that an STI does not lead to long-term health problems. If you learn that you are infected, you should immediately inform all of your sexual partners. Failing to tell a partner about an infection increases the risk of the spread of STIs to others.

Make sure you know...

> Avoiding sexual activity (abstinence) is the only absolute means of preventing sexually transmitted infections. If abstinence is not an option, then monogamy or limiting your sexual partners is the next best strategy. Be sure to discuss STIs and sexual history with all sexual partners.

> Using latex condoms will reduce the risk of contracting an STI.

> Avoid using drugs or alcohol prior to engaging in sexual activities.

Summary

1. Every year, millions of people in the United States are infected by one or more sexually transmitted infections (STIs).

2. Some of the most common sexually transmitted infections include HIV/AIDS, hepatitis B, human papillomavirus (which causes genital warts), genital herpes, chlamydia, gonorrhea, syphilis, trichomoniasis, pubic lice, and scabies.

3. AIDS is a fatal disease that develops from infection caused by the human immunodeficiency virus (HIV).

4. STIs caused by viruses are not curable and will reside in the body of the host for life. Hepatitis B is a liver disease caused by a viral infection and can be transmitted by sexual activity. Genital warts result from the spread of human papillomaviruses by sexual contact. Herpes is caused by a virus that can be transmitted through any form of sexual contact.

5. Chlamydia, gonorrhea, and syphilis are STIs caused by bacterial infections. They can be treated with antibiotics.

6. Trichomoniasis, pubic lice, scabies, and yeast infections are other infections that can be spread through vaginal, oral, and anal contact.

7. Most STIs can be avoided by abstaining from sex and/or following "safe sex" guidelines, including limiting your number of sexual partners, using condoms, and avoiding high-risk behaviors, such as drug or alcohol abuse.

Study Questions

1. Hepatitis B affects which internal organ?
   a. heart
   b. brain
   c. kidney
   d. liver

2. Genital warts are caused by
   a. human papillomavirus (HPV).
   b. hepatitis B.
   c. herpesvirus.
   d. a single-celled protozoan parasite.

3. Which of the following STIs is not caused by a virus?
   a. HPV
   b. hepatitis B
   c. genital herpes
   d. syphilis

4. Which stage of syphilis is characterized by a skin lesion called a chancre?
   a. stage 1—primary stage
   b. stage 2—secondary stage
   c. stage 3—latent stage
   d. stage 4—tertiary stage

5. What is the common characteristic of trichomoniasis, scabies, and pubic lice?
   a. These STIs can be prevented by using a condom during sexual activity.
   b. These STIs are caused by parasites.
   c. These STIs are found in men only.
   d. Once you have had one of these STIs, you can never get it again.

6. Name the seven most common STIs in the United States.

7. Which of the most common STIs are currently incurable?

8. Discuss the relationship between HPV, genital warts, and uterine or cervical cancer.

9. Discuss the three stages of AIDS, beginning with infection with HIV and leading to the final stage.

10. Outline the symptoms of chlamydia, trichomoniasis, hepatitis B, and gonorrhea. Do gender differences exist in symptoms of these STIs?

11. List the common symptoms of genital warts, herpes, and syphilis. Are symptoms for these STIs similar in men and women?

12. Identify the treatments available for all of the common STIs in the United States.

13. Outline ways to reduce your risk of contracting STIs.

14. Which STIs are becoming more common in the United States?

15. Discuss who should get tested for STIs.

Suggested Reading

Anderson, B. *Reproductive Health: Women and Men's Shared Responsibility*. Sudbury, MA: Jones and Bartlett, 2005.

Centers for Disease Control and Prevention. *HIV/AIDS in the United States*. Atlanta: Centers for Disease Control and Prevention, 2009.

Centers for Disease Control and Prevention. *Sexually Transmitted Disease Surveillance, 2007*. Atlanta: Centers for Disease Control and Prevention, 2008.

Donatelle, R. *Access to Health*, Green Edition. San Francisco: Benjamin Cummings, 2010.

Fields, R. *Drugs in Perspective*, 7th ed. St. Louis: McGraw-Hill, 2010.

Greenberg, J., C. Bruess, and D. Haffner. *Exploring the Dimensions of Human Sexuality*, 3rd ed. Sudbury, MA: Jones and Bartlett, 2007.

Pruitt, B., and J. Stein. *Decisions for Healthy Living*. San Francisco: Benjamin Cummings, 2004.

For links to the organizations and websites listed below, visit The Total Fitness and Wellness Website at www.pearsonhighered.com/powers.

Centers for Disease Control and Prevention
Provides information on a variety of disease-related topics, including the latest statistics on the incidence of and mortality from various diseases in the United States.

American Medical Association
Contains many sources of information about a wide variety of medical problems, including sexually transmitted infections.

WebMD
Contains information about a wide variety of diseases and medical problems, including sexually transmitted infections.

References

1. Eng, T., and W. Butler (Eds.). *The Hidden Epidemic: Confronting Sexually Transmitted Diseases*. Washington, DC: National Academy Press, 1997.

2. Centers for Disease Control and Prevention, National Prevention Information Network. STDs today. www.cdcnpin.org/scripts/std/std.asp. Accessed May 2009.

3. Centers for Disease Control and Prevention. Sexually transmitted diseases. www.cdc.gov/std. Accessed May 2009.

4. Centers for Disease Control and Prevention. CDC HIV/AIDS fact sheet: A glance at the HIV/AIDS epidemic. Revised August 2009. www.cdc.gov/hiv/resources/factsheets/PDF/us.pdf.

5. World Health Organization, UNAIDS Press Office. Press release, November 21, 2005. www.who.int/hiv/epiupdate2005.

6. UNAIDS. *UNAIDS 2008 Report on the Global AIDS Epidemic: Executive Summary*. Geneva, Switzerland: UNAIDS, 2008.

7. Daniels, D., R. Hillman, S. Barton, and D. Goldmeir. *Sexually Transmitted Disease and AIDS*. London: Springer-Verlag, 1993.

8. Watanabe, M. AIDS: 20 years later. *The Scientist* 15:1, 2001.

9. Nowak, T., and A. Handford. *Essentials of Pathophysiology*. St. Louis: McGraw-Hill, 1999.

10. Robbins, S., and M. Angell. *Basic Pathology*. Philadelphia: W. B. Saunders, 1997.

11. National Institute of Allergy and Infectious Diseases, National Institutes of Health. Human papillomavirus and genital warts. http://www3.niaid.nih.gov/topics/genitalWarts. Accessed May 2009.

12. Healthy People 2010. National health promotion and disease prevention objectives. PHS, 2001.

13. American Public Health Association. Condoms proved effective against HIV transmission. *The Nation's Health* 4, September 2001.

14. Centers for Disease Control and Prevention. Sexually transmitted diseases treatment guidelines. *Morbidity and Mortality Weekly Report* 51:1–80, 2002.

15. Centers for Disease Control and Prevention. MMWR recommendations and reports, sexually transmitted diseases treatment guidelines. May 10, 2002. www.cdc.gov/mmwr/preview/mmwrhtml/rr5106a1.htm.

16. Centers for Disease Control and Prevention. Cases of HIV infection and AIDS in the United States and Dependent Areas, 2007. *HIV/AIDS Surveillance Report* 19:(1), 2009. www.cdc.gov/HIV/topics/surveillance/resources/reports/2007report/default.htm.

17. Rosenberg, P., and M. Gail. Uncertainty in estimates of HIV prevalence derived by back calculation. *Annals of Epidemiology* 1:105–115, 1990.

18. Biggar, R., and P. Rosenberg. HIV infection/AIDS in the U.S. during the 1990's. *Clinical Infectious Diseases* 17(Suppl.):S219–S223, 1993.

19. Maynaud, P., and D. Mabey. Approaches to the control of sexually transmitted infections in developing countries. *Sexually Transmitted Infections* 80:174–182, 2004.

20. Fenton, K., and C. Lowndes. Recent trends in the epidemiology of sexually transmitted infections in European Union. *Sexually Transmitted Infections* 80:255–263, 2004.

21. Lowndes, C., and K. Fenton. Surveillance systems for STIs in the European Union: Facing a changing epidemiology. *Sexually Transmitted Infections* 80:264–271, 2004.

22. Brown, A. E., et al. Recent trends in HIV and other STIs in the United Kingdom. *Sexually Transmitted Infections* 80:159–166, 2004.

23. World Health Organization. Global AIDS epidemic continues to grow. 2006. www.who.int/hiv/mediacentre/news62.

24. Mullins, J., D. Nickle, L. Heath, A. Rodrigo, and G. Lerch. Immunogen sequence: The fourth tier of AIDS vaccine design. *Expert Reviews in Vaccines* 3:S151–S159, 2004.

25. Srivastava, I., J. Ulmer, and S. Barnett. Neutralizing antibody responses to HIV: Role of protective immunity and challenges for vaccine design. *Expert Reviews of Vaccines* 3:S33–S52, 2004.

26. UNAIDS/WHO. Press release: HIV infection rates decreasing in several countries but global number of people living with HIV continues to rise. 2005. www.who.int/hiv/epiupdate2005.

27. World Health Organization. UN High-Level Meeting on AIDS: Launch of the 2006 Report on Global AIDS Epidemic. 2006. www.who.int/hiv/mediacentre/news60.

Videos

Log on to www.pearsonhighered.com/powers to view these chapter-related videos.

Infectious Diseases and Sexually Transmitted Infections

Human Papillomavirus Vaccine Mandatory

Inventory of Attitudes and Behaviors toward Sexually Transmitted Infections

This laboratory is designed to help you identify attitudes and behaviors that increase your risk of contracting an STI. Remember, all STIs are preventable, and you determine your risk of being infected.

Read the following statements about sexual attitudes and behaviors, and identify whether each statement is true or false for you. Then, go to the key on the next page, and compute your level of risk for contracting an STI.

	True	False
1. I maintain a monogamous sexual relationship with a trusted partner.	___	___
2. I never engage in sexual activities without the use of a condom.	___	___
3. I never use alcohol or other drugs prior to sexual activities.	___	___
4. I am knowledgeable about the health risks associated with STIs.	___	___
5. I have a thorough knowledge about how all STIs are transmitted.	___	___
6. I do not share needles or syringes to inject drugs.	___	___
7. I am concerned about the risk of contracting an STI.	___	___
8. I always discuss STIs and "safe sex" with new partners prior to having sexual relations.	___	___
9. I always avoid sexual contact if I believe there is any risk of contracting an STI.	___	___
10. I believe that responsible "safe sex" is one of the best ways to reduce the chances of getting an STI.	___	___

Scoring and Interpretation

Count the number of "false" answers, and calculate your risk level for contracting an STI as follows:

0 "false" answers = low risk for infection with STI

1–3 "false" answers = high risk for infection with STI

4 or more "false" answers = very high risk for infection with STI

After calculating your risk, review all of the statements that you answered "false," and take action to correct this attitude or behavior so that you can respond "true" to these statements in the future. Answer the following questions to help you evaluate your sexual practices and think about STI prevention.

1. List three ways to bring up the subject of STIs with a new partner. How would you ask whether he or she has been exposed to any STIs or engaged in any risky behaviors?

_____

_____

_____

2. List three ways to bring up the subject of condom use with your partner. How might you convince someone to use a condom who does not want to?

_____

_____

_____

3. If you had an STI in the past that you might still possibly pass on (e.g., herpes), how would you tell your partner(s), and what precautions would you take during each act of sexual activity?

_____

_____

_____

Addiction and Substance Abuse

15

true or false?

1. A person can become addicted to a behavior.

2. Preventing an addiction is much easier than treating it.

3. Most college students binge drink at least once a week.

4. Nicotine is the addictive substance found in tobacco products.

5. Anabolic steroids promote the development of male sexual characteristics in both males and females.

Answers appear on the next page.

Have you smoked a cigarette, drunk alcohol to the point of intoxication, or gotten "high" sometime in the last month? If so, you may not think of yourself as addicted to these substances, and you may be right. However, regular use of substances such as these can lead to abuse of the substance, such that it affects a person's life and relationships. If you've ever had to skip class or call in sick at work because of a hangover, or if you've experienced a "blackout" where you were unable to remember what you did, said, or had done to you while you were drinking or using drugs, you have engaged in substance abuse. Many people think that such behaviors are a regular part of college life, but the reality is that not all college-aged individuals engage in these behaviors.

For those who do use and abuse alcohol, drugs, or tobacco, the short- and long-term consequences can directly affect health and, in some cases, can be deadly. In this chapter, we will discuss the nature of substance abuse and addiction, as well as specific, commonly used psychoactive drugs. We will also discuss strategies to avoid substance abuse. We begin by exploring the nature of addiction.

What Is Addiction?

The term **addiction** refers to a habitual psychological and physical dependence on a substance or practice that is beyond voluntary control (1). Specific addictive behaviors are often associated with the following traits (2):

- *Reinforcement leading to craving.* Repeated behaviors that produce pleasurable emotional states reinforce the behavior. This repeated reinforcement can lead to a craving to engage in a particular behavior.
- *Loss of control.* Addictive behaviors lead to a loss of self-control, and the individual loses the ability to resist engaging in the activity.
- *Escalation.* Many addictive behaviors are associated with an increased need for the behavior. That is, as the person repeats the addictive behavior, higher levels of the substance or activity are required to provide the same level of satisfaction.
- *Negative outcomes.* In all cases, addictive unhealthy behavior is associated with negative consequences, such as impairment in physical or mental health.

Because **denial** is often a characteristic of addiction, many people won't see their behaviors as destructive or seek treatment on their own. Family members, friends, or co-workers may need to persuade the user to undergo screening for addiction. In all cases, preventing an addiction is much easier than treating it.

Answers

1. **TRUE** Addiction is a state in which a person cannot control his or her actions. It is possible for a person to become addicted to behaviors such as gambling, shopping, or even playing video games.

2. **TRUE** Whether the addiction is to alcohol, tobacco, or gambling, abstaining in the first place is easier than treating the symptoms of physical and psychological dependence.

3. **FALSE** Although many people assume that all college students overindulge in alcohol, only about 20–28%—less than a third—of college students engage in binge drinking at all.

4. **TRUE** Nicotine, found in cigarettes, cigars, pipes, and other tobacco products, is a highly addictive substance that is absorbed in the lungs from the tobacco smoke or in the mouth from chewed tobacco.

5. **TRUE** Anabolic steroids are synthetic versions of the male sex hormone testosterone. For men, anabolic steroids can cause the testicles to shrink, reduce sperm count, increase the risk of prostate cancer, and lead to infertility, baldness, and the development of breasts. For women, anabolic steroids can cause the growth of facial hair, baldness, changes in or cessation of the menstrual cycle, enlargement of the clitoris, and a deepened voice.

Addiction Can Involve a Substance or Behavior

Almost anything can be addicting. In addition to substances such as drugs, alcohol, and tobacco (which we will discuss at length in the next section), people can become addicted to behaviors such as gambling, Internet usage, pornography, sex, gaming, eating, and exercising. The key is an inability to control their behavior. People addicted to exercise, for example, may struggle with guilt and anxiety if they miss a workout. Many compulsive exercisers do so to feel more in control of their lives.

Another potentially addictive behavior that has come under scrutiny in recent years is playing video games. Spending a lot of time playing video games does not necessarily qualify as an addiction, but an individual who cannot control the impulse for gaming has become addicted. Gaming becomes an escape from real-life problems, and the individual withdraws from other activities and social networks. The isolation that the person experiences can jeopardize jobs and relationships as he or she spends more and more time gaming.

An estimated 2 million American adults become compulsive gamblers at some point in their lifetime. Compulsive gambling is technically classified as an impulse-control disorder (3), but it is similar to gaming and other addictive behaviors because the individual cannot resist the temptation or drive to gamble. In men, compulsive gambling typically starts in adolescence, whereas women tend to start later in life (3).

Compulsive shoppers and spenders share the same characteristics as compulsive gamblers. They shop to feel better, but often the compulsive spending makes them feel worse. Women with this compulsive disorder often have clothing and possessions that they have never used, with the price tags still attached. They are often in denial about the problem, and if family or friends complain about their purchases, they hide the things they buy.

The emotional and psychological dependence on these impulses will affect relationships, finances, and possibly even one's career. Avoiding these behaviors is the best strategy for preventing addiction, but because this may not always be possible, anyone who experiences the first sign of a problem needs to seek help.

Addiction Can Be Physical and/or Psychological

Addictions to substances such as drugs or alcohol often begin when an individual experiences a problem, discomfort, or some form of emotional or physical pain and looks for something to make him or her feel better. For example, moving away from home to attend col-

Not being able to control the amount of time spent playing video games or surfing the Internet can indicate an addiction to these behaviors.

lege may cause you to miss your friends and family. Establishing new friendships on campus takes time and may involve an occasional rejection. Someone who feels like an outsider in a new environment or has been rejected by a group he or she wishes to join may turn to drugs or alcohol to ease the loneliness or the sting of rejection. At first, the drugs or alcohol seem to work because they dull the pain the person is trying to escape. As the person continues taking the substance, the drugs or alcohol may feel like the solution to their discomfort. Soon, a **dependence** on the substance is the individual's coping strategy for other painful or uncomfortable situations.

addiction Habitual psychological and physical dependence on a substance or practice that is beyond voluntary control.

denial An unconscious defense mechanism used to control anxiety by denying the existence of important troublesome information.

dependence The condition of being influenced by or subservient to a substance or practice.

TABLE 15.1
Specific Drugs and Their Potential for Dependence

Drug	Potential for Physical Dependence	Potential for Psychological Dependence
Morphine	High	High
Codeine	Moderate	Moderate
Heroin	High	High
Methadone	High	High
Barbiturates	High	Moderate
Cocaine	Possible	High
Amphetamines	Possible	High
Methamphetamine	Possible	High
LSD	None	Unknown
Mescaline, peyote	None	Unknown
Ecstasy	Unknown	Unknown
Marijuana	Unknown	Moderate
Alcohol	Possible	Possible
Steroids	Possible	Possible
Nicotine	High	High

Source: U.S. Department of Health and Human Services and SAMHSA's National Clearinghouse for Alcohol and Drug Information. http://ncadi.samhsa.gov/govpubs/rpo926.

When drugs or alcohol are used on a regular basis, the body builds up a **tolerance** to them and needs more of the substance to achieve the same effects. Eventually, addiction results as the body cannot feel "normal" (physically and/or psychologically) without the substance. Because addiction can be a chronic relapsing disorder, meaning you tend to fall back into old addictive behaviors even after treatment, it is important to seek help and break the cycle as soon as possible.

The most serious forms of addiction involve **chemical dependence** to drugs or alcohol. Such a dependence means the body will experience physical **withdrawal symptoms** once the substance is no longer being taken. By the time a user develops a physical dependence on a drug, his or her body craves the drug and needs it to maintain equilibrium. When the user ceases to take the drug, withdrawal symptoms may include restlessness, bone and muscle pain, vomiting, and diarrhea. Such symptoms peak between 24 and 48 hours of stopping intake and may last a week or several months. The severity of withdrawal symptoms depends on the health of the person. Drugs that are known to cause a high amount of physical dependence in users include nicotine, cocaine, and alcohol.

Causes of Addiction

Addictions often result from numerous causes. With substance addiction, the type of drug can also play a role. Drugs vary in their potential for dependence, and some drugs, such as alcohol, heroin, and cocaine, can result in an addiction more quickly than others. Similarly, using tobacco products poses a great risk for dependence, because nicotine is a highly addictive drug (Table 15.1). By contrast, drugs such as marijuana and codeine are relatively less addictive. Cocaine and morphine also affect how the brain communicates with the nerve cells (4). In some cases, addictive behaviors such as drug abuse or gambling trigger the release of chemicals (neurotransmitters such as dopamine) in the brain, leading to a psychological "rush," or the sensation of pleasure (5).

In addition to the type of drug used, genetics, psychological makeup, and social factors also influence the risk of developing drug dependence. Research indicates that differences in brain chemistry and metabolism make some individuals more vulnerable to drug dependence (5). At present, the precise differences in brain chemistry and metabolism that contribute to increased risk of drug dependence remain unclear, and this topic remains an active area of research.

Personal characteristics such as poor coping skills, social environment (spending time with people who use drugs), and heredity can also play a role in the development of an addiction. Psychological risk factors for drug dependence include an inability to cope with stress or rejection, a strong need for excitement, and a tendency toward impulsive behavior. In this regard, people may turn to drugs to avoid coping with stress, rejection, or depression. Social risk factors such as easy access to drugs, strong peer pressure to use drugs, drug use in your family, and a low education level increase your risk of developing a dependence on drugs.

Drug use and abuse occurs in people of all ages, education and income levels, and ethnic groups. However, research shows that some people are more likely to try illegal drugs and are consequently at greater risk for drug abuse. For example, young men with risk-taking personalities and a strong apathy toward school are at high risk for experimenting with drugs (6). In contrast, drug use is less common in individuals who are independent thinkers and are not easily influenced by their peers. Further, compared to individuals who are uninterested in schoolwork, individuals who attend school regularly and earn good grades are less likely to try illegal drugs.

Although brain chemistry, personality traits, and social factors do play a role in the development of some addictions, people are ultimately responsible for their own behavior, particularly in the early stages of experimentation with drugs, and must therefore take ownership of any addictive behaviors they exhibit. Making personal decisions not to experiment with potentially addictive substances or behaviors is the key to prevention. Further, recognizing the difference between a healthy habit and an addictive, unhealthy behavior is important to prevent addiction.

Substance Use versus Substance Abuse

An individual can abuse a substance even if there is no full-blown addiction. There are many substances that are misused and abused without necessarily leading to addiction. In fact, you can think of the levels of drug use as a continuum, with complete abstinence at one end, progressing to occasional use, then to abuse, and leading eventually to addiction. **Substance abuse** occurs when use of a drug interferes with other areas of one's life, for example, grades, work, relationships, or legal issues.

The American Psychiatric Association defines substance abuse as one or more of the following traits (2):

- Recurrent drug use, resulting in failure to perform major responsibilities at work, home, or school
- Continued drug use despite social or personal problems caused by the effects of the drug

- Recurrent drug use in a situation where the drug imposes physical danger to the individual (e.g., drug use before driving a car)
- Recurrent legal problems associated with drug use

Many people who engage in intermittent use of drugs may not exhibit any of the above traits on a regular basis. However, intermittent drug use has been shown to lead to drug abuse and is a warning sign to stop this type of behavior before the problem escalates.

Make sure you know...

> Addiction is a compulsive psychological need for a drug or other behaviors.
> In addition to drugs, alcohol, and tobacco, people can become addicted to video games, gambling, shopping, using the Internet, and other behaviors.
> Drugs vary in their potential for dependence. Highly addictive drugs include nicotine, cocaine, alcohol, and heroin.
> Addictions are often the result of several causes, including characteristics such as poor coping skills, environment, and heredity. Factors that determine risk for drug addiction are the type of drug used, genetics, psychological makeup, and social factors.
> Recognizing the difference between a healthy habit and an addictive, unhealthy behavior is important in preventing addiction.

What Substances Are Commonly Abused?

Alcohol abuse and the use of **illicit drugs** are two of the biggest substance problems in the United States today. Millions of Americans abuse alcohol and use illicit

tolerance The ability to endure the action of a drug continuously or in large doses without injurious effects.

chemical dependence A physical and psychological habituation to a mood- or mind-altering drug, such as alcohol or cocaine.

withdrawal symptoms Substance-specific symptoms that follow the cessation of, or reduction in, intake of a substance previously used regularly.

substance abuse The use of illegal drugs, the inappropriate use of legal drugs, and/or the repeated use of drugs to produce pleasure, to alleviate stress, or to alter or avoid reality.

illicit drugs Illegal drugs belonging to one of nine categories, including marijuana, cocaine, heroin, hallucinogens, inhalants; and the nonmedical use of prescription-type pain relievers, tranquilizers, stimulants, and sedatives.

Psychoactive drugs can be ingested, smoked, injected, or inhaled using a variety of devices. Drugs that are injected or inhaled enter the blood more quickly than drugs that are ingested, and therefore their effects are felt more quickly.

drugs, which include marijuana, cocaine, heroin, hallucinogens, inhalants, and prescription-type pain relievers, tranquilizers, stimulants, and sedatives (7). In addition to the psychological and/or physical dependence, abuse of alcohol or recreational drugs increases your risk of accidents and may damage your health.

Psychoactive Drugs

Any drug that causes a user to experience an altered state of consciousness—that is, to feel "high"—is a **psychoactive drug.** Soon after ingestion, injection, or inhalation, psychoactive drugs cross the blood–brain barrier. Users typically report feeling a surge of pleasurable sensation — a "rush." The intensity of the rush depends on how much drug is taken and how rapidly the drug enters the brain. Drugs that enter the brain rapidly, such as opiates (including heroin and morphine), can be particularly potent. Alcohol, nicotine, opiates, marijuana, hallucinogens (such as LSD and Ecstasy), and numerous other drugs are all psychoactive drugs (Table 15.2 on pages 420–421).

Examples of Psychoactive Drugs The most commonly abused drugs in the United States among individuals aged 18–25 are marijuana, prescription medications, cocaine, Ecstasy, alcohol, and tobacco (7). The physical effects associated with a **marijuana** "high" are produced by the chemical tetrahydrocannabinol (THC). The higher the THC concentration, the greater the effect. The THC content varies between 0.5% and 3%, with the average percentage of THC in marijuana sold in the United States at about 1% (8). Marijuana is most often smoked in pipes or in hand-rolled cigarettes (joints) or cigars (blunts). Effects are generally felt within 15 to 30 minutes and usually disappear within 2 to 3 hours.

Marijuana is classified as a stimulant, and its immediate effects are increased heart rate and blood pressure, bloodshot eyes, and dry mouth and throat. Evidence suggests that acute use of marijuana increases the risk of stroke in male adolescent users (9). Use of marijuana also impairs motor coordination and may increase your risk of accidents. Further, acute use of marijuana alters the normal function of memory centers in the brain. This memory loss resembles that observed in normal aging. However, whether these changes in function put long-term marijuana users at risk for early mental disorders is not clear.

The use of **cocaine** ("coke") in the United States increased dramatically during the 1980s, and today more than 5 million Americans use the drug annually. Between 1990 and 2000, Americans spent $35 billion to $70 billion yearly on cocaine (10). One survey suggests that as many as 6% of college students have experimented with cocaine, which makes cocaine the third most widely used drug by college students (1).

Cocaine is a powerful stimulant derived from the leaves of the coca shrub, which grows primarily in the Andes Mountains in South America. Cocaine is extracted from the coca leaves and produces a white powder that looks similar to sugar. Varying the extraction process can produce several different forms of cocaine, such as crack cocaine, rock cocaine, or freebase cocaine.

Common methods of taking cocaine include snorting, smoking, and intravenous injection. All routes of administration result in a rapid and short-lived high that generally lasts from 5 to 20 minutes. Cocaine is a highly addictive drug; when the cocaine high disappears, the user wants more. Spending over $1500 per day for cocaine is not uncommon for an addict. Cocaine addicts often suffer psychological damage, which eventually contributes to loss of jobs and financial ruin.

Cocaine is both an anesthetic and a central nervous system stimulant that increases heart rate and blood pressure. Other effects include a feeling of euphoria, heightened self-confidence, and increased alertness (11). In large doses, cocaine is extremely dangerous, and many people have died as a result of an overdose.

Another group of psychoactive drugs that have widespread popularity—the "club drugs"—includes several substances that young adults use at all-night dance parties ("raves" or "trances"), such as Ecstasy, gamma-hydroxybutyrate (GHB), ketamine, Rohypnol, methamphetamine, and LSD. The use of these drugs can cause serious health problems and in some cases can be fatal. Moreover, when club drugs are taken in combination with alcohol, the dangers are multiplied.

One particular club drug, methamphetamine, is a very addictive stimulant and is chemically related to amphetamines, but it is longer lasting, more potent, and more harmful to the central nervous system (CNS) (6). Methamphetamine is legally available only through a prescription that cannot be refilled. It has been manufactured in small, illegal laboratories, where its production endangers not only the people in the labs, but also neighbors and the environment. Short-term effects of methamphetamine include increased wakefulness, increased physical activity, decreased appetite, increased respiration, rapid heart beat, increased blood pressure, and hyperthermia. Cardiovascular collapse and death can occur from a single dose.

In addition to the "street drugs" that we often associate with drug abuse, there are numerous prescription medications that can also be highly addictive, on which people can become both psychologically and physically dependent. One example is the prescription painkiller OxyContin. The illegal use of this habit-forming drug, which was developed to ease the suffering of patients with painful diseases such as cancer, has grown markedly across the United States. Its addictive qualities have led to abuse among some recreational users; many have overdosed on this powerful painkiller, and others have turned to crime to feed their expensive habits.

Some people also misuse over-the-counter drugs to get a cheap high. Items such as cough suppressants and expectorants (which can contain as much as 40% alcohol) are sometimes ingested to achieve the same effects as derived from drinking alcohol. Cough and cold medications often contain dextromethorphan (DXM), a synthetic drug that is chemically similar to morphine. These medications are usually used successfully to treat cold symptoms and do not lead to addiction, but they can be misused to achieve other purposes. Chronic misuse of these substances may lead to dependence and have long-term adverse health effects.

Recovery from addiction to any psychoactive drug often requires professional help. For information on drug treatment programs, consult the National Institute on Drug Abuse website, www.nida.nih.gov.

Health Effects of Psychoactive Drug Use

Long-term use of marijuana can result in psychological dependence, and regular smoking of it causes lung damage similar to that caused by smoking tobacco (8). In fact, marijuana users usually inhale more deeply and hold their breath longer than tobacco smokers do, thereby increasing the lungs' exposure to carcinogenic smoke. The effect of long-term marijuana use on the heart is not well known; however, many investigators believe that marijuana increases the workload on the heart, which may eventually result in damage.

Some of the long-term complications from cocaine use are cardiovascular effects, including disturbances

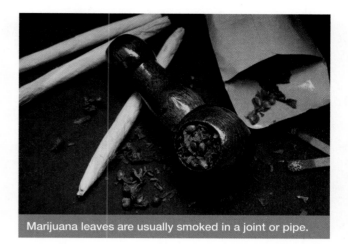

Marijuana leaves are usually smoked in a joint or pipe.

in heart rhythm and heart attacks; respiratory effects, such as chest pain and respiratory failure; neurological effects, including strokes, seizures, and headaches; and gastrointestinal complications, including abdominal pain and nausea. Long-term use of methamphetamines can result in paranoia, aggressiveness, extreme anorexia, memory loss, visual and auditory hallucinations, delusions, and severe dental problems.

Drug use by pregnant women can have serious health effects on the developing fetus. Prenatal exposure to marijuana results in the baby having weak responses to visual stimuli, increased tremulousness, and a high-pitched cry, which may indicate problems with neurological development. Many scientific studies have documented that babies born to mothers who abuse cocaine during pregnancy (so called "crack babies") are often delivered prematurely, have low birth weight, have smaller head circumference, and are shorter in length. Crack babies were once believed to suffer from severe, irreversible damage, such as reduced intelligence and social skills. Later research found that to be an exaggeration; however, crack babies do exhibit subtle, yet significant, deficits in cognitive performance, attention to tasks, and information processing. Babies born to women who used heroin and were treated with methadone while pregnant require treatment for withdrawal symptoms after birth.

psychoactive drugs   Pharmacological agents that alter mood, anxiety, behavior, cognitive processes, or mental tension.

marijuana   A psychoactive plant mixture (stems, leaves, or seeds) from either the *Cannabis sativa* or *Cannabis indica* (hemp) plants.

cocaine   A powerful stimulant derived from the leaves of the South American coca shrub.

TABLE 15.2
Commonly Abused Drugs and Their Effects

Drug (Classification)	How Administered	Intoxication Effects	Health Effects
Heroin (opiate)	Injected, smoked, snorted	Pain relief, euphoria, drowsiness, staggering gait	Nausea, constipation, confusion, sedation, respiratory depression and arrest, tolerance, addiction, unconsciousness, coma, death
Opium (opiate)	Swallowed, smoked	Same as for heroin	Same as for heroin
Cocaine (stimulant)	Injected, smoked, snorted	Increased heart rate, blood pressure, metabolism; feelings of exhilaration, energy; increased mental alertness; increased temperature	Rapid or irregular heart beat, reduced appetite, weight loss, heart failure, nervousness, insomnia
Methamphetamine (stimulant)	Injected, swallowed, smoked, snorted	Same as for cocaine, plus: aggression, violence, psychotic behavior	Same as for cocaine, plus: memory loss, cardiac and neurological damage; impaired memory and learning; tolerance, addiction
Nicotine (stimulant)	Smoked, snorted, taken in snuff and spit tobacco	Same as for cocaine	Same as for cocaine, plus: adverse pregnancy outcomes, chronic lung disease, cardiovascular disease, stroke, cancer, tolerance, addiction
Marijuana (cannabinoid)	Swallowed or smoked	Euphoria, slowed thinking and reaction time, confusion, impaired balance and coordination	Cough, frequent respiratory infections, impaired memory and learning, increased heart rate, anxiety, panic attacks, tolerance, addiction

Alcohol

Alcohol (ethyl alcohol) is the most widely used recreational drug in the United States, and the most popular drug on college campuses—it's used three times as much as marijuana and 20 times as much as cocaine (7). An estimated 64% of college students in the United States use alcohol, and some 38–44% abuse it (7). Full-time college students are more likely to use alcohol, binge drink, and drink heavily than are part-time college students and people of the same age who do not attend college (7).

Although many people consume alcohol to "get high," alcohol is actually a central nervous system depressant that slows down the function of the brain. This depressive effect results in impaired vision, slowed reaction time, and impaired motor coordination (12). Overconsumption of alcohol also impairs judgment. By decreasing the fear of dan-

CONSIDER THIS!

An estimated 1700 college students between 18 and 24 die each year from alcohol-related unintentional injuries, including motor vehicle crashes.

ger, it can encourage risk-taking behaviors (such as driving too fast), which increases the likelihood of accidents (12). Drinking too much can also increase the risk of poor judgment in social situations and in making decisions concerning sexual behavior.

The blood level of alcohol determines the magnitude of central nervous system depression by the drug. The **blood alcohol concentration (BAC)** is determined by the amount of alcohol consumed, body weight, and the rate of alcohol metabolism by the body. For example, if two men of different weights (e.g., 200 pounds versus 150 pounds) consume the same amount of alcohol, the smaller individual will have the higher BAC. This is also the reason that women feel the effects of alcohol sooner than men do. Their lighter body weights and higher percentages of body fat lead to greater concentrations of alcohol in their nervous systems.

TABLE 15.2   *(continued)*

Drug (Classification)	How Administered	Intoxication Effects	Health Effects
Lysergic acid diethylamide, also known as LSD (hallucinogen)	Swallowed, absorbed through mouth tissues	Altered state of perception and feeling	Persisting perception disorder (flashbacks); increased body temperature, heart rate, and blood pressure; loss of appetite; sleeplessness; numbness, weakness, tremors
Dextromethorphan, also known as DXM (narcotic)	Swallowed (found in some cough and cold medications)	Distorted visual perceptions to complete dissociative effects	At high doses, memory loss, numbness, nausea/vomiting
Anabolic steroids (hormones)	Injected, swallowed, applied to the skin	No intoxication	Hypertension, blood clotting, and cholesterol changes; liver cysts and cancer; kidney cancer; hostility and aggression; acne; in adolescents: premature stoppage of growth; in men: prostate cancer, reduced sperm production, shrunken testicles, breast enlargement; in women: menstrual irregularities, development of beard and other masculine characteristics
Laughing gas, whippets (inhalants)	Inhaled through nose or mouth	Stimulation, loss of inhibition; headache, nausea/vomiting, slurred speech, loss of motor coordination	Unconsciousness, cramps, weight loss, muscle weakness, depression, memory impairment, damage to cardiovascular and nervous systems, sudden death
Ecstasy, also known as MDMA (methylene dioxymethamphetamine) (stimulant)	Taken orally in tablet form	Feelings of well-being, mental stimulation; distortion in time and other sensory perceptions	Increase in body temperature, leading to kidney failure; increase in heart rate and blood pressure; heart wall stress

Source: Adapted from National Institute on Drug Abuse, Commonly abused drugs. www.drugabuse.gov/drugpages/dRugsofabuse.html.

Alcohol is metabolized in the liver, and, in general, the body can remove 0.3 ounce of alcohol per hour. In practical terms, this rate of removal is approximately half of one drink (Figure 15.1) per hour. An individual who drinks slowly, that is, less than one drink per hour, can maintain a relatively low BAC. In contrast, someone who drinks rapidly, consuming more than two drinks per hour, will increase his or her BAC to higher levels, leading toward intoxication.

Even low doses of alcohol can have significant behavioral and physical effects (Table 15.3). For instance, relatively small amounts of alcohol in your blood can decrease your level of alertness and increase your risk of injury (12). Higher doses can lead to impaired motor skills and slowed reaction times (13). These negative physical effects are the reason that state laws specify the legal level of blood alcohol for driving. Because

FIGURE 15.1
Ethyl alcohol is the psychoactive ingredient of all alcoholic beverages. A standard drink is defined as a 12-ounce beer, a 1.5-ounce cocktail drink, or a 5-ounce glass of wine. Each of these contains approximately 0.6 ounces of ethyl alcohol.

blood alcohol concentration (BAC)   The concentration of alcohol in the blood measured as a percentage by mass, by mass per volume, or a combination of both. A BAC of 0.20% can mean 2 grams of alcohol per 1000 grams of an individual's blood, or it can mean 0.2 gram of alcohol per 100 milliliters of blood.

TABLE 15.3
Behavioral and Physiological Effects of Alcohol

Blood Alcohol Concentration (BAC)	Behavioral and Physiological Effects	Hours Required to Metabolize Alcohol
0.0–0.5%	Increased relaxation, feeling of euphoria, and decreased alertness.	2–3
0.05–0.10%	Reduced social inhibition and impairment in reaction time and motor skills. This level of alcohol may significantly impact driving skills. Many states define legally drunk as a BAC of 0.08% or higher.	4–6
0.10–0.15%	Increased impairment in reaction time and motor skills. Loss of peripheral vision.	6–10
0.15–0.30%	Difficulty walking, slurred speech, impaired pain perception, and impairment in other sensory perceptions.	10–24
More than 0.30%	Can result in unconsciousness. Death possible at BAC levels of 0.35% or more. These levels of BAC are generally achieved by binge drinking.	More than 24

Source: Data from Ogden, E., and H. Moskowitz. Effects of alcohol and other drugs on driver performance. *Traffic Injury Prevention* 5(3):185–198, September 2004.

0.05–0.10% BAC results in significant impairment in reaction times and motor skills, all states have established 0.08% BAC as the legal definition for alcohol intoxication (13, 14).

Alcohol Abuse versus Alcohol Addiction
Not everyone who uses alcohol will abuse it or become addicted to it, and many Americans drink moderate amounts of alcohol occasionally, or on a regular basis, without suffering any ill health effects. However, because alcohol is widely available and affordable, it is one of the most significant drug problems in our society. Alcohol addiction is a very real problem for many people, and it can happen to anyone.

Alcohol abuse is a difficult phrase to define, because the abuse tends to be in the eye of the beholder. On the one hand, for many individuals whose religion requires abstinence, simply tasting an alcoholic beverage constitutes alcohol abuse. Similarly, anyone who drinks any amount of alcohol without being of legal drinking age is abusing it. On the other hand, some college students may believe that heavy drinking is simply a way of having a good time.

The American Psychiatric Association has defined *alcohol abuse* according to the following four abuse criteria: alcohol use in hazardous situations, alcohol-related school or work problems, recurrent interpersonal problems, and recurrent legal problems (2).

Drinking too much and/or drinking too often are major contributors to alcohol abuse.

Alcohol abuse is particularly harmful when it prevents the drinker from meeting work, school, or family responsibilities, and it can also be deadly. Approximately 1700 college students between the ages of 18 and 24 die each year as a result of alcohol abuse (15). In addition, consuming alcohol during pregnancy has been linked to alcohol-related birth defects, such as mental retardation.

Alcoholism, also known as *alcohol dependence*, is a disease that involves craving alcohol and not being able to control the impulse to drink — in other words, an addiction. Alcoholics develop a physical dependence on the alcohol as their tolerance to the drug increases over time. Addiction to alcohol may have hereditary, psychological, and environmental components. Treatment for alcoholism involves medication and counseling to help a person stop drinking. Three oral medications, disulfiram (Antabuse), naltrexone (Depade, ReVia), and acamprosate (Campral) are currently approved to treat alcohol dependence. These medications have been shown to help alcohol-dependent people reduce their drinking, avoid relapse, and achieve and maintain abstinence. They are not a "magic bullet," because no single medication works in every case and for every person. There is no cure for alcoholism, and once a person has stopped drinking, he must avoid all alcohol for life or suffer the possibility of a relapse with the next drink.

Unfortunately, alcohol abuse and alcohol addiction are not unknown among college students. A 2002 survey of more than 14,000 students at 119 four-year colleges showed that 31 percent of college students met the criteria for a diagnosis of alcohol abuse, and 6 percent for a diagnosis of alcohol dependence (16). Nearly 10% of college men under age 24 and nearly 5% of college women under age 24 met a 12-month diagnosis of alcohol dependence. Despite the prevalence of alcohol disorders on college campuses, few students reported having sought treatment for alcohol dependence.

Binge Drinking   One common type of alcohol abuse among college students is **binge drinking.** Binge drinking often begins around age 13, peaks between 18 and 22, and then gradually decreases over time (17). Binge drinking is associated with a wide array of social, emotional, behavioral, and health problems. Bars and alcohol distributors in college towns often provide easy access to cheap alcohol, which promotes binge drinking. In one study, binge drinking among college students aged 18–22 was reported to be around 44%, compared to 38% in people of the same age who were not enrolled full time in college (7). Students who live in fraternity or sorority houses tend to be the heaviest drinkers on campus, perhaps in response to the number of social events they host that include alcohol. Drinking games and tournaments, such as beer pong, encourage consumption of excessive amounts of alcohol over a short time period.

Alcohol poisoning, a severe and potentially fatal physical reaction to an alcohol overdose, is the most serious consequence of binge drinking. Approximately 300 deaths annually are due to alcohol-related injuries that include alcohol poisoning (16). A BAC of 0.35% or above can result in alcohol poisoning and death. Anyone who drinks to the point of unconsciousness may vomit and inhale the vomit, leading to asphyxiation, or may stop breathing. An individual whose breathing becomes too shallow (fewer than eight breaths per minute) or who cannot be awakened with shouting or shaking should be treated immediately by medical personnel, because this is a life-threatening medical emergency.

Drinking games, such as those played at many college parties, contribute to the incidence of binge drinking among this population.

CONSIDER THIS!

In a national study, 91% of women and 78% of men who were frequent binge drinkers considered themselves to be moderate or light drinkers.

Most people who binge drink are not alcohol dependent; however, a consistent pattern of alcohol abuse can result in a need to drink more in order to feel the effects of the drug, which can lead to dependence on the drug.

Use the Steps for Behavior Change box on page 424 to get a sense of your drinking habits and to determine whether you may be abusing alcohol. You can do a more detailed assessment of your drinking habits by answering the questions in Laboratory 15.1 on page 433. If you feel that you might be drinking too much, seek professional help from your health care provider or an organization such as Alcoholics Anonymous.

Health Effects of Alcohol Abuse   Chronic abuse of alcohol over a period of years can result in liver disease (e.g., cirrhosis), damage to the nervous system, and an increased risk of certain cancers (18). Development of liver disease due to years of drinking may eventually result in total liver failure and death. The damage to the nervous system that results from alcohol abuse is often localized to the left side of the brain, which is re-

alcoholism A chronic, progressive behavioral disorder characterized by a strong urge to consume alcohol and an inability to limit the amount of drinking despite adverse consequences.

binge drinking Drinking 5 or more drinks (for men) or 4 or more drinks (for women) at the same time or within a couple of hours of each other on at least 1 day in the past 30 days.

Children born with fetal alcohol syndrome exhibit several physical and mental effects.

sponsible for written and spoken language, logic, and mathematical skills. The degree of brain damage that occurs appears to be directly related to the amount of alcohol consumed (18). Further, repeated irritation of the gastrointestinal system by alcohol has been linked to cancers of the esophagus, pancreas, stomach, mouth, tongue, and liver. Another and often overlooked problem linked to chronic consumption of alcohol is malnutrition (see the Closer Look box on page 425).

Women who drink during pregnancy are subjecting the fetus to a wide range of preventable birth defects, including **fetal alcohol syndrome.** An estimated 1% of all live births show some alcohol-related prenatal damage, such as physical, behavioral, and learning problems. Babies born with fetal alcohol syndrome may have mild to severe learning disabilities and abnormal

STEPS FOR
BEHAVIOR CHANGE

Do you regularly abuse alcohol?

Take the following quiz to get a sense of your alcohol habits.

Y N

☐ ☐ Do you find it difficult to get through a week without drinking?

☐ ☐ Is going out with friends for the purpose of drinking a regular weekend event?

☐ ☐ Do you and/or your friends engage in foolish or dangerous behavior while intoxicated?

☐ ☐ Would your grades or class attendance be better if you drank less alcohol?

☐ ☐ Do you regularly "black out" from drinking too much, such that you don't remember periods of time?

If you answered yes to any of the above, you've engaged in at least one episode of alcohol abuse. Although this doesn't necessarily mean you will become addicted to alcohol, it does mean you should take measures to modify your behavior.

TIPS TO GAIN CONTROL OVER YOUR DRINKING HABITS

☑ Know your limits, and stay within them. If you are at a party and feel that you are drinking too much, learn to say no, dilute your drinks, or switch to a nonalcoholic beverage.

☑ When drinking, stick to the rule of less than 0.3 ounce (one drink) of alcohol per hour. This will reduce the likelihood that you will become physically or mentally impaired by alcohol.

☑ Wine, beer, and mixed drinks are less intoxicating than straight liquor. Stick to these more dilute drinks instead of the higher-alcohol beverages.

☑ Eating and drinking at the same time will slow the rate of alcohol absorption and reduce your chance of becoming impaired. Never drink on an empty stomach.

☑ When leaving a party or bar after drinking, don't drive; instead, call a cab, or have someone else—who is sober—drive you home.

A CLOSER LOOK

ALCOHOL ABUSE AND MALNUTRITION

Malnutrition is commonly associated with chronic alcohol abuse because the frequent presence of alcohol irritates the gastrointestinal system. An irritated gastric lining can result in impaired appetite, which in turn decreases food intake. A lowered food intake forces the body to function on a diet that is deficient in both calories and in essential nutrients such as protein and vitamins. In extreme cases, the resulting *undernutrition* can promote a loss of muscle mass and abnormal functioning of many body organs. Lack of vitamin A

may contribute to liver disease and other serious alcohol-related health problems. Lack of thiamin (vitamin B₁) has been associated with a degenerative brain disorder called Wernicke-Korsakoff syndrome. Alcohol abuse can also lead to *overnutrition*—and therefore contribute to overweight and obesity—because of its high calorie content. Remember, alcohol is not calorie-free, and mixed drinks in particular can approach the calorie levels of snacks and even desserts.

The best approach to dealing with alcohol-related malnutrition is to seek

professional help for alcoholism. In many cases, the cessation of alcohol abuse eliminates the alcohol-induced reduction in appetite, and the individual's return to normal eating habits provides the calories and nutrients needed for improved health. In severe cases of alcohol-related undernutrition, the advice of a physician and/or a nutritionist is required.

Source: National Institute of Neurological Disorders and Stroke. www.ninds.nih.gov; National Institute on Alcohol Abuse and Alcoholism (NIAAA). FAQs for the general public. www.niaaa.nih.gov/FAQs/General-English.

---

facial features (19). To prevent the effects of FAS, any woman who is pregnant, or thinks she may become pregnant, should abstain from consuming alcohol.

Tobacco

Nicotine, contained in tobacco products, is the most heavily used addictive drug in the United States. In 2006, 20.8% of all adults (45.3 million people) in the United States smoked cigarettes (20). Individuals aged 18–24 comprise an estimated 23.9% of all smokers (slightly more than 11 million people) (20). Cigarette smoking was found to be more common among men (23.9%) than women (18.0%). The good news is that smoking rates for young Americans are no longer climbing and have declined slightly from the peaks reached in the late 1990s. Nonetheless, a large number of Americans still use tobacco products.

Cigarette smoking has been the most popular method of nicotine use since the beginning of the 20th century (21). In 2007, cigarettes were by far the preferred tobacco product among youths aged 12–17, with 2.5 million (9.8%) having used cigarettes in the past month. Other tobacco usage included cigars (4.2%), smokeless tobacco (2.4%), and pipe tobacco (0.7%) (7). An average dose of nicotine is 1.8 mg per cigarette, compared to 3.6 mg in snuff, and 4.6 mg in chewing tobacco. A single cigar can contain nicotine levels ranging from the equivalent of one cigarette to an entire pack of cigarettes (22).

Cigarettes and other forms of tobacco, such as those found in snuff, chewing tobacco, pipes, and cigars, are associated with major health risks.

Nicotine Addiction   Nicotine provides an almost immediate "psychological kick" to the body because it causes the release of epinephrine from the adrenal cortex (located in an endocrine gland near the kidneys). This stimulates the central nervous system and increases both heart rate and blood pressure. This stimulation is lost rapidly, which leads to both depression and fatigue and causes the user to seek more nicotine.

Nicotine is absorbed readily from tobacco smoke in the lungs, and it does not matter whether the smoke comes from cigarettes, cigars, or pipes (21). Nicotine is also absorbed in the mouth when tobacco is chewed. With regular use of tobacco, nicotine can accumulate in the body and remain for several hours (21).

Clove cigarettes have been used as an alternative to tobacco products; however, clove cigarettes contain

fetal alcohol syndrome   A cluster of birth defects, which may include facial abnormalities, mental retardation, and growth problems, caused by alcohol consumption during pregnancy.

malnutrition   Poor nutrition due to an insufficient or poorly balanced diet or to faulty digestion or utilization of foods; can include *undernutrition,* or lack of sufficient nutrients, and *overnutrition,* or intake of too many calories.

nicotine   The addictive and psychoactive drug in tobacco plants.

Peer influence is one common reason that young people take up smoking.

about 60–70% tobacco and equal amounts of nicotine as do cigarettes (23). Exposure to tar, nicotine, and carbon monoxide is higher for smokers of clove cigarettes than for smokers of traditional tobacco cigarettes.

Addiction to nicotine results in withdrawal symptoms when a person tries to stop smoking. For example, studies indicate that when chronic smokers were deprived of cigarettes for 24 hours, they showed more anger, hostility, and aggression and less social cooperation (21). Further, people suffering from nicotine withdrawal take longer to regain emotional equilibrium following exposure to stress. Moreover, during periods of abstinence from smoking, smokers show a wide range of physical and mental impairments, such as impaired psychomotor skills (movement coordination) and impaired cognitive functions (21).

Studies have shown that some of the most successful long-term smoking cessation programs involve not only behavioral treatment (such as we discussed in Chapter 2) but also pharmacological treatment (21). Most pharmacological treatments involve nicotine gum or transdermal patches (placed on the skin) to deliver nicotine during the initial stages of smoking cessation. The success of smoking cessation treatment varies widely across studies. Generally, the rates of relapse for smoking cessation are highest in the first few weeks after smoking cessation and diminish greatly after about 3 months (21). So, if you smoke, it is possible to stop.

Secondhand Smoke   **Secondhand smoke** is a mixture of gases and particles from both burning tobacco products (also known as *sidestream smoke*) and smoke exhaled by smokers (also known as *mainstream smoke*). Secondhand smoke lingers in the air hours after cigarettes have been extinguished and contains toxic chemicals, more than 50 of which are known to

cause cancer. In addition to the absorption of nicotine from secondhand smoke, breathing secondhand smoke has immediate harmful effects on the cardiovascular system and can cause respiratory symptoms and slow lung growth in children. An estimated 150,000 to 300,000 new cases of bronchitis and pneumonia due to exposure to secondhand smoke have been diagnosed in American children under the age of 18 months (24). Additionally, secondhand smoke causes an estimated 3400 lung cancer deaths and 46,000 heart disease deaths in adult nonsmokers in the United States annually (25).

New legislation is being passed in almost every community in the United States to curb the exposure to secondhand smoke for all citizens. Smoking is banned in almost all government buildings, and many cities and states have passed legislation banning smoking in restaurants as well as bars. Because of these new laws, exposure rates to secondhand smoke have declined (20).

Health Effects of Tobacco Use   Tobacco smoking is the leading preventable cause of death in the United States and accounts for approximately one in every five deaths (438,000) per year (20). Cigarette smoking causes coronary heart disease, the leading cause of death in the United States, and doubles a person's chance for stroke (20). Regular tobacco use increases the risk of several forms of cancer, including cancers of the lung, larynx, esophagus, pancreas, bladder, and kidney (21). Compared to nonsmokers, men who smoke are 23 times more likely to develop lung cancer, and women who smoke are 13 times more likely (20). Tobacco use results in an annual cost of more than $96 billion in direct medical costs and $97 billion from loss of productivity (20).

Pregnant women who smoke are more likely to lose the baby during pregnancy or deliver the baby prematurely, before the lungs are fully developed. Children born to women who smoke are lower in birth weight and tend to develop more illnesses. The nicotine and other harmful chemicals in tobacco products are absorbed in the mother's bloodstream and pass through the placenta to the unborn child. Several of these chemicals may interfere with the developing baby's ability to get enough oxygen and nutrients in the womb, thus contributing to the low birth weight.

Caffeine

Caffeine is a bitter substance found in coffee, tea, soft drinks, chocolate, and certain medicines. Caffeine enters the bloodstream through the stomach and small intestine and can stimulate the central nervous system as soon as 15 minutes after it is consumed. For most people, the amount of caffeine in two to four cups of coffee a day is not harmful. When consumed in moderate doses, caffeine can increase alertness and give you an energy boost; however, too much caffeine can make you restless and irritable. Caffeine has also been associated with insomnia, headaches, and abnormal heart rhythms. Caffeine is eliminated slowly from the body and can remain in the body for hours. If you have trouble sleeping at night, try to avoid ingesting any product containing caffeine after 2:00 PM.

Some studies have shown that caffeine causes psychological dependence. However, there is no agreement on how much caffeine you would have to consume daily to become physically dependent on it. Even if you consume caffeine in moderate doses, you could get withdrawal symptoms when you stop using it. Typical withdrawal symptoms include headache, muscle pain, and fatigue. Some people may find that they are more sensitive to the effects of caffeine than others and should limit their use of caffeine. In addition, certain drugs and supplements may interact with caffeine. If you have questions about whether caffeine is safe for you, talk with your health care provider. See also the Closer Look box on page 428.

Make sure you know...

> Psychoactive drugs are those that cause a state of intoxication. Effects range from feelings of euphoria to increased heart rate, shallow breathing, a change in body temperature, and hallucinations.

> Commonly used psychoactive drugs include marijuana, cocaine, club drugs, alcohol, and tobacco. Common club drugs include Ecstasy, GHB, Rohypnol, ketamine, methamphetamine, and LSD.

> The most common recreational drug in the United States is alcohol, and it is estimated that over 85% of college students drink alcohol. Relatively low levels of blood alcohol (i.e., 0.05– 0.10%) can impair both reaction time and motor skills, resulting in a diminished ability to drive.

> Nicotine, the psychoactive drug in tobacco products, is one of the most addictive drugs available. Prolonged use of tobacco products can lead to numerous health problems, including an increased risk of heart disease and cancer. Babies born to mothers who smoked during pregnancy are at higher risk of having a low birth weight and developing more illnesses.

Anabolic Steroids

Anabolic steroids are the familiar name for synthetic substances related to male sex hormones (e.g., testosterone). Steroids are a class of drugs that are legally available only by prescription and are used primarily to treat conditions that occur when the body does not

produce enough testosterone, such as in delayed puberty and some types of impotence. Anabolic steroids can be taken orally in tablet or capsule form, injected directly into the muscle, or rubbed into the skin from ointment preparations.

During the 1930s, scientists discovered that anabolic steroids facilitated the growth of skeletal muscle in laboratory animals by mimicking the effect of naturally produced testosterone. This discovery led to abuse of these compounds first by bodybuilders and weight lifters and then by athletes in other sports. Doses taken by abusers for sports-related purposes can typically be 100 times more than the dosage used for treating legitimate medical conditions.

Long-term steroid use can have serious psychological side effects. Users become aggressive, developing extreme, uncontrolled bouts of anger known as "roid rage." Depression often results when the drugs are stopped and may contribute to dependence on anabolic steroids.

Anabolic steroids have been found to cause potentially fatal liver cysts and liver cancer, increased blood cholesterol levels, increased blood clotting, and increased hypertension, which can promote heart attack and stroke in both men and women. In boys and men, anabolic steroid abuse can reduce sperm production, shrink the testicles, lead to impotence, and cause baldness and irreversible breast enlargement (gynecomastia) (26). In girls and women, anabolic steroid abuse causes the development of masculine characteristics such as decreased body fat and breast size, deepened voice, excessive body hair growth, acne, male-pattern baldness, changes in the menstrual cycle, and enlargement of the clitoris (26).

About 3 million people use anabolic steroids, and one in four of these users started as a teenager (27). Some research has shown that 5% of teen boys and 2.5% of teen girls have used some form of anabolic steroids. Teenaged boys are more likely to use steroids to build muscle in the hopes that they will improve their athletic performance. Teenaged girls are more likely to use anabolic steroids as body-shaping drugs to increase their lean body mass (27). Regardless of the motive behind anabolic steroid use, these drugs are illegal and can do permanent damage to a person's health and negatively affect the reproductive system.

secondhand smoke The combination of smoke that comes from the burning end of a cigarette, cigar, or pipe and the smoke exhaled by the smoker.

caffeine A stimulant found in a wide variety of common foods such as coffee, tea, and chocolate.

anabolic steroids Synthetic hormones related to the male sex hormone testosterone.

A CLOSER LOOK

THE EFFECTS OF CAFFEINE

Caffeine is a stimulant found in a wide variety of common foods, including coffee, tea, and cocoa (see the table), and it is one of the most frequently ingested psychoactive drugs in the world (29). Caffeine affects the central nervous system by stimulating a variety of brain centers, increasing alertness and decreasing drowsiness (30). In fact, caffeine has been shown to reduce fatigue and improve performance during prolonged endurance exercise (e.g., running a marathon) (31, 32). Evidence that caffeine may improve endurance exercise performance has prompted the International Olympic Committee to consider banning high blood levels of caffeine during performance in the Olympic games.

As with other habit-forming drugs, chronic use of caffeine can lead to addiction (29, 30). Abrupt discontinuation of caffeine intake can result in severe headache, fatigue, irritability, and gastrointestinal distress. Nonetheless, cessation of caffeine use has been shown to be considerably easier than cessation of other stimulants, such as nicotine (28).

There is no consensus whether long-term use of caffeine poses a significant health risk. However, one review concluded that moderate daily intake of caffeine (less than 400 mg/day) is not associated with adverse health effects (29). Nonetheless, high doses of caffeine (500 mg or more) can increase both heart rate and blood pressure, and in some people, caffeine increases the risk of abnormal heart rhythms (30). Further, for people unaccustomed to caffeine or who consume caffeine in large doses, it can produce tremors, nervousness, restlessness, and insomnia. Therefore, people who consume caffeine should do so only in moderation.

Caffeine may have health effects during pregnancy. Some studies suggest that higher intake of caffeine (about three or more 8-ounce cups of coffee a day) may increase the risk of miscarriage and of low birth weight in the infant (33). However, small amounts of caffeine (about one to two 8-ounce cups of coffee a day) appear to be safe during pregnancy.

Caffeine Content of Popular Foods and Nonprescription Drugs

Food or Nonprescription Drug	Serving Size	Caffeine (mg)
Coffee (drip method)	8 fluid ounces	85
Coffee (instant)	8 fluid ounces	62
Coffee (decaffeinated)	8 fluid ounces	3
Espresso coffee (brewed)	8 fluid ounces	502
Tea (bag or loose)	8 fluid ounces	47
Tea (decaffeinated)	8 fluid ounces	3
Tea (herbal)	8 fluid ounces	0
Cocoa	8 fluid ounces	5
Chocolate milk	8 fluid ounces	5
Mountain Dew (soft drink)	12 fluid ounces	54
Coca Cola (soft drink)	12 fluid ounces	46
Dr. Pepper (soft drink)	12 fluid ounces	40
Pepsi Cola (soft drink)	12 fluid ounces	38
Root beer, ginger ale (soft drink)	12 fluid ounces	0
Red Bull (energy drink)	8.3 fluid ounces	80
SoBe No Fear (energy drink)	8 fluid ounces	83
Full Throttle (energy drink)	16 fluid ounces	144
Milk chocolate	1 ounce serving	6
Dark chocolate	1.45 ounce serving	31
NoDoz (Maximum Strength)	1 tablet or capsule	200
Vivarin	1 tablet or capsule	200
Excedrin (Extra Strength)	2 tablets	130

Sources: U.S. Department of Agriculture National Nutrient Database for Standard Reference, Release 18. November 2005; American Beverage Association, www.ameribev.org., accessed August 2007.

Make sure you know...

> Anabolic steroids are a class of synthetic substances related to the male sex hormone testerosterone.

> Although there are legitimate medical uses of anabolic steroids, abuse of them for bodybuilding or for improving sport performance can lead to harmful health effects, including psychological problems (e.g., rage and aggression) and physical side effects (e.g., changes in sexual characteristics and an impaired reproductive system).

Strategies to Avoid Drug Abuse

Avoiding drug use requires self discipline and control. Several steps can help protect you from the temptation to use drugs (28):

1. *Increase your self-esteem.* Take pride in yourself and your achievements. This will boost your confidence and improve your ability to say no to drugs.

2. *Learn how to cope with stress.* When you are stressed, use one or more of the stress management techniques discussed in Chapter 10 (such as exercise or progressive relaxation).

3. *Develop numerous interests.* Find and participate in new hobbies or sports that you enjoy.

4. *Practice assertiveness.* Becoming assertive is an important key to being able to decline drug use.

Summary

1. Alcohol, nicotine (tobacco products), marijuana, and cocaine are the most widely used and abused drugs in the United States. Alcohol is the single most common recreational drug used in the United States.

2. Use of alcohol, marijuana, and cocaine increases your risk of accidents, and prolonged use of these substances may result in psychological dependence, physical addiction, and damaged health.

3. Chronic abuse of alcohol can result in liver disease, damage to the nervous system, increased risk of certain cancers, and malnutrition. Blood alcohol concentrations of 0.05–0.10% can significantly reduce reaction time and impair motor skills.

4. Long-term use of marijuana may result in psychological dependence and may increase your risk of cardiopulmonary diseases.

5. Cocaine is a highly addictive drug that, when taken in large doses, can be lethal.

6. Use of tobacco can lead to an addiction to nicotine, and prolonged use of tobacco products can lead to numerous health problems, including increased risk of heart attack, stroke, and cancer.

7. Caffeine is a central nervous system stimulant found in numerous common foods and beverages. Whether chronic consumption of caffeine is a significant health risk is currently unclear.

8. Long-term use of anabolic steroids can cause psychological side effects, such as aggression and uncontrolled bouts of anger. In men, anabolic steroids also lead to shrunken testicles, reduced sperm count, breast development, infertility, and increased risk of prostate cancer. In women, use of anabolic steroids can cause the growth of facial hair, male-pattern baldness, changes in the menstrual cycle, enlargement of the clitoris, and a deepened voice.

9. You can decrease your risk of using drugs by increasing your self-esteem, learning how to cope with stress, developing numerous interests, and practicing assertiveness.

Study Questions

1. A key factor in preventing drug addiction is to
   a. know when to quit.
   b. use the drug only in a social setting.
   c. control the amount of drug you use.
   d. abstain from drug use.
   e. seek counseling.

2. Identify one trait that is *not* associated with addictive behavior.
   a. escalation of drug use
   b. loss of control
   c. craving the drug
   d. denying that there is a problem
   e. All of the above traits are associated with addictive behavior

3. Complete this sentence: One key factor that determines your risk for drug addiction is
   a. the type of drug used.
   b. how the drug enters your body.
   c. the cost of the drug.
   d. the time of day the drug is used.

4. Babies born to mothers who drink alcohol while pregnant tend to have
   a. autism.
   b. low birth weight.
   c. vision and hearing problems.
   d. respiratory problems.
   e. None of the above
5. Secondhand smoke is derived from
   a. exhaled smoke.
   b. smoke from burning tobacco products.
   c. smoke from industrial chimneys.
   d. smoke from wood-burning fireplaces.
   e. Both (a) and (b) are correct.
   f. Both (c) and (d) are correct.

6. Define and discuss the terms *substance abuse* and *addiction*.
7. Outline factors that determine the risk of developing an addiction to drugs.
8. Discuss the health effects of alcohol use.
9. Describe the changes in behavior and physical function that occur as blood alcohol levels increase.
10. What is the most widely used recreational drug in the United States?
11. List four steps that can help you feel less tempted to use drugs.
12. Discuss the health effects of marijuana use.
13. Describe the health effects of using anabolic steroids.

Suggested Reading

Donatelle, R. *Access to Health*, Green Edition. San Francisco: Benjamin Cummings, 2010.

Fields, R. *Drugs in Perspective*, 7th ed. St. Louis: McGraw-Hill, 2010.

Wilson, H. *Annual Editions: Drugs, Society, and Behavior*, 24th ed. St. Louis: McGraw-Hill, 2010.

For links to the organizations and websites listed below, visit The Total Fitness and Wellness Website at www.pearsonhighered.com/powers.

American Medical Association
Contains many sources of information about a wide variety of medical problems, including alcohol, tobacco, and drug use.

WebMD
Contains information about a wide variety of diseases and medical problems, including alcohol, tobacco, and drug use.

Higher Education Center for Alcohol and Other Drug Prevention
Presents information about alcohol and drug abuse on college campuses; also contains links to other related organizations.

National Institute on Drug Abuse
This comprehensive site contains information about commonly abused drugs, the incidence of drug abuse in the United States, and where to find help with rehabilitation from drug dependence.

References

1. *Stedman's Medical Dictionary for the Health Professions and Nursing*, 5th ed. Philadelphia: Lippincott Williams & Wilkins, 2005.
2. American Psychiatric Association. *Diagnostic and Statistical Manual of Mental Disorders*, 4th ed., Text revision. Washington, DC: American Psychiatric Association, 2000.
3. MayoClinic.com. Compulsive gambling. January 2009. www.mayoclinic.com/health/compulsive-gambling/DS00443.
4. MayoClinic.com. Drug addiction. October 2007. www.mayoclinic.com/health/drug-addiction/DS00183.
5. Cannon, C., and M. Bseikri. Is dopamine required for natural reward? *Physiology of Behavior* 81:741–748, 2004.
6. National Institute on Drug Abuse. Research Report Series. Updated July 2009. www.drugabuse.gov/ResearchReports.
7. Department of Health and Human Services. *Results from the 2007 National Survey on Drug Use and Health: National Findings,* Rockville, MD: Substance Abuse and Mental Health Services Administration, Office of Applied Studies, 2008.
8. Liska, K. *Drugs and the Human Body*, Englewood Cliffs, NJ: Prentice Hall, 2000.
9. Geller T., L. Loftis, and D. Brink. Cerebellar infarction in adolescent males associated with acute marijuana use. *Pediatrics* 113:e365–370, 2004.
10. Office of National Drug Control Policy. *National Drug Control Strategy Data Supplement 2009*, Washington, DC: Office of National Drug Control Policy, 2009.
11. White, S., and C. Lambe. The pathophysiology of cocaine abuse. *Journal of Clinical Forensic Medicine* 10:27–39, 2003.
12. Sindelar, H., N. Barnett, and A. Spirito. Adolescent alcohol use and injury: A summary and critical review of the literature. *Minerva Pediatrics* 56:291–309, 2004.
13. Ogden, E., and H. Moskowitz. Effects of alcohol and other drugs on driver performance. *Traffic Injury Prevention* 5:185–198, 2004.

14. MADD. .08 per se, 2004. www.MADD.org/Drunk-Driving/Drunk-Driving/laws/law.aspx?law=11.

15. Hingson, R., T. Heeren, M. Winter, and H. Wechsler. Magnitude of alcohol-related mortality and morbidity among U.S. college students ages 18–24: Changes from 1998 to 2001. *Annual Review of Public Health 26*: 259–279, 2005.

16. Knight, J. R., et al. Alcohol abuse and dependence among U.S. college students. *Journal of Studies on Alcohol* 63:263–270, May 2002.

17. National Institute on Alcohol Abuse and Alcoholism. *Trends in Underage Drinking in the United States, 1991–2007*. Surveillance Report no. 86. Bethesda, MD: U.S. Department of Health and Human Services, 2009.

18. Robbins, S., and M. Angell. *Basic Pathology*. Philadelphia: W. B. Saunders, 1997.

19. National Institute on Alcohol Abuse and Alcoholism. Frequently asked questions for the general public. Bethesda, MD: U.S. Department of Health and Human Services, February 2007. www.niaaa.nih.gov/FAQs/General-English.

20. Centers for Disease Control and Prevention, National Center for Chronic Disease Prevention and Health Promotion. Smoking and tobacco use: Fact sheets. 2009. www.cdc.gov/tobacco/data_statistics/fact_sheets/index.htm.

21. National Institute on Drug Abuse. NIDA Info Facts: Cigarettes and other tobacco products. 2009. www.drugabuse.gov/Infofacts/tobacco.html.

22. American Cancer Society. Secondhand smoke. www.cancer.org/docroot/PED/content/PED_10_2X _Secondhand_Smoke-Clean_Indoor_Air.asp. Revised May 2009.

23. Centers for Disease Control and Prevention. Epidemiologic notes and reports of illnesses possibly associated with smoking clove cigarettes. *Morbidity and Mortality Weekly Report*, May 1985. Available from www.cdc.gov/mmwr.

24. U.S. Department of Health and Human Services. The health consequences of involuntary exposure to tobacco smoke: A report of the Surgeon General. Atlanta, GA: U.S. Department of Health and Human Services, 2006. www.surgeongeneral.gov/library/secondhandsmoke/report.

25. American Lung Association. Quit smoking: Secondhand smoke fact sheet. www.lungusa.org. Updated 2009.

26. National Institute on Drug Abuse. Research Report Series—Anabolic Steroid Abuse. September 2006. www.drugabuse.gov/ResearchReports/Steroids.

27. Medline Plus. Many teen girls use steroids, June 2007. www.nlm.nih.gov/medlineplus.

28. Glantz, M., and C. Hartel (eds.). *Drug Abuse: Origins and Interventions*. Washington, DC: APA Publications, 1999.

29. Nawrot, P., S. Jordan, J. Eastwood, J. Rotstein, A. Hugenholtz, and M. Feeley. Effects of caffeine on human health. *Food Additives and Contamination* 20:1–30, 2003.

30. Maughan, R. Dietary supplements. *Journal of Sports Sciences* 22:95–113, 2004.

31. Powers, S., and S. Dodd. Caffeine and endurance performance: A review. *Sports Medicine* 2:165–174, 1985.

32. Dodd, S., R. Herb, and S. Powers. Caffeine and exercise performance: An update. *Sports Medicine* 15:14–23, 1993.

33. American College of Obstetricians and Gynecologists (ACOG). *Your Pregnancy and Birth*, 4th ed. Washington, DC: American College of Obstetricians and Gynecologists, 2005.

Videos

Log on to www.pearsonhighered.com/powers to view these chapter-related videos.

Addictions and Addictive Behavior

Kick Your Habit—Soft Addictions

Treating Addiction with Virtually Reality

Illicit Drugs

Eliminating Meth

Campus Drug Dealers

Alcohol

Spring Break Nightmare

Teen Drinking Test

Tobacco

Smash the Ash!

Second Hand Smoke

The Mitchell Report on Steroids in Baseball

NAME _____ DATE _____

Alcohol Abuse Inventory

This laboratory is designed to increase your awareness of your drinking habits. For this inventory to provide a valid assessment of your drinking behaviors, you must answer each question honestly. Check yes or no for each of the following questions regarding your use of alcohol.

	Yes	No
1. Do you often drink alone?	—	—
2. When drinking, do you often worry about running out of alcoholic beverages?	—	—
3. Do you drink alcohol daily?	—	—
4. Do you drink alcohol to reduce your stress levels?	—	—
5. Do you crave alcohol during all parts of the day?	—	—
6. Do you have trouble not drinking alcohol at a party?	—	—
7. After a night of drinking, do you sometimes have trouble remembering what you did?	—	—
8. Does your drinking impair your school or job performance?	—	—
9. Does your drinking impair your ability to use good judgment or cause you to have accidents?	—	—
10. Do you ever lie to friends or family about how much you drink?	—	—

Answering yes to only one of the questions above suggests that you may be drinking too much. Answering yes to two questions is a clear warning sign that you may have or are in the process of developing an alcohol abuse problem. Answering yes to three or more questions indicates that you have a serious alcohol abuse problem and that you should seek professional help.

Answer the following questions to help identify ways you can curb your alcohol consumption:

1. If you answered yes to question 1 and/or 2, try making access to alcohol an inconvenience. Identify two ways you can limit your access to alcohol in your home.

   * _____

   * _____

2. If you answered yes to question 3 and/or 4, try substituting a healthy behavior for the drinking behavior. What is a healthy behavior you could substitute for drinking alcohol? What are two stress management techniques you could try instead of drinking alcohol?

   * Healthy behavior: _____

   * Stress management technique: _____

   * Stress management technique: _____

3. If you answered yes to questions 5, 6, 7, 8, 9, and/or 10, recognize that alcohol is interfering with your life. Identify two campus resources and two community resources that you could use to address your alcohol-related behaviors.

   * _____

   * _____

   * _____

   * _____

NAME _____ DATE _____

Tobacco Usage Inventory

This laboratory is designed to increase your awareness of your tobacco habits. Habits are sometimes difficult to break because they become unconscious acts. Unrecognized triggers may cause the desire to smoke or use the product. Breaking a habit may be as easy as identifying the trigger and substituting a healthy behavior in place of the unhealthy one.

Over the next 24 hours, take an inventory of the tobacco products you use. Identify the number of tobacco products you use each hour, where you used the product (such as a certain room of the house or in the car), when you used the product (such as after a meal or first thing in the morning), and any other factors, such as being with friends, family, alone, and so on. You must answer each question honestly to provide a valid assessment of your tobacco usage behaviors.

Time of Day	Number of Tobacco Products Used	Location	What Were You Doing Before and During Usage?	Other Factors
12:00 AM				
1:00				
2:00				
3:00				
4:00				
5:00				
6:00				
7:00				
8:00				
9:00				
10:00				
11:00				
12:00 PM				
1:00				
2:00				
3:00				

LABORATORY

Time of Day	Number of Tobacco Products Used	Location	What Were You Doing Before and During Usage?	Other Factors
4:00				
5:00				
6:00				
7:00				
8:00				
9:00				
10:00				
11:00				
12:00 AM				

Analyze the above chart, noting any patterns to your use of tobacco. Answer the following questions:

1. Do you smoke or use more than 1 cigarette in any given hour of the day? When?

_____

_____

_____

2. Is there a particular location in your home, at school, or in a favorite restaurant or bar where you prefer to smoke? Where?

_____

_____

_____

3. Do you use tobacco products more often at certain times, such as around meal time, when talking on the phone, or driving in a car?

_____

_____

_____

4. Is there a friend or family member present or do you smoke alone?

_____

_____

_____

Now that you have identified a potential pattern to your tobacco usage, think about ways that you can change that pattern. For example:

- Look at the number of cigarettes that you used during 1 hour, and try cutting the number down by half over the next 2 weeks. Every 2 weeks, cut your usage in half.

- Identify one location from the above chart that you will make off-limits to any tobacco product over the next 2 weeks. Every 2 weeks, add another location to make off-limits. Do not add any new locations to the above list.

- Identify when you use the product and what might be the trigger event. For example, you may find that mealtime, studying, or talking on the telephone triggers your need to smoke. Try substituting a healthy behavior, such as taking a walk after a meal, eating a piece of fruit while studying, or drinking a glass of water when using the telephone.

- Examine the other factors that may influence your tobacco usage. You may find that you smoke only when you are alone or when you are with one particular individual or group of people. Identify a way in which you can continue to socialize with your friends without tobacco. For example, plan on meeting your friends in a smokeless restaurant, bar, or building. If you smoke when alone, try performing other tasks that will keep your hands occupied.

Note that these steps may help you cut down on smoking, but by themselves they may not be enough to kick the habit. Nicotine is a highly addictive substance and may require medical intervention, such as obtaining a prescription for the nicotine patch to help you quit.

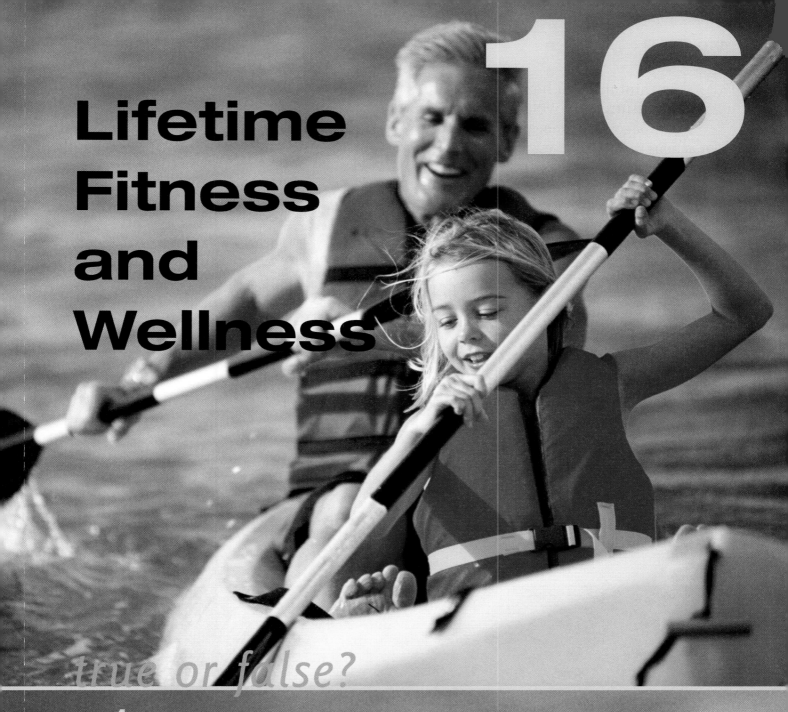

16

Lifetime Fitness and Wellness

true or false?

1. Older adults who maintain a regular exercise program can have fitness levels similar to younger adults.

2. All U.S. citizens have health insurance.

3. Pregnant women should not exercise.

4. Choosing a regular health care provider is an important part of maintaining good health.

5. There's not much you can do to slow the aging process after age 30.

Answers appear on the next page.

Maintaining a healthy level of fitness and wellness is an ongoing, lifelong process, and your actions today will have a significant impact on your health in 10, 20, 40, and 60 years. Similarly, your actions in the future will affect your health and wellness then and beyond. Think about the health and fitness levels of your parents, grandparents, or other older adults you know. Whatever their ages, they need to make healthy behavior choices across all the wellness dimensions to ensure good health now and in the years to come. Remember, fitness cannot be stored! As you recall from Chapter 2, the principle of reversibility states that if you stop being active, you lose fitness and those health and wellness benefits that you worked so hard to achieve.

In this chapter, we'll address fitness- and wellness-related considerations you are likely to experience throughout your lifetime. We will also discuss strategies for maintaining a lifetime fitness and wellness program.

Maintaining an Exercise Program during All Stages of Life

Rates of physical activity decline with age for most adults (1, 2). Throughout this text, we have discussed strategies for sticking with your exercise program and maintaining other health behavior changes. In this section, we want to bring to your attention times you are likely to experience a drop in your physical activity or find it more difficult to stick with a regular exercise program. Beginning a lifetime exercise program requires a strong personal commitment to physical fitness and application of the principles of behavior modification. Knowing when you are more likely to be less motivated or experience more personal barriers can help you plan ahead and maintain your physical activity.

You have already experienced one of the periods when we see declines in activity: starting college. Rates of physical activity tend to drop during periods of major life changes, such as when traditional and nontraditional students begin college life. (We hope the information you have learned in this course prevented you from experiencing the drop in activity or helped you to get back on track). Other periods during which people tend to lessen their physical activity are immediately after college (3), after moving, when starting a new job or graduate school, and when getting married or starting a family. In all these cases, people experience a lot of changes at once and can become overwhelmed. They may feel that they do not have time to fit in an exercise program with all their other commitments.

Graduating from college or beginning graduate school is generally a planned event, and you can prepare for it and the accompanying lifestyle changes ahead of time. As your income grows and your free time shrinks, you may find that morning or evening workouts in a health club are the most convenient way to incorporate physical activity into your daily routine. (See the box below for tips on keeping active as you transition to life after college). Thinking about and planning ahead for these times are key to staying active. Other life-changing periods, such as an unexpected death in the family or a sudden job loss, may come about without your having time to prepare.

Keep in mind that a lapse does not have to lead to failure. Scheduling a break and allowing a few extra days off during times when you feel overwhelmed is fine, as long as you also plan to get back on track. Planning for shortened or modified workouts is another option. Remember that people feel more relaxed and less anxious after exercise, so using those feelings as motivation can help some people stay active.

Some people report that as they get older, caring for a sick spouse or parent leaves them with less time for exercise. One possible solution is to hire outside help. Health care assistance can help you better manage your time and allow for scheduled exercise. It might also help with other wellness behaviors, such as getting adequate sleep and taking time for yourself.

Also, as you get older your interests and body will change, leading to changes in your workout choices. A long-time runner might have to shift to a lower-impact activity as his joints weaken with age. If you prefer an activity that requires more than one person, such as team sports or tennis, you might have difficulty finding others who share your interest as you move or age. Or, you might meet people who expose you to activities you had previously not considered. The important thing is to select activities you enjoy so you will be motivated to keep up a regular exercise routine. See Table 16.1 for examples of activities and the Consumer Corner on page 443 for tips on how to select a health club.

Make sure you know...

> Rates of physical activity decrease with age. Finding activities that you can maintain as lifetime activities is important to maintain regular exercise as you age.

> Many people find it difficult to maintain regular exercise during periods of change or transition. Recognizing and planning ahead for these periods can help you maintain your exercise program.

> The behavior change strategies you learned about earlier in the text will also help you maintain a lifetime activity program.

Fitness during Pregnancy

Can women exercise safely during a normal pregnancy? The answer is generally yes, but every pregnant woman should consult with her health care provider before starting a new program or continuing an existing program. Many women who exercise regularly may need to modify their workouts to adjust to the changes in their bodies during pregnancy. Exercise has been shown to have numerous benefits for pregnant women, including less weight gain, fewer discomforts, and shorter labor (4). There is also some evidence that exercise might help prevent and treat gestational diabetes (4, 5). Women who maintain their regular aerobic exercise during pregnancy can maintain cardiorespiratory fitness, have better posture, retain less weight, and have less back pain than women who remain sedentary. The risks associated with exercise during pregnancy tend to impact the fetus, so following the recommended exercise prescription and guidelines is very important.

The exercise prescription for pregnancy endorsed by the American College of Sports Medicine (ACSM) is 30–40 minutes of moderate-intensity aerobic exercise most days of the week. ACSM also recommends that the exercise be regular (6). So, women should

---

Sticking with an Exercise Program after Graduation

The following tips can help you maintain your activity level as you transition to life after college:

- Look for an apartment complex or housing development that has a fitness center on site.

- Check with your human resource department to see whether your company has a worksite fitness or wellness program. Some companies that do not have an onsite facility pay for or supplement your membership to a local fitness center.

- Continue to write out a schedule, and include your exercise time on your "to do" list.

- Look up the local recreation department to see where local parks are located.

- Look for clubs or groups that promote physical activity. Many areas have running, walking, golf, tennis, or other sport/activities groups. These are great ways to stay active and to meet people in a new city. If such a group does not already exist, consider starting one.

- Expect and plan for changes in your normal routine. You might have to play with different schedules or modify your existing exercise program to fit your new lifestyle.

TABLE 16.1
Fitness Evaluation of Various Activities and Sports

Sport/Activity	Cardiorespiratory Endurance	Upper Body Muscular Strength and Endurance	Lower Body Muscular Strength and Endurance	Flexibility	Caloric Expenditure (calories/min)
Aerobic Dance	Good	Good	Good	Fair	5–10
Badminton	Fair	Fair	Good	Fair	5–10
Baseball	Poor	Fair	Fair	Fair	4–6
Basketball	Good	Fair	Good	Fair	10–12
Bowling	Poor	Fair	Poor	Fair	3–4
Canoeing	Fair	Good	Poor	Fair	4–10
Golf (walking)	Poor	Fair	Good/Fair	Fair	2–4
Gymnastics	Poor	Excellent	Excellent	Excellent	3–4
Handball	Good	Good/Fair	Good	Fair	7–12
Karate	Fair	Good	Good	Excellent	7–10
Racquetball	Good/Fair	Good/Fair	Good	Fair	6–12
Running	Excellent	Fair	Good	Fair	8–15
Ice Skating	Good/Fair	Poor	Good/Fair	Good/Fair	5–10
Roller Skating	Good/Fair	Poor	Good/Fair	Fair	5–10
Downhill Skiing	Fair	Fair	Good	Fair	5–10
Cross-country Skiing	Excellent/Good	Good	Good	Fair	7–15
Soccer	Good	Fair	Good	Good/Fair	7–17
Tai chi	Good/Fair	Good/Fair	Good/Fair	Fair	5–9
Tennis	Good/Fair	Good/Fair	Good	Fair	5–12
Volleyball	Fair	Fair	Good/Fair	Fair	4–8
Waterskiing	Poor	Good	Good	Fair	4–7
Weight Training	Poor	Excellent	Excellent	Fair	4–6
Yoga	Poor	Poor	Poor	Excellent	2–4

Sources: From Getchell, B. *Physical Fitness: A Way of Life,* 5th ed. Copyright © 1998. Reprinted by permission of Pearson Education, Inc.; Lan, C., S. Chen, and J. Lai. Tai chi. *American Journal of Chinese Medicine* 32:151–160, 2004; Taylor-Pillae, R., and E. Foelicher. Effectiveness of tai chi in improving aerobic capacity: A meta analysis. *Journal of Cardiovascular Nursing* 19:48–57, 2004.

avoid skipping numerous consecutive days or weeks, but rather maintain a regular schedule each week throughout the pregnancy. Women should also avoid exercise or activities with a high risk for falling or that could cause trauma to fetus (4, 6). Women should also note that some activities they had done when they were not pregnant might have higher risk during pregnancy because of the changes that occur in their bodies. For example, joint laxity increases during pregnancy, and joints may feel less stable. Jogging might not normally be a problem, but if joints feel a little wobbly, women might consider walking or jogging on a treadmill to feel safer. Prolonged or high-intensity exercise may impair fetal development, and women should consult with their health care providers before continuing a more intense exercise program (4, 6).

Women who exercise during pregnancy should follow these guidelines (4, 6):

• Do not increase the amount of exercise you typically performed before your pregnancy.

• Do not participate in sports that have a high risk of injury (e.g., contact sports).

• Do not use exercises that require lying on the back for more than 5 minutes. The weight of the fetus may reduce blood flow through vessels supplying blood to the lower extremities. Also avoid standing without moving, because it can cause blood to pool in the extremities. Concentrate on non-weight-bearing exercises, such as cycling or swimming.

• During the last 3 months of pregnancy, avoid exercises that use quick jerking movements, because they may cause joint strains.

• Wear good supportive footwear and adequate breast support.

• Avoid exercise in the heat, and wear clothing that will allow your body to dissipate heat. The primary dangers of exercise during pregnancy are elevated body temperature and lack of blood flow to the baby. Aquatic exercise is an excellent means of

CONSUMER CORNER

HEALTH CLUBS: CHOOSING A FITNESS FACILITY

You don't need to join a fitness club to exercise, but it can be an appealing option for many people who want to stay active. Many people find that the social environment of a fitness club motivates them and helps them maintain their routine. The trained personnel on staff at fitness facilities can provide direction and instruction for beginners and others wanting to advance their programs. Additionally, fitness clubs can provide a safe, temperature-controlled environment for people who may be uncomfortable exercising outside.

Before choosing a fitness facility, consider the following recommendations:

- Check out all available options for fitness programs in your community before deciding to join any fitness club. Explore fitness facilities and programs offered by your local recreation department, YMCA, or university.

- Consider the club's location. You are more likely to visit the facility regularly if it is convenient to home, school, or work.

- Check the club's reputation with the Better Business Bureau (www.bbb.org). You can learn how long the club has been in business, whether complaints against it have been registered, and whether those complaints have been resolved.

- Visit the facility multiple times before you join to investigate the cleanliness of the locker rooms and the quality of exercise equipment. Try to visit the facility during your desired workout time, so you can see how crowded it becomes when you plan to workout.

- Inquire about the qualifications of the fitness instructors and personal trainers. It is important that the club's personnel be well trained. (See the Closer Look box on page 450).

- Consider the club's approach to fitness and training. Are routine fitness assessments and health screening (e.g., blood pressure measurement) available and recommended? Are instructors and trainers readily available to provide assistance, or do members have to seek out staff members for help?

- Avoid fitness clubs that require or recommend signing a contract committing you to multiple months of membership fees. Long-term contracts might seem more cost-effective, but month-to-month payments are actually your best option. You are less likely to lose money if the club closes or you need to terminate your membership before the end of the contract. Also, be wary of contract clauses that waive the club's liability for injury to you or your right to defend yourself in court.

- Avoid clubs that advertise overnight fitness results or quick weight loss. After having read this book, you know that these claims are false.

Sources: Balady, G. Health clubs: Are they right for you? *Harvard Men's Health Watch,* November 6, 1998; Health clubs: What to look for. *Consumer Reports,* February 1999.

Examine the features of a health club carefully before joining.

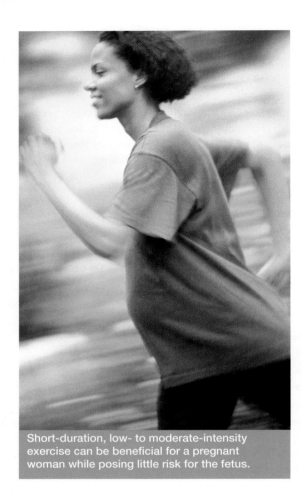

Short-duration, low- to moderate-intensity exercise can be beneficial for a pregnant woman while posing little risk for the fetus.

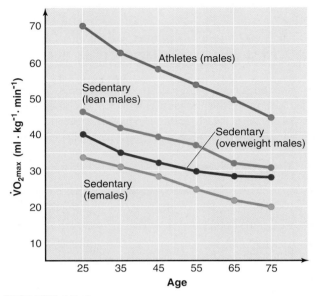

FIGURE 16.1

Changes in $\dot{V}O_2$max with advancing age. After age 25, the typical decline is approximately 10% per decade.

Source: Neiman, D. *Exercise Testing Prescription: A Health Related Approach,* 6th ed. Copyright © 2007. Reprinted by permission of the McGraw-Hill Companies.

preventing large gains of body heat, because water removes heat from the body better than air.

• Drink plenty of water to maintain hydration. Also, consider sports drinks or eating a small amount (30–50 g) of carbohydrates to maintain blood glucose levels during exercise.

• Monitor your exercise intensity using rating of perceived exertion (RPE). An RPE value of 11–13 is recommended.

• If you were sedentary or had a low activity level before pregnancy, start with a light-intensity, non-impact or low-impact exercise. ACSM recommends an exercise intensity of 20–39% of heart rate reserve.

• Stop exercising immediately and call your health care provider if you experience any of the following: shortness of breath, dizziness, numbness, tingling, abdominal pain, or vaginal bleeding.

Make sure you know...

> Exercise is safe for healthy pregnant women who are not experiencing complications with pregnancy.

> Pregnant women can do aerobic exercise up to 30–40 minutes at a moderate intensity (RPE 11–13).

> Pregnant women should avoid activities with high risk for falling or trauma to the fetus or that require lying down or standing without movement.

Fitness during Older Adulthood

The causes of aging have been studied for years, and there are numerous theories to explain why we age, but none completely explains all of the physical and mental changes that occur. Experts who study aging now believe the aging process results from a combination of genetics, environment, diet, and lifestyle factors (7, 8).

For older adults (age 65 and older—those who are typically nearing retirement age), exercise is just as important as it is for the rest of the adult population. Everyone experiences a significant decline in $\dot{V}O_2$max with age (Figure 16.1) regardless of their level of exercise participation. However, research has shown that older adults who engage in a regular, vigorous physical activity program can have levels of aerobic fitness that are similar to someone much younger (9). So as you can see in Figure 16.1, a 75-year-old male athlete can have an aerobic capacity similar to that of a 25-year-old sedentary man! Let's take a look at some of the typical biological changes that are a part of the aging process.

Exercise is beneficial for people of all ages.

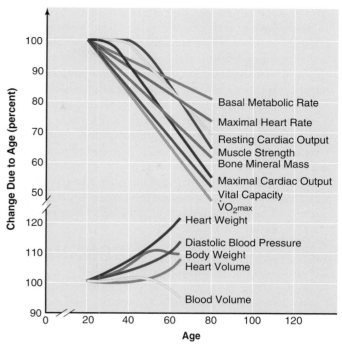

FIGURE 16.2
Physiological changes that accompany aging.

Source: Neiman, D. *Exercise Testing Prescription: A Health Related Approach,* 6th ed. Copyright © 2007. Reprinted by permission of the McGraw-Hill Companies.

Physical and Mental Changes of Aging

As we age, we all experience a gradual decline in biological function, including numerous changes in both the body and mind. During youth, the organ systems in healthy bodies function at a higher level than is required for optimal function. Because of the high level of functioning, gradual and small age-related changes in organ systems do not impair their function. However, over a period of time, the decline is more drastic and has a noticeable impact on functional ability. We begin to see many of the age-related changes in the body as young as 30 to 40 years (10). The physiological changes that happen as we age are similar to those seen with physical inactivity or the prolonged weightlessness experienced by astronauts (Figure 16.2).

The most common functional age-related changes are decreased cardiorespiratory function, increased body fat, and a more fragile musculoskeletal system (10). Approximately one-half of the decline in functional capacity results from a decrease in physical activity (10). Maintaining a regular exercise program as you age can help to maintain a higher level of cardiovascular functioning during the aging process. For sedentary adults, beginning a regular exercise program can improve cardiorespiratory function (6). Additionally, regular exercise can help maintain a healthy body composition and the mineral content of bone during the aging process.

Maximal heart rate decreases with age. (Recall that you can estimate your maximal heart rate by subtracting your age from 220). Because maximal heart rate decreases, maximal cardiac output also decreases (Chapter 3). An additional cardiovascular change is a progressive buildup of fatty plaque in blood vessels, resulting in "hardening of the arteries," or the atherosclerotic process. The hardening of the arteries can also contribute to a gradual increase in blood pressure, resulting in age-related high blood pressure (hypertension).

Both bone and joint health are affected in the aging process. We gradually lose bone strength as a result of a decrease in bone mineral density (osteoporosis). These changes increase the risk for falls and fractures. We typically achieve peak bone mass in our early 20s, so developing adequate bone mass when we are young is important to prevent osteoporosis. Weight-bearing exercise and resistance training can help strengthen muscle and bone (11, 12). The loss of bone mass in women is greatly accelerated after menopause because of the decline in estrogen. Aging also results in a loss of connective tissue between joints that can result in arthritis, inflammation, and pain during movement.

A loss of skeletal muscle mass and function, called **sarcopenia,** is a major age-related health problem for both men and women. Muscular strength lost during aging is directly related to loss of skeletal muscle mass. Total muscle mass declines by approximately 40% between the ages of 20 and 80 years. The loss of muscle mass is a significant issue because it results in reduced mobility and independence and increases the risk of falls. Skeletal muscles generate the force required to maintain bone mass, and loss of bone mass is associated with increased risk for falling and fractures. Therefore, age-related loss of muscle results in a vicious cycle as it contributes to the loss of bone mass in older adults.

Numerous other changes take place during the aging process. Some of the changes we can slow with our behavior choices, as we will discuss in the next section. The following list includes the commonly experienced changes that are part of normal aging.

- The skin changes during aging. Oil production declines, changes occur in connective tissue, and skin pigmentation changes. As a result, the skin can appear dry, spotted, and/or wrinkled.

- Many people experience changes in their vision around age 40. The inability to focus on close objects **(presbyopia),** impaired night vision, and a loss of depth perception are common changes.

- Changes in the cells on the tongue and in the nose lead to a decline in taste and smell. These changes can contribute to a loss of appetite associated with older age.

- The brain and central nervous system also experience age-related changes. There is a loss of brain cells (neurons) and a decrease in neurotransmitters. One of the more obvious age-related changes in brain function is a gradual loss of memory.

- Hair begins to thin after about age 20. Also, as cells at the base of hair follicles age, they produce less pigment, so hair color begins to fade and turn gray.

CONSIDER THIS!

Studies have shown that mortality rates are 20–30% lower in a given time period among people who expend 1000 kilocalories in physical activity per week.

Successful Aging

We cannot stop the aging process, but we can sustain good physical fitness and wellness through older age by making healthy choices about our behaviors. Good nutrition, regular exercise, and many other healthy behavior choices that have been described throughout this book (e.g., not smoking, getting regular medical screenings, and having healthy relationships) are the keys for successful aging. Neglect and abuse of our body and mind can accelerate the aging process and result in a faster decline in function. A few simple lifestyle choices that you can make every day will make a significant difference in your ability to slow down aging and maintain wellness.

Maintain Lifelong Regular Physical Exercise

Regular aerobic exercise will maintain a healthy cardiovascular system. A program of weight training will maintain muscular strength and help keep your bones healthy, which will help to reduce the increased age-related risk of CVD, osteoporosis, and falls. Regular exercise also helps to maintain a healthy body weight, which is important because risk for many obesity-related diseases also increases with age.

Eat a Healthy Diet   A varied diet, low in calories and fat, is essential to maintain a healthy body weight and to reduce the risk of both heart disease and cancer. As we discussed in Chapter 7, a healthy diet should focus on fresh fruits and vegetables, whole grains, and lean portions of poultry and fish.

Exercise Your Mind   The brain is a "plastic organ" that is enhanced with increased mental activity. Conversely, lack of mental activity can result in a decline in brain function. To keep your mind sharp and your brain functioning at a high level, you should challenge your mind with a lifelong program of learning. Reading, thinking, problem solving, and intelligent conversation can all keep your mind active as you age.

Avoid Substance Abuse   As discussed in Chapter 15, abuse of alcohol and other drugs can have very negative consequences on health and wellness. Smoking and the use of other tobacco products greatly increase your risk of cardiovascular disease and certain cancers. Choosing to use alcohol only in moderation and avoiding substance abuse can greatly improve your ability to achieve successful aging and maintain wellness.

Reduce Stress   Recognizing, managing, and reducing stress in your daily life is essential to maintain wellness. Get adequate amounts of sleep, take time for yourself, and practice the stress management and relaxation techniques discussed in Chapter 10.

Protect Your Skin and Eyes from Sun Damage   Chronic exposure to ultraviolet (UV) rays from the sun can damage your skin and lead to premature aging and also increase the risk of skin cancer. Further, UV exposure can damage your eyes and impair your vision by increasing the risk of cataracts. It is important to protect your skin from sun damage by using sunscreen and wearing protective clothing (e.g., long sleeves and hats). Protect your eyes from UV damage by wearing sunglasses with UV protection within the lens.

Get Regular Medical Checkups   Regular visits with your health care provider are important for early detection and treatment of disease. We will discuss medical checkups and screenings in more detail in the next section.

Exercise Prescription for Older Adults
Older adults can safely participate in aerobic, resistance, and flexibility exercises, but they might have to modify the exercise prescriptions presented earlier in the text. An older adult who has exercised regularly her entire adult life may continue with the same exercise prescription she followed during middle age. Keep in mind that exercise prescriptions are typically made relative to the individual's maximal capacity. The absolute levels of heart rate or resistance will change, but the prescription will still be based on a percentage of maximal heart rate or resistance.

An older person with a history of inactivity will likely have low cardiorespiratory functioning and weak muscles. For individuals who have a lower level of functioning, a lower intensity than typically recommended can produce significant improvements (6). Older adults should consult with their health care providers before beginning an exercise program. Using rating of perceived exertion or percentage of maximal heart rate to monitor exercise intensity is preferred when the person is taking medications that alter heart rate. Older adults also need to consider safety when planning their exercise program. Considering the risk for falling and the amount of strength, balance, and coordination needed for the exercise is important. Activities such as walking, cycling, swimming, and light

weight training are generally recommended. Water exercises are a good choice for older adults just starting an exercise program.

The following guidelines outline some specific considerations for exercise after age 45 for men and after age 55 for women (6).

• Because the risks of heart disease increases with age, men over age 45 and women over age 55 should perform a physician-supervised, graded exercise stress test before engaging in any vigorous physical fitness program.

• Non-weight-bearing exercises are recommended to reduce the risk of musculoskeletal problems. Weight-bearing exercises are beneficial but should be performed with balance support to avoid falls.

sarcopenia Loss of skeletal muscle mass that occurs with aging.

presbyopia Farsightedness that results from weakening of the eye muscles.

Keys to Success in Lifetime Wellness

Maintaining a regular program of good health behavior, exercise, and healthy dietary practices to achieve "total wellness" requires motivation and a lifetime commitment to a healthy lifestyle. Keys to success in adhering to a lifetime wellness program include the following:

• A desire to achieve wellness
• Establishing both short- and long-term wellness goals
• Maintaining a regular schedule of wellness activities (e.g., exercise, healthy diet, and relaxation)
• Scheduling routine medical checkups and screening tests as recommended by your physician or health care provider
• Remaining informed about changing medical opinion about good health behaviors, nutrition, and exercise programs to sustain wellness
• Scheduling time for exercise and relaxation every day
• Associating with peers who are positive "wellness" role models
• Forgiving yourself when you commit wellness lifestyle errors; when these events occur, simply make the necessary behavioral adjustments to get back on the correct path to sustain wellness
• Expecting to be successful in achieving a lifetime of wellness; a positive attitude is essential for lifetime wellness

- Exercise intensity should be at the lower end of the target heart rate range.
- Exercise frequency should be limited to 3 to 4 days per week to reduce the risk of injury.
- Exercise duration should be modified to meet the needs (and abilities) of each individual. For example, in the beginning stages of the exercise program, many unconditioned older adults cannot exercise for more than 5 to 10 minutes per exercise session. In this case, individuals may exercise several times per day for short durations (e.g., three 10-minute sessions per day). As the program progresses, individuals can slowly increase the duration of each session and begin to have fewer daily sessions (e.g., two 15-minute sessions per day).

Make sure you know...

> Aging is a slow, gradual decline in biological function. The most common functional changes seen with both aging and inactivity are decreased cardiorespiratory function, increased body fat, and musculoskeletal fragility.
> Approximately one-half of the decline in functional capacity observed with aging is due to a decrease in physical activity.
> Regular exercise and medical screenings, not smoking, protecting your eyes and skin from the sun, and keeping your mind active are examples of healthy behavior choices that contribute to successful aging.
> Exercise capacity decreases with age, but older adults who remain active can maintain a high level of cardiovascular functioning.
> Older adults who start an exercise program can improve their fitness levels and enjoy health benefits.
> Men over age 45 and women over age 55 should have a physician supervised exercise test before beginning a vigorous program.

Being a Savvy Fitness Consumer

Over the course of your lifetime, you will have the opportunity to buy thousands of fitness-related products and consume countless amounts of fitness information. You will see advertisements, infomercials, websites, and magazine covers that claim to hold the keys to better performance or improved physical appearance. Some of these items may be written by experts and become useful, but many will be provided by individuals with little or no formal training in exercise science. Unfortunately, nonexperts often convey misinformation, and some have created or perpetuated exercise myths.

As a lifetime consumer of fitness and wellness information, you will need to evaluate continually the validity of various claims and marketing messages. Part of this evaluation involves critically analyzing the credibility of your information source. You should also be aware of some of the most common misperceptions that exist about fitness and wellness products. We discuss some of these next.

Hand Weights

Some manufacturers claim that using hand weights during your aerobic exercise workouts will greatly increase arm and shoulder strength. Although carrying hand weights will increase the energy expenditure during exercise, 1- to 3-pound hand weights do not promote significant strength gains, particularly in college-aged individuals.

Additionally, there are some concerns about the use of hand weights with aerobic exercise. First, gripping them may increase blood pressure (13). Individuals with high blood pressure should seek a physician's advice about using hand weights during exercise. Hand weights may also aggravate existing elbow or shoulder arthritis. Some aerobics instructors have banned hand weights in classes because of the danger of hitting someone with an outstretched hand.

Ergogenic Aids

Numerous manufacturers market **ergogenic aids** that they claim promote strength and cardiovascular fitness. These products are usually endorsed by champion athletes or feature testimonials from "regular" people who achieved unbelievable results. The key concerns for the consumer are whether ergogenic aids promote fitness and whether they are healthy.

Only limited scientific evidence supports the notion that nutritional ergogenic aids (such as nutritional and herbal supplements) promote fitness or increase athletic performance in humans. Anabolic steroids and the drug clenbuterol have proved to increase muscle mass (14, 15), but both drugs have harmful effects on health. Studies have shown that use of these drugs can result in serious organ damage and, in some cases, death (8, 16–18). The gains that can be achieved are not worth the health risks. Their cost and health risks make ergogenic aids an unwise choice if you want to improve strength and fitness.

Exercise Equipment

Every week, magazine and television ads promote a "new" exercise device designed to trim waistlines and build huge muscles overnight. As you learned in your class and from reading this text, there are no "miracle" exercise devices that will produce these changes in a healthy way. A well-rounded fitness program can be designed without exercise equipment, but many people like to use exercise equipment in their workouts. If you decide to purchase exercise equipment, do your research first to make sure the device will help you accomplish your health and fitness goals. Buy from a reputable and well-established company. Beware of mail-order products, and examine the product before you buy. When in doubt about the usefulness of an exercise product, consult a fitness expert.

Hot Tubs, Saunas, and Steam Baths

Hot tubs, saunas, and steam baths are popular at many health clubs. Although they might promote relaxation, they do not promote fat loss or improve physical fitness. Water loss due to perspiration will reduce your body weight temporarily, but the weight loss does not result from fat loss. The weight returns when you replace the lost fluids by eating and drinking.

One of the major concerns about the use of hot tubs and saunas is how they affect the regulation of blood pressure. These forms of heat stress increase blood flow to the skin to promote cooling, which reduces blood return to the heart and may reduce blood flow to the brain, thereby causing fainting. When using a sauna, hot tub, or steam bath, take the following precautions:

- Talk with your health care provider before using hot baths if you suffer from heart disease, hypertension, diabetes, kidney disease, or chronic skin problems or if you are pregnant.
- Don't use these facilities when you are alone; someone should be readily available to get emergency help if you develop a health problem, such as fainting.
- Don't wear jewelry in hot baths. The metal will absorb heat and may burn your skin.
- Don't drink alcohol prior to or while using these facilities. Alcohol can increase your risk of fainting during heat exposure.
- Don't exercise in a sauna, hot tub, or steam bath. The combination of exercise and a hot environment may result in overheating.
- Do not use a sauna, hot tub, or steam bath immediately after vigorous exercise. Using a steam bath without cooling down after exercise increases your risk of fainting.
- The duration of stay and recommended temperatures of saunas, steam baths, and hot tubs are as follows:

Sauna. Air temperature should not exceed 190°F (~88°C), and you should not stay in the sauna more than 15 minutes.

Steam bath. Air temperature should not exceed 120°F (~38°C), and you should not stay in the steam bath more than 10 minutes.

Hot tub (or whirlpool). Water temperature should not exceed 100°F (~38°C), and you should not stay in the hot tub more than 15 minutes.

Fitness Books and Magazines

When you read a book or magazine article about health and fitness, you need to consider the credibility of the source. Although many fitness books have been written by exercise science experts, others have been written by models, movie stars, body builders, and even professional or Olympic athletes who have no academic training in exercise science. Having athletic talent or a good physique does not make someone a fitness expert. Likewise, the letters MD or PhD after a person's name do not mean he or she is an expert in everything related to health and fitness. Consider doing an Internet search on the authors of magazine articles you read to see whether they are qualified to give information on that topic. Be aware that even reputable magazines can feature articles that are not written by the most qualified sources.

How do you evaluate the credibility of a fitness or weight control book? After reading and studying this book, you should be able to distinguish between fitness facts and fiction. For example, you know that articles that promise overnight results or quick, effortless weight loss are not good plans. You can also use the guidelines provided in the Closer Look box on page 450 to help identify fitness experts. If you have doubts about the information in a new fitness book, talk to your instructor, or contact a local fitness expert for advice.

Making Informed Health Care Choices

Making good decisions about managing your personal health care is another factor that will be very important to maintaining wellness over your lifetime. You need to know when to seek advice from medical and health professionals, and you need to be able to make informed health care decisions. Being an informed

ergogenic aid A drug or nutritional product that improves physical fitness and exercise performance.

WHAT IS A FITNESS EXPERT?

There is no standard definition of a *fitness expert*, but anyone who has earned an advanced degree (such as an MS or a PhD) in exercise science, kinesiology, or exercise physiology from a reputable university can generally be considered a fitness expert. Many trained professionals in health education, physical education, and nutrition also may qualify as fitness experts. Individuals with bachelor's degrees in exercise science may have a sufficient background to answer many fitness-related questions, but professionals with more advanced degrees should be more knowledgeable about exercise and fitness.

Exercise scientists who are actively conducting research in their area of specialty and are active in professional organizations such as the American Physiological Society or the American College of Sports Medicine are generally the best sources for the most up-to-date information, especially for technical information. Physicians with postgraduate training in exercise science or a strong interest in preventive medicine also are good sources of scientifically based fitness information.

Many fitness clubs advertise that their employees are certified trainers or instructors. However, certification does not equate to expertise. Some certifications can be obtained online by individuals with little to no formal training in exercise science, whereas others require a college degree and practical experience. You can locate fitness professionals with reputable certifications through the American College of Sports Medicine website (www.acsm.org).

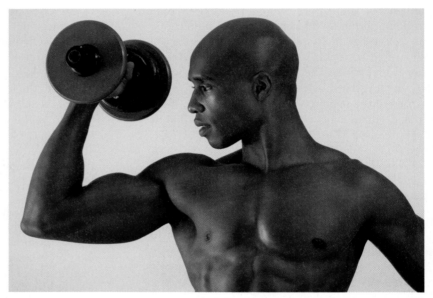

Having a championship physique does not make an individual a fitness expert.

health care consumer is the key to intelligent use of the health care system. In the following sections, we discuss several important health care issues, including how to choose a personal health care provider, deciding when to seek professional medical treatment instead of treating yourself, and the timing of regular checkups and tests.

Understanding Health Insurance

Maintaining regular health insurance coverage is extremely important for avoiding a potentially disastrous financial situation should you become ill or injured. Unfortunately, there are more than 43 million people in the United States without health insurance (19). As a responsible health consumer, your best interest is to avoid falling into this category.

Many students are covered by their parents' or spouse's **health insurance** plan. Other students have their own plans, possibly through a student health center. At some point, such as after graduation or when starting a new job, you are likely to have to make decisions about the health insurance you carry. How do you choose the best health insurance plan for your needs? There are many factors to consider regarding the various options of different insurance plans.

Many people get health insurance plans through their employer. Fortunately, most companies have human resource departments with personnel who can explain the options and answer your questions to help you pick the best plan. However, you should have some information before meeting with your human resources representative so you know what questions to ask. Insurance through your employer is called *group insurance*, and this type of insurance is usually very affordable because the employer pays some or all of the costs (20). You can usually include your spouse and children on your group plan. Because rates of insurance, coverage, and co-pay differ, couples who both have insurance available through an employer should compare plans before choosing one for their family.

If your company does not offer group insurance or does not have good plans available, you can get your own insurance plan, called *individual insurance* (20). Because you do not have the benefit of getting assistance from a human resources representative, you need to examine the details of the potential plans very carefully. Many plans offer a brief trial period for you to examine the policy and cancel if it does not fit your needs.

Regardless of whether you have group or individual health insurance, you typically have three options: fee-for-service, health maintenance organization (HMO), and preferred provider organization (PPO). A fee-for-service plan provides more options for doctors and hospitals than the other types of plans (20). With this plan, you pay a premium and a deductible for services. After the deductible is reached, you will have to pay a predetermined portion of the medical charges (20). Many plans have an upper limit on the amount you pay in one year. A fee-for-service plan offers a lot of choices, but it can be more costly and requires more record keeping by you.

With HMOs, many basic services are covered by the cost of the premium. This type of plan is less expensive and requires less paperwork than the fee-for-service plan, but your choices of doctors and hospitals are limited (20). Also, coverage of advanced medical procedures frequently is limited.

The PPO combines the best of fee-for-service and HMO plans. You have greater choice of physicians and hospitals than with an HMO, but if you choose one outside the preferred provider list, the coverage will be lower (20). With a PPO, you will typically have a small co-pay for routine medical and preventive care and a deductible for other services. You can use Laboratory 16.4 at the end of this chapter to help you determine the best type of plan for your needs.

Choosing a Health Care Provider

Choosing a personal health care provider is an important decision. Everyone, regardless of age, needs a good, reliable health care provider for common med-

ical problems. The benefits of having a regular provider are that the person will be familiar with your medical history and that you are more likely to develop a relationship that will make you more comfortable when discussing your medical issues.

Although your health care provider will likely often be a primary care physician, other medical professionals may sometimes address your health care needs. For example, many women see a nurse practitioner or midwife for annual exams and/or during a pregnancy. Physician's assistants also sometimes conduct routine tests and screenings. Although these medical professionals can help you with many routine and preventive health care needs, they might need to refer you to a physician for some medical concerns.

Using the emergency room or walk-in medical clinics for basic medical care, rather than contacting your regular health care provider, is often a mistake and can be expensive (21). Emergency room physicians are trained to take care of emergencies, but they are not the best choice for routine health care. Walk-in medical clinics are well prepared to take care of day-to-day health care problems, but these clinics will not have your medical history. Choosing a regular health care provider who will maintain your medical history on file and who is competent to recognize and treat a range of medical problems is important for optimal use of the health care system.

There are two basic types of doctors people choose as their general physician: family practitioners and internists. Family practitioners are physicians who have completed a 3-year residency (training after medical school) and are trained in a wide variety of medical topics. Family practitioners are capable of treating most acute and chronic illnesses for people of all ages. However, for complicated illnesses, family practitioners often refer patients to the appropriate medical specialist (see the Closer Look box on the next page for details on medical specialists).

Internists specialize in adult medical problems. Like family practitioners, internists complete a 3-year residency after medical school and pass a rigorous examination to receive specialty certification (21). Internists receive advanced medical training in areas such as heart disease, cancer, diabetes, and arthritis. However, complicated diseases might require that an internist refer patients to a specialist for further evaluation.

Once you select the type of physician you want, you should do some investigating before selecting a

health insurance A contractual relationship with an insurance company in which the company pays medical and health care costs in exchange for a paid premium for the service.

A CLOSER LOOK

GLOSSARY OF MEDICAL SPECIALISTS

Medical specialists are doctors who have received focused training in a specific area of medicine. These doctors have several years of training in addition to a normal residency and have passed rigorous board exams in their area of expertise. The following list describes the most common types of medical specialists.

Anesthesiologist Administers anesthesia during surgery and monitors the patient's immediate recovery following surgery.

Cardiologist Diagnoses and treats diseases of the heart and blood vessels.

Dermatologist Specializes in care and treatment of skin diseases.

Emergency room specialist Specializes in the care and treatment of trauma patients and acute illnesses.

Gastroenterologist Diagnoses and treats diseases of the digestive system and liver.

Hematologist Specializes in disorders of the blood.

Internist Specializes in the nonsurgical treatment of adults. Major areas of medical interest may include heart disease, cancer, diabetes, and arthritis.

Neurologist Diagnoses and treats disorders of the brain and nervous system.

Neurosurgeon Specializes in surgical treatment of disorders of the brain and nervous system.

Obstetrician/gynecologist A gynecologist specializes in the treatment of the reproductive systems of women, whereas an obstetrician specializes in the treatment of pregnant women and delivering babies.

Oncologist Specializes in the treatment of cancer.

Otorhinolaryngologist Specializes in diagnosis and treatment of problems in the ear, nose, and throat.

Pediatrician Specializes in the treatment of children.

Physiatrist Specializes in physical medicine and rehabilitation.

Psychiatrist Treats behavior and mental health disorders using both psychotherapy and medications.

Radiologist Specializes in the use of imaging technology (e.g., X-ray imaging, ultrasound) to diagnose diseases (e.g., cancer) and injuries (e.g., broken bones).

Surgeon Specializes in the use of surgery to diagnose and treat diseases. A general surgeon may perform a wide variety of surgical procedures, whereas other surgeons specialize in a specific area of surgery (e.g., cardiovascular surgery, plastic surgery).

Urologist Diagnoses and treats problems associated with the urinary tract in men and women, and in reproductive disorders in men.

---

specific doctor. In making your choice, consider the following factors (21):

- *Medical training and background.* You should know the physician's education and professional background, including board certification. Get personal recommendations about the physician's technical skills, if possible. Also, find out which hospitals the physician uses.

- *Physician availability.* How available is the doctor of your choice? If you have an urgent medical need, will he or she make arrangements to see you the day you call the office? Will the doctor be available to take phone calls and return phone calls promptly?

- *Medical philosophy.* What is the physician's medical philosophy? Will he or she treat each illness seriously or dismiss any of your medical problems? Will he or she prescribe medication every time you have a medical complaint?

- *Is the doctor with a group or solo?* If your doctor is in a solo practice, are other doctors available to treat your medical problems when your personal physician is away?

- *Bedside manner.* Finding a personal physician that you are comfortable with is very important. Most people seek someone who shows an obvious concern about the patient's health. You should have complete confidence that you will receive an

STEPS FOR
BEHAVIOR CHANGE

Are you a savvy health care consumer?

Do you make optimal use of the health care resources that are available to you? Take the following quiz to find out.

Y N

☐ ☐   Do you have a regular health care provider?

☐ ☐   Do you have health insurance?

☐ ☐   Do you consult with a pharmacist if you do not know which over-the-counter medication to purchase for minor illnesses?

☐ ☐   Do you know which Internet sources are reputable for health information?

☐ ☐   Do you ask about medication side effects and interactions when given a prescription?

TIPS TO BECOME A BETTER HEALTH CARE CONSUMER

☑   Request the same health care provider when you make appointments at your student health center or doctor's office. Remember that developing a relationship with your health care provider will be beneficial over time.

☑   Learn about the services at your student health center. Some colleges provide basic services free of charge if your student fees are paid.

☑   Check with your parents or spouse to see whether you are covered under their insurance policy. If you're not covered, check with your student health center to see what type of insurance policies they have available for students.

☑   Ask your health care provider or pharmacist about drug interactions and side effects for any medications you take, including over-the-counter medications and herbal supplements. Throw away over-the-counter and prescription medications when they are past the expiration date.

☑   Consult the Web resources listed at the end of each chapter for recommended, credible sources of health information.

---

informed and carefully considered opinion from your doctor. Your physician also should be comfortable with your wanting a second opinion for diagnosis and for treatment options. Again, get personal recommendations if possible.

- *Medical payment requirements.*   What kind of payment is required? Do you have to pay the fee directly, or will the doctor's office bill your insurance company? Sometimes you will need to check with your insurance company for a list of health care providers that accept your policy.

Deciding When to See a Health Care Provider

How do you know when it's time to see a health care provider? You know your body, and you can tell when something is not quite right. However, that does not mean you need to run to the doctor's office every time something bothers you. Often you can call your physician or health care provider and get information by phone. Some insurance companies also have information call centers where you can talk to a doctor, nurse, or other health care professional to get information and to find out whether you should see your personal health care provider.

TABLE 16.2

Medical Checkups: Your Examination Timetable

This chart provides general guidelines for physical exams and routine medical tests for men and women. Note that these guidelines are for people of average health risks only and do not replace the advice of your health care provider.

Age	Sex	Test	Frequency
18 and over	M/F	Complete physical	Every 1–3 years
	M/F	Blood pressure	Every 1–2 years
	M/F	Blood lipid (cholesterol) profile	Every 1–5 years
	F	Pelvic exam	Annually
	F	Pap smear	Every 1–3 years
	F	Breast exam	Annually
40 and over	M/F	Visual acuity, glaucoma	Every 2–4 years
	M	Fecal occult blood test	Annually
	M	Digital rectal exam	Annually
	F	Mammogram	Annually
50 and over	M/F	Sigmoidoscopy	Every 5 years
	M/F	Colonoscopy	Every 10 years
	F	Fecal occult blood test	Annually
65 and over	M/F	Visual acuity, glaucoma	Annually
	M/F	Hearing	Annually

Sources: Margen, S. (Ed.). *The Wellness Encyclopedia*. Boston: Houghton Mifflin Company, 1995; *Mayo Clinic Family Health Book.* New York: HarperResource, 2003; Thomas, M., S. Habermann, S. Rajkumar, S. Randall, M. Edson, C. Scott, M. Litin, K. Amit, M. Ghost, and D. McCallum. *Mayo Clinic Internal Medicine Board Review.* Philadelphia: Lippincott Williams and Williams, 2004; American Heart Association (www.americanheart.org); Prevent Blindness America (www.preventblindness.org/eye_tests/near_vision_recom.html).

In general, the decision to see your health care provider should be guided by your medical history and the nature and duration of the symptoms. For example, if you take regular medication for an existing medical condition and you get a head cold or the flu, you might need to see, or at least call, your health care provider to find out what type of medication you can take without causing a drug interaction. However, for someone else, taking over-the-counter medication and resting for a few days might be fine.

If you are generally healthy and develop symptoms of an illness but are unsure of their significance, call your health care provider and ask for medical advice over the phone. Medical professionals can often help you determine whether you need an office visit or can monitor your symptoms at home.

For any symptom that is severe, persistent, or recurring, you should see your health care provider immediately. You should seek immediate medical attention if you have any of the following injuries or symptoms: suspicion of a broken bone, severe bleeding, deep wound, severe burns, chest pain, shortness of breath, poisoning or drug overdose, and/or sudden loss of consciousness (22).

Timing of Regular Medical Checkups and Medical Tests

The frequency with which you schedule your physical exams and other routine medical screening tests will vary according to your age, occupation, lifestyle, risk factors, and medical history. General guidelines for both men and women are presented in Table 16.2. The recommendations provided are for individuals of average risk and do not replace the advice of your health care provider (22). In general, most medical experts believe that routine physical exams should include checks of blood pressure, height, weight, blood lipids, and pulmonary and cardiovascular function. Adults should begin routine physicals at age 18 and continue throughout the life span (21, 22).

Communicating Effectively with Your Health Care Provider

The relationship between a patient and health care provider plays an important role in the quality and effectiveness of medical care. Here are some guidelines for getting the most from your visit to the health care provider.

- Prepare for your appointment in advance. Studies show that 70% of correct medical diagnoses depend on what you tell your medical professional about your symptoms (22). Prior to your visit, write down a list of your symptoms. Try not to leave anything out of your list, even if you think it seems minor. Something you think is a minor detail might be very important.

- Bring any medications that you are taking to your appointment, including over-the-counter medications, supplements, and herbal treatments, and mention any current medical treatments you are using. You might think they are not important, but they can have side effects and can interact with medications.

- Remember, no question is a dumb question. Write out a list of questions before your appointment, and feel free to ask them. Let your health care provider know if you do not understand the answers to your questions or any other information you were given. If you are unclear about any part of your diagnosis and treatment options, ask for another explanation of your problem and the proposed treatment.

- If you want to know more about your condition, ask your doctor to recommend resources where you can find additional information. Finally, prior to leaving the doctor's office, make certain that you understand the next steps for your treatment (i.e., return for another visit, more tests, and/or obtaining a prescription).

Make sure you know...

> Maintaining regular insurance coverage is extremely important to avoid a potentially disastrous financial situation should you become ill or injured. You have options for health insurance plans, and the plan you choose will depend on your individual needs and preferences.

> Choosing a regular health care provider is an important part of maintaining wellness. You should choose one with whom you have good rapport and who can provide the services you need.

> Knowing when to see a health care provider will depend on your symptoms and medical history. Often, advice for minor illness can be provided over the phone. You should visit the emergency room only in true emergency situations.

> Maintaining wellness includes getting regular checkups and medical screenings at the recommended intervals.

> For cases in which medical attention is necessary, prepare for the visit by writing down a list of your symptoms and questions. Ask questions during the exam so that you fully understand your condition and the necessary treatment.

Summary

1. Exercise must be performed regularly throughout life to achieve the benefits of physical fitness, wellness, and disease prevention. Maintaining a regular program of good health behaviors, exercise, and healthy dietary practices requires motivation and a lifetime commitment to a healthy lifestyle.

2. Exercise is safe for healthy pregnant women. However, all pregnant women should consult with their health care providers about exercise during their pregnancies. There are modifications for exercise prescriptions for pregnant women.

3. Older adults can safely participate in regular exercise, and they will gain fitness and reduce their disease risk with an exercise program. Older adults should see their health care providers before beginning an exercise program to determine what modifications may be needed.

4. Numerous changes take place in the body and mind during the aging process. The cardiovascular and muscular systems decline in function, bones become more fragile, and hearing, eyesight, skin, and memory are all affected with age. Healthy behavior choices contribute to successful aging

5. After studying this book, you should be able to distinguish credible fitness information from common misperceptions. If you have doubts about the validity of a new fitness product or textbook, contact a fitness expert for advice.

6. There are several choices for health insurance, including group plans obtained through employers and individual plans. Fee-for-service, HMO, and PPO are the common types of group and individual plans available.

7. When selecting your personal health care provider, consider your needs, payment options, and the characteristics and qualifications of the health care provider before making a decision.

8. Knowing whether to see a health care provider for an illness will depend on your symptoms and medical history. When you meet with your health care provider, you should have with you a written list of symptoms and questions.

Study Questions

1. Which is not a recommended exercise for pregnant women?
   a. water aerobics
   b. abdominal toning class performed on the floor
   c. walking on a treadmill
   d. light- or moderate-intensity resistance training

2. Which of the following is not a change experienced during the aging process?
   a. decline in maximal heart rate
   b. decline in cardiorespiratory fitness
   c. decrease in muscle mass
   d. all are changes that occur with aging

3. Which of the following is not a recommended behavior for successful aging?
   a. taking vitamin and herbal supplements daily
   b. regular exercise
   c. getting regular screenings
   d. not smoking

4. Which of the following is a common misconception about fitness?
   a. Using a sauna can result in fat loss.
   b. Using hand-held weights while walking will not significantly increase arm strength.
   c. Even reputable fitness magazines can contain fitness myths.
   d. All are common misconceptions.

5. Which type of health insurance plan provides the most freedom when selecting a physician or hospital?
   a. PPO
   b. HMO
   c. fee-for-service
   d. group plan

6. Outline the key factors that play a role in maintaining a regular program of exercise.

7. List five points to consider when choosing a health club.

8. Give your definition of a fitness expert.

9. Numerous exercise misconceptions exist. Discuss the misconceptions associated with saunas, the use of hand weights, and nutritional ergogenic aids.

10. What factors should you consider when purchasing exercise equipment?

11. List several precautions you should take when using hot tubs, saunas, or steam baths.

12. List five activities that are considered to be good or excellent modes of promoting cardiorespiratory fitness.

13. Discuss the major age-related changes in fitness and wellness, and describe actions that you can take to maintain fitness and wellness throughout the life span.

14. Describe strategies for choosing a personal physician.

15. List nine keys to success for achieving lifetime wellness.

Suggested Reading

Booth, F. W., and M. V. Chakravarthy. Cost and consequences of sedentary living: New battleground for an old enemy. *President's Council on Physical Fitness and Sports Research Digest* 3:16, 2002.

Howley, E., and B. D. Franks. *The Fitness Professional's Handbook*, 5th ed. Champaign, IL: Human Kinetics, 2007.

Mayo Clinic Family Health Book, 4th ed. New York: Time, Inc. Home Entertainment, 2009.

Nieman, D. *Exercise Testing and Prescription*, 6th ed. St. Louis: McGraw-Hill, 2007.

Powers, S. and E. Howley. *Exercise Physiology: Theory and Application to Fitness and Performance*, 7th ed. New York: McGraw-Hill, 2009.

For links to the organizations and websites listed below, visit The Total Fitness and Wellness Website at www.pearsonhighered.com/powers.

American College of Sports Medicine
Contains information about aging, exercise, health, and fitness.

WebMD

Includes the latest information on a variety of health-related topics, including diet, exercise, and stress; also contains links to other sites on nutrition, fitness, and wellness topics.

American Council on Exercise

A nonprofit organization that provides information on a variety of topics related to exercise and fitness.

President's Council on Physical Fitness and Sports

Provides information concerning a wide range of subjects related to exercise and fitness.

American Medical Association

Contains many sources of information about a wide variety of medical and health issues.

Mayo Clinic

Contains information about a wide variety of diseases and medical issues. Also a good source for information about aging, nutrition, and choosing health care providers.

Fit Pregnancy

Provides expert information for moms-to-be on prenatal nutrition and exercise.

References

1. Caspersen, C. J., M. A.Pereira, and K. M. Curran. Changes in physical activity patterns in the United States, by sex and cross-sectional age. *Medicine and Science in Sports and Exercise* 32:1601–1609, 2000.

2. Sallis, J. F. Age-related decline in physical activity: A synthesis of human and animal studies. *Medicine and Science in Sports and Exercise* 32:1598–1600, 2000.

3. Sparling, P. B., and T. K.Snow. Physical activity patterns in recent college alumni. *Research Quarterly for Exercise and Sport* 73:200–205, 2002.

4. American College of Obstetricians and Gynecologists. Exercise during pregnancy and during the postpartum period. *Clinical Obstetrics and Gynecology* 46:496–499, 2003.

5. Artal, R. Exercise: The alternate therapeutic intervention for gestational diabetes. *Clinical Obstetrics and Gynecology* 46:479–487, 2003.

6. American College of Sports Medicine. *ACSM's Guidelines for Exercise Testing and Prescription*, 7th ed. Philadelphia: Lippincott Williams and Wilkins 2006.

7. Harman, D. The free radical theory of aging. *Antioxidants and Redox Signaling* 5:557–561, 2003.

8. Powers, S., and E. Howley. *Exercise Physiology: Theory and Application to Fitness and Performance*, 7th ed. New York: McGraw-Hill, 2009.

9. Spirduso, W. W., and D. L. Cronin. Exercise dose-response affects on quality of life and independent living in older adults. *Medicine and Science in Sports and Exercise* 33(6 Suppl):S598–S608, 2001.

10. Marcell, T. J. Sarcopenia: Causes, consequences, and preventions. *Journal of Gerontology* 58(10): M911–M916, 2003.

11. Hellekson K. L. NIH releases statement on osteoporosis prevention, diagnosis, and therapy. *American Family Physician* 66:161–162, 2002.

12. Houtkooper, L. B., V. A. Stanford, L. L. Metcalfe, T. G. Lohman, and S. B. Going. Preventing osteoporosis the bone estrogen strength training way. *ACSM's Health and Fitness Journal* 11:21–27, 2007.

13. Evans, B. W., J. A. Potteiger, M. C. Bray, and J. L. Tuttle. Metabolic and hemodynamic responses to walking with hand weights in older individuals. *Medicine and Science in Sports and Exercise* 26:1047–2052, 1994.

14. Criswell, D., S. Powers, and R. Herb. Clenbuterol-induced fiber type transition in the soleus of adult rats. *European Journal of Applied Physiology* 74:391–396, 1996.

15. Aagaard, P. Making muscles "stronger": Exercise, nutrition, drugs. *Journal of Musculoskeletal and Neuronal Interactions* 4:165–174, 2004.

16. Palmer, R., M. Delday, D. McMillan, B. Noble, P. Bain, and C. Maltin. Effects of the cyclo-oxygenase inhibitor, fenbufen, on clenbuterol-induced hypertrophy of cardiac and skeletal muscle of rats. *British Journal of Pharmacology* 101:835–838, 1990.

17. Taylor, W., S. Snowball, C. Dickson, and M. Lesna. Alterations in liver architecture in mice treated with anabolic androgens and dimethylnitrosamine. *NATO Advanced Study Institute Series*, Series A 52:279–288, 1982.

18. Lamb, D., and M. Williams. *Ergogenics: Enhancement of Performance in Exercise and Sport*. Vol. 4. Madison, WI: Brown and Benchmark, 1991.

19. National Center for Health Statistics. FastStats: Health insurance coverage. April 2009. www.cdc.gov/nchs/fastats/hinsure.htm.

20. Agency for Healthcare Research and Quality, Department of Health and Human Services. *Questions and Answers about Health Insurance: A Consumer Guide.* AHRQ Publication No. 07-0043. Rockville, MD: Agency for Healthcare Research and Quality, 2007.

21. Margen, S. (Ed.). *The Wellness Encyclopedia*. Boston: Houghton Mifflin Company, 1995.

22. *Mayo Clinic Family Health Book*. New York: HarperResource, 2003.

Videos

Log on to www.pearsonhighered.com/powers to view these chapter-related videos.

Healthy Aging

Seniors Say No to Retirement

Caring for Elderly Parents

Consumerism

Dr. Web's Credentials

Holistic Health Care (with Dr. Northrup)

Complementary and Alternative Medicine

NAME _____ DATE _____

Wellness Profile

After reading *Total Fitness and Wellness,* you will be equipped with the knowledge and skills you need to lead a healthy, fit lifestyle. Take the opportunity now to reexamine your strengths in the six areas of wellness. Write your top three strengths for each component of wellness below.

Physical Wellness

Maintaining overall physical health and participating in physical activities. Examples of strengths include cardiorespiratory endurance, balance, and flexibility.

1. _____
2. _____
3. _____

Emotional Wellness

Possessing a positive self-concept and dealing appropriately with your feelings. Strengths may include self-confidence, trust, and optimism.

1. _____
2. _____
3. _____

Intellectual Wellness

Retaining knowledge, thinking critically about issues, making sound decisions, and finding solutions to problems. Examples include inquisitiveness, curiosity, and dedication.

1. _____
2. _____
3. _____

Social Wellness

Developing lasting relationships with family and friends and contributing to the community. Strengths in this area may include compassion and friendliness.

1. _____
2. _____
3. _____

Environmental Wellness

Protecting yourself from environmental hazards and minimizing your negative impact on the environment. Behaviors such as recycling and carpooling are examples of strengths in this aspect of wellness.

1. _____
2. _____
3. _____

Spiritual Wellness

Having a sense of meaning and purpose in life. Behaviors such as prayer, meditation, helping others, and enjoying nature are examples of strengths along this dimension.

1. _____
2. _____
3. _____

Is there an aspect of wellness that you need to develop more fully? If so, which one? What are some specific behaviors you can do now to improve this wellness component in your life?

_____
_____
_____
_____
_____
_____

NAME _____ DATE _____

Evaluating Fitness Products

Complete this activity to evaluate fitness advertisements you see or hear regularly. Find three examples (from magazines, TV or radio ads, or online) of misleading or false claims on fitness or health products. Answer the following questions for each of your products.

1. What are two specific things (images or statements) that are false or misleading in the ad?

   _____

   _____

2. What makes them false? Support your answer with information you learned in class.

   _____

   _____

   _____

3. What are the credentials of the author or person endorsing the project? Is the information provided by an expert in the field of exercise science or physical fitness?

   _____

   _____

   _____

4. Are the benefits of the product realistic?

   _____

   _____

   _____

5. Does the ad contain gimmick words, such as "quick," "spot reduce," or "just minutes a day"?

   _____

   _____

   _____

6. Is the main purpose of the ad to provide useful information or only to sell a product?

   _____

   _____

   _____

LABORATORY

NAME _____ DATE _____

Exercise Training during Pregnancy

Use the following laboratory to design an exercise prescription for a pregnant woman.

Pregnancy and Exercise

Pregnancy places special demands on a woman's body because of the developing fetus's need for calories, protein, vitamins, minerals, and a stable physiological environment. To protect mother and fetus, consult a physician or other health care provider prior to initiating an exercise program.

Design a regular exercise program (at least 3 days per week) for a woman in her second trimester. Keep in mind that she should avoid exercises on her back and should emphasize non-weight-bearing activities. Describe the type of activity and duration of the exercise session. (*Example:* Monday could be lap swimming at a moderate pace for 20 minutes). Don't forget to include specific rest days.

Sunday	Monday	Tuesday	Wednesday	Thursday	Friday	Saturday

NAME _____ DATE _____

Selecting the Best Health Insurance Plan

The Agency for Healthcare Research and Quality suggests answering the following questions about your health care needs and wants to determine whether a fee-for-service, HMO, or PPO is best for you. This quiz won't answer all of your questions, but it will get you on track to making a sound decision for your health care needs.

For each group, circle the number of the statement (1 or 2) that best describes how you feel:

1. Having complete freedom to choose doctors and hospitals is the most important thing to me in a health plan, even if it costs more.

2. Holding down my costs is the most important thing to me, even if it means limiting some of my choices.

1. I travel a lot or have children that live away from me, and we may need to see doctors in other parts of the country.

2. I do not travel a lot and almost all care for my family will be needed in our local area.

1. I don't mind a health insurance plan that includes filling out forms or keeping receipts and sending them in for payment.

2. I prefer not to fill out forms or keep receipts. I want most of my care covered without a lot of paperwork.

1. In addition to my premiums, I am willing to pay for the cost of routine and preventive care, such as office visits, checkups, and shots. I also like knowing that I can get an appointment for these services when I want one.

2. I want a health plan that includes routine and preventive care. I don't mind if I have to wait for these services to be scheduled or for an available appointment with my doctor.

1. If I need to see a specialist, I probably will ask my doctor for a recommendation, but I want to decide whom to go to and when. I don't want to have to see my primary care doctor each time before I can see a specialist.

2. I don't mind if my primary care doctor must refer me to specialists. If my doctor doesn't think I need special services, that is fine with me.

If your answers are mostly 1's: You want to make your own health care choices, even if it costs you more and takes more paperwork. Fee-for-service may be the best plan for you.

If your answers are mostly 2's: You are willing to give up some choices to hold down your medical costs. You also want help in managing your care. Consider a health maintenance organization.

If your answers are some 1's and some 2's: You might want to look for a plan such as a preferred provider organization that combines some of the features of fee-for-service and those of a health maintenance organization.

1. According to your responses, what type of plan is best for you? Is this the type of plan you currently have?

   _____

   _____

   _____

2. Are there services with your current plan that do not meet your needs? If so, what are they?

   _____

   _____

   _____

3. What type of plan would better meet your needs?

   _____

   _____

   _____

Source: Agency for Healthcare Research and Quality, Department of Health and Human Services. Checkup on health insurance. www.ahrq.gov/consumer/insuranceqa.

NAME _____ DATE _____

An Exercise Interview with an Older Adult

Interview a friend or family member over age 60 about his or her physical activity and exercise habits. Use the following questions to assess their physical activity habits and to evaluate their activity status.

Interview Questions

1. Do you perform some type of exercise at least 3 times per week? (Be sure to provide the interviewee with some examples of exercise, based on what you've learned in this course.)

   _____

2. If you answered yes to question 1, what types of exercise do you do? How long is each exercise session? What are some benefits you get from your exercise program?

   _____

   _____

   _____

3. If you answered no to question 1, what are some reasons you do not exercise? How do you think an exercise program could affect your health?

   _____

   _____

   _____

4. Do you do things that are not exercise, but that keep you active, such as gardening, other yard work, or heavy housework? If so, what do you do, and how often do you do these activities?

   _____

   _____

   _____

5. How have your exercise and activity habits changed throughout your lifetime? Are you more or less active than you were in the past? How have your choices of activities changed? How has your exercise prescription changed?

   _____

   _____

   _____

Assessment Questions

1. Does the person you interviewed meet the current physical activity recommendations? If no, what are some changes he or she could make?

   _____

   _____

   _____

2. Does the person you interviewed have an accurate perception of exercise and activity for older adults? If not, what information would you give that person to clarify his or her misperceptions?

   _____

   _____

   _____

3. Does the person you interviewed have a lifetime pattern that is similar to what we see in the general population?

   _____

   _____

   _____

Appendix A Answers to Study Questions

Chapter 1

1. c. Physical activity is any type of occupational, leisure, or lifestyle related physical movement. Exercise is one example of leisure physical activity.

2. a. Although exercise is not a component of wellness, it can help you achieve physical health, which is one of the components of total wellness.

3. c. Agility may be important for sport performance, but it is not linked to improved overall health and therefore is not considered a major component of health-related physical fitness.

4. d. Reduced risk for osteoporosis and heart disease, as well as improved mental health are all benefits of regular physical activity.

5. a. Current goals of Healthy People 2010 seek to improve the quantity and quality of life for all Americans. Eliminating health disparities is also a key objective to meet these goals.

6. b. An individual in the action stage of change has been participating in a new health behavior for 6 months or less, but once this individual has moved beyond 6 months, he or she will be in the maintenance stage of change.

7. d. Developing a plan, getting the support of friends and family, and seeking outside help from others are all important actions to take in initiating a health behavior change.

8. d. Assessing your current behavior—including number and effort of behaviors you want to change, your motive for behavior change and current behaviors patterns—is an important step to take when planning a change.

Chapter 2

1. d. Supercompensation is not one of the five key principles of exercise training.

2. c. Current guidelines indicate that a minimum of 30 minutes of moderate exercise each day can produce numerous health benefits.

3. a. A few minutes of low intensity exercise (a warm-up) at the beginning of an exercise training session benefits the body by increasing both muscle temperature and blood flow to active muscles.

Chapter 3

1. c. Aerobic exercises include activities that promote cardiorespiratory fitness, such as jogging, swimming, and cycling.

2. a. Activities that promote muscle strength and endurance, such as wrestling, utilize the anaerobic energy pathway to create ATP and provide energy to muscles.

3. b. As an individual's cardiorespiratory fitness level increases, resting heart rate will decrease because the heart becomes more efficient at pumping blood throughout the body. This allows the heart to beat fewer times per minute to pump the same amount of blood.

4. c. You should exercise at a level of at least 50% of your heart rate reserve in order to improve health-related physical fitness and cardiorespiratory endurance.

5. d. Increases in heart rate, cardiac output, and breathing are normal physical changes you will experience during cardiorespiratory exercise.

6. a. Arteries are the blood vessels that move oxygen-rich blood away from your heart. Veins return oxygen-depleted blood back to the heart.

Chapter 4

No multiple choice questions in chapter 4.

Chapter 5

1. d. The shape of the bones, and tight skin and tendons can all affect one's flexibility at a joint. Bone length is typically not a factor.

2. e. The two types of proprioceptors are Golgi organs and muscle spindles, and they are found in tendons and muscles, respectively. Motor units are not a type of proprioceptor.

3. b. False. Most people, including athletes and non athletes, would benefit from the improved flexibility that results from regular static stretching.

4. b. A few minutes of light exercise before stretching will minimize your risk of injury. Where and when you stretch is not likely to affect your risk. Stretching to the point of pain is more likely to result in injury than stretching to the point of mild discomfort.

5. d. An imbalance in muscle strength caused by weak hamstrings or abdominal muscles (or a combination of both) can result in a forward curve (or hyperextension) of the lower back, resulting in back pain. Stretching and strengthening these muscles are important for avoiding LBP.

Chapter 6

1. b. Essential fat, necessary fat the body requires to maintain certain functions, should be at least 3 percent of total body weight in men and 12 percent in women.

2. d. Anemia is not a health consequence of overweight or obesity.

3. b. False. Excess fat in the abdomen or waist can put one at greater risk for heart disease and diabetes than an individual who stores body fat in their hips and thighs and lower part of the body.

4. a. While skinfold testing, underwater weighing, and bioelectrical impendence analysis are reliable methods for assessing body composition, the waist-to-hip ratio is the technique used to determine disease risk associated with body fat distribution.

5. c. A BMI of 30 kg/m² or greater is considered obese. A healthy BMI is less than 25 for men and less than 27 for women.

6. b. A Skinfold test is an easy measure to obtain and can provide good estimates when done properly.

7. d. Type 1 diabetes is not a health consequence of being underweight or having an eating disorder. Being underweight is associated with health problems such as malnutrition and osteoporosis.

8. a. True. Your BMI is a good estimate of your weight status, however, BMI does not give you a direct measure of percent fat. The method can over- or underestimate body fatness

Chapter 7

1. b. Carbohydrates provide the main source of fuel for your brain, and are the main source of energy during exercise.

2. c. Protein is used by the body to build muscle, skin, connective tissues, and other structural body tissues.

3. c. While water doesn't provide energy or build bone or protein, it is involved in numerous metabolic and other body processes, including blood formation.

4. d. A well-balanced diet consists of 58 percent carbohydrates, 30 percent fats, and 12 percent protein.

5. c. Antioxidants neutralize free radicals in the body, which prevent them from causing damage to cells.

Chapter 8

1. b. Optimal body fat percentages for health and fitness in men range from 10–20%, and from 15%–25% in women. The ranges allow for individual differences in physical activity and appearance.

2. f. Leptin and ghrelin are hormones that play a role in appetite. Leptin depresses appetite, while ghrelin contributes to appetite.

3. d. Energy balance occurs when the amount of calories you consume is equal to the amount of calories you consume, and therefore your weight will not change. If you consume more calories then you burn, you will gain weight. If you consume fewer calories than you burn, you will lose weight.

4. c. Physical activity that uses large muscle groups, such as cardiovascular and strength training is best to achieve weight loss. While flexibility training, yoga and Pilates can be part of a physical fitness program, cardiovascular training improves muscles' ability to burn fat as energy, resulting in weight loss.

5. d. Using the MyPyramid plan is a healthy way to eat for nutrition and overall health. Drastic measures for weight loss such as anorexia, bulimia, or using diet pills can be harmful to your health and constitute disordered eating.

Chapter 9

1. d. Smoking, hypertension, and high blood cholesterol are major risk factors for cardiovascular disease. Resting pulse rate is not a risk factor.

2. d. Normal blood pressure is 120/80 mm/Hg, so a blood pressure reading of 140/90 would be considered high blood pressure, or hypertension.

3. b. HDL is "good" cholesterol and LDL is "bad" cholesterol. When your LDL is high you are at increased risk for CHD, but if your HDL is high, your risk for developing CHD decreases.

4. c. Cardiovascular disease is leading cause of death in the United States for all ages.

5. b. Obesity, hypertension, and stress can all be modified by healthy lifestyle changes, however heredity, or the genes you are born with, cannot be changed.

Chapter 10

1. d. There are a variety of physical symptoms associated with stress, including headaches, anxiety, and muscle tension.

2. c. Eustress is positive stress that motivates and energizes us. Distress is the type of stress that can have a negative impact on our mental and physical health.

3. a. Epinephrine, cortisol, and norepinephrine are hormones released into the bloodstream during the stress response. Dopamine does not play a role in the body's response to stress.

4. d. Every day life situations can contribute our stress levels. These situations can include financial responsibilities, interpersonal relationship problems, and academic pressures.

5. b. Alcohol is not an effective way to cope with stress. Using alcohol to cope may eventually increase your stress level by affecting your ability to sleep, be productive, and may even lead to alcohol abuse.

Chapter 11

1. c. Evaporation is the body's major mechanism of heat loss during exercise. It is the only method that can dissipate enough heat during exercise to maintain a core temperature close to normal.

2. b. High humidity inhibits sweat evaporation. So, along with high heat, high humidity can cause a rapid rise in body temperature.

3. d. Layering clothing is the best method to insulate your body. Air is an excellent insulator, and layering clothing traps air between layers to insulate the body.

4. b. In cold weather the body's core temperature can decrease to dangerous levels, causing hypothermia.

5. b. At high alitudes, there is less oxygen available in the air, and thus, there is a reduced level of oxygen in the blood. In order to compensate, breathing increases to maximize the available oxygen.

Chapter 12

1. d. Any abnormal stress in the form of improper shoes, training techniques, or alignment abnormalities can impact muscles, tendons, joints, etc., and cause injury to a runner.

2. a. Because back pain is often associated with muscle weakness, exercise plays a role in prevention. In particular, core strength training, including your abdominal muscles, can readily prevent such damage.

3. b. Acute muscle soreness immediately after exercise is usually due to overuse or injury.

4. d. Because shin splints are typically caused by stress on the soft tissues, each of the listed precautions can reduce the stress on the tissues and reduce the risk of injury.

5. d. Ligaments cannot withstand much movement without injury. Thus, refraining from exercises that place a strain on joints is the best way to prevent damage.

Chapter 13

1. b. Lung cancer is the leading cause of cancer deaths for women in United States. While more women are diagnosed with breast cancer per year than lung cancer, breast cancer is typically detected earlier and is more treatable than lung cancer.

2. d. When a malignant tumor (one that is cancerous) metastasizes this means that the cancer cells have spread to other parts of the body. A benign tumor is not cancer.

3. c. Performing regular breast self exams is one thing you can do to prevent your cancer risk. However, behaviors such as poor diet, physical inactivity, and excessive alcohol consumption can increase your risk.

4. a. Skin cancer is the most common type of cancer, but is highly treatable if detected early. For people under the age of 30 melanoma is the most common type of skin cancer.

5. d. A nagging cough or hoarseness, a sore that does not heal, and unusual bleeding or discharge are three of the seven warning signs of cancer. If you have any one of these, make an appointment to see your doctor right away.

Chapter 14

1. d. Hepatitis B promotes an inflammatory response in the liver that results in a decrease in normal liver function. For this reason, Hepatitis B, which can be transmitted via bodily fluids, is a serious disease.

2. a. There are over 30 strains of human papillomavirus (HPV), and while many infected individuals do not experience noticeable symptoms, some strains of HPV are responsible for genital warts.

3. d. Syphilis is a bacterial infection. If it is treated early, it can be cured with antibiotics.

4. a. Stage 1, primary syphilis, generally includes a dime-sized, painless sore, called a chancre, located at the initial site of infection.

5. b. These infections are all caused by parasites

Chapter 15

1. d. A key factor in preventing an addiction is to abstain from the addictive behavior in the first place.

2. e. Each trait is associated with an addiction. Addictive behaviors begin as a single use of the drug, but over time cravings become stronger and an individual can lose control. This results in an escalation of drug use. When confronted, most addicts will deny that they have a drug problem.

3. a. Some drugs are more addictive than others. Each drug affects the brain in different ways.

4. b. Babies born to mothers who drink alcohol while pregnant may be born with fetal alcohol syndrome. One effect of FAS is low birth weight; however, a newborn can have low birth weight without having FAS.

5. e. Secondhand smoke is derived from a smoker's exhaled smoke (mainstream smoke) and the smoke given off from burning tobacco products (sidestream smoke).

Chapter 16

1. b. Pregnant women should avoid exercises that require them to lie on their backs for five minutes or more. For this reason, pregnant women should avoid floor-based abdominal toning exercises.

2. d. As you age, your maximal heart rate, cardiorespiratory fitness, and muscle mass all decrease.

3. a. Taking a daily vitamin or herbal supplement is not proven to ensure successful aging; however, regular exercise, regular medical screenings, and not smoking are all ways to age successfully.

4. a. Spending time in a sauna or steam bath to lose weight is a common fitness misconception. You may lose weight temporarily due to water loss, but as soon as you eat or drink, you will replace the lost fluids and your weight will return.

5. c. A fee for service plan provides the most freedom, but this type of health plan can be more costly than PPOs or HMOs.

APPENDIX B Nutritive Value of Selected Foods and Fast Foods

This section presents nutritional information about a wide array of foods, including many fast foods. Values are given for calories, protein, carbohydrates, fiber, fat, saturated fat, and cholesterol for common foods and serving sizes. Use this information to assess your diet and make improvements. This is only a sampling of the most common foods. See the MyDietAnalysis database for a more extensive list of foods.

MDA Code	Food Name	Amt	Wt (g)	Ener (kcal)	Prot (g)	Carb (g)	Fiber (g)	Fat (g)	Sat (g)	Chol (g)
Beverages										
Alcoholic Beverages										
22831	Beer	12 fl. oz	360	157	1	13		0	0	
34053	Beer, light	12 fl. oz	353	105	1	5	0	0	0	
22606	Beer, non alcoholic	12 fl. oz	353	73	1	14	0	0	0	
22884	Wine, red	1 fl. oz	29	24	0	1		0	0	
22861	Wine, white	1 fl. oz	29.3	24	0	1		0	0	
22514	Gin, 80 proof	1 fl. oz	27.8	64	0	0	0	0	0	
22593	Rum, 80 proof	1 fl. oz	27.8	64	0	0	0	0	0	
22515	Tequila, 80 proof	1 fl. oz	27.8	64	0	0	0	0	0	
22594	Vodka, 80 proof	1 fl. oz	27.8	64	0	0	0	0	0	
22670	Whiskey, 80 proof	1 fl. oz	27.8	64	0	0	0	0	0	
Coffee, Tea and Dairy Drink Mixes										
20012	Coffee, brewed	1 cup	237	2	0	0	0	0	0	0
20686	Coffee, decaffeinated, brewed	1 cup	237	0	0	0	0	0	0	0
20439	Coffee, espresso	1 cup	237	5	0	0	0	0	0.2	0
20402	Coffee, from mix, French vanilla, sugar & fat free	1 ea	7	25	0	5	0	0	0.1	0
85	Chocolate milk, prepared w/syrup	1 cup	282	254	9	36	1	8	4.7	25
46	Hot cocoa, w/aspartame, sodium, vitamin A, prepared w/water	1 cup	256	74	3	14	1	1	0	0
48	Hot cocoa, prep from dry mix with water	1 cup	275	151	2	32	1	2	0.9	3
166	Hot cocoa, w/marshmallows, from dry packet	1 ea	28	112	1	24	1	1	0.4	2
39	Chocolate flavor, dry mix, prepared w/milk	1 cup	266	226	9	32	1	9	4.9	24
41	Strawberry flavor, dry mix, prepared w/milk	1 cup	266	234	8	33	0	8	5.1	32
20014	Tea, brewed	1 cup	237	2	0	1	0	0	0	0
20036	Tea, herbal (not chamomile) brewed	1 cup	237	2	0	0	0	0	0	0
Fruit and Vegetable Beverages and Juices										
71080	Apple juice, canned or bottled, unsweetened	1 ea	262	123	0	31	0	0	0	0
20277	Capri Sun All Natural Juice Drink, Fruit Punch	1 ea	210	99	0	26	0	0	0	0
5226	Carrot juice, canned	1 cup	236	94	2	22	2	0	0.1	0
3042	Cranberry juice cocktail	1 cup	253	137	0	34	0	0	0	0
20024	Fruit punch, canned	1 cup	248	117	0	30	0	0	0	0
20035	Fruit punch, from frozen concentrate	1 cup	247	114	0	29	0	0	0	0
20101	Grape drink, canned	1 cup	250	153	0	39	0	0	0	0
3053	Grapefruit juice, from frozen concentrate, unsweetened	1 cup	247	101	1	24	0	0	0	0
20045	Lemonade flavor drink, from dry mix	1 cup	266	112	0	29	0	0	0	0
20047	Lemonade w/aspartame, low kcal, from dry mix	1 cup	237	5	0	1	0	0	0	0

Ener = energy (kilocalories); **Prot** = protein; **Carb** = carbohydrate; **Fiber** = dietary fiber; **Fat** = total fat; **Sat** = saturated fat; **Chol** = cholesterol.

°This food composition table has been prepared for Pearson Education, Inc. and is copyrighted by ESHA Research in Salem, Oregon, the developer of the MyDietAnalysis software program.

MDA Code	Food Name	Amt	Wt (g)	Ener (kcal)	Prot (g)	Carb (g)	Fiber (g)	Fat (g)	Sat (g)	Chol (g)
20070	Orange drink, canned	1 cup	248	122	0	31	0	0	0	0
20004	Orange flavor drink, from dry mix	1 cup	248	122	0	31	0	0	0	0
71108	Orange juice, canned, unsweetened	1 ea	263	110	2	26	1	0	0	0
3090	Orange juice, fresh	1 cup	248	112	2	26	0	0	0.1	0
3091	Orange juice, from frozen concentrate, unsweetened	1 cup	249	112	2	27	0	0	0	0
5397	Tomato juice, canned w/o salt	1 cup	243	41	2	10	1	0	0	0
20849	Vegetable and fruit, mixed juice drink	4 oz	113	33	0	8	0	0	0	0
20080	Vegetable juice cocktail, canned	1 cup	242	46	2	11	2	0	0	0
Soft Drinks										
20006	Club soda	1 cup	237	0	0	0	0	0	0	0
20685	Low-calorie cola, with aspartame, caffeine free	12 fl. oz	355	4	0	1	0	0	0	0
20843	Cola, with higher caffeine	12 fl. oz	370	152	0	39	0	0	0	0
20008	Ginger ale	1 cup	244	83	0	21	0	0	0	0
20032	Lemon-lime soft drink	1 cup	246	98	0	25	0	0	0	0
20027	Pepper-type soft drink	1 cup	246	101	0	26	0	0	0.2	0
20009	Root beer	1 cup	246	101	0	26	0	0	0	0
Other										
20033	Soy milk	1 cup	245	127	11	12	3	5	0.6	0
20041	Water, tap	1 cup	237	0	0	0	0	0	0	0
Breakfast Cereals										
40095	All-Bran/Kellogg	0.5 cup	30	78	4	22	9	1	0.2	0
40032	Cap'n Crunch/Quaker	0.75 cup	27	108	1	23	1	2	0.4	0
40297	Cheerios/Gen Mills	1 cup	30	111	4	22	4	2	0.4	0
40126	Cinnamon Toast Crunch/Gen Mills	0.75 cup	30	127	2	24	1	3	0.5	0
40195	Corn Flakes/Kellogg	1 cup	28	101	2	24	1	0	0.1	0
40089	Corn Grits, instant, plain, prepared/Quaker	1 pkg	137	93	2	21	1	0	0	0
40206	Corn Pops/Kellogg	1 cup	31	117	1	28	0	0	0.1	0
40179	Cream of Rice, prepared w/salt	1 cup	244	127	2	28	0	0	0	0
40182	Cream of Wheat, instant, prepared w/salt	1 cup	241	149	4	32	1	1	0.1	0
40104	Crispix/Kellogg	1 cup	29	109	2	25	0	0	0.1	0
40218	Froot Loops/Kellogg	1 cup	30	118	2	26	1	1	0.5	0
40217	Frosted Flakes/Kellogg	0.75 cup	31	114	1	28	1	0	0	0
11916	Frosted Mini-Wheats, bite size/Kellogg	1 cup	55	189	6	45	6	1	0.2	0
40209	Raisin Bran/Kellogg	1 cup	61	195	5	47	7	2	0.3	0
40210	Rice Krispies/Kellogg	1.25 cup	33	128	2	28	0	0	0.1	0
60887	Shredded wheat, large biscuit	2 ea	37.8	127	4	30	5	1	0.2	0
40211	Special K/Kellogg	1 cup	31	117	7	22	1	0	0.1	0
Dairy and Cheese										
500	Cream, half & half	2 Tbs	30	39	1	1	0	3	2.1	11
11	Milk, condensed, sweetend, canned	2 Tbs	38.2	123	3	21	0	3	2.1	13
19	Milk, lowfat, 1% fat, chocolate	1 cup	250	158	8	26	1	2	1.5	8
218	Milk, 2%, w/added vitamins A & D	1 cup	245	130	8	13	0	5	3	
6	Milk, nonfat/skim, w/added vitamin A	1 cup	245	83	8	12	0	0	0.1	5
1	Milk, whole, 3.25%	1 cup	244	146	8	11	0	8	4.6	24
20	Milk, whole, chocolate	1 cup	250	208	8	26	2	8	5.3	30
72088	Yogurt, fruit variety, nonfat	1 cup	245	230	11	47	0	0	0.3	5
1287	American Cheese, nonfat slices	1 pce	21.3	32	5	2	0	0	0.1	3
13349	Cheez Whiz cheese sauce/Kraft	2 Tbs	33	91	4	3	0	7	4.3	25

MDA Code	Food Name	Amt	Wt (g)	Ener (kcal)	Prot (g)	Carb (g)	Fiber (g)	Fat (g)	Sat (g)	Chol (g)
1014	Cottage cheese, 2% fat	0.5 cup	113	102	16	4	0	2	1.4	9
1015	Cream cheese	2 Tbs	29	101	2	1	0	10	6.4	32
1452	Cream cheese, fat free	2 Tbs	29	28	4	2	0	0	0.3	2
1016	Feta, crumbled	0.25 cup	37.5	99	5	2	0	8	5.6	33
47887	Mozzarella, whole milk, slice	1 ea	34	102	8	1	0	8	4.5	27
1075	Parmesan, grated	1 Tbs	5	22	2	0	0	1	0.9	4
1024	Ricotta, part skim	0.25 cup	62	86	7	3	0	5	3.1	19
1064	Ricotta, whole milk	0.25 cup	62	108	7	2	0	8	5.1	32
Eggs and Egg Substitutes										
19525	Egg substitute, liquid	0.25 cup	62.8	53	8	0	0	2	0.4	1
19506	Egg, white, raw	1 ea	33.4	17	4	0	0	0	0	0
19509	Egg, whole, fried	1 ea	46	92	6	0	0	7	2	210
19515	Egg, whole, hard boiled	1 ea	37	57	5	0	0	4	1.2	157
19521	Egg, whole, poached	1 ea	37	54	5	0	0	4	1.1	156
19516	Egg, whole, scrambled	1 ea	61	101	7	1	0	7	2.2	215
19508	Egg, yolk, raw, fresh	1 ea	16.6	53	3	1	0	4	1.6	205
Fruit										
72101	Apricots, canned, heavy syrup, drained	1 cup	182	151	1	39	5	0	0	0
3164	Fruit cocktail canned in juice	1 cup	237	109	1	28	2	0	0	0
71079	Apple w/skin, raw	1 cup	125	65	0	17	3	0	0	0
3331	Applesauce, canned, sweetened w/added Vit C	0.5 cup	128	97	0	25	2	0	0	0
3657	Apricot, raw	1 cup	165	79	2	18	3	1	0	0
3210	Avocado, California, peeled, raw	1 ea	173	289	3	15	12	27	3.7	0
71082	Banana, peeled, raw	1 ea	81	72	1	19	2	0	0.1	0
71976	Grapefruit, fresh	0.5 ea	154	60	1	16	6	0	0	
3055	Grapes, Thompson seedless, fresh	0.5 cup	80	55	1	14	1	0	0	4
3642	Melon, fresh, wedge	1 pce	69	23	1	6	1	0	0	5
3168	Mixed fruit (prune, apricot & pear) dried	1 oz	28.4	69	1	18	2	0	0	0
3216	Nectarine, raw	1 cup	138	61	1	15	2	0	0	0
3726	Peach, peeled, raw	1 ea	79	31	1	8	1	0	0	0
3106	Pear, raw	1 ea	209	121	1	32	6	0	0	0
3766	Raisins, seedless	50 ea	26	78	1	21	1	0	0	0
72113	Pineapple, fresh, slice	1 pce	84	38	0	10		0		5
3085	Orange, fresh	1 ea	184	86	2	22	4	0	0	
3135	Strawberries, halves/slices, raw	1 cup	166	53	1	13	3	0	0	0
Grain Products										
Breads, Rolls, and Bread Crumbs										
71170	Bagel, cinnamon-raisin	1 ea	26	71	3	14	1	0	0.1	0
71167	Bagel, egg	1 ea	26	72	3	14	1	1	0.1	6
71152	Bagel, plain/onion/poppy/sesame, enriched	1 ea	26	67	3	13	1	0	0.1	0
42433	Biscuit, w/butter	1 ea	82	280	5	27	0	17	4	0
71192	Biscuit, Plain or Buttermilk, refrig dough, baked, reduced fat	1 ea	21	63	2	12	0	1	0.3	0
42004	Bread crumbs, dry, plain, grated	1 Tbs	6.8	27	1	5	0	0	0.1	0
49144	Bread, crusty Italian w/garlic	1 pce	50	186	4	21	10	2.4	6	
70964	Bread, garlic, frozen/Campione	1 pce	28	101	2	12	1	5	0.8	
42069	Bread, oat bran	1 pce	30	71	3	12	1	1	0.2	0

MDA Code	Food Name	Amt	Wt (g)	Ener (kcal)	Prot (g)	Carb (g)	Fiber (g)	Fat (g)	Sat (g)	Chol (g)
42095	Bread, wheat, reduced kcal	1 pce	23	46	2	10	3	1	0.1	0
71247	Bread, white, commercially prepared, crumbs/cubes/slices	1 pce	9	24	1	5	0	0	0.1	0
42084	Bread, white, reduced kcal	1 pce	23	48	2	10	2	1	0.1	0
26561	Buns, hamburger, Wonder	1 ea	43	117	3	22	1	2	0.4	
42021	Hamburger/hot dog bun, plain	1 ea	43	120	4	21	1	2	0.5	0
42115	Cornbread, prepared from dry mix	1 pce	60	188	4	29	1	6	1.6	37
71227	Pita bread, white, enriched	1 ea	28	77	3	16	1	0	0	0
71228	Pita bread, whole wheat	1 ea	28	74	3	15	2	1	0.1	0
71368	Roll, dinner, plain, homemade w/reduced fat (2%) milk	1 ea	43	136	4	23	1	3	0.8	15
42161	Roll, French	1 ea	38	105	3	19	1	2	0.4	0
71056	Roll, hard/kaiser	1 ea	57	167	6	30	1	2	0.3	0
42297	Tortilla, corn, w/o salt, ready to cook	1 ea	26	58	1	12	1	1	0.1	0
90645	Taco shell, baked	1 ea	5	23	0	3	0	1	0.2	0
Crackers										
71451	Cheez-its/Goldfish crackers, low sodium	55 pce	33	166	3	19	1	8	3.2	4
43507	Oyster/soda/soup crackers	1 cup	45	193	4	32	1	5	0.7	0
70963	Ritz crackers/Nabisco	5 ea	16	79	1	10	0	4	0.6	0
43587	Saltine crackers, original premium/Nabisco	5 ea	14	59	2	10	0	1	0.3	0
43545	Sandwich crackers, cheese filled	4 ea	28	134	3	17	1	6	1.7	1
43546	Sandwich crackers, peanut butter filled	4 ea	28	138	3	16	1	7	1.4	0
44677	Snackwell Wheat Cracker/Nabisco	1 ea	15	62	1	12	1	2		
43581	Wheat Thins, baked/Nabisco	16 ea	29	136	2	20	1	6	0.9	0
43508	Whole wheat cracker	4 ea	32	142	3	22	3	6	1.1	0
Muffins and Baked Goods										
42723	English muffin, plain	1 ea	57	132	5	26		1	0.2	
62916	Muffin, blueberry, commercially prepared	1 ea	11	30	1	5	0	1	0.2	3
44521	Muffin, corn, commercially prepared	1 ea	57	174	3	29	2	5	0.8	15
44514	Muffin, oat bran	1 ea	57	154	4	28	3	4	0.6	0
44518	Toaster muffin, blueberry	1 ea	33	103	2	18	1	3	0.5	2
Noodles and Pasta										
38048	Chow mein noodles, dry	1 cup	45	237	4	26	2	14	2	0
38047	Egg noodles, enriched, cooked	0.5 cup	80	110	4	20	1	2	0.3	23
38060	Spaghetti, whole wheat, cooked	1 cup	140	174	7	37	6	1	0.1	0
38251	Egg noodles, enriched, cooked w/salt	0.5 cup	80	110	4	20	1	2	0.3	
38102	Macaroni noodles, enriched, cooked	1 cup	140	221	8	43	3	1	0.2	
38118	Spaghetti noodles, enriched, cooked	0.5 cup	70	111	4	22	1	1	0.1	4
Grains										
38076	Couscous, cooked	0.5 cup	78.5	88	3	18	1	0	0	0
38080	Oats	0.25 cup	39	152	7	26	4	3	0.5	0
38010	Rice, brown, long grain, cooked	1 cup	195	216	5	45	4	2	0.4	0
38256	Rice, white, long grain, enriched, cooked w/salt	1 cup	158	205	4	45	1	0	0.1	0
38019	Rice, white, long grain, instant, enriched, cooked	1 cup	165	193	4	41	1	1	0	0
Pancakes, French Toast, and Waffles										
42156	French Toast, homemade w/reduced fat (2%) milk	1 pce	65	149	5	16	1	7	1.8	75
45192	Pancake/waffle, buttermilk/Eggo/Kellogg	1 ea	42.5	99	3	16	0	3	0.6	5

MDA Code	Food Name	Amt	Wt (g)	Ener (kcal)	Prot (g)	Carb (g)	Fiber (g)	Fat (g)	Sat (g)	Chol (g)
45117	Pancakes, plain, homemade	1 ea	77	175	5	22	1	7	1.6	45
45193	Waffle, lowfat, homestyle, frozen	1 ea	35	83	2	15	0	1	0.3	9

Meat and Meat Substitutes

Beef

MDA Code	Food Name	Amt	Wt (g)	Ener (kcal)	Prot (g)	Carb (g)	Fiber (g)	Fat (g)	Sat (g)	Chol (g)
10093	Beef, average of all cuts, lean & fat (1/4″ trim) cooked	3 oz	85.1	260	22	0	0	18	7.3	75
10705	Beef, average of all cuts, lean (1/4″ trim) cooked	3 oz	85.1	184	25	0	0	8	3.2	73
10133	Beef, whole rib, roasted, 1/4″ trim	3 oz	85.1	305	19	0	0	25	10	71
58129	Ground beef (hamburger), 25% fat, cooked, pan-browned	3 oz	85.1	236	22	0	0	15	6	76
58119	Ground beef (hamburger), 15% fat, cooked, pan-browned	3 oz	85.1	218	24	0	0	13	5	77
58109	Ground beef (hamburger), 5% fat, cooked, pan-browned	3 oz	85.1	164	25	0	0	6	2.9	76
10791	Porterhouse steak, lean & fat (1/4″ trim) broiled	3 oz	85.1	280	19	0	0	22	8.7	61
58257	Rib eye steak, small end (ribs 10-12), 0″ trim, broiled	3 oz	85.1	210	23	0	0	13	4.9	94
58094	Skirt steak, trimmed to 0″ fat, broiled	3 oz	85.1	187	22	0	0	10	4	51
58328	Strip steak, top loin, 1/8″ trim, broiled	3 oz	85.1	171	25	0	0	7	2.7	67
10805	T-Bone steak, lean & fat (1/4″ trim) broiled	3 oz	85.1	260	20	0	0	19	7.6	55
11531	Veal, average of all cuts, cooked	3 oz	85.1	197	26	0	0	10	3.6	97

Chicken

MDA Code	Food Name	Amt	Wt (g)	Ener (kcal)	Prot (g)	Carb (g)	Fiber (g)	Fat (g)	Sat (g)	Chol (g)
15057	Chicken breast, w/o skin, fried	3 oz	85.1	159	28	0	0	4	1.1	77
15080	Chicken, dark meat, w/skin, roasted	3 oz	85.1	215	22	0	0	13	3.7	77
15026	Chicken, dark meat, w/o skin, fried	3 oz	85.1	203	25	2	0	10	2.7	82
15042	Chicken drumstick, w/o skin, fried	3 oz	85.1	166	24	0	0	7	1.8	80
15048	Chicken, wing, w/o skin, fried	3 oz	85.1	180	26	0	0	8	2.1	71
15059	Chicken, wing, w/o skin, roasted	3 oz	85.1	173	26	0	0	7	1.9	72

Turkey

MDA Code	Food Name	Amt	Wt (g)	Ener (kcal)	Prot (g)	Carb (g)	Fiber (g)	Fat (g)	Sat (g)	Chol (g)
51151	Turkey bacon, cooked	1 oz	28.4	108	8	1	0	8	2.4	28
51098	Turkey patty, breaded, fried	1 ea	42	119	6	7	0	8	2	26
16110	Turkey breast w/skin, roasted	3 oz	85.1	130	25	0	0	3	0.7	77
16038	Turkey breast, no skin, roasted	3 oz	85.1	115	26	0	0	1	0.2	71
16101	Turkey, dark meat w/skin, roasted	3 oz	85.1	155	24	0	0	6	1.8	100
16003	Turkey, ground, cooked	1 ea	82	193	22	0	0	11	2.8	84

Lamb

MDA Code	Food Name	Amt	Wt (g)	Ener (kcal)	Prot (g)	Carb (g)	Fiber (g)	Fat (g)	Sat (g)	Chol (g)
13604	Lamb, average of all cuts (1/4″ trim) cooked	3 oz	85.1	250	21	0	0	18	7.5	83
13616	Lamb, average of all cuts, lean (1/4″ trim) cooked	3 oz	85.1	175	24	0	0	8	2.9	78

Pork

MDA Code	Food Name	Amt	Wt (g)	Ener (kcal)	Prot (g)	Carb (g)	Fiber (g)	Fat (g)	Sat (g)	Chol (g)
12000	Bacon, broiled, pan-fried, or roasted	3 pcs	19	103	7	0	0	8	2.6	21
28143	Canadian bacon	1 ea	56	68	9	1	3	1	27	
12211	Ham, cured, boneless, regular fat (11% fat) roasted	1 cup	140	249	32	0	0	13	4.4	83
12309	Pork, average of retail cuts, cooked	3 oz	85.1	232	23	0	0	15	5.3	77
12097	Pork, ribs, backribs, roasted	3 oz	85.1	315	21	0	0	25	9.4	100
12099	Pork, ground, cooked	3 oz	85.1	253	22	0	0	18	6.6	80

Nutritive Value of Selected Foods and Fast Foods

MDA Code	Food Name	Amt	Wt (g)	Ener (kcal)	Prot (g)	Carb (g)	Fiber (g)	Fat (g)	Sat (g)	Chol (g)
Lunchmeats										
13000	Beef, thin slices	1 oz	28.4	42	5	0	0	2	0.8	20
58275	Bologna, beef and pork, low fat	1 ea	14	32	2	0	0	3	1	5
13157	Chicken breast, oven roasted deluxe	1 oz	28.4	29	5	1	0	1	0.2	14
13306	Corned beef, cooked, chopped, pressed	1 ea	71	101	14	1	0	5	2	46
13264	Ham, slices, regular (11% fat)	1 cup	135	220	22	5	2	12	4	77
13101	Pastrami, beef, cured	1 oz	28.4	41	6	0	0	2	0.8	19
13215	Salami, beef, cotto	1 oz	28.4	59	4	1	0	4	1.9	24
16160	Turkey breast slice	1 pce	21	22	4	1	0	0	0.1	9
58279	Turkey ham, sliced, extra lean, prepackaged or deli-sliced	1 cup	138	163	27	2	0	5	1.8	92
Sausage										
13070	Chorizo, pork & beef	1 ea	60	273	14	1	0	23	8.6	53
57877	Frankfurter, beef	1 ea	45	148	5	2	0	13	5.3	24
13012	Frankfurter, turkey	1 ea	45	102	6	1	0	8	2.7	48
57890	Italian sausage, pork, cooked	1 ea	83	286	16	4	0	23	7.9	47
13021	Pepperoni sausage	1 pce	5.5	26	1	0	0	2	0.9	6
13185	Pork sausage links, cooked	2 ea	48	165	8	0	0	15	5.1	37
58227	Sausage, pork, pre-cooked	3 oz	85	321	12	0	0	30	9.9	63
58007	Turkey sausage, breakfast links, mild	2 ea	56	132	9	1	0	10	4.4	34
Meat Substitutes										
7509	Bacon substitute, vegetarian, strips	3 ea	15	46	2	1	0	4	0.7	0
7722	Garden patties, frozen/Worthington, Morningstar	1 ea	67	119	11	10	4	4	0.5	1
7674	Harvest burger, original flavor, vegetable protein patty	1 ea	90	138	18	7	6	4	1	0
90626	Sausage, vegetarian, meatless	1 ea	28	72	5	3	1	5	0.8	0
7726	Spicy Black Bean Burger/Worthington, Morningstar	1 ea	78	115	12	15	5	1	0.2	1
Nuts										
4519	Cashews, dry roasted w/salt	0.25 cup	34.2	196	5	11	1	16	3.1	0
4728	Macadamia nuts, dry roasted, unsalted	1 cup	134	962	10	18	11	102	16	0
4592	Mixed nuts, w/peanuts, dry roasted, salted	0.25 cup	34.2	203	6	9	3	18	2.4	0
4626	Peanut butter, chunky w/salt	2 Tbs	32	188	8	7	3	16	2.6	0
4756	Peanuts, dry roasted w/o salt	30 ea	30	176	7	6	2	15	2.1	0
4696	Peanuts, raw	0.25 cup	36.5	207	9	6	3	18	2.5	0
4540	Pistachio nuts, dry roasted, salted	0.25 cup	32	182	7	9	3	15	1.8	0
Seafood										
17029	Bass, freshwater, cooked w/dry heat	3 oz	85.1	124	21	0	0	4	0.9	74
17037	Cod, Atlantic, baked/broiled (dry heat)	3 oz	85.1	89	19	0	0	1	0.1	47
19036	Crab, Alaskan King, boiled/steamed	3 oz	85.1	83	16	0	0	1	0.1	45
17090	Haddock, baked or broiled (dry heat)	3 oz	85.1	95	21	0	0	1	0.1	63
17291	Halibut, Atlantic & Pacific, baked or broiled (dry heat)	3 oz	85.1	119	23	0	0	3	0.4	35
17181	Salmon, Atlantic, farmed, cooked w/dry heat	3 oz	85.1	175	19	0	0	11	2.1	54
17099	Salmon, Sockeye, baked or broiled (dry heat)	3 oz	85.1	184	23	0	0	9	1.6	74
71707	Squid, fried	3 oz	85.1	149	15	7	0	6	1.6	221
17066	Swordfish, baked or broiled (dry heat)	3 oz	85.1	132	22	0	0	4	1.2	43
56007	Tuna salad, lunchmeat spread	2 Tbs	25.6	48	4	2	0	2	0.4	3
17151	White tuna, canned in H_2O, drained	3 oz	85.1	109	20	0	0	3	0.7	36
17083	White tuna, canned in oil, drained	3 oz	85.1	158	23	0	0	7	1.1	26

MDA Code	Food Name	Amt	Wt (g)	Ener (kcal)	Prot (g)	Carb (g)	Fiber (g)	Fat (g)	Sat (g)	Chol (g)
Vegetables and Legumes										
Beans										
7038	Baked beans, plain or vegetarian, canned	1 cup	254	239	12	54	10	1	0.2	0
5197	Bean sprouts, mung, canned, drained	1 cup	125	15	2	3	1	0	0	0
7012	Black beans, boiled w/o salt	1 cup	172	227	15	41	15	1	0.2	0
5862	Beets, boiled w/salt, drained	0.5 cup	85	37	1	8	2	0	0	0
90018	Cowpeas, cooked w/salt	1 cup	171	198	13	35	11	1	0.2	0
7081	Hummus, garbanzo or chickpea spread, homemade	1 Tbs	15.4	27	1	3	1	1	0.2	0
7087	Kidney beans, canned	1 cup	256	210	13	37	11	2	0.2	0
7006	Lentils, boiled w/o salt	1 cup	198	230	18	40	16	1	0.1	0
7051	Pinto beans, canned	1 cup	240	206	12	37	11	2	0.4	0
6748	Snap green beans, raw	10 ea	55	17	1	4	2	0	0	0
5320	Snap yellow beans, raw	0.5 cup	55	17	1	4	2	0	0	0
90026	Split peas, boiled w/salt	0.5 cup	98	116	8	21	8	0	0.1	0
7054	White beans, canned	1 cup	262	307	19	57	13	1	0.2	0
Fresh Vegetables										
9577	Artichokes (globe or French) boiled w/salt, drained	1 ea	20	10	1	2	1	0	0	0
6033	Arugula/roquette, raw	1 cup	20	5	1	1	0	0	0	0
90406	Asparagus, raw	10 ea	35	7	1	1	1	0	0	0
5558	Broccoli stalks, raw	1 ea	114	32	3	6	4	0	0.1	0
5036	Cabbage, raw	1 cup	70	17	1	4	2	0	0	0
90605	Carrots, baby, raw	1 ea	15	5	0	1	0	0	0	0
5049	Cauliflower, raw	0.5 cup	50	12	1	3	1	0	0	0
90436	Celery, raw	1 ea	17	2	0	1	0	0	0	0
7202	Corn, white, sweet, ears, raw	1 ea	73	63	2	14	2	1	0.1	0
5900	Corn, yellow, sweet, boiled w/salt, drained	0.5 cup	82	89	3	21	2	1	0.2	0
5908	Eggplant (brinjal) boiled w/salt, drained	1 cup	99	35	1	9	2	0	0	0
5087	Lettuce, looseleaf, raw	2 pcs	20	3	0	1	0	0	0	0
51069	Mushrooms, brown, Italian, or crimini, raw	2 ea	28	6	1	1	0	0	0	0
90472	Onions, chopped, raw	1 ea	70	29	1	7	1	0	0	0
5116	Peas, green, raw	1 cup	145	117	8	21	7	1	0.1	0
7932	Peppers, jalapeno, raw	1 cup	90	27	1	5	2	1	0.1	0
90493	Peppers, sweet green, chopped/sliced, raw	10 pcs	27	5	0	1	0	0	0	0
6990	Pepper, sweet red, raw	1 ea	10	3	0	1	0	0	0	0
9251	Potatoes, red, flesh and skin, baked	1 ea	138	123	3	27	2	0	0	0
9245	Potatoes, russet, flesh and skin, baked	1 ea	138	134	4	30	3	0	0	0
5146	Spinach, raw	1 cup	30	7	1	1	1	0	0	0
90525	Squash, zucchini w/skin, slices, raw	1 ea	118	19	1	4	1	0	0	0
6924	Sweet potato, baked in skin w/salt	0.5 cup	100	90	2	21	3	0	0.1	0
5180	Tomato sauce, canned	0.5 cup	123	39	2	9	2	0	0	0
90532	Tomato, red, ripe, whole, raw	1 ea	15	3	0	1	0	0	0	0
5306	Yam, peeled, raw	0.5 cup	75	88	1	21	3	0	0	0
Soy and Soy Products										
7564	Tempeh	0.5 cup	83	160	15	8	9	1.8	0	
7015	Soybeans, cooked	1 cup	172	298	29	17	10	15	2.2	0
7542	Tofu, firm, silken, 1″ slice	3 oz	85.1	53	6	2	0	2	0.3	0
Meals and Dishes										
92216	Tortellini with cheese filling	1 cup	108	332	15	51	2	8	3.9	45
57658	Chili con carne w/beans, canned entree	1 cup	222	269	16	25	9	12	3.9	29

Nutritive Value of Selected Foods and Fast Foods

MDA Code	Food Name	Amt	Wt (g)	Ener (kcal)	Prot (g)	Carb (g)	Fiber (g)	Fat (g)	Sat (g)	Chol (g)
57703	Chili, vegetarian chili w/beans, canned entree/Hormel	1 cup	247	205	12	38	10	1	0.1	0
57068	Macaroni and cheese, unprepared/Kraft	1 ea	70	259	11	48	1	3	1.3	10
70958	Stir fry, rice & vegetables, w/soy sauce/Hanover	1 cup	137	130	5	27	2	0		
70943	Beef & bean burrito/Las Campanas	1 ea	114	296	9	38	1	12	4.2	13
16195	Chicken & vegetables/Lean Cuisine	1 ea	297	252	19	32	5	6	1	24
70917	Hot Pockets, beef & cheddar, frozen	1 ea	142	403	16	39		20	8.8	53
70918	Hot Pockets, croissant pocket w/chicken, broccoli, & cheddar, frozen	1 ea	128	301	11	39	1	11	3.4	37
56757	Lasagna w/meat sauce/Stouffer's	1 ea	215	277	19	26	3	11	4.7	41
11029	Macaroni & beef in tomato sauce/Lean Cuisine	1 ea	283	249	14	37	3	5	1.6	23
5587	Mashed potatoes, from granules w/milk, prep w/water & margarine	0.5 cup	105	122	2	17	1	5	1.3	2
70898	Pizza, pepperoni, frozen	1 ea	146	432	16	42	3	22	7.1	22
56703	Spaghetti w/meat sauce/Lean Cuisine	1 ea	326	313	14	51	6	6	1.4	13

Snack Foods

MDA Code	Food Name	Amt	Wt (g)	Ener (kcal)	Prot (g)	Carb (g)	Fiber (g)	Fat (g)	Sat (g)	Chol (g)
10051	Beef jerky	1 pce	19.8	81	7	2	0	5	2.1	10
63331	Breakfast bars, oats, sugar, raisins, coconut	1 ea	43	200	4	29	1	8	5.5	0
61251	Cheese puffs and twists, corn based, low fat	1 oz	28.4	123	2	21	3	3	0.6	0
44032	Chex snack mix	1 cup	42.5	181	5	28	2	7	2.4	0
23059	Granola bar, hard, plain	1 ea	24.5	115	2	16	1	5	0.6	0
23104	Granola bar, soft, plain	1 ea	28.4	126	2	19	1	5	2.1	0
44012	Popcorn, air-popped	1 cup	8	31	1	6	1	0	0.1	0
44076	Potato chips, plain, no salt	1 oz	28.4	152	2	15	1	10	3.1	0
5437	Potato chips, sour cream & onion	1 oz	28.4	151	2	15	1	10	2.5	2
44015	Pretzels, hard	5 pcs	30	114	3	24	1	1	0.1	0
44021	Rice cake, brown rice, plain, salted	1 ea	9	35	1	7	0	0	0.1	0
44058	Trail mix, regular	0.25 cup	37.5	173	5	17	2	11	2.1	0

Soups

MDA Code	Food Name	Amt	Wt (g)	Ener (kcal)	Prot (g)	Carb (g)	Fiber (g)	Fat (g)	Sat (g)	Chol (g)
50398	Beef barley, canned/Progresso Healthy Classics	1 cup	241	142	11	20	3	2	0.7	19
50081	Chicken noodle, chunky, canned	1 cup	240	175	13	17	4	6	1.4	19
50085	Chicken rice, chunky, ready to eat, canned	1 cup	240	127	12	13	1	3	1	12
50088	Chicken vegetable, chunky, canned	1 cup	240	166	12	19	0	5	1.4	17
90238	Chicken, chunky, canned	1 cup	240	170	12	17	1	6	1.9	29
50697	Cup of Noodles, ramen, chicken flavor, dry/Nissin	1 ea	64	296	6	37	14	6.3		
50009	Minestrone, canned, made w/water	1 cup	241	82	4	11	1	3	0.6	2
92163	Ramen noodle, any flavor, dehydrated, dry	0.5 cup	38	172	4	25	1	6	2.9	0
50043	Tomato vegetable, from dry mix, made w/water	1 cup	253	56	2	10	1	1	0.4	0
50028	Tomato, canned, made w/water	1 cup	244	85	2	17	0	2	0.4	0
50014	Vegetable beef, canned, made w/water	1 cup	244	78	6	10	0	2	0.9	5
50013	Vegetarian vegetable, canned, made w/water	1 cup	241	72	2	12	0	2	0.3	0

Desserts

MDA Code	Food Name	Amt	Wt (g)	Ener (kcal)	Prot (g)	Carb (g)	Fiber (g)	Fat (g)	Sat (g)	Chol (g)
62904	Brownie, commercially prepared, square, lrg, 2-3/4″ × 7/8″	1 ea	56	227	3	36	1	9	2.4	10
46062	Cake, chocolate, homemade, w/o icing	1 pce	95	340	5	51	2	14	5.2	55
46091	Cake, yellow, homemade, w/o icing	1 pce	68	245	4	36	0	10	2.7	37

MDA Code	Food Name	Amt	Wt (g)	Ener (kcal)	Prot (g)	Carb (g)	Fiber (g)	Fat (g)	Sat (g)	Chol (g)
71337	Doughnut, cake, w/chocolate icing, lrg, 3 1/2"	1 ea	57	270	3	27	1	18	4.6	35
45525	Doughnut, cake, glazed/sugared, med, 3"	1 ea	45	192	2	23	1	10	2.7	14
47026	Animal crackers/Arrowroot/Tea Biscuits	10 ea	12.5	56	1	9	0	2	0.4	0
90636	Chocolate chip cookie, commercially prepared 3.5" to 4"	1 ea	40	196	2	26	1	10	3.1	0
47006	Chocolate sandwich cookie, creme filled	3 ea	30	140	2	21	1	6	1.1	0
62905	Fig bar, 2 oz	1 ea	56.7	197	2	40	3	4	0.6	0
90640	Oatmeal cookie, commercially prepared, 3-1/2" to 4"	1 ea	25	112	2	17	1	5	1.1	0
47010	Peanut butter cookie, homemade, 3"	1 ea	20	95	2	12	0	5	0.9	6
62907	Sugar cookie, refrigerated dough, baked	1 ea	23	111	1	15	0	5	1.4	7
57894	Pudding, chocolate, ready to eat	1 ea	113	158	3	26	1	5	0.8	3
2612	Pudding, vanilla, ready-to-eat	1 ea	113	147	3	25	0	4	1.7	8
2651	Rice pudding, ready-to-eat	1 ea	142	231	3	31	0	11	1.7	1
57902	Tapioca pudding, ready-to-eat	1 ea	113	135	2	22	0	4	1.1	1
71819	Frozen yogurt, chocolate, nonfat	1 cup	186	199	8	37	2	1	0.9	7
72124	Frozen yogurt, flavors other than chocolate	1 cup	174	221	5	38	0	6	4	23
2010	Ice cream, light, vanilla, soft serve	0.5 cup	88	111	4	19	0	2	1.4	11
90723	Ice popsicle	1 ea	59	47	0	11	0	0	0	0
42264	Cinnamon rolls w/icing, refrigerated dough/Pillsbury	1 ea	44	150	2	24	5	1.2		
71299	Croissant, butter	1 ea	67	272	5	31	2	14	7.8	45
45572	Danish, cheese	1 ea	71	266	6	26	1	16	4.8	11
45593	Toaster pastry, Pop Tart, apple-cinnamon/Kellogg	1 ea	52	205	2	37	1	5	0.9	0
23014	Chocolate syrup, fudge-type	2 Tbs	38	133	2	24	1	3	1.5	1
510	Whipped cream topping, pressurized	2 Tbs	7.5	19	0	1	0	2	1	6
54387	Whipped topping, frozen, low fat	2 Tbs	9.4	21	0	2	0	1	1.1	0

Fats, Oils, and Condiments

MDA Code	Food Name	Amt	Wt (g)	Ener (kcal)	Prot (g)	Carb (g)	Fiber (g)	Fat (g)	Sat (g)	Chol (g)
90210	Butter, unsalted	1 Tbs	14	100	0	0	0	11	7.2	30
8084	Oil, vegetable, canola	1 Tbs	14	124	0	0	0	14	1	0
8008	Oil, olive, salad or cooking	1 Tbs	13.5	119	0	0	0	14	1.9	0
8111	Oil, safflower, salad or cooking, greater than 70% oleic	1 Tbs	13.6	120	0	0	0	14	0.8	0
44483	Shortening, household	1 Tbs	12.8	113	0	0	0	13	2.6	0
1708	Barbecue sauce, original	2 Tbs	36	63	0	15	0			
27001	Catsup	1 ea	6	6	0	2	0	0	0	0
53523	Cheese sauce, ready-to-eat	0.25 cup	63	110	4	4	0	8	3.8	18
54388	Cream substitute, powdered, light	1 Tbs	5.9	25	0	4	0	1	0.2	0
50939	Gravy, brown, homestyle, canned	0.25 cup	60	25	1	3	1	0.3	2	
23003	Jelly	1 Tbs	19	51	0	13	0	0	0	0
25002	Maple syrup	1 Tbs	20	52	0	13	0	0	0	0
44476	Margarine, regular, 80% fat, with salt	1 Tbs	14.2	102	0	0	0	11	1.8	0
8145	Mayonnaise, safflower/soybean oil	1 Tbs	13.8	99	0	0	0	11	1.2	8
8502	Miracle Whip, light/Kraft	1 Tbs	16	37	0	2	0	3	0.5	4
435	Mustard, yellow	1 tsp	5	3	0	0	0	0	0	0
23042	Pancake syrup	1 Tbs	20	47	0	12	0	0	0	0
23172	Pancake syrup, reduced kcal	1 Tbs	15	25	0	7	0	0	0	0
53524	Pasta sauce, spaghetti/marinara	0.5 cup	125	92	2	14	1	3	0.4	0
53646	Salsa picante, mild	2 Tbs	30.5	8	0	1	0	0		0
504	Sour cream, cultured	2 Tbs	28.8	62	1	1	0	6	3.8	13
53063	Soy sauce	1 Tbs	18	11	2	1	0	0	0	0

Nutritive Value of Selected Foods and Fast Foods

MDA Code	Food Name	Amt	Wt (g)	Ener (kcal)	Prot (g)	Carb (g)	Fiber (g)	Fat (g)	Sat (g)	Chol (g)
53652	Taco sauce, red, mild	1 Tbs	15.7	7	0	1	0	0		0
53004	Teriyaki sauce	1 Tbs	18	15	1	3	0	0	0	0
8024	1000 Island, regular	1 Tbs	15.6	58	0	2	0	5	0.8	4
8013	Blue/Roquefort cheese, regular	2 Tbs	30.6	154	1	2	0	16	3	5
90232	French, regular	1 Tbs	12.3	56	0	2	0	6	0.7	0
44498	Italian, fat-free	1 Tbs	14	7	0	1	0	0	0	0
44696	Ranch, reduced fat	1 Tbs	15	33	0	2	0	3	0.2	3
8035	Vinegar & oil, homemade	2 Tbs	31.2	140	0	1	0	16	2.8	0
Fast Food										
6177	Baked potato, topped w/cheese sauce	1 ea	296	474	15	47		29	10.6	18
56629	Burrito w/beans & cheese	1 ea	93	189	8	27		6	3.4	14
66023	Burrito w/beans, cheese & beef	1 ea	102	165	7	20	2	7	3.6	62
66024	Burrito w/beef	1 ea	110	262	13	29	1	10	5.2	32
56600	Biscuit w/egg sandwich	1 ea	136	373	12	32	1	22	4.7	245
66029	Biscuit w/egg, cheese & bacon sandwich	1 ea	144	477	16	33	0	31	11.4	261
66013	Cheeseburger, double, condiments & vegetables	1 ea	166	417	21	35		21	8.7	60
56649	Cheeseburger, large, one meat patty w/condiments & vegetables	1 ea	219	563	28	38		33	15	88
15063	Chicken, breaded, fried, dark meat (drumstick or thigh)	3 oz	85.1	248	17	9	1	15	4.1	95
15064	Chicken, breaded, fried, light meat (breast or wing)	3 oz	85.1	258	19	10	1	15	4.1	77
56000	Chicken filet, plain	1 ea	182	515	24	39		29	8.5	60
56635	Chimichanga w/beef & cheese	1 ea	183	443	20	39		23	11.2	51
5461	Cole slaw	0.75 cup	99	147	1	13		11	1.6	5
56606	Croissant w/egg & cheese sandwich	1 ea	127	368	13	24		25	14.1	216
56607	Croissant w/egg, cheese & bacon sandwich	1 ea	129	413	16	24		28	15.4	215
66021	Enchilada w/cheese	1 ea	163	319	10	29		19	10.6	44
66020	Enchirito w/cheese, beef & beans	1 ea	193	344	18	34		16	7.9	50
66031	English muffin w/cheese & sausage sandwich	1 ea	115	393	15	29	1	24	9.9	59
66010	Fish sandwich w/tartar sauce	1 ea	158	431	17	41	0	23	5.2	55
90736	French fries fried in vegetable oil, medium	1 ea	134	427	5	50	5	23	5.3	0
56638	Frijoles (beans) w/cheese	0.5 cup	83.5	113	6	14		4	2	18
56664	Ham & cheese sandwich	1 ea	146	352	21	33		15	6.4	58
56662	Hamburger, large, double, w/condiments & vegetables	1 ea	226	540	34	40		27	10.5	122
56659	Hamburger, one patty w/condiments & vegetables	1 ea	110	279	13	27		13	4.1	26
66007	Hamburger, plain	1 ea	90	274	12	31		12	4.1	35
5463	Hash browns	0.5 cup	72	151	2	16		9	4.3	9
66004	Hot dog, plain	1 ea	98	242	10	18		15	5.1	44
2032	Ice cream sundae, hot fudge	1 ea	158	284	6	48	0	9	5	21
6185	Mashed potatoes	0.5 cup	121	100	3	20		1	0.6	2
56639	Nachos w/cheese	7 pcs	113	346	9	36		19	7.8	18
6176	Onion rings, breaded, fried	8 pcs	78.1	259	3	29		15	6.5	13
6173	Potato salad	0.333 cup	95	108	1	13		6	1	57
56619	Pizza w/pepperoni 12" or 1/8	1 pce	108	275	15	30		11	3.4	22
66003	Roast beef sandwich, plain	1 ea	139	346	22	33		14	3.6	51
56671	Submarine sandwich, cold cuts	1 ea	228	456	22	51	2	19	6.8	36
57531	Taco	1 ea	171	369	21	27		21	11.4	56
71129	Shake, chocolate 12 fl. oz	1 ea	250	317	8	51	5	9	5.8	32
71132	Shake, vanilla, 12 fl. oz	1 ea	250	369	8	49	2	16	9.9	57

Index

NOTE: A *t* following a page number indicates tabular material, an *f* following a page number indicates an illustration, and a *b* following a page number indicates a boxed feature.

Aspirin, in heart disease prevention, 280b
Atherosclerosis, 270, 271b, 271f
    aging and, 445
    coronary heart disease and, 271, 271f,
        272f, 280b
    smoking and, 274
Atherosclerotic plaque, 270, 271b, 271f
    in coronary arteries, 271, 271f, 272f
ATP (adenosine triphosphate), 55, 55b
    production of, 55–56, 55b, 56f
Atypical mycobacterial infection, in HIV
    infection/AIDS, 396t
Autonomic nervous system, 295, 295b
    in stress response, 295–296

BAC. See Blood alcohol concentration
Back extension exercise, 115, 167
Back muscles
    flexibility/stretching exercises for, 45, 152,
        154, 157, 158, 167
    isotonic exercises for, 112–113, 115, 117
Back pain, 345–346
    assessing risk of, 365–366
    causes/risk factors for, 143b
    prevention of, 143
        flexibility/stretching exercises in, 143,
            167
        spinal alignment and, 142f
Back to wall test, 365
Bacteria, 401b. See also specific organism
    sexually transmitted infection caused by,
        400, 401b
Balance, decisional, in behavior modification,
    12
Balanced diet. See Diet, healthy/balanced
Balanced low-calorie diet, 246t
    aging/longevity affected by, 248b
Ballistic stretching, 144, 145b
Barbiturates, dependence potential of, 416t
Bardet-Biedl syndrome, 241
Barriers, behavior change, identifying, 13
Basal metabolic rate, 244. See also Resting
    metabolic rate
Behavior(s), addictive, 414, 415. See also
    Addiction
Behavior change, 11–16, 13b, 14b, 25
    alcohol use/abuse and, 424b
    assessing habits and, 12–13
    behavior modification strategies and, 12,
        15–16
    cardiorespiratory endurance and, 70,
        70b
    cardiovascular disease risk and, 281b
    goals for, 14
        realistic, 12, 37
    health care consumer improvement and,
        453b
    identifying barriers to, 13
    injury prevention and, 356b
    physical activity in daily routine and, 41b
    skin protection and, 383b
    sleep habits and, 302b, 303
    smoking cessation and, 15
    Stages of Change Model and, 11–12, 11b
    steps in, 13b

STI prevention and, 407b
strength/endurance/weight training and,
    106b
time management and, 301b, 303
unhealthy behaviors and, 14
in weight control/nutrition, 15–16, 242b,
    251–252
    body composition assessments and,
        183
    eating triggers and, 241, 242b,
        267–268
    fast food and, 216b
    sugar consumption and, 212b
Behavior change contracts, 12, 13b
Behavior modification, 12, 15–16. See also
    Behavior change
    for smoking cessation, 15
    for weight loss, 15–16, 251–252
Bench press, 116
Benign tumor, 368, 369b
BIA. See Bioelectrical impedance analysis
Biceps curl, 111
Biceps femoris, isotonic exercises for, 114
Biceps muscle
    flexibility exercises for, 156
    isotonic exercises for, 111
Bicycle, stationary
    for cycle ergometer fitness test, 60, 60f,
        61b, 79, 79–81t
    for spinning, 69b
Bicycle accidents, reducing risk of, 358b
Binge drinking, 423, 423b, 423f
Binge eating
    in bulimia, 255
    stress and, 307
Binge eating disorder, 255–256, 255b
Bioelectrical impedance analysis (BIA), in
        body fat measurement, 181–182, 181b
    "at home" devices based on, 182b
Biopsy, in cancer diagnosis, 368, 369b
Biotin
    DRI for, 213b
    RDA for, 211t
Bleeding, treatment of, 357–358
Blood alcohol concentration, 420–421, 421b,
        422t
    alcohol poisoning and, 423
Blood pressure, 272
    exercise affecting, 59, 59b
    in hypertension, 272. See also
        Hypertension
    lowering, coronary heart disease risk and,
        279, 286
    measurement of, 272
    normal, 272
Blood transfusion, HIV transmission and,
    395
Blood vessels, 53
BMI. See Body mass index
BodPod, in body fat measurement, 180,
    181f
Body composition, 10–11, 11b, 169–194,
    171b. See also Body fat
    assessment of, 178–182, 182b, 187–192,
        189t, 190t, 192t, 259
        behavior change and, 183

field methods for, 178–180, 179t
laboratory measurements and,
    180–182, 180f, 181f
behavior change and, 183
definition of, 170, 171b
exercise affecting, 58
goals for, 183
ideal (healthy/optimal) body weight and,
    170, 171, 172f, 182–183, 193–194,
    240–241, 259
overweight/obesity and, 170, 171, 172f,
    173
relationship to health, 171–178, 171f
underweight and, 176–177
Body fat, 170
    losing. See Weight control
    need for, 171–173, 171f, 172f
    percentage of, 170, 171. See also Body
        composition
        assessment of, 178–182, 182b,
            187–192, 189t, 190t, 192t, 259
        behavior change and, 183
        exercise affecting, 58
        health and, 171, 172, 172f
        ideal (healthy/optimal) body weight
            and, 170, 171, 172f, 182–183,
            193–194, 240–241, 259
        overweight/obesity and, 170, 171,
            172f, 173
        underweight and, 176–177
    regional storage/distribution of, 171–173,
        171f, 172f
        coronary heart disease risk and, 173,
            277
Body image
    assessing, 265–266
    healthy weight and, 173
Body mass index (BMI), 178–179, 179b,
    179t, 187, 194, 259–260
Body temperature regulation, 326, 327f
Body weight. See also Obese/obesity
    ideal (healthy/optimal), 182–183, 193–194,
        240–241, 259–260
        benefits of, 173
        body composition/percent of body fat
            and, 170, 171, 172, 172f, 182–183,
            193–194, 240–241, 259
        body mass index and, 178–179, 179t,
            194, 259–260
        energy balance and, 243–245, 243f,
            244f, 245t
    losing. See Weight control
Bone(s)
    aging affecting, 445–446, 445f
    movement limitations and, 141
Bone mass
    age-related changes in, 7, 445–446, 445f
    exercise affecting, 7–8, 7f, 8f, 59
    loss of (osteoporosis), 7, 7b, 445–446
Borg Rating of Perceived Exertion, 62, 62f,
    63b, 93–94
Boron, DRI for, 213b
Botulism, 222
Bovine somatotropin, milk from animals
    treated with, 223
Brachialis muscle, isotonic exercises for, 111

Rectus abdominus muscle, isotonic exercises for, 115

Rectus femoris muscle, isotonic exercises for, 114

Recuperation, principle of, 34–35, 35b, 35f

Rehabilitation, after exercise-related injury, 353, 353f

Relapse prevention, in behavior modification, 12

weight loss and, 16

Relationships. See Interpersonal relationships

Relaxation techniques, 303f, 304–306, 306f

progressive relaxation and, 304–305, 305b

stress-related coronary heart disease and, 279–281

Repetition(s) (reps), strength gains and, 107–108, 107f

Repetition maximum (RM), 107

muscular strength evaluation and, 103, 103b, 107, 123–128

Resistance exercise. See also Strength/endurance training; Weight training

in weight control, 249

Resistance stage, of general adaptation syndrome, 300

Respiratory system, response to exercise by, 56–57

Rest/ice/compression/elevation (RICE), 352–353, 353b

Resting metabolic rate (resting energy expenditure), 97b, 244, 245b

strength training affecting, 96–97, 249

Rest/sleep, stress management and, 302b, 303, 303f

Reversibility, principle of, 35, 35b, 35f

ReVia. See Naltrexone

Rhomboid muscles, isotonic exercises for, 112

Riboflavin (vitamin B2), 202t

DRI for, 213b

RDA for, 211t

RICE (rest/ice/compression/elevation), 352–353, 353b

Risk-taking behavior(s)

alcohol use/abuse and, 420

unintentional injury and, 354–355

RM. See Repetition maximum

RMR. See Resting metabolic rate

Road rage, 299, 300b

Rohypnol, 418

RPE. See Rating of Perceived Exertion

"Runner's knee" (patellofemoral pain syndrome), 350–351, 350f, 351b

Running shoes, selecting, 34b

Safety issues, for strength/endurance/weight training program, 105

Saliva, HIV transmission and, 396

Salmonella food poisoning, 222

Salt. See Sodium

Sarcopenia, 446, 447b

Saturated fatty acids, 199t, 200, 201b

cholesterol and, 199t, 200, 201

Saunas, 449

Scabies, 404, 405b

Seafood, consumption of during pregnancy, 200b

Secondhand smoke, 426, 427b

cancer risk and, 381

coronary heart disease risk and, 274

Sedentary lifestyle

coronary heart disease risk and, 276–277

exercise affecting, 276–277, 277f, 279, 280b

obesity and, 10

Selenium, 204t

DRI for, 213b

RDA for, 210t

Self-esteem, healthy body weight and, 173

Self-examination

breast, 373, 374b

skin, 376, 377b

testicular, 375, 376b

Self-monitoring, in behavior change, 12

Self-reinforcement, in behavior modification, 12

achieving fitness goal and, 38

weight loss and, 16

Selye, Hans, 296, 299–300

Semimembranosus muscle, isotonic exercises for, 114

Semitendinosus muscle, isotonic exercises for, 114

Set(s), 107, 107b

strength gains and, 107–108, 107f

Sex (gender)

coronary heart disease risk and, 277, 278t

strength/endurance/weight training differences and, 105

stress levels and, 298

Sexually transmitted infection(s), 391–412, 393b. See also specific disease

definition of, 392–393, 393b

incidence of, 392, 393f, 406b

worldwide distribution of, 397b

inventory of attitudes/behaviors about, 411–412

questions about, 406b

reducing risk of, 404–407, 405f, 407b

Sexual partners, STI risk reduction and

discussing high-risk behavior and, 405–406

limiting number and, 405, 405f

Shaping, as behavior change strategy, 14, 15b

Shin muscles, flexibility exercises for, 151

Shin splints, 351, 351b, 351f

Shin stretch, 151

Shoes, running/exercise

injuries and, 344

selecting, 34b

Shoppers, compulsive, 415

Shoulder

flexibility exercises for, 156

isotonic exercises for, 112, 116, 117

Shoulder flexibility test, 144, 145b, 163–164, 164t

Sidestream smoke, 426. See also Secondhand smoke

Side stretch, 45, 155

Sigmoidoscopy, in colorectal cancer screening, 372

Silicon, DRI for, 213b

Simple carbohydrates (simple sugars), 197–198. See also Carbohydrate(s)

in balanced/healthy diet, 197, 197f, 206

reducing intake of, 206, 212b

Sit-and-reach test, 144, 145b, 163–164, 164t

Sitting hamstring stretch, 158

Sitting toe touch, 45

Sit-up (hand behind head), injury and, 158

Sit-up test, 103, 103b, 132, 134t

Skeletal muscle, 97–98, 97f, 98f. See also under Muscle

Skin

aging affecting, 446

movement limitations and, 141, 141t

poisons on, treatment of, 357

protection of

cancer prevention and, 376, 382–383, 383b

successful aging and, 447

Skin cancer, 371f, 375–376, 377b

self-examination/early detection of, 376, 377b

ultraviolet radiation exposure and, 376, 382–383, 383b

Skinfold test, 179, 179b, 187–188, 189t, 190t

Sleep apnea, obesity and, 176

Sleep deprivation, exercise affecting, 59, 59b

Sleep/rest

changes in, burnout and, 304b

stress management and, 302b, 303, 303f

Slow progression phase, 109b

for flexibility/stretching routine, 146–147, 147t

for strength/endurance/weight training program, 109, 109b, 109t

Slow-twitch fibers, 100, 101b, 101t

exercise intensity and, 101, 102f

individual variations/genetics and, 101

Smell sensation, aging affecting, 446

Smoking, 15, 425–426, 426f

addiction to nicotine and, 15, 416, 416t, 420t, 425–426

assessment (inventory) of, 435–437

cancer risk and, 371, 381–382, 426

cessation of, 15

behavior modification strategies for, 15

cancer risk affected by, 371, 381–382

coronary heart disease risk and, 278–279

coronary heart disease risk and, 274, 274f, 278t, 286, 426

health effects of, 426

stress and, 307

Social health, 3, 4f

assessment of, 22, 459

Social support, stress management and, 306

Socioeconomic status, wellness issues and, 5b

Sodium, 203, 204t, 275t

DRI for, 213b

in healthy/balanced diet, 207, 207f, 214t

hypertension and, 274–275, 275t

reducing intake of, 207, 207f, 275, 275t

Soft tissues, flexibility/movement limitations and, 141, 141t

Soleus muscle
  flexibility/stretching exercises for, 45, 150, 152
  isotonic exercises for, 117
Soluble fiber, 198, 199b
Somatotropin, bovine, milk from animals treated with, 223
Specificity of exercise, 33–34, 33b, 34b, 105b
  strength/endurance/weight training and, 104, 105b
Spenders, compulsive, 415
Spermicides, with nonoxynal 9, STI risk and, 406–407
SPF (sun protection factor), 376, 377b
Spinning, 69b
Spiritual health/wellness, 3–4, 3f, 4f
  assessment of, 23, 460
  development of in stress management, 306
Sports activities
  HIV transmission and, 396
  injuries and. See Exercise-related injuries
Sports drinks/gels, 217, 218f
Spot reduction, 254t
Sprains, 348–349, 348f, 349b
Stability, measuring, 137–138
Stages of Change Model, 11–12, 11b
Standing toe touch, injury and, 158
Starch(es), 198, 199b
Starter phase, 109b
  for flexibility/stretching routine, 146, 147t
  for strength/endurance/weight training program, 109, 109b, 109t
Static (isometric) exercise, 99, 99b
  weight-training program/exercises and, 106–107
Static stretching, 144, 145b
Statin drugs (statins), for cholesterol lowering, 280
Stationary bikes
  for cycle ergometer fitness test, 60, 60f, 61b, 79, 79–81t
  for spinning, 69b
Steambaths, 449
Step stretch, 45
Step test, 60, 83–84, 83f, 84f, 85t
Sternocleidomastoid muscle, flexibility exercises for, 156
Steroids, anabolic, 102b, 421t, 427–428, 427b
  dependence potential of, 416t
Sterol(s), 200, 201b
STI(s). See Sexually transmitted infection(s)
Stiff muscle, movement limitations and, 141
St. John's Wort, 220t
Storage fat, 171–173, 171b, 171f, 172f
  heart disease risk and, 173, 277
Straight leg lift, 365
Strain (muscle), 347–348, 347b, 347f
Strength, muscular, 10, 95–138. See also Muscular strength; Strength/endurance training
Strength/endurance training. See also Weight training
  adaptation to, 104–105
  benefits of, 96, 104
  designing program for, 105–107, 106b, 109t

principles for, 102–104
dietary/protein requirements and, 108b, 217
exercise prescription for, 107–108, 107f, 109–110, 109t, 110t
  individualization of, 109, 109t
gender differences and, 105
goals for, 108–109
guidelines/precautions for, 109b
maintenance phase for, 109, 109b, 109t
  motivation and, 110
muscle mass gain and, 252
for older adults, 118b
physiological changes caused by, 104
progressive resistance exercise (PRE) and, 104, 105b
protein needs and, 108b, 217
rate of improvement and, 104–105
safety concerns and, 105
sample exercises and, 111–117
slow progression phase for, 109, 109b, 109t
specificity of training and, 104, 104f, 105b
starter phase for, 109, 109b, 109t
starting and maintaining, 108–110, 109b, 109t, 110t
training log for, 129
types of programs for, 105–107
Stress, 294–302, 295b, 295f
  accidents/unintentional injury and, 355
  allostasis/allostatic load and, 301, 301b
  assessment of, 311–313
  burnout and, 304b, 305b
  chronic, 296
    health affected by, 299–302, 300f
      assessing risk for illness and, 321–323
  college students and, 298–299, 299f
  common causes of, 298–299
  coronary heart disease risk and, 278, 278t
    stress management/relaxation techniques and, 279–281
  definition of, 294–295, 295b, 295f
  excessive, 304b
  factors affecting levels of, 297–299, 297t
  gender and, 298
  health and, 299–302, 300f
    assessing risk for illness and, 321–323
  management of. See Stress management
  negative (distress), 295, 295b, 295f, 304b
  nutritional supplements and, 307b
  past experiences and, 298
  personality type and, 297–298, 297t, 319–320
  positive (eustress), 295, 295b, 295f
  response to, 294, 295–296, 295b, 296f
    emotional health and, 3
Stress diary, 313
Stress fractures, 351–352, 351b, 352f
Stress index questionnaire, 311–312
Stress management, 301b, 302–307, 302b, 303f
  breathing exercises and, 305
  coronary heart disease risk and, 279–281
  counterproductive behaviors in, avoidance of, 306–307
  exercise and, 303–304, 303f

meditation and, 303f, 306, 306f, 307b
nutritional supplements and, 307b
reducing stressors and, 303
relaxation techniques and, 303f, 304–306, 306f
rest and sleep and, 302b, 303, 303f
spiritual wellness and, 306
successful aging and, 447
support network and, 306
time management and, 301b, 303, 315–317
visualization (imagery) and, 306, 307b
Stressor(s), 294, 295b
  reducing, in stress management, 303
Stress response, 294, 295–296, 295b, 296f
Stretches. See also Flexibility
  back pain prevention and, 143, 167
  ballistic, 144, 145b
  for cool-down after cardiorespiratory workout, 64
  designing program of, 144–149
  dynamic, 144, 145b
  injury prevention/hazardous exercises and, 147, 149b
    contraindicated and substitute exercises and, 157–159
  intensity of, 39
  joint health and, 142
  passive and active, 146, 146f, 147f
  progression log for, 165–166
  proprioceptive neuromuscular facilitation and, 144, 145–146, 145b, 146f, 147f
  sample, 150–159
  static, 144, 145b
  for warm-up, 39, 45
Stretch reflex, 141–142, 141b
Stroke, 271–272, 271b, 272f
  heat, 330
Stroke volume, 53, 53b
  exercise affecting, 56, 57
"Structure/function rule," 219
Subcutaneous fat, 171, 171b, 171f
Submaximal cycle test (cycle ergometer fitness test), 60, 60f, 61b, 79, 79–81t
Substance abuse, 417, 417b. See also Substance use/abuse
Substance use/abuse, 413–437
  accidents/unintentional injury and, 355
  addiction and, 414–417, 415b
  avoiding, 429
    STI risk reduction and, 406
    successful aging and, 446–447
  causes/risk of addiction and, 416–417, 416t
  chemical dependence and, 416, 417b
  drugs commonly used, 416t, 417–429
  stress and, 307
  use versus abuse and, 417
  withdrawal and, 416, 417b
Sucrose (table sugar), 198
  reducing intake of, 206, 212b
Sudden cardiac death, exercise and, 280b
Sugar (sucrose), 198
  reducing intake of, 206, 212b
Sugar substitutes, 206, 212b
Sulfate, DRI for, 213b
Sun exposure, protecting skin from

Photo Credits

All photos by Creative Digital Visions, Pearson Benjamin Cummings, except the following:

p. 1: Carl Schneider/Taxi/Getty Images; p. 3: Giantstep/Photonica/Getty Images; p. 4: DAJ/Getty Images; p. 8: MIXA/Getty Images; p. 9: David Stoecklein/Corbis; p. 10: Tim de Waele/Corbis; p. 11: Mark Dadswell/Getty Images; p. 15: Stone/Getty Images; p. 32: Daniel Hurst/Daniel Hurst Photography/images.com; p. 33 (top) JGI/Getty Images; p. 33 (second from top) David Madison/Getty Images; p. 33 (third from top) Tom Kola/Jupiter Images; p. 33 (bottom) John Kelly/Getty Images; p. 34: Richard Price/Taxi/Getty Images; p. 35: Comstock/Jupiter Images; p. 38 (left) Arthur Tilley/Stone/Getty Images; p. 38 (right) Strauss/Curtis/Masterfile; p. 49: Bubbles Photolibrary/Alamy; p. 51: altrendo images/Getty Images; p. 53: David Sacks/Image Bank/Getty Images; p. 58: Comstock/Jupiter Images; p. 60: Angelika Schwarz; p. 61: Paul Hill/iStockphoto; p. 83 (left) Elena Dorfman, Pearson Benjamin Cummings; p. 60: (right) Kristin Piljay, Pearson Benjamin Cummings; p. 95: Alan Jacubek/Corbis; p. 111: Elena Dorfman, Pearson Benjamin Cummings; p. 132 (bottom a&b): Elena Dorfman, Pearson Benjamin Cummings; p. 137: Elena Dorfman, Pearson Benjamin Cummings; p. 139: Anthony Redpath/Corbis; p. 144: Spike Mafford/Getty Images; p. 148: Spencer Grant/PhotoEdit; p. 155 (bottom) Elena Dorfman, Pearson Benjamin Cummings; p. 169: Patrik Giardino/Corbis; p. 171: Gregg Adams/Getty Images; p. 172 (left): Mike Brinson/Image Bank/Getty Images; p. 172 (right): Jeff Green-Martin/PhotoEdit; p. 173: Guryanov Oleg/Shutterstock, Tom McNemar/iStockphoto; p. 176 (top): David Freund/iStockphoto; p. 176 (bottom): Janet Duran/Black Star; p. 180: Fitness Institute of Texas/University of Texas; p. 181 (left & right): David Young-Wolff/PhotoEdit; p. 182: Kristin Piljay, Pearson Benjamin Cummings; p. 188 (all): Elena Dorfman, Pearson Benjamin Cummings; p. 195: Brooke Fasani/Corbis; p. 198: Brian Hagiwara/Foodpix/Jupiter Images; p. 203: Philip Harvey/Corbis; p. 206: Alice Edward/Getty Images; p. 207:Lew Robertson/Getty Images; p. 218: Kristin Piljay, Pearson Benjamin Cummings; p. 222: Pascal Broze/age footstock; p. 239: Corbis; p. 244: Larry Dale Gordon/Getty Images; p. 246: Comstock/Corbis; p. 249: Elizabeth Etienne/Alamy; p. 253: Nancy Kaszerman/ZUMA/Corbis; p. 255 (top): Rootstein; p. 255 (bottom): Nina Berman/Sipa Press; p. 269: John Henley/Corbis; p. 272: NiKreationS/Alamy; p. 274: David Bishop/Phototake; p. 277: Getty Photodisc; p. 279: Jeff Boyle/Asia Images/Jupiter Images; p. 293: Jonathan Andrew/Corbis; p. 294: Jeffrey Coolidge/Corbis; p. 298: Ryan McVay/Getty Images; p. 299: Andersen Ross/Getty Images; p. 306: PatitucciPhoto/Aurora Photos; p. 307: Scott K. Powers; p. 325: John Kelly/Image Bank/Getty Images; p. 329: Owen Franken/Corbis; p. 332: Dorling Kindersley Media Library; p. 333: Mike Powell/Corbis; p. 335: S. P. Gillette/Corbis; p. 343: Corbis; p. 349: Princess Margaret Rose Orthopedic Hospital/SPL/Photo Researchers; p. 355: David Crausby/Alamy; p. 357: Dorling Kindersley Media Library; p. 369: Syracuse Newspapers/The Image Works; p. 370: vario images GmbH & Co.KG/Alamy; p. 376: Kristin Piljay, Pearson Benjamin Cummings; p. 377 (top left): ISM/Phototake; p. 377 (top right/bottom right): CNRI/Photo Researchers; p. 377 (bottom left): P. Marazzi/Photo Researchers; p. 379: Tony Freeman/PhotoEdit; p. 391: Tony Freeman/PhotoEdit; p. 395: sgame/Shutterstock; p. 402: Photo Researchers; p. 403: Eye of Science/Photo Researchers; p. 405: Ronnie Kaufman/Corbis; p. 413: Stockbyte/Getty Images; p. 415: Wang Leng/Asia Images/Jupiter Images; p. 418: Tom Croke/Acclaim Images; p. 419: Comstock/Jupiter Images; p. 420: Leonid Smirnov/Shutterstock; p. 423: Don Farrall/Getty Images; p. 423 (top): David Young-Wolff/PhotoEdit; p. 424: David H. Wells/Corbis; p. 426: Bananastock/Jupiter Images; p. 439: Larry Williams/Corbis; p. 443: Jeffrey Aaronson/Network Aspen; p. 444: Leland Bobbe/Stone/Getty Images; p. 445: Steven Peters/Stone/Getty Images; p. 446: Photodisc/Getty Images; p. 450: Comstock Images/agefotostock